# Health

## The Basics

Fourth Canadian Edition

# Health

## Fourth Canadian Edition

## The Basics

Rebecca J. Donatelle
Oregon State University

Anne Johnson Munroe
Sheridan College

Alex Munroe
Wilfrid Laurier University

Angela M. Thompson
St. Francis Xavier University

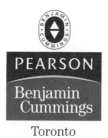

PEARSON

Benjamin
Cummings

Toronto

To my husband Kelly and our children Rhett and Kassandra—you three are my inspiration.

*Angie*

**Library and Archives Canada Cataloguing in Publication**

Health: the basics/Rebecca J. Donatelle ... [et al.].—4th Canadian ed.

Includes index.
ISBN-13: 978-0-205-53558-3
ISBN-10: 0-205-53558-5

1. Health—Textbooks.    I.  Donatelle, Rebecca J., 1950–

RA776.H42 2008      613      C2006-905096-1

ISBN-13: 978-0-205-53558-3
ISBN-10: 0-205-53558-5

Editor-in-Chief: Gary Bennett
Marketing Manager: Colleen Gauthier
Acquisitions Editor: Michelle Sartor
Developmental Editors: Pamela Voves and Madhu Ranadive
Production Editor: Marisa D'Andrea
Copy Editor: Kelli Howey
Proofreader: Trish O'Reilly
Production Coordinator: Andrea Falkenberg
Indexer: Sheila Flavel
Compositor: Integra
Photo and Permissions Researcher: Christina Beamish
Art Director: Julia Hall
Interior and Cover Design: Anthony Leung
Cover Image: Masterfile

1 2 3 4 5     12 11 10 09 08

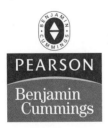

PEARSON

Benjamin Cummings

# BRIEF CONTENTS

# CONTENTS

# PREFACE

Most of today's university and college students already know more about their health than any previous generation. Part of the reason is that we, as a nation, simply know more about our health and what we can do to obtain optimal health and wellness and preserve it than Canadians did in the past. Still, understanding health requires constant critical thinking because we are bombarded by information from various media outlets—the Internet, newspapers, magazines, television, radio, and movies—and we have to learn how to make sense of the information presented, determine if it is valid or useful, then apply it to ourselves. This latter point is particularly difficult; that is, translating the basic facts into a meaningful, personally relevant plan of action can be a difficult task. There are many more decisions about their health that students are required to make. With so many choices available, how can they be sure their everyday decisions will ultimately lead to optimal health? What *is* optimal health? With this in mind, we have placed increasing emphasis in this text on developing skills to help students make informed, responsible lifestyle choices related to their health.

Achieving good health includes recognizing the importance of a particular health outcome, understanding the factors that contribute to the positive and negative aspects of health, contemplating how personal actions affect our health, and choosing to change or modify risky behaviours and develop new and improved behaviours. *Health: The Basics* is an important source of reliable health information. As you use the latest information, the special features, and the learning aids in the book and its supplements, we hope to engage your students in the process with the long-term result of increased self-responsibility regarding health, as well as improved overall health and wellness.

In setting out to revise the Fourth Canadian Edition for post-secondary students, we listened to the comments and concerns of Canadian personal health educators. We learned that we share the following goals for a personal health text:

- To prepare students to lead healthy lives, now and in the future, providing tools and strategies to make responsible health decisions and to effect positive behaviour change.

- To include "high-interest" topics traditionally left out of health texts, such as multicultural and sex-specific perspectives on health.

- To provide current Canadian material and statistics that include the latest health research and citations.

- To recognize that students learn visually and require strong pedagogical elements to help them synthesize information and build healthy behaviour skills.

- To include practical, real-life applications of the material presented in the text that encourage students to think critically and apply the material to their own lives.

## NEW TO THE FOURTH CANADIAN EDITION

The first Canadian edition of *Health: The Basics* was adapted to reflect the unique Canadian context as it applies to health. The second and third Canadian editions were updated with new research and current information to assist Canadian students in learning about their health. New sections included Focus on Canada, Your Spiritual and Emotional Health, and Health in the Media boxes. In this fourth Canadian edition, revisions were made to once again update research, statistics, and report on new developments in the field of health and wellness in Canada. Some specific examples include the Integrated Pan-Canadian Healthy Living Strategy and SuPeR SMART goal setting added to Chapter 1; the new dietary reference intakes along with a review of and update on Canada's Food Guide to Healthy Eating in Chapter 7; an increased focus on physical activity as a necessary part of a healthy lifestyle in Chapter 9; and the re-introduction of the topic of caffeine to Chapter 11. In keeping with new movements across Canada, a greater emphasis was placed on spiritual health throughout the textbook. Finally, several Focus on Canada and Health in the Media boxes were updated.

## ORGANIZATION

- Beginning with the introduction of the **DECIDE model for decision making, Prochaska and DiClemente's Stages of Change model, and SuPeR SMART goal setting** in Chapter 1, decision making through critical thinking is a cornerstone of every chapter—from the **What Do You Think?** scenarios, reflective questions, and boxed features throughout the chapter to the **Taking Charge** sections at the end of each chapter.

- **Heart disease and cancer coverage** emphasizes prevention and treatment of the major killers in Canada. A revised section on the primary, controllable risk factors for heart disease and lifestyle (controllable) risks for cancer are new additions.

- **Coverage of sex issues** in health is integrated throughout the text. Topics include sex bias in mental health treatment; women and heart disease; and how sex and gender roles may affect stress, stress management, and a person's ultimate health status.

- The book highlights **the role of the community** and how to improve a community's health. Community coverage appears throughout the text and in special community-focused "Checklists for Change" within the Taking Charge boxes.

- **Prevention** is emphasized in the context of making healthy lifestyle choices and changing not-so-good health behaviours. For example, the text covers how early intervention allows more options, how prevention eases the burden on the healthcare system, and how prevention can positively influence the quality and quantity of life.

- A **pedagogical framework** that stresses building health skills is integrated consistently throughout the text. Students will learn specific applications through the colourful Rate Yourself, Skills for Behaviour Change, Building Communication Skills, and Taking Charge boxes.

*Health: The Basics* includes the following special feature boxes designed to help build health behaviour skills and to encourage students to think about and apply the concepts:

**Skills for Behaviour Change** boxes suggest specific skills students can develop and use in improving their lifestyle behaviours related to health and wellness.

**Building Communication Skills** boxes strengthen the emphasis on using communication as a tool to better health. These boxes provide practical suggestions for improving communication, interpersonal relationships, and social interactions—essential components of good health.

**Focus on Canada** boxes highlight health issues specifically related to Canadians.

**Your Spiritual and Emotional Health** boxes introduce stories, practices, and techniques that will help students to understand, build, and strengthen their spiritual and emotional health.

**Health in the Media** boxes report on high-interest health issues and encourage students to assess the mainstream media sources' interpretation of each health issue.

**Rate Yourself** (self-assessment) boxes give students the chance to evaluate their behaviours and determine ways to improve their lifestyle and, ultimately, their health.

**Taking Charge** boxes encourage students to apply the chapter material to their own lives. This highly acclaimed feature includes the following sections: "Making Decisions for You," which outlines steps and strategies for making and implementing health decisions; "Checklists for Change," which outline specific actions to be taken to change unhealthy behaviours, on a personal and a community level; and "Critical Thinking," which presents a hypothetical situation in which students must make a decision (we encourage the use of the DECIDE model to make this decision).

Other features in the book include:

**Chapter Objectives:** Each chapter begins with a list of objectives tied to the major sections of the chapter to emphasize important topics.

**What Do You Think? chapter-opening scenarios:** These scenarios can be used to prompt stimulating discussions that introduce the concepts presented in the chapters.

**What Would You Do? reflective questions:** These questions appear throughout each chapter to encourage students to think critically about the concepts presented and how they may relate to them. They can also be used as discussion questions in class.

**Running Glossary of Key Terms:** For convenience and added emphasis, key terms are boldfaced in the text and defined at the bottom of the page spread where they first appear.

**Chapter Summary:** Linked to the chapter-opening learning objectives, these summaries provide a quick, at-a-glance review of key points presented in each chapter.

**Discussion Questions:** Tied to major sections of the chapter, these new questions encourage critical thinking of the important concepts presented from varying angles.

**Application Exercises:** These exercises are linked to the chapter-opening scenarios and expand discussion and critical reflection.

**Health on the Net:** This section gives students a list of useful websites related to each chapter. The sites have been researched and tested for quality and relevance.

**Notes:** Extensive listings of the references cited in each chapter are provided in the Notes section at the end of the text. Canadian references are indicated in red.

# SUPPLEMENTS

Available with *Health: The Basics,* Fourth Canadian Edition, is a comprehensive set of ancillary material designed to facilitate classroom preparation and enhance student learning.

**Instructor's Resource CD-ROM (ISBN 0-205-51981-4):** The Instructor's Resource CD-ROM (IRCD) contains everything you need for efficient course preparation. All the supplements on the IRCD have been revised to reflect changes made to the

Canadian edition. The Instructor's CD-ROM contains the following four supplements:

■ **Instructor's Manual:** This comprehensive manual, filled with material to enhance the course, includes the following: what's new in this edition; chapter objectives; detailed chapter outlines; discussion questions; student activities including individual, community, and diverse population/non-traditional categories; additional references for further information; and a list of applicable media resources for classroom presentation.

■ **Test Generator:** The Test Generator is composed of more than 1,400 questions made up of multiple-choice, true/false, fill-in-the-blank, matching, and essay formats. Each question is rated for difficulty level and for skill type as factual, applied, or conceptual. Answers and page references to the text also are provided with each question as feedback. TestGen test-generating software allows instructors to custom design, save, and generate classroom tests. The test program permits instructors to edit, add, or delete questions from test banks; edit existing graphics and create new graphics; analyze test results; and organize a database of tests and student results. This new software allows for greater flexibility and ease of use.

■ **PowerPoint Slides:** The PowerPoint Lecture Slides provide instructors with lecture notes to supplement their in-class lessons. More than 400 PowerPoint presentation slides provide an indispensable teaching tool for instructors.

■ **Image Library:** Almost all of the figures and tables from the text are available to instructors in the Image Library. Instructors can download these images to include in their own classroom presentations.

**CBC Videos (DVD—ISBN 0-205-53671-9 and VHS—ISBN 0-205-53672-7):** Current information from such CBC series as *The National* and *Marketplace* complement the text and enhance learning by bringing to life practical applications and issues. With the latest news and information on health, these videotapes provide an excellent vehicle for launching lectures, showing additional examples, and sparking classroom discussion.

The CBC videos are also available for viewing to both students and instructors on Pearson Education Canada's Online Video Central website (accessed through **www.pearsoned.ca**).

Available to instructors only—the Instructor's Manual, PowerPoints, and Test Generator are available for download from a password-protected site on the Pearson Education Online Catalogue (**www.pearsoned.ca**).

Follow the online instructions to create a password and download the available supplements.

**Companion Website** (**www.pearsoned.ca/donatelle**): This student resource site offers practice quiz quesions and case scenarios. Students can submit their answers for grading and receive instant feedback. Access to current topics and research in the health-related disciplines is made easy with a chapter-by-chapter list of weblinks. To complete this set of study tools offered to students, an online glossary with all key terms and definitions from the text is available for easy reference.

# ALSO AVAILABLE— ADDITIONAL STUDENT SUPPLEMENTS

**Take Charge of Your Health! Worksheets (ISBN 0-8053-6037-9):** This pad of worksheets includes 38 self-assessment activities.

**Behavior Change Log Book and Wellness Journal (ISBN 0-8053-7844-8):** This assessment tool helps students track daily exercise and nutritional intake and create a long-term nutrition and fitness prescription plan. It also includes a Behavior Change Contract and topics for journal-based activities.

# ACKNOWLEDGMENTS

We thank the following people at Pearson Education Canada for their part in the fourth Canadian edition of *Health: The Basics:* editor-in-chief Gary Bennett; developmental editors Pamela Voves, Maurice Esses, and Madhu Ranadive; production editor Marisa D'Andrea; production coordinator Andrea Falkenberg; copy editor Kelli Howey; proofreaders Trish O'Reilly and Laurel Sparrow; and technical reviewer Ken Brooks.

We also thank the following reviewers:

Jacquie Cottingham, Confederation College

Shawn N. Fraser, Athabasca College

Iris Gravel, Sir Sandford Fleming College

Peter Katzmarzyk, Queen's University

Madelyn P. Law, Brock University

Mark Lund, Grant MacEwan College

Anne MacGregor, Kwantlen College

Linda McDevitt, Algonquin College

David Thomas, Fanshawe College of Applied Arts and Technology

Patti Thorne, Memorial University

## A Great Way to Learn and Instruct Online

The Pearson Education Canada Companion Website is easy to navigate and is organized to correspond to the chapters in this textbook. Whether you are a student in the classroom or a distance learner you will discover helpful resources for in-depth study and research that empower you in your quest for greater knowledge and maximize your potential for success in the course.

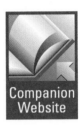
Companion Website

[**www.pearsoned.ca/donatelle**] Enter

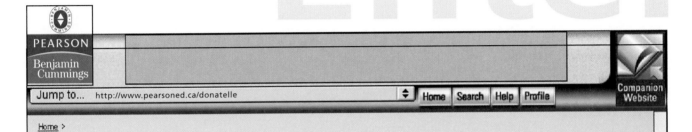

Jump to... | http://www.pearsoned.ca/donatelle | Home | Search | Help | Profile

Home >

### Companion Website

*Health: The Basics*, Fourth Canadian Edition
by Donatelle/Munroe/Munroe/Thompson

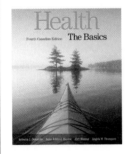

#### Student Resources

The modules in this section provide students with tools for learning course material. Some of these modules include:

- Review of Learning Objectives and the What Do You Think? chapter-opening scenarios
- Self-Tests
- Critical Thinking Questions
- Practice Quizzes, including multiple-choice (with and without feedback), true and false, short-answer, and matching
- Case Studies in Health
- Accessing Your Health
- Glossary Flashcards

In the quiz modules students can send answers to the grader and receive instant feedback on their progress through the Results Reporter. Coaching comments and references to the textbook may be available to ensure that students take advantage of all available resources to enhance their learning experience.

#### Instructor Resources

The modules in this section provide instructors with additional teaching tools. Downloadable PowerPoint Presentations, Test Generator, and an Instructor's Manual are just some of the materials that may be available in this section. Where appropriate, this section will be password protected. To get a password, simply contact your Pearson Education Canada Representative or call Faculty Sales and Services at 1-800-850-5813.

# CHAPTER 1

# PROMOTING HEALTHY BEHAVIOUR CHANGE

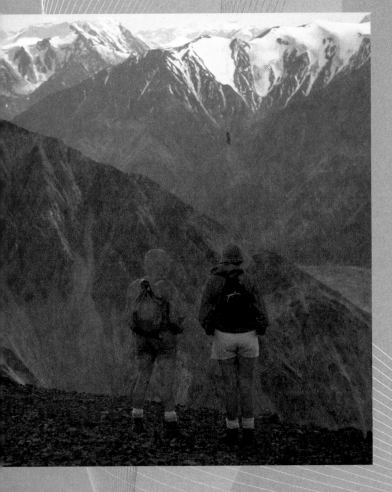

## CHAPTER OBJECTIVES

- Define health and wellness, and explain the interconnected roles of the physical, social, mental, occupational, emotional, environmental, and spiritual dimensions of health.

- Describe the health status of Canadians, the factors that contribute to health, and the national goals for promoting health and preventing premature death and disability.

- Identify the leading causes of death and the lifestyle patterns associated with them.

- Examine how predisposing factors, beliefs, attitudes, and significant others affect your behaviour changes.

- Survey behaviour-change techniques and learn how to apply them to personal situations.

- Apply decision-making techniques to behaviour changes.

Tim is a 22-year-old second-year university student who is 35 kilograms overweight and does not like physical activity. A sensitive, caring young man, he has many close friends and is a volunteer at various health-related agencies that help people in need. He enjoys nature and the inner peace he derives sitting on the beach listening to the waves or a quiet night by a campfire in the wilderness. He is a strong advocate for human rights, animal rights, and the preservation of the environment.

Kim is a 20-year-old first-year student who lives off campus. She tries to eat well most of the time, thinks she is five kilograms overweight, and walks two to four kilometres per day. She is shy and hasn't made many friends since coming to college. During a typical day, she goes to class, studies, watches TV, and writes letters to her high-school friends and family. She likes cycling, but finds time to get out for a short ride only on weekends. She is tired much of the time and wonders why she is in school.

■ Do you know people similar to either Tim or Kim? Who do you think is healthier? Why? Who is less healthy? Why? What factors contribute to their current attitudes and behaviours? What actions could you take to help these people achieve a more balanced "healthstyle"? Where else could they go for help at your school? In your community?

If you and your close friends were to list the most important things in your lives, you might be surprised at the differences in the responses. Some of you would probably list family, love, financial security, significant others, and happiness. Others might list health. Raised on a steady stream of clichés and slogans—"If you have your health, you have everything," "Be all that you can be," "Use it or lose it," "Just do it"—most of us readily acknowledge that good health is a desirable attribute. But what does it really mean to be healthy? How can you "get healthy" if you aren't doing so well right now? How can you maintain and enhance the positive attitudes and behaviours you already have? How can you change the not-so-good attitudes and behaviours you have?

This text will provide you with access to health information consistent with who you are and what you want to become. You can make many changes in your attitude and behaviours that may significantly reduce your risk factors. For the risk factors beyond your control, you must learn to react, adapt, and make optimal use of the resources available to you to create the best situation for yourself. By making informed, rational decisions, you will be able to improve the quality—and quantity—of your life.

# WHAT IS HEALTH?

Although we use the term *health* almost unconsciously, few people understand the broad scope of the word. For some, health simply means the antithesis of sickness. To others, it means being in good physical shape and the ability to resist disease and illnesses. Still others use the terms *wellness* or *well-being* to include a wide array of factors that lead to positive health status. Why all the variations? Partly because of the different perceptions of an increasingly enlightened way of health that have evolved over time. As our understanding of illness has improved, so has our ability to understand the many nuances of health. Although our current understanding has evolved over centuries, we have a long way to go in achieving a truly comprehensive view of this very complex term.

## Health and Sickness: Defined by Extremes

Before the late 1800s, people viewed health simply as the opposite of sickness. A person was healthy if he or she wasn't suffering from a life-threatening infectious disease. When deadly epidemics such as bubonic plague, pneumonic plague, influenza, tuberculosis, and cholera killed millions of people, survivors were considered healthy and congratulated themselves on their good fortune. In the late 1800s and early 1900s, researchers began to discover that the victims of these epidemics were not simply unhealthy people, but victims of microorganisms found in contaminated water, air, and human waste. Public health officials moved swiftly to sanitize the environment and, as a result, many people began to think of health as good hygiene. Practices such as sanitary disposal of wastes, hand washing, and other behaviours that promoted hygiene then became the harbingers of good health.

## Health: More Than a Statistic

Once scientists began to learn about the microorganisms that cause infectious diseases, dramatic changes occurred in the sickness profile of the Canadian public. In the early 1900s, the leading causes of death were infectious diseases, such as tuberculosis, pneumonia, and influenza, and the average life expectancy was only 58.8 years for males and 60.6 years for females.[1]

Improved sanitation brought about dramatic changes in life expectancy, and the development of vaccines and antibiotics added years to the average life span. According to **mortality** (death rate) statistics, people are now living longer than in any previous time in our history. Further, **morbidity** (illness) rates indicate that people are also sick less often from the common infectious diseases that devastated previous generations. Today, because most childhood diseases are curable and because multiple public health efforts are aimed at reducing the spread of infectious diseases, many people are living well into their 70s, 80s, and even 90s. The average Canadian child born in 2003 (the latest data available) has a life expectancy of 79.9 years—77.4 years for males and 82.4 for females.[2]

However, just because we're living longer and not getting sick as often doesn't mean we're necessarily healthier. If you and your classmates were asked to define the term *health,* there would be many different views. In 1947, the World Health Organization (WHO), whose objective is "the attainment by all peoples of the highest possible level of health,"[3] defined health this way: "Health is the state of complete physical, mental, and social well-being, not merely the absence of disease or infirmity."[4] For the first time, health was defined as more than the absence of disease or a vital statistic indicating low mortality or morbidity rates. However, critics argued that complete health is much more than just a measure of physical, social, and intellectual aspects of life, given the growing recognition of how mental, occupational, environmental, and spiritual health contribute to the quality of life as well as to the number of years a person lives. Health is also limited by such factors as income, education, occupation, access to medical care, environmental pollution, age, and sex. Since education is known to be one of the determinants of health, increasing your knowledge is one way to lessen risks to your health.

## Health as Wellness: Putting Quality into Years

Rene Dubos, a biologist and philosopher, expanded the WHO's definition of **health**. We have adopted Dubos's definition: "Health involves social, emotional, mental, spiritual, and biological fitness on the part of the individual, which results from adaptations to the environment." [5] The concept of adaptability or the ability to successfully cope with life's ups and downs became a key element of the overall health definition. Eventually the term **wellness** became popular. It includes the previously mentioned elements and implied there were levels of health in each category. To achieve a high level of wellness, a person attempts to move progressively higher on a continuum of positive health indicators. Today, *health* and *wellness* are often used interchangeably to mean the dynamic, ever-changing process of trying to achieve one's individual potential in each of the interrelated dimensions. These dimensions typically include those presented in Figure 1.1.

- **Physical health.** Includes physical characteristics such as body size and shape, sensory acuity, susceptibility to disease and disorders, body functioning, and recuperative ability. Newer definitions of physical health include our ability to perform activities of daily living, such as getting out of bed in the morning, bending over to tie our shoes, and shoulder checking while driving.

- **Social health.** Refers to the ability to have satisfying interpersonal relationships, interact with others, and adapt to various social situations and to daily behaviours.

- **Mental health.** Refers to the ability to think clearly, reason objectively, analyze critically, and use brain power effectively to meet life's challenges. It means learning from successes and failures and making responsible decisions that take into consideration all aspects of a situation.

- **Occupational health.** Refers to the personal satisfaction people get from their careers or stages of career development. It also involves attaining

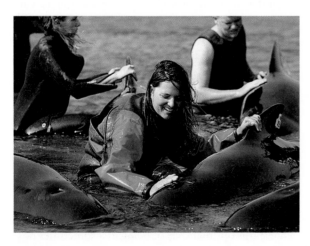

*Responsiveness to the physical, social, mental, occupational, emotional, environmental, and spiritual dimensions of life—not merely the presence or absence of illness—determines health status.*

**Mortality:** Death rate.

**Morbidity:** Illness rate.

**Health:** Dynamic, ever-changing process of trying to achieve individual potential in the physical, social, mental, occupational, emotional, environmental, and spiritual dimensions.

**Wellness:** An ongoing, active process of trying to achieve the highest level of health possible in each dimension.

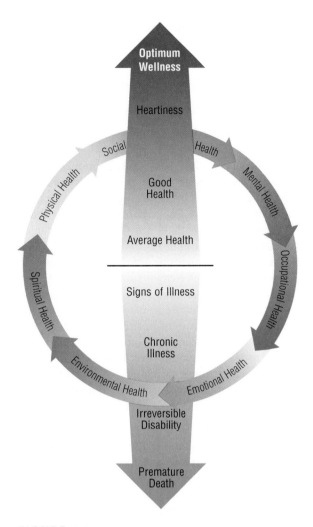

## FIGURE 1.1

### The Dimensions of Health and the Wellness Continuum

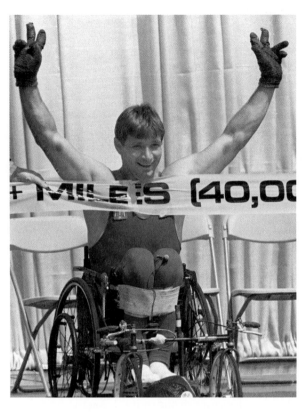

*Having the motivation to improve the quality of life within the framework of your unique capabilities and limitations is crucial to achieving optimal health and wellness.*

and maintaining a satisfying balance between work and leisure. Occupational health includes a work environment that accommodates personal strengths and weaknesses while minimizing stress and health risk.

- **Emotional health.** Refers to the "feeling" component and to the ability to express emotions when appropriate and to control inappropriate expressions of emotion. Feelings of self-esteem, self-confidence, self-efficacy, trust, love, and many other emotional reactions and responses are part of emotional health.

- **Environmental health.** Refers to an appreciation of the external environment and the role individuals play in preserving, protecting, and improving environmental conditions. Environmental health can include the student's personal studying environment—the desk, room, lighting, noise level, comfortable emotional atmosphere, and so on.

- **Spiritual health.** Refers to a feeling of unity with the environment—a feeling of oneness with others and with nature—and a guiding sense of meaning or value in life. It may also include the ability to understand and express one's purpose in life; to feel a part of a greater spectrum of existence; to experience love, joy, pain, sorrow, peace, contentment, and wonder over life's experiences; and to care about and respect all living things. Spiritual health may involve a belief in a supreme being or a specified way of living prescribed by a particular religion.

Whether contemporary definitions are of health or wellness, they focus on individual attempts to achieve optimal well-being within a realistic framework of individual potential. In Figure 1.1, a continuum from illness to optimal well-being describes health and wellness. Where you are on this continuum may vary from day to day, but if you persist in your attempts to change attitudes and behaviours to reduce risk, your chances of remaining on the positive end of the continuum will greatly improve. Each of us must try to achieve this optimal level of being in a sometimes hostile environment and come to terms with obstacles by focusing on our positive attributes whenever possible, changing negative aspects that we can, and learning to recognize and deal with the aspects we can't change.

## Breast Cancer Hope: Yukon River Quest

Many of us have heard of dragon boat races. More importantly, we are aware of the reasoning behind them. Participants of dragon boat races are most often survivors of breast cancer or are individuals paddling in memory or support of a wife, mother, sister, daughter, aunt, grandmother, cousin, or friend who has had the illness. What do you do if you can't find a body of water that's available or suitable for a dragon boat race? What if you don't have a dragon boat? You adjust or adapt to your natural terrain and find a boat that works, just as the Yukon River Quest does for a number of breast cancer survivors in the Yukon.

Inaugurated in 1999 with kayaks and small canoes as the only participating vessels, the Yukon River Quest is the world's longest annual canoe and kayak race that begins in Whitehorse and ends approximately 740 kilometres later in Dawson City. Many of the 11 women who came together to compete in 2001 had never paddled before. They paddled in a Voyageur canoe under the team name of "Paddlers Abreast" and finished their first race in just under 86 hours. In 2005, the team whittled their time down to 60 hours and 25 minutes, placing fourth behind the winning team that came in at just over 55 hours.

The teams that form the Yukon River Quest develop a camaraderie that goes beyond their similarities in experiences with breast cancer. This camaraderie reflects the hope these women have for their future—one without cancer. The women (and their friends) who choose to participate in the Yukon River Quest take part because of their need to share hope, to live beyond their experiences with breast cancer, and to grab a hold of life again.

A Yukon filmmaker, Werner Walcher, created a documentary about the paddlers and their experiences. He tells the story of all breast cancer survivors who participated for five years in the Yukon River Quest. In this documentary, Walcher shows that women with breast cancer lead full and active lives. Further, he attempts to present the male partner's view because he feels that as a male, it is difficult to understand what a woman with breast cancer really goes through. Walcher's wife had a breast cancer scare, and experienced the procedures of being tested and waiting for results. It was this experience that fuelled his interest in a documentary on women's and their partners' experiences with breast cancer. He hopes that national interest will develop as a result of the film and that it will provide hope to those who are diagnosed with the disease in the future.

Source: Adapted from N. Reveler, "Paddlers Abreast—Yukon River Quest," *Network News: Essential News for Canadians Affected by Breast Cancer* 10 (Winter/Spring 2006). Accessed on December 18, 2006, from www.cbcn.ca/en/?page=7181&section=4.

---

Well individuals take an honest look at their personal capabilities and limitations and make an effort to change factors within their control. They try to achieve a balance in each of the health and wellness dimensions while trying to achieve a positive position on the imaginary wellness continuum. Many people believe that wellness can best be achieved by adopting a holistic approach in which a person emphasizes integrating and balancing mind, body, and spirit. Persons on the illness and disability end of the continuum may have failed to achieve this integration and balance, and may be seriously deficient in one or more of the wellness dimensions.

The disability component of the wellness continuum does not imply that a person with physical or mental disabilities cannot achieve wellness. Such a person may in fact be very healthy in terms of relationships with others, level of self-confidence, and environmental sensitivity; have a meaningful and satisfying occupation; and maintain an overall attitude toward life including reaching his or her physical or mental potential within his or her limitation. In contrast, a person who spends hours in front of a mirror lifting weights to perfect the size and shape of each muscle may be unhealthy in these same terms. Appearance and physical performance indicators are only two signs of a person's overall health and provide a very limited indication of how well or healthy a person is.

Typically, the closer you get to your potential in the seven components, the healthier or more well you are. Keep in mind that optimal health and wellness is not a static state that one can achieve but rather an ongoing, active process that includes the positive attitudes and behaviours in each of the dimensions. By completing the appraisal in the Rate Yourself box, you may gain a better perspective on how you measure up in each of the dimensions discussed previously.

# How Healthy Are You?

Although many of us recognize the importance of healthy attitudes and behaviours, we often don't maintain a healthy regimen. Rate your health status in each of the following dimensions by circling the number that best describes you.

|  | Very Unhealthy | Somewhat Unhealthy | Somewhat Healthy | Very Healthy |
|---|---|---|---|---|
| Physical Health | 1 | 2 | 3 | 4 |
| Social Health | 1 | 2 | 3 | 4 |
| Emotional Health | 1 | 2 | 3 | 4 |
| Environmental Health | 1 | 2 | 3 | 4 |
| Spiritual Health | 1 | 2 | 3 | 4 |
| Mental Health | 1 | 2 | 3 | 4 |
| Occupational Health | 1 | 2 | 3 | 4 |

After completing the above section, how healthy do you think you are? Which area(s), if any, do you think you should work on improving? Now answer the following set of questions regarding each dimension of health. Indicate how often you think the statements describe you.

## PHYSICAL HEALTH

|  | Rarely, If Ever | Sometimes | Most of the Time | Always |
|---|---|---|---|---|
| 1. I maintain a desirable weight. | 1 | 2 | 3 | 4 |
| 2. I engage in vigorous exercises such as brisk walking, jogging, swimming, or running for at least 30 minutes per day, 3–4 times per week. | 1 | 2 | 3 | 4 |
| 3. I do exercises designed to strengthen my muscles and joints. | 1 | 2 | 3 | 4 |
| 4. I warm up and cool down by stretching before and after vigorous exercise. | 1 | 2 | 3 | 4 |
| 5. I feel good about the condition of my body. | 1 | 2 | 3 | 4 |
| 6. I get 7–8 hours of sleep each night. | 1 | 2 | 3 | 4 |
| 7. My immune system is strong and I am able to avoid most infectious diseases. | 1 | 2 | 3 | 4 |
| 8. My body heals itself quickly when I get sick or injured. | 1 | 2 | 3 | 4 |
| 9. I have lots of energy and can get through the day without being overly tired. | 1 | 2 | 3 | 4 |
| 10. I listen to my body; when there is something wrong, I seek professional advice. | 1 | 2 | 3 | 4 |

## SOCIAL HEALTH

|  | Rarely, If Ever | Sometimes | Most of the Time | Always |
|---|---|---|---|---|
| 1. When I meet people I feel good about the impression I make on them. | 1 | 2 | 3 | 4 |
| 2. I am open, honest, and get along well with other people. | 1 | 2 | 3 | 4 |
| 3. I participate in a wide variety of social activities and enjoy being with people who are different from me. | 1 | 2 | 3 | 4 |

| | Rarely, If Ever | Sometimes | Most of the Time | Always |
|---|---|---|---|---|
| 4. I try to be a "better person" and work on behaviours that have caused problems in my interactions with others. | 1 | 2 | 3 | 4 |
| 5. I get along well with the members of my family. | 1 | 2 | 3 | 4 |
| 6. I am a good listener. | 1 | 2 | 3 | 4 |
| 7. I am open and accessible to a loving and responsible relationship. | 1 | 2 | 3 | 4 |
| 8. I have someone I can talk to about my private feelings. | 1 | 2 | 3 | 4 |
| 9. I consider the feelings of others and do not act in hurtful or selfish ways. | 1 | 2 | 3 | 4 |
| 10. I consider how what I say might be perceived by others before I speak. | 1 | 2 | 3 | 4 |

## EMOTIONAL HEALTH

| | Rarely, If Ever | Sometimes | Most of the Time | Always |
|---|---|---|---|---|
| 1. I find it easy to laugh about things that happen in my life. | 1 | 2 | 3 | 4 |
| 2. I avoid using alcohol as a means of helping me forget my problems. | 1 | 2 | 3 | 4 |
| 3. I can express my feelings without feeling silly. | 1 | 2 | 3 | 4 |
| 4. When I am angry, I try to let others know in non-confrontational and non-hurtful ways. | 1 | 2 | 3 | 4 |
| 5. I am a chronic worrier and tend to be suspicious of others. | 4 | 3 | 2 | 1 |
| 6. I recognize when I am stressed and take steps to relax through exercise, quiet time, or other activities. | 1 | 2 | 3 | 4 |
| 7. I feel good about myself and believe others like me for who I am. | 1 | 2 | 3 | 4 |
| 8. When I am upset, I talk to others and actively try to work through my problems. | 1 | 2 | 3 | 4 |
| 9. I am flexible and adapt or adjust to change in a positive way. | 1 | 2 | 3 | 4 |
| 10. My friends regard me as a stable, emotionally well-adjusted person. | 1 | 2 | 3 | 4 |

## ENVIRONMENTAL HEALTH

| | Rarely, If Ever | Sometimes | Most of the Time | Always |
|---|---|---|---|---|
| 1. I am concerned about environmental pollution and actively try to preserve and protect natural resources. | 1 | 2 | 3 | 4 |
| 2. I report people who intentionally hurt the environment. | 1 | 2 | 3 | 4 |
| 3. I recycle my garbage. | 1 | 2 | 3 | 4 |
| 4. I reuse plastic and paper bags and tin foil. | 1 | 2 | 3 | 4 |
| 5. I vote for pro-environmental candidates in elections. | 1 | 2 | 3 | 4 |
| 6. I write my elected leaders about environmental concerns. | 1 | 2 | 3 | 4 |
| 7. I consider the amount of packaging covering a product when I buy groceries. | 1 | 2 | 3 | 4 |
| 8. I try to buy products that are recyclable. | 1 | 2 | 3 | 4 |
| 9. I use both sides of the paper when taking class notes or doing assignments. | 1 | 2 | 3 | 4 |
| 10. I try not to leave the tap running too long when I brush my teeth, shave, or bathe. | 1 | 2 | 3 | 4 |

## SPIRITUAL HEALTH

| | Rarely, If Ever | Sometimes | Most of the Time | Always |
|---|---|---|---|---|
| 1. I believe life is a precious gift that should be nurtured. | 1 | 2 | 3 | 4 |
| 2. I take time to enjoy nature and the beauty around me. | 1 | 2 | 3 | 4 |
| 3. I take time alone to think about what's important in life—who I am, what I value, where I fit in, and where I'm going. | 1 | 2 | 3 | 4 |
| 4. I have faith in a greater power, be it a God-like force, nature, or the connectedness of all living things. | 1 | 2 | 3 | 4 |
| 5. I engage in acts of caring and goodwill without expecting something in return. | 1 | 2 | 3 | 4 |
| 6. I feel sorrow for those who are suffering and try to help them through difficult times. | 1 | 2 | 3 | 4 |
| 7. I feel confident that I have touched the lives of others in a positive way. | 1 | 2 | 3 | 4 |
| 8. I work for peace in my interpersonal relationships, in my community, and in the world at large. | 1 | 2 | 3 | 4 |
| 9. I am content with who I am. | 1 | 2 | 3 | 4 |
| 10. I go for the gusto and experience life to the fullest. | 1 | 2 | 3 | 4 |

## MENTAL HEALTH

| | Rarely, If Ever | Sometimes | Most of the Time | Always |
|---|---|---|---|---|
| 1. I tend to let my emotions get the better of me and I act without thinking. | 1 | 2 | 3 | 4 |
| 2. I learn from my mistakes and try to act differently the next time. | 1 | 2 | 3 | 4 |
| 3. I follow directions or recommended guidelines and act in ways likely to keep myself and others safe. | 1 | 2 | 3 | 4 |
| 4. I consider the alternatives before making decisions. | 1 | 2 | 3 | 4 |
| 5. I am alert and ready to respond to life's challenges in ways that reflect thought and sound judgment. | 1 | 2 | 3 | 4 |
| 6. I tend to act impulsively without thinking about the consequences. | 1 | 2 | 3 | 4 |
| 7. I actively try to learn all I can about products and services before making decisions. | 1 | 2 | 3 | 4 |
| 8. I manage my time well, rather than time managing me. | 1 | 2 | 3 | 4 |
| 9. My friends and family trust my judgment. | 1 | 2 | 3 | 4 |
| 10. I think about my self-talk (the things I tell myself) and then examine the real evidence for my perceptions and feelings. | 1 | 2 | 3 | 4 |

## OCCUPATIONAL HEALTH

| | Rarely, If Ever | Sometimes | Most of the Time | Always |
|---|---|---|---|---|
| 1. I am happy with my career choice. | 1 | 2 | 3 | 4 |
| 2. I look forward to work. | 1 | 2 | 3 | 4 |
| 3. My work responsibilities are consistent with my values. | 1 | 2 | 3 | 4 |
| 4. The advantages in my career are consistent with my values. | 1 | 2 | 3 | 4 |
| 5. I am happy with the balance between my work and leisure time. | 1 | 2 | 3 | 4 |
| 6. I am happy with the amount of control I have in my work. | 1 | 2 | 3 | 4 |
| 7. My work gives me personal satisfaction and stimulation. | 1 | 2 | 3 | 4 |
| 8. I am happy with the professional and personal growth provided by my job. | 1 | 2 | 3 | 4 |
| 9. I feel my work allows me to make a difference in the world. | 1 | 2 | 3 | 4 |
| 10. My work contributes positively to my overall well-being. | 1 | 2 | 3 | 4 |

## PERSONAL CHECKLIST

Now, total your scores in each of the health dimensions and compare them to the ideal score. Which areas do you need to work on? How does your score compare with how you rated yourself in the first part of the questionnaire?

|  | Ideal Score | Your Score |
|---|---|---|
| Physical Health | 40 | _____ |
| Social Health | 40 | _____ |
| Emotional Health | 40 | _____ |
| Environmental Health | 40 | _____ |
| Spiritual Health | 40 | _____ |
| Mental Health | 40 | _____ |
| Occupational Health | 40 | _____ |

## WHAT YOUR SCORES MEAN

Scores of 35–40: Outstanding! Your answers show you are aware of the importance of this component of your health. More important, you are putting your knowledge to work for you by practising good health habits. As long as you continue to do so this component will not pose a serious health risk. It's likely that you are setting an example for your family and friends to follow.

Scores of 30–35: Your health practices in this area are good, but there is room for improvement. Look again at the items you answered that scored one or two points. What changes could you make to improve your score? Even a small change in behaviour can help you achieve better health.

Scores of 20–30: Your health risks are showing! Would you like more information about the risks you are facing and why it is important for you to change these behaviours? Perhaps you need help in deciding how to make the changes you desire. In either case, help is available from this book, from your professor, and from your student health services.

Scores below 20: You may be taking serious and unnecessary risks with your health. Perhaps you are not aware of the risks and what to do about them. In this book you will find the information you need to help you improve your scores and your health.

Source: Adapted from the U.S. Health and Human Services, *Health Style: A Self Test* (Washington, DC: Public Health Service, 1981).

## Health Promotion: Helping You Stay Healthy

In discussions of health and wellness, the term **health promotion** is often used. Health promotion requires educational, organizational, environmental, and financial supports to help individuals and groups build positive health behaviours and to change negative ones. In other words, health promotion programs don't just tell people to lose weight and to eat better: they help them learn more (*educational supports*), provide programs and services that encourage them to participate (*organizational supports*), establish rules governing their attitudes and behaviours and supporting their decisions to change (*environmental supports*), and provide monetary incentives to motivate them toward healthful decision making (*financial supports*). In short, health promotion enhances the likelihood that, once a person decides to change a behaviour, conditions are optimal for success. In health promotion healthy people at risk for disease are identified and efforts are made to motivate them to improve their health. Further, various health promotion efforts encourage those whose health and wellness are already sound to maintain and improve their relevant health-enhancing activities.

In 2005, the Pan-Canadian Healthy Living Strategy was released (see the Focus on Canada box).[6] Actions proposed through this Strategy should improve the health status and health outcomes of the Canadian population.[7] Further, the proposed actions should reduce the current burden and contribute to the efficiency and sustainability of Canada's universal health-care delivery system. Rather than focusing on individual behaviour change, the Healthy Living Strategy takes a population health approach, recognizing that sustainable changes in individual behaviours are difficult without addressing living and working conditions. Thus, one of the key elements of the Strategy is to recognize and address linkages between lifestyle choices and the social, economic, and environmental influences on them.[8]

**Health promotion:** Combines educational, organizational, policy, financial, and environmental supports to help people change negative health behaviours.

# The Integrated Pan-Canadian Healthy Living Strategy 2005

An extensive pan-Canadian consultation process resulted in the release of the *Integrated Pan-Canadian Healthy Living Strategy 2005.* This first strategy focuses on healthy eating, physical activity, and their relationship to healthy weights; plans exist for future strategies to cover topics such as mental health and injury prevention. The federal, provincial, and territorial Ministers of Health noted a need for a pan-Canadian healthy living approach in 2002. Various consultations followed across the country, and the Strategy is the culmination of these discussions.

## THE HEALTHY LIVING STRATEGY

The Healthy Living Strategy provides a conceptual framework for sustained action that focuses on improving the health of all Canadians as a group. With all the population rather than individuals as the focus of the strategy, it is necessary to address the inequalities in health status among various population groups. The Healthy Living Strategy visualizes Canada as a healthy nation, with conditions that support the attainment of optimal health and wellness. Thus, the goals of the Healthy Living Strategy are to improve overall health outcomes and to reduce health disparities.

## HEALTHY LIVING TARGETS

Given the current overweight and obesity epidemic, along with Canadians' eating and physical activity habits, the proposed pan-Canadian Healthy Living targets "seek to obtain a 20 percent increase in the proportion of Canadians who are physically active, eat healthily, and are at healthy body weights." The year 2015 is considered the first marker for ongoing monitoring and evaluation to assess progress and allow for adjustments as appropriate. Specifically, the targets of the Healthy Living Strategy are:

*Healthy Eating:* By 2015, increase by 20 percent the proportion of Canadians who make healthy food choices according to the Canadian Community Health Survey (CCHS) and Statistics Canada (SC)/Canadian Institute for Health Information (CIHI) health indicators. This target would measure the food insecurity index and the consumption of vegetables and fruits, among other things.

*Physical Activity:* By 2015, increase by 20 percent the proportion of Canadians who participate in regular physical activity based on 30 minutes per day of moderate to vigorous activity as measured by the CCHS and the Physical Activity Benchmarks/Monitoring Program.

*Healthy Weights:* By 2015, increase by 20 percent the proportion of Canadians at a "normal" body weight based on a Body Mass Index (BMI) of 18.5 to 24.9, as measured by the National Population Health Survey (NPHS), CCHS, and SC/CIHI health indicators.

The *Integrated Pan-Canadian Healthy Living Strategy 2005* is available from www.phac-aspc.gc.ca/hl-vs-strat/pdf/hls_e.pdf. Information about the *Canadian Community Health Survey* can be obtained from www.hc-sc.gc.ca/fn-an/surveill/nutrition/commun/index_e.html.

*Canadian Guidelines for Body Weight Classification in Adults, 2003* is available from www.hc-sc.gc.ca/fn-an/nutrition/weights-poids/guide-ld-adult/cg_quick_ref-ldc_rapide_ref_e.html.

Information from *Statistics Canada* is available from www.statcan.ca.

Information from the *Canadian Institute for Health Information* is available from www.cihi.ca.

Information about the *Canadian Community Health Survey* can be obtained from www.hc-sc.gc.ca/fn-an/surveill/nutrition/commun/index_e.html.

## QUESTIONS

1. Identify problems that affect the health of Canadians. How many of these problems are directly (or indirectly) a result of poor dietary practices, physical inactivity, or overweight?

2. Do you think the Healthy Living targets are reasonable? Why or why not? What targets would you choose? Why?

3. Why are integrated efforts among the various sectors a critical component in the pursuit of public health? What contributions to population health could these other sectors provide? How would these other sectors benefit from improvements in health and the conditions that influence health?

Source: Adapted from The Secretariat for the Intersectoral Healthy Living Network in partnership with the F/P/T Healthy Living Task Group and the F/P/T Advisory Committee on Population Health and Health Security (ACPHHS), "The Integrated Pan-Canadian Healthy Living Strategy 2005," retrieved on May 31, 2006, from www.phac-aspc.gc.ca/hl-vs-strat/pdf/hls_e.pdf.

# Social Marketing: Creating Change

Social marketing is very much like advertising, but instead of pushing a product, social marketers push ideas: they promote social change to encourage positive attitudes, behaviours, and healthy living, using the principles of market analysis, planning, and control to persuade people to embrace a healthy way of living: discouraging smoking, unsafe sex, and substance and alcohol abuse, and encouraging active living and healthy eating. The goal of social marketing in health promotion is to persuade a target audience to move from one way of thinking and acting to another, healthier one.

Social marketers have to understand the attitudes and behaviours of target audiences, populations, or groups of people they want to reach and find ways to change these attitudes and behaviours by a strategic mix of traditional marketing tactics: special events with corporate sponsorship, special promotions, information, skills-development and communication resources, direct marketing, and public or media relations.

Health Canada often uses tracking studies to monitor the impact of its campaigns to determine if the time and money spent developing a resource has been put to good use. Attitudes and perceptions are, by their very nature, slow to change, so the vast majority of tracking studies are conducted at three- and sometimes six-month intervals. Information from such studies often forms the basis of mid-campaign changes in marketing strategy.

Many health promotion campaigns have been launched in areas such as anti-smoking, safety, drug abuse, drinking and driving, AIDS, nutrition, and physical fitness. Which campaigns do you think have been effective in changing unhealthy behaviours among Canadians? Which campaigns have been less effective? What is the difference in these campaigns? in the attitudes and behaviours they are trying to change?

Source: Adapted from the Social Marketing Network Website, www.hc-sc.gc.ca/hppb/socialmarketing/resources/primer.html, Health Canada, 2001.

---

The Strategy primarily emphasizes healthy eating, physical activity, and their relationship to healthy weights. Other healthy living priorities will be addressed in upcoming initiatives. As mentioned, a population health approach guides the Healthy Living Strategy. Using this approach, healthy living at a population level refers to the attitudes and behaviours that improve or maintain the health of the entire population and its subgroups. [9] When this approach is applied to individuals, healthy living refers to enhancing healthy behaviours, making healthy choices, and living in healthy ways. At all levels, the social, economic, political, cultural, and environmental conditions must be supportive of healthy living.

Whether we use the term health or wellness, we are talking about a person's overall responses to the challenges of living. Occasional dips into the ice cream bucket and other dietary slips, a missed daily walk, or an outburst of anger—and other deviations from optimal behaviours—should not be viewed as major failures to maintain wellness. In fact, the ability to recognize that each of us is an imperfect being trying to adapt in an imperfect world signals individual well-being.

We must also remember to be tolerant of others trying to improve their health. Rather than being warriors against pleasure in our zeal to change the health behaviours of others, we need to be supportive, understanding, and nonjudgmental in our interactions with them. *Health bashing*—intolerance or negative feelings, words, or actions aimed at people who fail to meet our expectations of health—may indicate our deficiencies in the psychological, social, or spiritual dimensions of the health continuum.

## Prevention: The Key to Future Health

**Prevention** means taking positive actions now to avoid becoming sick or less well later. Getting immunized against diseases such as polio, not smoking or chewing tobacco, practising safer sex, eating well, engaging in regular physical activity, and taking similar preventive measures constitute **primary prevention**—actions designed to stop health problems before they start. **Secondary prevention** is the early recognition of

**Prevention:** Actions or behaviours designed to keep you from getting sick or less well.

**Primary prevention:** Actions designed to stop problems before they start.

**Secondary prevention:** Intervention early in the development of a health problem to reduce symptoms or to halt its progression.

a health problem and intervention to eliminate or reduce its underlying causes before a more serious illness develops. Attending health education seminars in order to stop smoking is an example of secondary prevention. Another example of secondary prevention is modifying one's dietary intake and inactivity in response to a blood-cholesterol or blood-glucose test.

Two-thirds of deaths in Canada are a result of cardiovascular diseases, cancer, type 2 diabetes, and respiratory diseases. [10] These chronic diseases share common preventable factors—physical inactivity, unhealthy dietary intake, and tobacco use. Further, these preventable factors are influenced by the following environmental determinants: income, employment, education, geographic isolation, and social exclusion. Common sense would suggest that health promotion dollars should focus on the primary and secondary prevention of these and other lifestyle-related diseases. Instead, government money is primarily allocated for research and so-called **tertiary prevention**, treatment or rehabilitation efforts made after a person has become sick. This is clearly a misnomer—even though the intent of tertiary prevention is to prevent the further development of the disease (for example, chemotherapy and radiation therapy for individuals with cancer, or coronary bypass surgery for people with cardiovascular disease), it is more costly and less effective in promoting health than any other method.

when a study explores issues for one sex but generalizes the findings to both sexes. (The same thing can be said for age bias; that is, conducting research on 20-year-olds and applying the results to all age groups.) In the past, studies that examined the precise effects of a drug or treatment did not include women because researchers did not want to deal with variations caused by women's menstrual cycles. *Gender insensitivity* means overlooking sex as an important variable. An example of gender insensitivity might be research on symptoms of heart disease that looks at men and women but does not analyze data separately to determine if there are similarities or differences. When differences do not exist between men and women, the data can be collapsed and analyzed together; otherwise, sex should be a controlled variable. The term *double standards* refers to the "evaluation, treatment or measurement of the identical behaviours, traits or situations by different means."[13] In 1996, a policy on clinical trials stated that if the product is likely to be used by women then the testing must also be done on women. There has been increasing pressure placed on government to provide a more balanced approach to funding women's health programs. One example of increased activism is in the area of breast cancer. In Canada one in ten women will be diagnosed with breast cancer, yet it wasn't until the mid-1990s that much research was conducted on the causes, treatments, and social and psychological concerns of women diagnosed with it.

# SEX DIFFERENCES AND HEALTH STATUS

Although much of male and female anatomy is identical, it's clear that many major medical differences exist. Many diseases—osteoporosis, arthritis, headaches, thyroid disease, lupus, and Alzheimer's disease, for example—are far more common in women than in men. Further, diseases may appear differently in men than in women—for example, symptoms of a heart attack in women are more vague than they are in men. Finally, although women live longer than men, they don't necessarily have a better quality of life.[11]

## Sex and Gender

Sex bias has been identified as a serious weakness in medical research. In one study that reviewed medical journals in Canada and the United States, four factors reflecting bias were identified: androcentricity, overgeneralization, gender insensitivity, and double standards.[12] *Androcentricity* means viewing the world from a male perspective. *Overgeneralization* occurs

# IMPROVING YOUR HEALTH

## Benefits of Achieving Optimal Health

Figure 1.2 provides an overview of the leading causes of death in Canada, and Figures 1.3 to 1.5 give estimated incidence and mortality rates for heart disease, stroke, and cancers in men and women. Heart disease and cancer continue to be the leading causes of death. As Figure 1.3 shows, deaths from cardiovascular disease are declining among men and women. The Atlantic provinces have higher mortality rates than the western provinces, and these rates are consistent with the relative prevalence of smoking, high blood pressure, and obesity in these regions. Figure 1.4 provides estimated new cases and deaths from cancer for men. (The Canadian Cancer Society updates its estimates each year; see www.cancer.ca.) Incidence rates have declined for most forms of cancer, but there have been sizeable increases in the detection of prostate cancer through PSA testing. New cases of lung cancer have

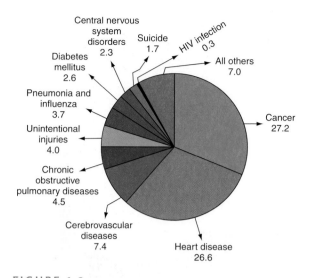

FIGURE 1.2

**Causes of Death in Canada, 1997**

Source: "Selected Leading Causes of Death, by Sex," adapted from Statistics Canada, www40.statcan.ca/l01/cst01/health36.htm.

been declining since the 1980s, likely because of the decrease in the number of males smoking.

Figure 1.5 shows estimated new cases and deaths from cancer for women. The incidence of new cancers has been relatively stable since the 1980s. Breast cancer is estimated to be the most common newly diagnosed cancer among women, but the leading cause of cancer death is still expected to be lung cancer. Breast and lung cancer have been increasing among women since the 1970s. While prevention and control strategies are making an impact on death rates from breast and prostate cancer, the increasing number of women who smoke is of concern since rates of lung cancer death are linked to the prevalence of smoking.

For example, you may be predisposed to a less healthy lifestyle if medical services are scarce in your area or if family members or friends smoke, drink heavily, or abuse drugs. While you can't change your genetic history, and improving your environment and the health-care system can be difficult, you can influence your future health status by the behaviours you choose today.

As previously mentioned and illustrated in Figure 1.2, heart disease and cancer are the leading causes of death in Canada. Reduction in risk for these and other major diseases is a benefit that you can hope to achieve when choosing healthy behaviours. Other benefits are:

- improved quality of life, in addition to an increased life span

- greater energy levels and increased capacity for and interest in having fun

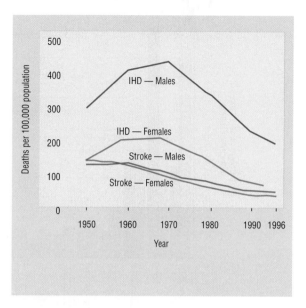

FIGURE 1.3

**Death Rates Due to Ischemic Heart Disease and Stroke, Canada, 1950 to 1996***

* Age-standardized to the 1991 Canadian population.

Source: "Death Rates due to Ischemic Heart Disease and Stroke, Canada 1950–1996," adapted from the Statistics Canada publication "Health Indicators," Catalogue No. 82-221, 1999.

- a stronger immune system, which enhances your ability to fight infections

- improved self-confidence, self-concept and self-esteem, and self-efficacy

- enhanced relationships with others due to better communication and "quality" time spent with them

- an improved ability to control and manage stress

- a reduced reliance on the health-care system

- improved cardiovascular functioning

- increased muscle tone, strength, flexibility, and endurance, which results in improved physical appearance, performance, and self-esteem

- a more positive outlook on life, fewer negative thoughts, and an ability to view life as challenging and to see negative events as an opportunity for growth

- improved environmental sensitivity, responsibility, and behaviours

- enhanced levels of spiritual health, awareness, and feelings of oneness with yourself, others, and the environment

**Tertiary prevention:** Treatment or rehabilitation efforts aimed at limiting the effects of the disease.

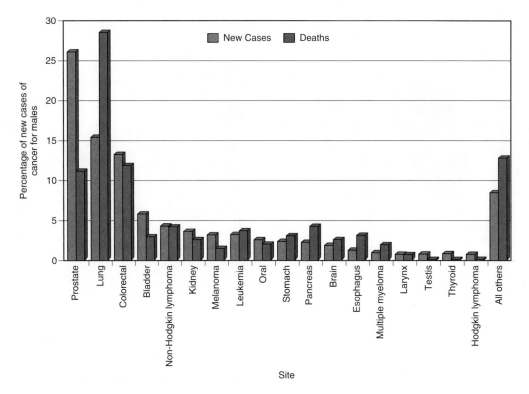

FIGURE 1.4

**Percentage Distribution of Estimated New Cases and Deaths for Selected Cancer Sites, Males, 2006**

Source: Canadian Cancer Society/National Cancer Institute of Canada, *Canadian Cancer Statistics 2006* (Toronto, Canada, 2006).

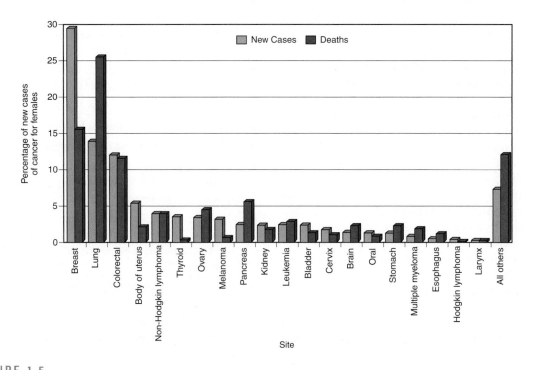

FIGURE 1.5

**Percentage Distribution of Estimated New Cases and Deaths for Selected Cancer Sites, Females, 2006**

Source: Canadian Cancer Society/National Cancer Institute of Canada, *Canadian Cancer Statistics 2006* (Toronto, Canada, 2006).

## Making Health-Wise Choices

Although mounting evidence indicates significant benefits to being healthy, many people find it difficult to become and remain healthy. Most experts believe that several key behaviours will help people live longer, such as:

- getting a good night's sleep (minimum of seven hours)
- maintaining healthy eating habits and maintaining weight
- participating in regular physical activities
- practising safer sex
- avoiding tobacco products
- limiting intake of alcohol
- keeping up with regular self-exams and medical checkups

Although health professionals can statistically assess the health benefits of these behaviours, there are several other actions that may not cause quantifiable "years added to life" but may significantly result in "life added to years." These include:

- controlling the real and imaginary stressors in life
- maintaining meaningful relationships with family and friends
- making time for yourself and being as kind to yourself as you are to others
- participating in at least one fun activity each day
- respecting the environment and the people in it
- considering alternatives when making decisions and assessing how actions affect others
- valuing each day and making the best of each opportunity
- viewing mistakes as opportunities to learn and grow
- understanding the health-care system and using it wisely

While it's easy to list things that one *should* do and even things that one may really *want* to do, change is not easy. All people, no matter where they are on the health and wellness continuum, have to start somewhere. The key is to decide what needs to change, determine the major actions necessary for the accomplishment of goals, set up a plan of action, and get started. But first it is important to take a close look at the factors that may contribute to current behaviours.

## Preparing for Behaviour Change

Mark Twain said that "habit is habit, and not to be flung out the window by anyone, but coaxed downstairs a step at a time." Changing negative behaviours into healthy ones is a time-consuming and difficult process. The chances of successfully changing negative behaviours improve when you make gradual changes that give you time to unlearn negative patterns and substitute positive ones. We have not yet developed a foolproof method for effectively changing behaviours, but we do know that certain behaviour changes can benefit individuals and society. To understand how the process of behaviour change works, we must first identify specific behaviour patterns and try to understand the reasons for them.

## Factors Influencing Behaviour Change

Figure 1.6 identifies the major factors that influence behaviours and behaviour-change decisions. These factors can be divided into three general categories: predisposing, enabling, and reinforcing factors.

### Predisposing Factors

Our life experiences, knowledge, cultural and ethnic inheritance, and current beliefs and values are all *predisposing factors* influencing behaviours and behaviour change. Factors that may predispose us to certain conditions include our age, sex, race, income, family, education, environment, and access to health care. For example, if your parents smoked, you are 90 percent more likely to start smoking than someone whose parents didn't. If your peers smoke, you are 80 percent more likely to smoke than someone whose friends don't.

### Enabling Factors

Skills or abilities, physical, emotional, and mental capabilities, and resources and accessible facilities that make health decisions more convenient or difficult are *enabling factors*. Positive enablers encourage you to carry through on your intentions. Negative enablers work against your intentions to change. For example, if you would like to join a local fitness centre but discover that the closest one is 10 kilometres away and that the membership fee is $600, those negative enablers may deter you from joining. On the other hand, if your school's fitness centre is two blocks away, is open until midnight, and has a reduced rate for students, those positive enablers will probably convince you to use the centre. Identifying these positive and negative enabling

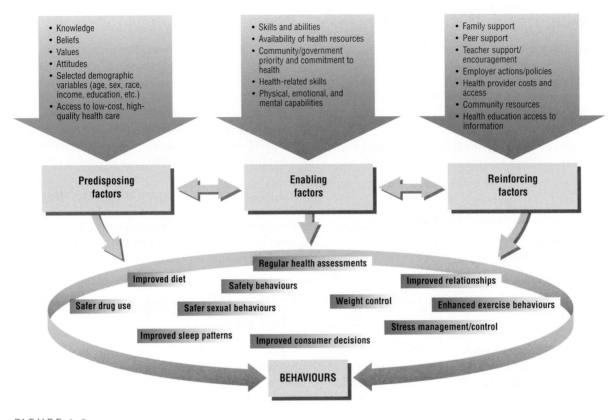

FIGURE 1.6
Factors That Influence Your Behaviour-Change Decisions

factors and devising alternative plans when the negative factors outweigh the positive ones is part of a necessary planning strategy for behavioural change.

## Reinforcing Factors

The presence or absence of support, encouragement, or discouragement that significant people in your life bring to a situation are *reinforcing factors*. For example, if you decide to stop smoking and your family and friends smoke in your presence, you may be tempted to start smoking again. In other words, your smoking behaviour is reinforced. If, however, you are trying to stop smoking and you have cut down from a pack to half a pack a day and all your friends tell you how great you're doing, your positive behaviour will be reinforced and you will be more likely to continue the reduction. Reinforcing factors also include policies and services that make it easier for you to maintain a particular behaviour. Policies such as smoke-free public buildings reinforce the behaviour of individuals who stop smoking. Reinforcing factors, which may influence you toward positive or negative behaviours, include money, popularity, support and appreciation from friends, and family interest and enthusiasm for what you are doing.

The way you reward or punish yourself for your successes and failures may affect your chances of adopting healthy behaviours. Learning to accept small failures and to concentrate on your successes may foster further successes. Berating yourself because you ate ice cream, argued with a friend, or didn't jog because it was raining may create an internal environment in which failure becomes almost inevitable. Telling yourself that you're worth the extra time and effort and giving yourself a pat on the back for small accomplishments is an often-overlooked factor in positive behaviour change.

It is not our intention to blame you if you are struggling with personal health behaviours or to suggest that all the variables that affect health are within your control. Our goal is to help you realize which factors are within your personal control and to show you how to maximize your decision-making powers to take that control—to maintain or improve your current health or to prevent premature deterioration of your health status.

Major changes in health behaviours are not made by following easy, one-step recipes. Lasting behaviour changes that ultimately improve your overall health and well-being require careful thought, individual analysis, and considerable effort. Changing beliefs, attitudes, values, actions, and behaviours that have been developing from infancy is difficult. Even the most strong-willed people discover that willpower alone is not enough to get them through the many adjustments needed to make lifelong behaviour changes.

Wanting to change is a prerequisite of the change process, but there is much more to the process than motivation. Motivation must be combined with common sense, commitment, and a realistic understanding of how best to move from point A to point B. *Readiness* is the state of being that precedes behaviour change. People who are ready to change possess the knowledge, attitudes, skills, and internal and external resources that make change a likely reality. For someone to be ready for change, certain basic steps and adjustments in thinking must occur. See also the Skills for Behaviour Change box.

## WHAT WOULD YOU DO?

What lifestyle behaviours would you like to change? Why? What predisposing, enabling, and reinforcing factors will help you to make this change? What predisposing, enabling, and reinforcing factors could make this change difficult? What can you do to avoid (or limit the effect of) these difficulties? Whom do you think you could ask to help support you in your behaviour-change efforts?

## Your Beliefs and Attitudes

Even if you know why you should make a specific behaviour change, your beliefs and attitudes about the value of your actions in making a difference will significantly affect what you do. We assume that when rational people realize there is a risk in what they are doing, they will act to reduce that risk. But this is not necessarily true. Consider the number of physicians and other health professionals who smoke, fail to manage stress, consume high-fat diets, are inactive, and act in other unhealthy ways. Surely they know better, but their "knowing" is disconnected from their "doing." Why? Two strong influences on our actions are beliefs and attitudes.

A **belief** is an appraisal of the relationship between some object, action, or idea (for example, smoking) and some attribute of that object, action, or idea (for example, smoking is expensive, dirty, and causes cancer—or, it is a sexy, cool, adult activity). Beliefs develop from direct experience (for example, if you have trouble breathing after smoking for several years) or from secondhand experience or knowledge conveyed by other people (for example, if you see your

grandfather die of lung cancer or emphysema after he smoked for years).[14] Although most of us have a general idea of what constitutes a belief, we may be a bit uncertain about what constitutes an attitude. We often hear or make such comments as, "He's got a rotten attitude," or, "She needs an attitude adjustment," but may still be unable to define *attitude*. An **attitude** is a relatively stable set of beliefs, feelings, and behavioural tendencies in relation to something or someone.

## Do Beliefs and Attitudes Influence Behaviours?

It seems logical to conclude that your beliefs will influence your behaviours. If you believe (make the appraisal) that taking drugs (an action) is harmful for you (attribute of that action), you will choose not to use drugs. If you believe that drinking and driving are incompatible, you will choose not to drink and drive.

Or will you? Psychologists studying the relationship between beliefs and health behaviours determined that although beliefs may subtly influence behaviours, they may not actually cause people to change them. The **health belief model (HBM)** explains how beliefs may or may not influence subsequent behaviours (see Figure 1.7).[15] Although many other models attempt to explain the influence of beliefs on behaviours, the HBM is one of the most widely accepted models. According to the HBM, several factors must support a belief in order for change to be likely:

- *Perceived seriousness of the health problem.* First, a person needs to consider how severe the medical and social consequences would be if the health problem were to develop or be left untreated. The more serious a person believes the effects will be, the more likely he or she is to take action. For example, heart disease is the number-one killer of Canadians; therefore, a person is likely to perceive it as a serious health problem.

- *Perceived susceptibility to the health problem.* Next, a person needs to evaluate the likelihood of developing the health problem. Those who perceive themselves as more likely to develop the health problem are more likely to take preventive action. For example, if your mother and sister were recently diagnosed with breast cancer, you are likely to consider yourself highly susceptible.

**Belief:** Appraisal of the relationship between some object, action, or idea and some attribute of that object, action, or idea.

**Attitude:** Relatively stable set of beliefs, feelings, and behavioural tendencies in relation to something or someone.

**Health belief model (HBM):** Model for explaining how beliefs may influence behaviours.

# Are You "Staged" for Change?

Have you ever come up with a great New Year's (or Monday-morning) resolution about something you are going to "do differently" only to have your good intention fall by the wayside a few days later? As most people discover at one time or another, changing established behaviours is not an easy task. Much of what we do is influenced by an entire host of variables, including our past history, reward systems, values, and culture. If you are in your 20s, you've been doing the same sorts of things for years, and these behaviours seem to be a part of who you are. Changing that part of you will not be easy.

A number of theories or models help explain why some people are successful in their attempts at behaviour change and others are not. One popular theory is the Stages of Change or Transtheoretical model developed by James Prochaska and Carlo DiClemente in the early 1980s. Developed from research on smoking cessation and drug and alcohol addiction, the Stages of Change model has been applied to a wide range of health behaviours over the years, including HIV prevention. Essentially, the Stages of Change model asks:

1. Are you ready for change? and

2. Where are you on the readiness scale?

This probably sounds a bit familiar to you. Like other behavioural models discussed in this chapter, the Stages of Change model indicates that the readier you are to change and the greater your motivation to change, the more likely your success. From their research, Prochaska and DiClemente concluded that an individual proceeds through distinctive stages during the change process. Those stages are:

1. **Precontemplation.** People in the precontemplation stage have no current intention of changing. They may have tried to change a behaviour before and given up, or they may be in denial and unaware of any problem.

   *Strategies for Change:* Sometimes a few frank yet kind words from friends may be enough to make precontemplators take a closer look at themselves. This is not to say that you should become a "warrior against pleasure" or tell people what to do when they haven't asked for advice. Recommending readings or making tactful suggestions, however, can help precontemplators consider making a change.

2. **Contemplation.** In this phase, people recognize that they have a problem and begin to contemplate the need to change. Acknowledgment usually results from increased awareness, often due to feedback from family and friends or access to information or increased knowledge. Despite this acknowledgment, people can languish in this stage for years, realizing that they have a problem but lacking the time or energy to make the change.

   *Strategies for Change:* Often, contemplators need a little push to get them started. This may come in the form of helping them set up a change plan (for example, an exercise routine), buying a helpful gift (such as a low-fat cookbook), sharing articles about a particular problem, or inviting them to go with you to hear a speaker on a related topic. People often need time to think about a course of action or to build skill. Your assistance can help them move off the point of indecision.

3. **Preparation.** Most people at this point are close to taking action. They've thought about what they might do and may even have come up with a plan. Rather than thinking about why they can't begin, they have started to focus on what they can do.

   *Strategies for Change:* People in the preparation stage can benefit from following a few simple guidelines. Set realistic goals (large and small), take small steps toward change, change only one thing at a time, reward small milestones, and seek support from friends and family. Identify factors that have enabled success or served as a barrier to success in the past, and modify them where possible. Fill out a Behaviour Change Contract to help you commit to making these changes.

4. **Action.** In this stage, people begin to follow their action plans. Those prepared for change who have thought about alternatives, engaged social support, and made a realistic plan of action are more ready than those who have given it little thought. Unfortunately, too many people start behaviour change here rather than going through the first three stages. Without a plan, without enlisting the help of others, or without a realistic goal, failure is likely.

   *Strategies for Change:* Publicly stating the desire to change helps ensure success. Encourage friends who are making a change to share their plans with you. Offer to help, and try to remove potential obstacles from their intended action plan. Social support and the buddy system can motivate even the most reluctant person.

5. **Maintenance.** Maintenance requires vigilance, attention to detail, and long-term commitment. Many people reach a goal, only to relax and slip back into the undesired behaviours. In this stage, it is important to be aware of the potential for relapses and develop strategies for dealing with such challenges. Common causes of relapse include overconfidence, daily temptations, stress or emotional distractions, and self-deprecation.

   *Strategies for Change:* During maintenance, continue taking the same actions that led to success in the first place. Find fun and creative ways to maintain positive behaviours. This is where a willing and caring support group can be vital. Knowing where on campus to turn for help when you don't have a close support network is also helpful.

6. **Termination.** By this point, the behaviour is so ingrained that the current level of vigilance may be unnecessary. The new behaviour has become an essential part of daily living. Can you think of someone you know who has made a major behaviour change that has now become an essential part of that person's life?

■ *Cues to action.* Those who are reminded or alerted about a potential health problem are more likely to take preventive action. For example, having your doctor tell you that your blood sugar levels are indicative of a prediabetic state may be the cue you need to get physically active and lose weight.

Three other factors are linked to perceived risk for health problems: *demographic variables,* including age, sex, race, and ethnic background; *sociopsychological variables,* including personality traits, social class, and social pressure; and *structural variables,* including knowledge about or prior contact with the health problem.

The health belief model is followed many times every day. Take smokers, for example. Older smokers are likely to know other smokers who developed serious heart or lung problems as a result of smoking. They are thus more likely to perceive a threat to their health connected with the behaviour of smoking than is a young person who just started. The greater the perceived threat of health problems caused by smoking, the greater the chance a person will quit smoking. However, many chronic smokers know that they have serious health problems, yet they continue to smoke. Why do people fail to take actions to avoid further harm? Some people do not believe that they will be affected by a severe problem—they act as if they have

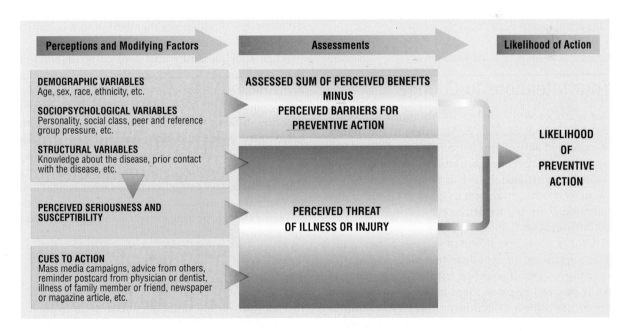

## FIGURE 1.7
### Health Belief Model

Source: Adapted by permission from Edward P. Sarafino, *Health Psychology: Biopsychosocial Interactions* (New York: John Wiley & Sons, 1990) 190. © 1990 by John Wiley & Sons.

some kind of immunity—and are unlikely to change their behaviours. In some cases, they think that, even if they get cancer or have a heart attack, the health-care system and improving technologies will be able to take care of them. For these individuals, a cue such as a friend or family member having a heart attack or being diagnosed with lung cancer may be the thing to put them into action.

Other HBM factors that affect the likelihood of behaviour change are assessments about whether the benefits outweigh the costs and whether actions will actually work. If you are so addicted to smoking that the thought of quitting is not acceptable to you, or if you enjoy smoking too much, you will probably keep smoking, particularly if the consequences won't be felt for some time and the pleasure is there at the moment. Similarly, you are not likely to make the effort to do something (for example, go for a jog) if you won't feel the benefits right away.

## WHAT WOULD YOU DO?

Is there a health behaviour you should change? What could happen if you do not change this health behaviour (perceived seriousness of the health problem)? How likely are you to develop the health problem (perceived susceptibility)? What made you aware of this potential health problem (cues to action)? What steps will you take today to start the behaviour-change process?

## Your Intentions to Change

Our attitudes tend to reflect our emotional responses and follow from our beliefs. According to the **theory of reasoned action**, our behaviours result from our intentions to perform actions. An intention is a result of our attitude toward an action and our beliefs about what others may want us to do. [16] A behavioural intention, then, is a written or stated commitment to perform an action.

If, for example, you are out of shape and your health is important to you, you may take steps to improve your fitness level. If your best friend tells you that you really do need to get in shape and you want to gain his or her respect or admiration, your intention to become more physically active may become stronger. In brief, the more consistent and powerful your attitudes about an action and the more you are influenced by others to take that action, the greater will be your stated intention to do so—in this example, to get more

physically active. The more you verbalize your commitment to physical activity, the more likely it is that you will do some sort of physical activity.

## Significant Others as Change Agents

Many people are highly influenced by the approval or disapproval (real or imagined) of close friends and loved ones and of the social and cultural groups to which they belong. Such influences can offer support for health actions, making healthy behaviours all the more possible to attain; they can also affect behaviours negatively, interfering with even the best intentions of making a positive change.

### Your Family

From the time of your birth, your parents have influenced your behaviours by giving you strong cues about which actions are socially acceptable and which are not. Brushing your teeth, bathing, wearing deodorant, and chewing food with your mouth closed are probably behaviours that your family instilled in you long ago. Your family culture influenced your food choices, your religious and political beliefs, and your other values and actions. If you deviated from your family's norms, a family member probably let you know fairly quickly. Good family units share unconditional love and trust, dedication to the healthy development of all family members, and a commitment to work out difficulties.

When a loving family unit does not exist, when it does not provide for basic human needs, or when dysfunctional, irresponsible individuals try to build a family under the influence of drugs or alcohol, it becomes difficult for a child to learn positive health behaviours. Healthy behaviours get their start in healthy homes; unhealthy homes breed unhealthy habits. Healthy families provide the foundation for a clear and necessary understanding of what is right and wrong, what is positive and negative. Without this fundamental grounding, many young people have great difficulties.

### The Influence of Others

Just as your family influences your actions during your childhood, your friends and significant others influence your behaviours as you grow older. Most of us desire to fit the "norm" and avoid hassles in our daily interactions with others. If you deviate from the actions expected in your hometown or among your friends, you may suffer ostracism, strange looks, and other negative social consequences. Understanding the subtle and not-so-subtle ways in which other people influence our actions is an important step in changing our behaviours.

The behaviour choices we make can be explained by the *theory of planned behaviour.*[17] This theory outlines three reasons for how we choose to behave:

- *Our attitudes toward the behaviour,* for example what we think about the positive or negative effects of our actions and the importance of each.

- *Our level of perceived behavioural control,* or our beliefs about the constraints and opportunities we might have concerning the behaviour.

- *Our subjective norms,* or whether or not we think our actions will meet the approval or disapproval of people important to us.

For example, if you want to lose weight because you believe it will make you more desirable to a romantic partner, you will have strong intentions to a weight-loss program (*attitudes* toward the behaviour). Intentions are powerful indicators of successful behaviour change. If there is a convenient, affordable fitness centre near you, and if the schedule works for you, you will be more motivated and believe you can make the change (*control beliefs*). Finally, if friends offer encouragement (*subjective norms* ), you are more likely to remain motivated to change your behaviours. On the other hand, if you perceive that your friends think you're a nerd for going to the gym, or if the gym is inconvenient or expensive, you may quickly lose your motivation. The opinions of key people play a powerful role in our motivation to change behaviours.

The influence of others can serve as a powerful social support for our positive behaviour changes. At other times, we are influenced to drink too much, party too hard, eat too much, or engage in some other negative action because we don't want to be left out or because we fear criticism. Learning to understand the subtle and not-so-subtle ways in which our families, friends, and other people have influenced and continue to influence our behaviours is an important step toward changing our behaviours.

If you are engaged in an abusive relationship, having friends you trust and can confide in can give you the strength to walk away from the situation—to change your behaviours. Someone who will accept you unconditionally and be there for you can be a wonderful asset and give you the support to deal with life's challenges. The more social support options you have, and the closer the relationship or social bonds, the greater the chances that you will be able to deal with crises in healthy ways. If you expand your social support network to include counsellors, spiritual advisers, and others, you will further increase your likelihood of success. Whom would you call if you were stranded in the middle of a cold, snowy night on a remote road? Who would get out bed, without question, to come and get you? Surprisingly, many people have no one to call under any circumstances, let alone when they are in crisis. The importance of cultivating and maintaining close ties is an important part of overall health.

# BEHAVIOUR-CHANGE TECHNIQUES

Once you have analyzed the factors influencing your current behaviours, as well as the factors that may influence the direction and potential success of the behaviour change you are considering, you must decide which of several possible behaviour-change techniques will work best for you.

## Shaping: Developing New Behaviours in Small Steps

Regardless of how motivated and committed you are to change, some behaviours are almost impossible to change immediately. To reach your goal, you may need to take a number of individual steps, each designed to change one small piece of the larger behaviour. This process is known as **shaping**.

For example, suppose you have been inactive for a while. You decide that you want to become more physically active and physically fit. Your long-term goal is to be able to run five kilometres. You realize that it is not wise—and it will hurt—to simply start running, so you decide to build up your fitness gradually. During week one, you will walk for 30 minutes every other day at a moderate pace. During week two, you will increase the time to 45 minutes. In week three, you will increase the intensity of your walk and still go for 45 minutes. In week four, you will alternate 5 minutes of walking with 5 minutes of jogging. These gradual steps—and more like them—will help you to reach your goal.

---

**Theory of reasoned action:** Model for explaining the importance of our intentions in determining behaviours.

**Shaping:** Using a series of small steps to get to a particular goal gradually.

Whatever the desired behaviour change, all shaping involves:

- starting slowly and trying not to cause undue stress during the early stages of the program
- keeping the steps small and achievable
- being flexible and ready to change if the original plan proves uncomfortable
- refusing to skip steps or to move to the next step until the previous step has been mastered; behaviours don't develop overnight, so they won't change overnight.
- rewarding yourself for meeting short- and long-term goals

## Visualizing: The Imagined Rehearsal

Mental practice and rehearsal can help change unhealthy behaviours into healthy ones. Athletes and others have used a technique known as **imagined rehearsal** to reach their goals. By visualizing their planned action ahead of time, they were better prepared when they put themselves to the test.

For example, suppose you want to ask a classmate out on a date. Imagine the setting, (walking together to class). Then, in your mind and out loud, practise exactly what you want to say ("There's a great concert this Sunday, and I was wondering if . . ."). Mentally anticipate different responses ("Oh, I'd love to, but . . .") and what you will say in response ("How about I give you a call some time this week?"). Careful mental and verbal imagined rehearsal will greatly improve your likelihood of success.

## Modelling

**Modelling**, or learning behaviours by carefully observing other people, is one of the most effective strategies for changing behaviours. If you carefully observe behaviours you admire, and isolate their components, you can model the steps of your behaviour-change strategy on a proven success. For example if you have trouble talking to people you don't know very well, one of the easiest ways for you to improve your communication skills is to observe someone whose social skills you admire. Do they talk or listen more? How do they listen? How do people respond to them? What makes them good communicators? What is their body language like? If you observe the behaviours you admire and isolate their components, you can model the steps

in your behaviour-change technique based on a proven success.

## Controlling the Situation

Sometimes, putting yourself in the right setting or with the right group of people will positively influence your behaviours directly or indirectly. Many situations and occasions trigger similar behaviours by different people. For example, in libraries, churches, and museums, most people talk softly. Few people laugh at funerals. The term **situational inducement** refers to an attempt to influence a behaviour by using situations and occasions that are structured to exert control over that behaviour. If you are trying to reduce the fat in your diet, an example could be choosing to eat at a vegetarian restaurant rather than a fast-food chain.

## Reinforcement: "Different Strokes for Different Folks"

A **positive reinforcement** seeks to increase the likelihood that a behaviour will occur by presenting something positive as a reward for that behaviour. Each of us is motivated by different reinforcers. While a special T-shirt may be a positive reinforcer for young adults entering a fun run, it may not be for a 50-year-old runner who dislikes message-bearing T-shirts, or for someone with a drawer full of them. Most positive reinforcers can be classified under five headings:

- *Consumable reinforcers* are delicious edibles such as candy, cookies, or gourmet meals.
- *Activity reinforcers* are opportunities to watch TV, go on a vacation, go swimming, or do something else enjoyable.
- *Manipulative reinforcers* are such incentives as lower rent in exchange for mowing the lawn or the promise of a better grade for doing an extra-credit project.
- *Possessional reinforcers* are tangible rewards such as a new TV or a sports car.
- *Social reinforcers* are such things as loving looks, affectionate hugs, and praise.

## Changing Self-Talk

*Self-talk*, or the way you think and talk to yourself, can also play a role in modifying your health-related behaviours. Here are some cognitive procedures for changing self-talk.

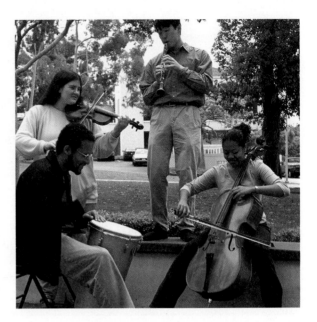

*The support and encouragement of friends with similar interests will strengthen your commitment to develop and maintain positive health behaviours.*

### Rational-Emotive Therapy

This form of cognitive therapy or self-directed behaviour change is based on the premise that there is a close connection between what people say to themselves and how they feel. Most everyday emotional problems and related behaviours stem from irrational statements that people make to themselves when events in their lives are different from what they would like them to be.[18]

### Meichenbaum's Self-Instructional Methods

In Meichenbaum's behavioural therapies, clients are encouraged to give *self-instructions* ("Slow down, don't rush") and *positive affirmations* ("My speech is going fine—I'm almost done!") to themselves instead of thinking self-defeating thoughts ("I'm talking too fast—my speech is terrible") when a situation seems to be getting out of control. Meichenbaum is perhaps best known for a process known as *stress inoculation*, in which clients are subjected to extreme stressors in a laboratory environment. Before a stressful event (for example, going to the doctor), clients practise individual coping skills (for example, deep breathing exercises) and self-instructions (for example, "I'll feel better once I know what's causing my pain"). Meichenbaum demonstrated that clients who practised coping techniques and self-instruction were less likely to resort to negative behaviours in stressful situations.

### Blocking or Thought Stopping

By purposely blocking or stopping negative thoughts, a person can concentrate on taking positive steps toward necessary behaviour change. For example, suppose you are preoccupied with your ex-partner, who recently deserted you for someone else. In blocking or thought stopping, you consciously stop thinking about the situation and force yourself to think about something more pleasant (for example, dinner tomorrow with your best friend). By refusing to dwell on negative images and by forcing yourself to focus elsewhere, you can save wasted energy, time, and emotional resources and move on to positive change.

# MAKING BEHAVIOUR CHANGE

## Self-Assessment: Antecedents and Consequences

Behaviours, thoughts, and feelings always occur in a context—the situation. Situations can be divided into two components: the events that come before a

**Imagined rehearsal:** Practising through mental imagery, to become better able to perform an event.

**Modelling:** Learning specific behaviours by watching others perform them.

**Situational inducement:** Attempts to influence a behaviour by using situations and occasions structured to exert control over that behaviour.

**Positive reinforcement:** Presenting something positive following a behaviour being reinforced.

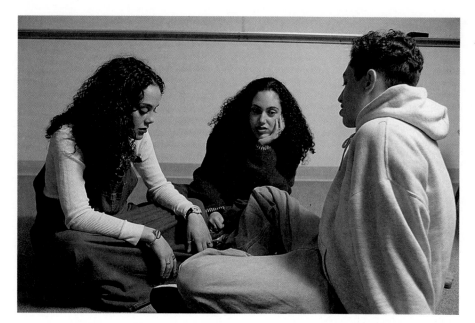

*Talking with friends or family can help you clarify your thinking about behaviours you want to change and provide ongoing support as you attempt to reach your goals.*

behaviour and those that come after it. *Antecedents* are the setting events for a behaviour; they cue or stimulate a person to act in certain ways. Antecedents can be physical events, thoughts, emotions, or the actions of other people. *Consequences*—the results of behaviours—affect whether a person will repeat a behaviour.[19] Consequences also include physical events, thoughts, emotions, or the actions of other people.

Learning to recognize the antecedents of behaviours and acting to modify them is one method of changing our behaviours. A diary noting your undesirable behaviours and identifying the settings in which they occur can be a useful tool. For example, if you are gaining weight, keep a diary of when, where, why, how, and with whom you eat. If you are shovelling in the potato chips while studying, you may need to study in the library, where food isn't allowed, or keep only low-calorie snacks in the house. If you eat more when you are angry, upset, depressed, or stressed, try to deal directly with your stressors or engage in an alternative activity, such as going for a walk or swim. The positive consequences of these changes will be that you will maintain your weight and feel better about yourself.

## Analyzing the Behaviours You Want to Change

Successful behaviour change requires a careful assessment of exactly what it is that you want to change. All too often we berate ourselves by using generalities: "I am not a good person, I'm lousy to my friend, I need

to be a better person." Before you can begin to change a negative behaviour, you must take a hard look at its specifics. Determining the specific behaviours you would like to change—in contrast to the general problem—will allow you to set clear goals for change. What are you doing that makes you a lousy friend? Are you gossiping about your friends? Are you lying to them? Have you been a "taker" rather than a "giver" in the friendship? Or are you really a good friend most of the time? What specifically do you do that makes you a not-so-good friend?

Let's say the problem is gossiping. You can analyze this behaviour by examining the following components:

- *Frequency*. How often are you gossiping? All the time, or only once in a while?

- *Duration*. Have you been gossiping about your friend for a long period of time? How long?

- *Seriousness*. Is your gossiping just idle chatter, or are you really getting down and dirty and trying to injure the other person? What are the consequences for you? for your friend? for your friendship? for the person listening to you?

- *Basis for the problem behaviour*. Is your gossip based on facts, on your perceptions of facts, or on deliberate embellishments of facts? Are you trying to make yourself look or feel better? to discredit your friend?

- *Antecedents*. What kinds of situations trigger your gossiping? Do some settings or people bring out the gossip in you more than other settings and people? What triggers your feelings of dislike for or irritation toward your friend? Why are you talking behind your friend's back?

# Decision Making: Choices for Change

You've assessed the antecedents and consequences of the behaviour you want to change and analyzed its components. Now comes the real crunch: deciding what to do when faced with choices. Decision making is a skill you must consciously develop. Choosing among alternatives is difficult when you are consciously and unconsciously pressured by internal and external influences. For example, "just saying no" is, of course, one choice when you are handed a glass of beer or wine at a party. However, if you are trying desperately not to be considered a dweeb, if people with whom you identify all drink, or if you like the taste of beer or wine, the decision becomes harder. By practising the following decision-making skills prior to having that drink put into your hands, you will increase your chances of making the choice you really want to make. This set of skills, referred to by the acronym DECIDE, can be applied to many situations in which you have to make a decision.[20]

**D** *Decide in advance what the problem is.* By defining the problem in advance, you will have time to decide how important it is. If you have really decided that drinking is not for you, or that drinking in certain situations could put you at risk, you will have your basic criteria for acting in specific situations.

**E** *Explore the alternatives.* List the possible alternatives, ranging from not drinking to drinking heavily. If any of these alternatives is unacceptable to you, cross it off and work with those remaining.

**C** *Consider the consequences.* Think about each of the alternatives remaining. What are the possible positive and negative consequences of each? Think about what will probably happen, not just what may happen in the best and worst scenarios. How risky is each alternative? Are the consequences of losing the friendship of a group because you refuse to drink as serious as the risk of drinking heavily and getting into trouble sexually or drinking and driving? Is there another alternative that could reduce your risks?

**I** *Identify your values.* Your beliefs and feelings about certain behaviours represent your values, which influence the majority of your behaviours. When choosing to drink or not to drink in a social setting, or when choosing how much to drink, you should base your choice on an analysis of your values.

**D** *Decide and take action.* If you have seriously thought about the first four DECIDE skills and decided that it's okay to have one or two drinks over the course of the evening and that is the absolute limit, this may be a reasonable decision for you. Now you must take action based upon your decision—you must actively resist temptation and stick to your limit.

**E** *Evaluate the consequences.* A key component of the decision-making process is a careful look backward at your decision and your resulting behaviours, how you felt about them, and whether you want to do anything differently in the future. You may add other alternatives at the second step, for instance. The secret to success is to think about the problem in advance, consider your values and wants, and anticipate the choices you will have.

## WHAT WOULD YOU DO?

How often do you have to make decisions that relate to your health? Are many of these decisions difficult? Which ones? Why is it sometimes hard for you to make decisions? What things influence your decisions?

# Goal Setting and Behaviour Change: SuPeR SMART

Goal setting is a critical part of the behaviour-change process. As noted previously, creating realistic short- and long-term goals provides a target for your efforts. One practical method of goal setting is called SuPeR SMART.[21]

**Self-controllable.** The goals you set must be within your control. If eating healthier is a goal, a more specific appropriate goal would be to ensure that you consume at least two fruits and three vegetables each day. If becoming more physically active is something you would like to do, an example of a self-controllable goal is to add 15 minutes of walking each day after dinner.

**Public.** If you make your goal visible—for you and others to see—it will be a constant reminder of what you are trying to achieve. Using the examples above, keep a calendar on the refrigerator or somewhere else in your kitchen where you can tick off the number of fruits and vegetables you consume each day. Similarly, indicate on the calendar with a checkmark that you walked your 15 minutes after dinner.

**Rewards.** Rewarding yourself for accomplishments is important and helps to motivate you to stay on track. The reward, however, should not contradict what you are trying to achieve (for example, treating yourself to a bag of chips when you are trying to eat healthier). Instead, reward yourself with a new workout T-shirt or a new book. Rewards should occur frequently enough that they are attainable and do provide the needed motivation.

# Managing Your Behaviour: Change Strategies

Having read this chapter, you should realize that health involves many dimensions of your life. Changing negative health-related behaviours is a complicated, multifaceted process requiring a great deal of commitment, personal insight, and knowledge. Very few of us could ever "just do it" (at least not on the first try), as the advertisements may lead you to believe. As you read this book, you will find that each chapter lists specific activities and choices that enable you to adopt or maintain healthy behaviours. It may be helpful for you to consider the following activities and questions as you begin planning your best course of action.

## MAKING DECISIONS FOR YOU

1. List a specific behaviour that you want to change. Although there may be many behaviours you would like to change, list only one to increase your chance of success.

2. Outline the steps you will take to achieve this change.

3. What reinforcers can you give yourself along the way? Whom could you call upon to help keep you motivated? Is that person willing to help?

4. What techniques do you think will be most useful (positive reinforcement, shaping, modelling, imagined rehearsal, situational inducement, changes in self-talk, others)?

## CHECKLIST FOR CHANGE: MAKING PERSONAL CHOICES

- Are you ready to make this change? Are you in a healthy emotional state? Are you doing it for you, or to please someone else?

- Have you completed a personal health history to assess your risks from various sources?

- Have you developed an action plan with short- and long-term goals? Have you set priorities?

- Have you assessed your personal resources? Whom can you call on to help you? Where can you go for support and advice?

- Have you planned alternative actions in case you run into obstacles or begin to self-sabotage?

- Have you set up a list of reinforcers and supports that will keep you motivated along the way?

- Have you established a set of guidelines for success? Will you have small goals to achieve at selected intervals or will you consider yourself successful only if you have met your ultimate goal?

## CHECKLIST FOR CHANGE: MAKING COMMUNITY CHOICES

- Have you taken time to become educated about issues or concerns affecting others in your community?

- Have you prioritized the actions that you can take to make a difference in changing community behaviours? Do you have a particular goal?

- Do you act responsibly to preserve the environment by consuming fewer resources? Using fewer packaged items? Do you reuse, recycle, and reduce consumption whenever possible?

- Do you analyze what is happening in your school, community, province, and nation by reading about issues, actively discussing problems and possible solutions, and developing personal opinions?

- Do you listen carefully to what your elected officials say and let them know in writing or by calling if you disagree with them?

- Do you volunteer your time to help less fortunate others at least once during every term?

- Do you purchase products and services from companies that have proven records of protecting the environment, providing safe foods and products, and supporting the health and well-being of others through their organizational practices?

## CHECKLIST FOR CHANGE: MAKING CRITICAL THINKING CHOICES

Each chapter of this text will end with a decision-making situation. You may wish to use the DECIDE model introduced in this chapter to develop decision-making skills. For your first decision, let's return to the situation described when we introduced the model: To drink or not to drink. Let's assume that you are attending a major floor party tonight where alcohol will be served—and you have a test tomorrow afternoon. Using the decision-making model, will you drink? If so, will you set a limit? How will you respond if you're offered more than your limit?

**Specific.** Your goals should be clear and precise. "Eating healthier" is not very precise. Meeting the guidelines set out in Canada's Food Guide to Healthy Eating is more precise. "Getting more active" is not very precise. Engaging in 30 minutes of physical activity every day is much more clear.

**Measurable.** Your goals should be measurable. Thus, a goal of meeting the guidelines set in the Food Guide (consuming minimally 5 servings from grain products, 5 servings from vegetables and fruits, 2 servings from milk products, and 2 servings from meat and alternatives), or of accumulating 30 minutes of physical activity every day, can be easily measured.

**Adjustable.** Your short- and long-term goals need to be adjustable. Life can be unpredictable, and if you start to fall behind because of one stressor or another it is important to recognize that it's okay to not reach your goals, so long as you can get on track as soon as possible. Using our examples, even though you did not meet the Food Guide requirements over your holidays or engage in 30 minutes of physical activity every day, you can resume with your healthier eating or getting more active once you return. You may also learn more about yourself and why it was that you were not able to stay on track such that you can adjust the next time and more successfully keep up with your goals.

**Realistic.** To successfully change your behaviours, your goals must be realistic. In determining the reality of your goals, you should evaluate your financial, environmental, physical, and emotional situations. A goal to climb Mount Everest in the next year, although admirable, may not be realistic if you do not have the financial means to get there or the family or social networks to support your efforts.

**Time-based.** Again, your goals should be quantifiable and include a specific date or timeline for achievement. Setting a realistic timeline requires accountability for your choices and actions. Thus, in the first week of changing your behaviours you may add 10 minutes of physical activity each day. The next week you may increase the time to 15 minutes, and so forth until you reach your goal of 30 minutes each day. Be careful to set a realistic and achievable timeline to avoid failure and maintain motivation. Similarly, if your timeline is too long, you may lose sight of what you are trying to achieve.

Whether your behaviour change is to become more socially active, eat healthier, become physically active, or enhance your spiritual health, your goal setting should be guided by the SuPeR SMART components and aimed at improving your overall well-being.

## SUMMARY

- Health is defined as a dynamic process of trying to achieve your individual potential in the physical, social, mental, occupational, emotional, environmental, and spiritual dimensions. Wellness involves actively trying to achieve the highest level of health possible along each dimension.

- Although Canadians have an increased average life span, we need to increase our span of *quality* life— in other words, to add life to our years.

- Sex continues to play a major role in health status and care. Women have longer lives but more medical problems than men. The political support to include women in medical research and training attempts to close the gap in health care.

- The leading causes of death are heart disease, cancer, and stroke. Many of the risks associated with these leading killers can be reduced through lifestyle changes.

- Several factors contribute to your health status, but not all of them are within your control. Your beliefs and attitudes, your intentions to change, support from significant others, and your readiness to change are factors over which you have some degree of control. Access to health care, genetic predisposition, health policies, and other factors are potential reinforcing, predisposing, and enabling factors that may influence your health decisions.

- Applying to your personal situation behaviour-change techniques such as shaping, visualizing, modelling, controlling the situation, reinforcing, and changing self-talk will help you to be successful in making behaviour changes.

- Decision making has several key components: Defining the problem, Exploring alternatives, Considering consequences, Identifying your values, Deciding and acting, and Evaluating the consequences of your choices. Following the DECIDE model can assist you to make behaviour changes.

# DISCUSSION QUESTIONS

1. How are the terms *health* and *wellness* similar? What, if any, are important distinctions between these terms?

2. How healthy are Canadians today? How will health promotion and illness and injury prevention improve quantity and quality of life?

3. What are some of the major differences in the way males and females are treated in the health-care system? Why do you think these differences exist? What can be done to change this?

4. What are the leading causes of death in Canada? What lifestyle changes can you make to lower your risks for major diseases?

5. What is the health belief model? The theory of reasoned action? The theory of planned behaviour? How may each of these models be working when a young man decides to smoke his first cigarette? his last cigarette?

6. Explain the predisposing, reinforcing, and enabling factors influencing the decision of a young mother on social support to sell drugs to support her children.

7. Describe how you could use each of the behaviour-change techniques to change your couch-potato behaviour and become physically active on a regular basis.

8. What are the key components of the decision-making process? Why is it important that you be ready to change before you try to start changing?

# APPLICATION EXERCISE

Reread the What Do You Think? scenarios at the beginning of the chapter and answer the following questions.

1. From what you learned in this chapter, what steps would Tim and Kim have to take to change their behaviours?

2. On your campus, where could students having similar problems go for help?

3. As a friend, what can you do to be more supportive of the health of someone you know who is trying to make a change?

# HEALTH ON THE NET

World Health Organization
**www.who.int**

Health Canada
**www.hc-sc.gc.ca**

Canadian Institute for Health Information
**www.cihi.ca**

Canadian Health Network
**www.canadian-health-network.ca**

Statistics Canada: Canadian Health Statistics
**www40.statcan.ca/l01/cst01/**

Canadian Institutes of Health Research
**www.cihr-irsc.gc.ca**

Medbroadcast Health News
**www.medbroadcast.com**

# CHAPTER 2

# PSYCHOSOCIAL HEALTH

*Achieving Mental, Emotional, Social, and Spiritual Wellness*

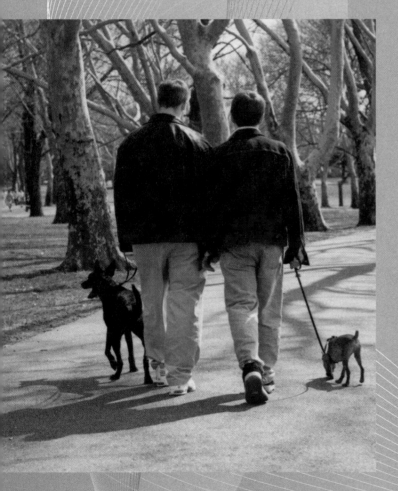

## CHAPTER OBJECTIVES

- Define psychosocial health in terms of its mental, emotional, social, and spiritual components, and identify the basic elements shared by psychosocially healthy people.

- Identify the external and internal factors influencing psychosocial health.

- Describe positive steps you can take to enhance your psychosocial health.

- Identify and describe common psychosocial problems, and explain their causes and available treatments.

- Evaluate the role sex plays in diagnoses and treatment of mental health.

- Identify the warning signs of suicide and know what actions can be taken to help an individual who is suicidal.

- Identify the different types of mental health professionals and the most common types of therapy.

Marisol is a 19-year-old first-year student majoring in liberal arts. She has become increasingly bored with her classes, finds little excitement in her days, and doesn't have the energy or desire to go out with friends. One recent weekend she stayed in bed for two days "resting," and when she got up on Monday she was still so tired that she could barely stay awake in class. She can't concentrate, finds herself lounging on the couch watching TV every evening, and doesn't care whether her apartment is a mess. She has gone to the student health centre, but after several tests the doctor tells her that there is nothing physically wrong with her.

■ Have you ever felt like Marisol does? What do you think is wrong with her? What do you think contributed to her present condition? Do you have any friends showing similar characteristics? Why might a typical student health professional miss such obvious symptoms? What do you think Marisol should do to help herself get better? As a friend, what could you do to help her? What services and programs are available on your campus or in your community for helping someone like her?

Most of us have felt "down" occasionally, but we are typically able to get through the day in a reasonably productive, if not altogether exciting, way. We eventually sort through seemingly overwhelming problems, suppress our anxieties, and use our social support system (families, friends, and significant others) to help us through the low times. But for some of us, these down times become persistent, nagging experiences that vary from small "downers" to "black holes" that are increasingly difficult to emerge from. Whether caused by temporary setbacks or major blows, these miserable moods sap our energy, reduce our physical reserves, waste our time, diminish our spirit, and take the joy out of our lives. They may even lead to a serious mental illness. Eventually, they may result in a shortened life span—reduced quantity as well as quality of life. How we feel and think about ourselves, those around us, and our circumstances can tell us a lot about our psychosocial health. Similar to our physical health, our psychosocial health can have a profound impact on the quality and quantity of our lives. Again, like our physical health, we can enhance our psychosocial health by becoming aware of and working toward modifying our relevant attitudes and behaviours.

# DEFINING PSYCHOSOCIAL HEALTH

**Psychosocial health** encompasses the mental, emotional, social, and spiritual dimensions of health. Psychosocially healthy people have managed to develop these dimensions to optimal levels (see Figure 2.1). They seem to have an endless reserve for facing the ups and downs of life. They respond to challenges, disappointments, joys, frustrations, and pain by summoning up personal resources acquired through years of experience. Their resiliency is strong and they are actively involved in the process of living rather than trapped in despondency caused by the negative events in their lives.

Psychosocial health is the result of a complex interaction of a person's history and conscious and unconscious thoughts about and interpretations of the past. Although definitions of psychosocial health vary, psychosocially healthy people share several basic elements:[1]

■ *They feel good about themselves.* Psychosocially healthy people are not overwhelmed by fear, love, anger, jealousy, guilt, or worry. They know who they are, have a realistic sense of their capabilities, and respect themselves even though they realize they are not perfect.

■ *They feel comfortable with other people.* Pychosocially healthy people have satisfying and lasting personal relationships and do not take advantage of others; nor do they allow others to take advantage of them. They can give and receive love, consider others' interests, respect personal differences, and feel responsible for their fellow human beings.

■ *They control tension and anxiety.* Psychosocially healthy people recognize the underlying causes and symptoms of stress in their lives and consciously avoid illogical or irrational thoughts, unnecessary aggression, hostility, excessive excuse making, and blaming others for their problems. They use resources and learn skills to control reactions to stressful situations including constructively expressing positive and negative feelings and learning to tolerate their frustrations.

■ *They are able to meet the demands of life.* Psychosocially healthy people try to solve problems as they arise, to accept responsibility, and to plan ahead. They break problems down into manageable bits and work through them one piece at a time. They set realistic goals, think for themselves, and make independent decisions.

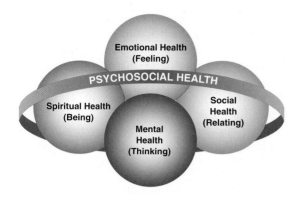

## FIGURE 2.1

Psychosocial Health as a Complex Interaction of Mental, Emotional, Social, and Spiritual Health

Acknowledging that change is inevitable, they welcome new experiences. They are flexible and willing to change while accepting the inevitable when they must.

- *They curb hate and guilt.* Psychosocially healthy people acknowledge and combat their tendencies to respond with hate, anger, thoughtlessness, selfishness, vengeful acts, or feelings of inadequacy. They do not try to knock others aside to get ahead but rather reach out to help others—even those they don't particularly care for.

- *They maintain a positive outlook.* Psychosocially healthy people approach each day with a presumption that things will go well. Since they believe that life is a gift, they are determined to enjoy it on a moment-to-moment basis rather than wander through it aimlessly. They block out most negative and cynical thoughts, give the good things in life star billing, and look to the future with enthusiasm.

- *They enrich the lives of others.* Psychosocially healthy people recognize that there are others whose needs may be greater than their own. They seek to ease these others' burdens by doing such simple things as giving a ride to an elderly neighbour who can't drive, bringing flowers to someone in pain, making dinner for someone too grief-stricken to cook, volunteering at a community agency, and making charitable donations. They generally trust others and themselves.

- *They cherish the things that make them smile.* Psychosocially healthy people make a special place in their lives for memories of the past. Family pictures, high-school mementos, souvenirs of past vacations, and other reminders of

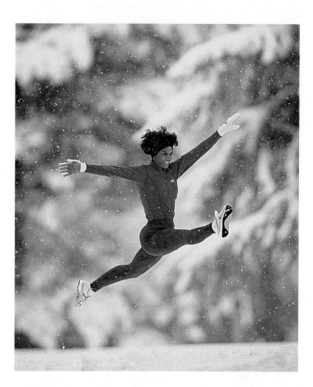

*A joyful spirit and the resiliency to face life's ups and downs are measures of psychosocial health.*

good experiences brighten their day. Fun is an integral part of their lives. So is making time for themselves.

- *They value diversity.* Psychosocially healthy people don't fear difference; they are not threatened by people of a different race, sex, religion, sexual orientation, ethnicity, or political party. They are not judgmental and do not force their beliefs and values on others.

- *They appreciate and respect nature.* Psychosocially healthy people enjoy and respect natural beauty and wonders. They take the time to enjoy their surroundings, act responsibly, and are conscious of their place in the universe.

Of course, few of us ever achieve perfection in all these areas. Attaining psychosocial health and wellness involves many complex processes. This chapter will help you to understand not only what it means to be psychosocially healthy, but also how you may run into difficulties in attaining psychosocial health. Learning how to assess and monitor your health and taking action to improve it are important parts of psychosocial health.

**Psychosocial health:** The mental, emotional, social, and spiritual dimensions of health.

## Mental Health: The Thinking You

The term **mental health** is used to describe the "thinking" or "rational" part of psychosocial health. It describes your ability to perceive things happening around you in realistic ways, to use reasoning when approaching problems, to interpret what is happening, and to evaluate your situation effectively and react appropriately. In short, you are able to sort through the clutter of events, contradictory messages, and uncertainties of a situation and attach meaning (either positive or negative) to it based upon your experiences, attitudes, behaviours, and environmental cues. Your values, attitudes, and beliefs about your health, relationships with your family and others, and life in general are usually—at least in part—a reflection of your mental health.

A mentally healthy person is likely to respond to disappointment or frustration without throwing things, outbursts of rage, excessive drug or alcohol use, or blaming others. For example, suppose you decide to spend your spring break with friends on the beaches of Cuba, Mexico, or the Dominican Republic, knowing you have a major term paper and an exam when you return from your vacation. When you return from your holiday and quickly throw together a paper and study for your exam, you should not fall off the deep end when you get a "D" for your efforts, blame the instructor or your study-partners for your low grade, and start drinking to drown your sorrows. A mentally healthy student would act responsibly for the choices made, learn from the mistakes, and plan differently next time.

Similarly, people going through a difficult break-up in a relationship often have difficulty picking themselves up and moving on in healthy ways. Learning to acknowledge that it is okay to feel sad, unhappy, disappointed, or frustrated and getting help through counselling or talking with trusted friends is part of a healthy process in adapting and coping. Unfortunately too many of us get caught up in our emotional upheavals and are unable to pull ourselves out of the deep funks we find ourselves in.

When a person's mental health deteriorates, he or she may experience sharp declines in rational thinking and increasingly distorted perceptions. Then a person may become cynical and distrustful, experience volatile mood swings, or choose to be isolated from others. These negative reactions to events may threaten the life and health of others. People showing such signs of extreme abnormal behaviours or mental disorders are classified as having mental illnesses, discussed later in this chapter.

## Emotional Health: The Feeling You

**Emotional health** is a term that's often used interchangeably with mental health. Although closely related, emotional health more accurately refers to the "feeling," or subjective, side of psychosocial health and includes emotional reactions to life. **Emotions** are intensified feelings or complex patterns of feelings that we experience on a minute-by-minute, day-to-day basis. Love, hate, hurt, despair, release, joy, anxiety, fear, frustration, and intense anger are some of the many emotions we experience. Typically, emotions are described as the interplay of four components: *physiological arousal, feelings, cognitive (thinking) processes,* and *behavioural reactions*. Each time you are in a stressful situation you react physiologically as you consciously or unconsciously interpret the situation.

There are four basic types of emotions: (1) emotions resulting from harm, loss, or threats; (2) emotions resulting from benefits; (3) borderline emotions, such as hope and compassion; and (4) more complex emotions, such as grief, disappointment, bewilderment, and curiosity.[2] Each of us may experience these emotions in combination at any time. As rational beings, it is our responsibility to evaluate our individual emotional responses, the environment causing these responses, and the appropriateness of our actions or reactions to these responses.

Emotionally healthy people are usually able to respond appropriately to upsetting events. When threatened, they are not likely to react in an extreme fashion, behave inconsistently, or adopt an offensive-attack mode. Emotionally unhealthy people are much more likely to let their feelings overpower them. How many times have you seen someone react with extreme anger by shouting, slamming a door, or punching a wall? Emotionally unhealthy people may be highly volatile and prone to unpredictable emotional outbursts and to inappropriate, sometimes frightening, responses to events. An ex-boyfriend who becomes so angry that he begins to hit and push you around because he is jealous of your new relationship is showing an extremely unhealthy and dangerous emotional reaction.

Emotional health may also affect social health. Someone feeling hostile, withdrawn, or displaying other mood fluctuations may be avoided by others. People in the midst of emotional turmoil may be grumpy, nasty, irritable, or overly quiet; they may cry easily or demonstrate other disturbing emotional responses. Since they are not much fun to be around, their friends may avoid them at the very time they most need emotional support. Social isolation is just one of the many potentially negative consequences of unstable emotional responses.

For students, a more immediate concern is the impact of emotional trauma or turmoil on academic performance. Have you ever tried to study for an exam after a fight with a close friend or family member? Emotional turmoil may seriously affect your ability to think, reason, or act in a rational way. Many otherwise rational people do ridiculous things when they are going through a major emotional upset. Mental functioning and emotional responses are intricately connected.

## Social Health: Interactions with Others

Social health is the part of psychosocial health dealing with our interactions with others on an individual and group basis, our ability to use social resources and support in time and need, and our ability to adapt to a variety of social situations. Socially healthy individuals have a wide range of social interactions with family, friends, and acquaintances, and are able to have a healthy interaction with an intimate partner. They are able to listen, to express themselves, to form healthy relationships, to act in socially acceptable and responsible ways, and to find a best fit for themselves in society. Numerous studies document the importance of social health in promoting physical and mental health as well as enhanced longevity. Two factors, in particular, are key:[3]

- *Presence of strong social bonds.* **Social bonds**, or social linkages, reflect the general degree and nature of interpersonal contacts and interactions. Social bonds generally provide six major functions: (1) intimacy, (2) feelings of belonging to or integration with a group, (3) opportunities for giving or receiving nurturance, (4) reassurance of one's worth, (5) assistance and guidance, and (6) advice. In general, people more "connected" to others manage stress more effectively and are much more resilient when bombarded by life's crises.

- *Presence of key social supports.* **Social supports** refer to relationships that bring positive benefits to

the individual. Social supports can be either expressive (emotional support, encouragement) or structural (housing, money). Families provide structural and expressive support to children. Social support can be provided informally by friends and family, or formally by professionals in hospitals, agencies, and clinics. Adults need to develop their social supports. Psychosocially healthy people create a network of friends and family to whom they can give and receive informal support.

Social health also reflects the way we react to others around us. In its most extreme forms, a lack of social health may be represented by aggressive acts of prejudice and bias toward other individuals or groups. **Prejudice** is a negative evaluation of an entire group of people that is typically based on unfavourable (and wrong) ideas about the group.[4] In its most obvious manifestations, prejudice is reflected in acts of discrimination against others, in overt acts of hate and bias, and in purposeful intent to harm individuals or groups.

## Spiritual Health: An Inner Quest for Well-Being

Although mental, emotional, and social health are key factors in your overall psychosocial functioning, it is possible for you to be mentally, emotionally, and socially healthy and still not achieve optimal levels of psychosocial well-being. What is missing? For many people, that difficult-to-describe element that gives zest to life is the spiritual dimension. What does it mean to be spiritually healthy? Spiritual health reflects our values, beliefs, and perceptions of the world and all living things. It refers to the belief in some unifying force that gives life purpose or meaning or to a sense of belonging to a scheme of existence greater than the merely personal. For some people, this unifying force is nature; for others, it is a feeling of connection to other people coupled with a recognition of the eternal

**Mental health:** The "thinking" part of psychosocial health. Includes values, attitudes, and beliefs.

**Emotional health:** The "feeling" part of psychosocial health. Includes emotional reactions to life.

**Emotions:** Intensified feelings or complex patterns of feelings we experience.

**Social bonds:** Degree and nature of interpersonal contacts.

**Social supports:** Structural and expressive aspects of social interactions.

**Prejudice:** A negative evaluation of an entire group of people typically based on unfavourable and often wrong ideas about the group.

nature of the human race; for still others, the unifying force is a god or other spiritual symbol.

Many of us live on a rather superficial material plane throughout our formative years. We have basic human needs that must be satisfied according to a set hierarchical order. We tend to be rather egocentric, or self-oriented, during these formative years and seek immediate material and emotional gratification while denying or ignoring the spiritual aspect of our lives. Worrying about the clothes you wear, the car you drive, the appearance of your apartment, and other material possessions are examples of this type of preoccupation. According to many psychologists and psychoanalysts our materialistic Western civilization leads us to deny our spiritual needs for much of our lives. But there comes a point, usually around midlife, when we discover that material possessions do not bring a sense of happiness or self-worth.[5] Crisis may move us to this realization earlier. A failed relationship, a serious accident, the death of a close friend or family member, or other loss often prompts us to look for meaning in what is happening around us. We then recognize that material things, prestige, money, power, and fame count for little in the larger scheme of existence, and that if we were to die tomorrow these would not give meaning to our lives. We question "Is that all there is?" Whatever the reason, the search for an answer brings new opportunities for understanding ourselves and to grow spiritually. As we develop into spiritually healthy beings, we begin to recognize we are unique individuals. We reach a better understanding of our strengths and shortcomings and of our place in the universe. Many of us find that our families, the environment, animals, friends, strangers who are suffering, and religion assume greater significance in our lives. We become more willing to sacrifice for others or to improve the world around us. People do not have to wait until their middle years to experience spiritual growth. While the media regularly report horrible stories of hate, crime, violence, and global destruction, they frequently ignore the heartening stories of young people with humanistic concerns who volunteer to work with others in need and are seriously searching for meaning in life.

Spiritual health takes time and experience to acquire. The longer you live, the more you experience. The more you ponder the meaning of your experiences, the greater your chances of achieving spiritual health. In its purest sense, spirituality addresses four main themes: interconnectedness, the practice of mindfulness, spirituality as a part of everyday life, and living in harmony with the community (Figure 2.2).

- *Interconnectedness.* **Interconnectedness** refers to a sense of belonging and connecting with oneself, with others, and with a larger meaning or purpose

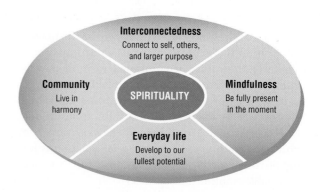

**FIGURE 2.2**

**Four Major Themes of Spirituality**

of life. Connecting with oneself involves exploring feelings, assessing your reactions to people and experiences, and taking mental notes when things or people cause you to lose equilibrium. It also involves considering your values and achieving congruence between your goals and what you can do to achieve them without compromising your values.

- *Practice of mindfulness.* **Mindfulness** refers to the ability to be fully present in the moment. It has been described as a way of nurturing greater awareness and clarity. It is a form of inner flow—a holistic sensation you feel when totally involved in the present.[6] You can achieve this inner flow through an almost infinite range of opportunities for enjoyment and pleasure, either through the development and practice of physical and sensory skills in sport, music, dance, or yoga, or through the development of symbolic skills in areas such as poetry, philosophy, or mathematics.

- *Spirituality as a part of daily life.* Spirituality is embodied in the ability to discover and articulate our basic purpose in life; to learn how to experience love, joy, peace, and fulfillment; and to help ourselves and others achieve their full potential.[7] This ongoing process of growth fosters three convictions: faith, hope, and love. **Faith** is the belief that helps us realize our unique purpose in life; **hope** is the belief that allows us to look confidently and courageously to the future; and **love** involves accepting, affirming, and respecting self and others regardless of who they are.[8]

- *Living in harmony with our community.* Our values are an extension of our beliefs about the world and attitude toward life. These values are formed over time through a series of life experiences, and are reflected in our hopes, dreams, desires, goals, and ambitions.[9] Though most people have some idea of what is important to them, many spend life largely unaware of how their values impact them or those around them until a life-altering event shakes up their perspective on life.

## Spirituality: A Key to Better Health

Although the specific impact of spirituality on health remains elusive, many experts affirm the importance of this dimension in achieving health and wellness. A recent study of spirituality among post-secondary students from 46 diverse universities and colleges indicated that spirituality played a role in student health, grades, and other aspects of student life.[10] The study found a correlation between spirituality and health achievement, with more spiritually oriented students having better health, better grades, more involvement in charitable organizations or volunteerism, and more interest in helping others. Other studies also indicated a correlation between spirituality and positive health outcomes. For example, mindfulness therapies have been used effectively to treat depression, to reduce stress in outpatient therapy and in the nursing profession, with anxiety and heart disease treatments, and other problems.[11]

## A Spiritual Resurgence

An increase in spiritual awareness does not necessarily equate to an increase in beliefs in God or other religious figures. Many people find spiritual fulfillment in music, poetry, literature, art, nature, and intimate relationships.[12] For some, spirituality means a quest for self and selflessness—a form of therapy and respite from a sometimes challenging personal environment. This quest for a life force, which helps people deeply experience the moments of their lives rather than just living through them, has received much scholarly and popular attention. Self-help books that focus on spirituality consistently top the bestseller lists; writers and psychologists such as William James, Carl Jung, Gordon Allport, Erich Fromm, Viktor Frankl, Abraham Maslow, and Rollo May have made spirituality a major focus of their work.

### WHAT WOULD YOU DO?

What do mental, emotional, social, and spiritual health each mean to you? What are your strengths and weaknesses in each of these components? What can you do to enhance your strengths? How can you improve areas that are not so strong? What will you do differently this week to improve your mental, emotional, social, or spiritual health?

# FACTORS INFLUENCING PSYCHOSOCIAL HEALTH

Although it's relatively easy to say what psychosocial health is, it is much more difficult to assess why some people are psychosocially well virtually all the time, others are some of the time, and still others almost never are. What factors have influenced your patterns of mental, emotional, social, and spiritual health? Are these factors changeable? Can you do anything to improve your health if you have problems? How can you enhance the positive qualities you already possess?

Most of our mental, emotional, social, and spiritual reactions to life are a direct outcome of our experiences and social and cultural expectations. Each of us is born with the innate capacity to experience emotions. Some of us apparently have a predisposition toward more emotionality than others. But how we express our emotions has a lot to do with our mental interpretations of events. These interpretations are often learned reactions to certain environmental and social stimuli.

## External Influences

Our psychosocial health is based on how we perceive our life's experiences. While some experiences are under our control, others are not. External influences are those factors in our life that we do not control, such as who raised us and the physical environment in which we live.

## Influences of the Family

Our families have a significant influence on our psychosocial development. Children raised in healthy, nurturing, happy families are more likely to become well-adjusted, productive adults. Children raised in **dysfunctional families** in which violence, sexual,

**Interconnectedness:** A web of connections, including our relationship to ourselves, to others, and to a larger meaning or purpose in life.

**Mindfulness:** Awareness and acceptance of the reality of the present moment.

**Faith:** Belief that helps each person realize a unique purpose in life.

**Hope:** Belief that allows us to look confidently and courageously to the future.

**Love:** Acceptance, affirmation, and respect for self and others.

**Dysfunctional families:** Families in which there is violence; physical, emotional, or sexual abuse; parental discord; or other negative family interactions.

physical, or emotional abuse, negative behaviours, distrust, anger, dietary deprivation, drug abuse, parental discord, or other negative characteristics are present may have a harder time adapting to life. In dysfunctional families, security and unconditional love and trust are lacking and the children are often confused and psychologically bruised. Yet not all people raised in dysfunctional families become psychosocially unhealthy. Conversely, not all people from healthy family environments become well adjusted. Obviously more factors are involved in our "process of becoming" than just our family.

### Influences of the Wider Environment

While isolated negative events may do little damage to psychosocial health, persistent stressors, uncertainties, and threats may cause significant problems. Children raised in environments where crime is rampant and daily safety is in question, for example, run an increased risk of psychosocial problems. Drugs, crime, violent acts, school failure, unemployment, and a host of other bad things can happen to good people. But it is believed that certain protective factors—such as having a positive role model in the midst of chaos, or a high level of self-esteem—may help children from even the worst environments remain healthy and well adjusted.

Another important influence on psychosocial health is access to health services and programs designed to support the maintenance or enhancement of psychosocial health. Going to a support group or seeing a trained counsellor or therapist is often a crucial first step in prevention and intervention efforts. Individuals from poor socioeconomic environments who have difficulty accessing such services often find it difficult to secure help in positively influencing their psychosocial health.

# Internal Influences

Although your life experiences influence you in fairly obvious ways, many internal factors are also working more subtly to shape who you are and whom you become. Some of these factors are your hereditary traits, your hormonal functioning, your physical health status (including neurological or nervous system functioning), your physical fitness level, and selected elements of your mental and emotional health. If problems occur with any of these factors, overall psychosocial health declines.

### Self-Efficacy and Self-Esteem

During our formative years, our successes and failures in school, in sports, in friendships, in our intimate relationships, in our jobs, and in every other aspect of life subtly shape our perceptions and beliefs about our personal worth and ability to act to help ourselves. These perceptions and beliefs in turn become internal influences on our psychosocial health.

**Self-efficacy** describes a person's belief about whether he or she can successfully engage in and execute a specific behaviour. If one has already been successful in academics, sports, or achieving popularity, one will undoubtedly expect to be successful in these events in the future. If one has always been the last chosen to play on a team or has never been able to make friends easily, one may tend to believe that failure is inevitable. In general, the more self-efficacious a person is and the more his or her past experiences have been positive, the more likely he or she will be to keep trying to execute a specific behaviour successfully. People who have a high level of self-efficacy are also more likely to feel that they have **personal control** over situations, or, in other words, believe their own internal resources allow them to control events. On the other hand, a person with low self-efficacy may give up easily or never even try to change a behaviour. Learning new skills and having successful experiences can help improve confidence and add to a "can-do" attitude.

**Self-esteem** refers to one's sense of self-respect or self-worth. It can be defined as an evaluation of oneself and one's personal worth as an individual. People with high self-esteem tend to feel good about themselves and express a positive outlook on life. People with low self-esteem often do not like themselves, constantly demean themselves, and doubt their ability to succeed.

Our self-esteem is a result of the relationships we have with our parents and family during our formative years, with our friends as we grow older, with our significant others as we form intimate relationships, and with our teachers, co-workers, and others throughout our lives. If we felt loved and valued as children, our self-esteem allows us to believe that we are inherently loveable individuals.

### Learned Helplessness versus Learned Optimism

People who continually experience failure may develop a pattern of responding known as **learned helplessness**, in which they give up and fail to take any action to help themselves.[13] These attitudes and resultant behaviours are due in part to society's tendency toward *victimology*, blaming one's problems on other people and circumstances versus taking ownership of the situation. Although viewing ourselves as victims may help us to feel better temporarily, it does not address the underlying causes of a problem. Ultimately, it can erode self-efficacy and foster learned helplessness by making us feel that we cannot do anything to improve the situation or the outcome.

Countering learned helplessness is the theory that we can also learn to be optimistic; that is, **learned optimism**.[14] Research on learned optimism provides growing evidence for the central place of mental health in overall positive development.

## Personality

Our personality is the unique mix of characteristics that distinguishes us from others. Hereditary, environmental, cultural, and experiential factors influence how we develop. For each of us, the amount of influence exerted by any of these factors differs. Our personality determines how we react to the challenges of life. It also determines how we interpret the feelings we experience and how we resolve the conflicts we feel on being denied the things we need or want.

Most of the recent schools of psychosocial theory promote the idea that we have the power not only to understand our behaviours but also to actively change it and thus to mould our personalities. Although much has been written about the importance of a healthy personality, there is little consensus on what exactly it is. In general, people who possess the following traits appear to be psychologically healthy:[15]

- *Extroversion*: The ability to adapt to a social situation and demonstrate assertiveness as well as power or interpersonal involvement.
- *Agreeableness*: The ability to conform, be likeable, and demonstrate friendly compliance as well as love.
- *Openness to experience*: The willingness to demonstrate curiosity and independence (also referred to as *inquiring intellect*).
- *Emotional stability*: The ability to maintain social control.
- *Conscientiousness*: The qualities of being dependable and demonstrating self-control, discipline, and a need to achieve.

## Life Span and Maturity

Although the exact determinants of personality are impossible to define, researchers do know that they are not static. Rather, our personalities change as we move through the stages of our lives. Our temperaments also change as we grow, as illustrated by the extreme emotions experienced by many in early adolescence. Most of us learn to control our emotions as we advance toward adulthood.

The college or university years mark a critical transition period for young adults and their parents. During this time, many move away from their families and establish themselves as independent adults. For most, this step toward maturity entails changing the nature of their relationship with their parents. The transition to independence is easier if they have successfully accomplished earlier developmental tasks such as learning how to solve problems, to make and evaluate decisions, to define and adhere to personal values, and to establish casual and intimate relationships. Management of personal finances, career management strategies, interpersonal communication skills, and parenting skills (for those who choose to become parents) are among the developmental tasks postsecondary students must accomplish. Older students often have to balance the responsibilities of family, career, and school. Parents of students must accept their children's greater independence and, in some cases, adjust to being alone after years of family interaction.

If you have not fulfilled earlier tasks, you will continue to grow but may find your life interrupted by recurrent "crises" left over from earlier stages. For example, if you did not learn to trust others in childhood, you may have difficulty establishing intimate relationships in late adolescence or early adulthood.

## Resiliency and Developmental Assets

Over the last decade, it has become well established that some people are much better prepared to meet the challenges of life than others are. The combination of certain personality traits coupled with a supportive environment can equip one to deal effectively with life's many challenges. These individuals are able to cope and even thrive in times of great stress or pressure. **Resiliency**, or *protective factors*, is a term used to describe those traits or characteristics that protect an individual or community from threat or harm. In a sense, these traits may serve to inoculate one against potential ill health. People with assets, whether financial, emotional, spiritual, physical,

---

**Self-efficacy:** Belief in your ability to perform a task successfully.

**Personal control:** Belief that your internal resources allow you to control a situation.

**Self-esteem:** One's sense of self-respect or self-worth.

**Learned helplessness:** Pattern of responding to situations by giving up because you have always failed in the past.

**Learned optimism:** Pattern of responding that is optimistic, because you choose to view each situation positively.

**Resiliency:** Those traits or characteristics that protect an individual or community from threat or harm.

# Tips for Building Self-Esteem and Self-Efficacy

How can you build self-esteem? Many things you do daily can have a significant impact on the way you feel about yourself. Practise these tips regularly to bolster your self-esteem and self-efficacy.

- *Pay attention to your needs and wants.* Listen to what your body, your mind, and your heart are telling you.
- *Take good care of yourself.* Eat healthy foods, limit junk foods, be physically active on a regular basis, manage your stress, and get adequate sleep.
- *Take time to do things you enjoy.* Make a list of things you enjoy doing. Then do one thing from that list every day.
- *Do something that you have been putting off.* Cleaning out your closet, going to a fitness class, or paying a bill that you've been putting off will make you feel like you've accomplished something.
- *Give yourself rewards.* Acknowledge that you are a good person by rewarding yourself occasionally.
- *Spend time with people.* People who make you feel better about yourself are great self-esteem boosters. Avoid, or limit your time with, people who treat you badly or make you feel bad about yourself.
- *Display items that you like.* You may have items that remind you of your achievements, your friends, or of special times. Keep those special items close by.

- *Make your meals a special time.* Get rid of distractions like the television and really concentrate on enjoying your meal, whether by yourself or with others.
- *Learn something new every day.* Take advantage of any opportunity to learn something new every day—you'll feel better about yourself and be more productive.
- *Do something nice for another person.* There is no greater way to feel better about yourself than to help someone in need. Check out local volunteer opportunities or make a special effort to be nice to those around you such as your parents, siblings, or roommates.

Sources: A. L. Story, "Self-Esteem and Self-Certainty: A Mediational Analysis," *European Journal of Personality 18*.2 (2004): 115; M. E. Copeland, "Building Self-Esteem: A Self-Help Guide," Center for Mental Health Services [online booklet], accessed May 2004, www.mentalhealth.org/publications/ allpubs/SMA-3715/default.asp.

---

mental, or social, and other positive forces in their lives are likely to be resilient and bounce back when facing life's challenges.

## WHAT WOULD YOU DO?

Which factors of psychosocial health have had the greatest positive impact on your life? Any negative influences? Which are influencing your life most now? How resilient are you? How can you build resiliency?

# ENHANCING PSYCHOSOCIAL HEALTH

You may believe that your psychosocial health is fairly well developed by the time you reach college or university. However, attaining self-fulfillment is a lifelong, conscious process that involves building self-efficacy

and self-esteem, understanding and controlling emotions, maintaining support networks, and learning to solve problems and make decisions.

## Developing and Maintaining Self-Esteem and Self-Efficacy

There are several ways to build self-esteem and self-efficacy. These include finding a support group, trying to be a support for others, completing required tasks, forming realistic expectations, making time for yourself, maintaining your physical health, and examining your problems and seeking help. See the Skills for Behaviour Change box for other ideas.

### Finding a Support Group

One of the best ways to gain self-esteem and self-efficacy is through a support group—peers who share your values. A support group can make you feel good about yourself and help you to take an honest look at your actions and choices. Although you might seek support in a wholly new group, remember that old ties are often the strongest. Keeping in contact with old friends and family members can provide a foundation of unconditional love that will help you through the many life transitions ahead.

### Trying to Be a Support for Others

Feel better about yourself by helping others to feel good about themselves. Write more postcards and "thinking of you" notes to people who matter. This will build your self-esteem and that of your friends. Become more interesting by being more interested (in people, current events, and so on). Send news clippings to friends. Join a discussion, political action, or recreational group.

### Completing Required Tasks

Another way to boost your self-esteem or self-efficacy is to complete required tasks successfully and on time. You are not likely to succeed in your studies if you leave term papers until the last minute, fail to keep up with the reading for your courses, and do not ask for clarification of points confusing you. Some university and college campuses provide study groups for various content areas. Your school's student services department may offer tips for managing time, understanding assignments, dealing with professors, and preparing for test taking. Poor grades, or grades that do not meet a student's expectations, are major contributors to diminished self-esteem and to emotional distress among post-secondary students.

### Forming Realistic Expectations

Having realistic expectations of yourself—and others—is another method of boosting self-esteem and self-efficacy. College or university is a time to explore your potential. If you expect perfect grades, a steady stream of Saturday-night dates and a soap opera-type romantic involvement, a good job, and a beautiful home and car, you may be setting yourself up for failure. Assess your current resources and the direction in which you are heading. Set small, incremental goals that are possible for you to meet. Don't decide, "I'm going to turn my life around and get better grades" without some realistic actions or goals to support your intentions. Decide also that tomorrow you will spend at least two hours studying for a class or going to the library to do research on a paper, or decide to talk to your professor to see what he or she recommends to help you to better understand a topic.

### Taking and Making Time for You

Taking time to enjoy yourself is another way to boost your psychosocial health. For some people, participating in a sport improves self-esteem and self-efficacy by creating a sense of achievement. For others, meditating, doing volunteer work, getting a massage, or meeting a new challenge, such as successfully auditioning for a play, can all enhance your psychosocial growth. Viewing each new activity as something to look forward to and an opportunity to grow is an important part of keeping the excitement in your life.

### Maintaining Physical Health

Maintaining physical health also contributes to self-esteem. Regular physical activity fosters a sense of well-being. Nourishing meals can help you to feel good about yourself and help to avoid the weight gain experienced by many college or university students. Getting adequate sleep and managing your stress are two other behaviours critical to maintaining your physical health.

### Examining Problems and Seeking Help

Examining your problems and seeking help when needed will also boost your self-esteem and self-efficacy. Facing and solving problems can be one of life's most satisfying experiences. You do not necessarily have to deal with your problems alone. Help can come in the form of a friend, a group, or a mental health professional.

### WHAT WOULD YOU DO?

Which of the above tasks have you actively pursued in the past month, past six months, and past year? Are you actively involved in enhancing your self-esteem and self-efficacy? Why or why not?

## Getting Adequate Rest

Getting adequate sleep is a key contributor to positive physical and psychosocial functioning. Many of us never seem to get enough sleep. Either we don't make enough time to sleep or we can't seem to fall asleep once our heads hit the pillow. An estimated 20 to 40 percent of adults have trouble sleeping. Known as insomnia, this sleep disorder affects almost everyone at one time or another. Insomnia is more common in women than in men, and its prevalence correlates with age and socioeconomic class. Though many people turn to over-the-counter sleeping pills, barbiturates, or tranquillizers to get some sleep, the following methods for conquering sleeplessness are less harmful:[16]

- *Go to bed and rise on a regular schedule.* Keep this schedule no matter how much you have or haven't slept in the recent past. If sleep difficulties persist, sleep clinics are available to help diagnose sleep disorders.

- *Don't drink alcohol or smoke before bedtime.* Alcohol can disrupt sleep patterns while nicotine is a stimulant that can disrupt the ability to fall asleep.

- *Avoid eating a heavy meal in the evening, particularly at bedtime.* Don't drink large amounts of liquids before retiring, either.

- *Engage in regular physical activity.* However, not right before bed; physical activity acts as a stimulant, speeding the body's metabolism and making it harder to fall asleep immediately after.

- *Eliminate or reduce consumption of caffeinated beverages* (coffee, tea, hot chocolate, and some soft drinks) and foods (chocolate, cocoa) except in the morning or early afternoon.

- *Limit daytime naps, even if you're tired.* If you must nap, make it a "cat-nap," no longer than 20 minutes.

- *Establish a relaxing nighttime ritual that puts you in the mood to sleep.* Spend an hour or more reading, listening to music, watching TV, or taking a warm bath.

- *Don't bring work to bed.*

- *If you're unable to fall asleep after 30 minutes, get up and do something rather than lie there.* If you wake up in the middle of the night and can't fall asleep again, try reading for a short time. Counting sheep or reconstructing a happy event or narrative in your mind may lull you to sleep. Try imagining yourself relaxing on a beach with the waves rolling in, or in a favourite tranquil place.

- *Avoid reproaching yourself.* Don't make your sleeplessness a cause for additional worry. Insomnia is not a crime. Not everyone needs eight hours of sleep. You can feel well—and be quite healthy—on fewer.

- *Don't watch the clock at night.* Turn it to the wall to avoid the temptation to worry about the night slipping away.

## Understanding the Mind–Body Connection

Can negative emotions and stress make a person physically sick? Can positive emotions and happiness help a person feel well? Do positive emotions boost the immune system? Although considerable research has attempted to conclusively answer these questions, much remains unknown. For decades, research focused primarily on negative emotions and disease; however, little is known about the role of positive emotions in preserving health and protecting against disease. Many believe that this end of the emotions continuum may hold the key to future advances in health and that mind–body health science may be elevated to new heights as a result of recent findings. One emotion that appears to have particularly positive benefits is *happiness.*

### Happiness and Physical Health

**Happiness** refers to a number of positive states in which individuals actively embrace the world around them.[17] As researchers examined characteristics of happy people, they found that this emotion had a profound impact on the body. Specifically, researchers found that happiness or related mood states like hopefulness, optimism, and contentment reduced the risk or limited the severity of cardiovascular disease,

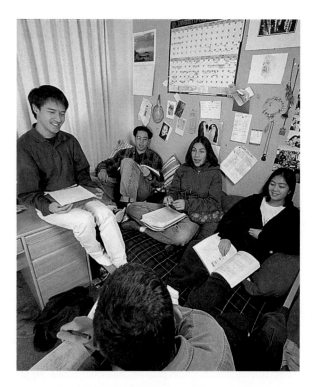

*Past successes and happy experiences, often recalled through photos, mementos, and recollections, contribute to a person's psychosocial health.*

## How happy are you?

Read the following statements, and then rate your level of agreement with each one using the 1–7 scale.

| 1 | 2 | 3 | 4 | 5 | 6 | 7 |
|---|---|---|---|---|---|---|
| Strongly disagree | Disagree | Slightly disagree | Neither agree nor disagree | Slightly agree | Agree | Strongly agree |

1. In most ways, my life is close to my ideal. _____
2. The conditions of my life are excellent. _____
3. I am satisfied with my life. _____
4. So far I have gotten the important things I want in life. _____
5. If I could live my life over, I would change almost nothing. _____

Total score: _____

Scoring:
31–35: You are very satisfied with your life  26–30: Satisfied  21–25: Slightly satisfied
20: You are neither satisfied nor dissatisfied  15–19: Slightly dissatisfied  10–14: Dissatisfied  5–9: Very dissatisfied

FIGURE 2.3

Satisfaction with Life Scale

Source: W. Pavot and E. Diener, "Review of the Satisfaction with Life Scale," *Psychological Assessment 5* (1993): 164–172.

pulmonary disease, diabetes, hypertension, colds, and other infections. Laughter increases heart and respiration rates, and reduces stress hormones in the same way as physical activity does. For this reason, it has been promoted as a possible risk reducer for those with hypertension and other forms of cardio-vascular disease.[18]

If happiness is good for your health, how does one "get happy"? **Subjective well-being (SWB)** refers to that uplifting feeling of inner peace or overall "feel-good state," which includes happiness. SWB is defined by three central components:[19]

1. *Satisfaction with present life.* People high in SWB tend to like their work and are satisfied with their current personal relationships. They are sociable, outgoing, and willing to open up to others. They also like themselves and enjoy good health and self-esteem.
2. *Relative presence of positive emotions.* People with high SWB more frequently feel pleasant emotions, mainly because they perceive the world around them in a generally positive way. They have an optimistic outlook, and they expect success in what they undertake.
3. *Relative absence of negative emotions.* Individuals with a strong sense of SWB experience fewer and less severe episodes of negative emotions, such as anxiety, depression, and anger.

Researchers also suggest that people may be biologically predisposed to happiness. In fact, happiness may be related to actual differences in brain physiology—*neurotransmitters*, the chemicals that transfer messages between neurons, may function more efficiently in happy people.[20] Others suggest that we can develop happiness by practising positive psychological actions.[21]

You do not have to be happy all the time to achieve overall subjective well-being. Everyone experiences disappointments, unhappiness, and times when life seems unfair. But people with SWB are typically resilient, able to look on the positive side, able to get themselves back on track fairly quickly, and less likely to fall into despair over setbacks. There are several myths about happiness: that it depends on age, sex, race, and socioeconomic status. Take the quiz on happiness and see how satisfied you are with life (Figure 2.3).

Humans are remarkably resourceful creatures. We respond to great loss, such as the death of a loved one or a traumatic event, with an initial period of grief, mourning, and sometimes rage. Yet, with time and the support of loving family and friends, we brush off the bad times and find satisfaction and peace. Typically, humans learn from suffering and emerge stronger and ready to deal with the next crisis. Most find some measure of happiness after the initial shock and pain of loss. Those who are otherwise healthy, in good physical condition, and part of a strong social support network can adapt and cope effectively.

**Happiness:** Feeling of contentment created when one's expectations and physical, psychological, and spiritual needs have been met and one enjoys life.

**Subjective well-being (SWB):** That uplifting feeling of inner peace and overall feel-good state.

## Does Laughter Enhance Psychosocial Health?

Remember the last time you laughed so hard that you cried? Remember how relaxed you felt afterward? Researchers are beginning to understand the role of humour in our lives and health. For example, laughter has been shown to have the following effects:

- Stressed people with a strong sense of humour become less depressed and anxious than those whose sense of humour is less well developed.
- Students who use humour as a coping mechanism report that it predisposes them to a positive mood.
- Telling a joke, particularly one that involves a shared experience, increases one's sense of belonging and social cohesion.

Clearly, laughter enhances mental and emotional health. It also promotes social health: people like to be around others who are fun and laugh easily. Learning to laugh puts more joy into everyday experiences and increases the likelihood that people will keep company with us.

Positive emotions such as joy, interest, and contentment serve valuable life functions. Joy is associated with playfulness and creativity. Interest encourages us to explore our world, which enhances knowledge and cognitive ability. Contentment allows us to savour and integrate experiences, an important step in achieving mindfulness and insight. By building our physical, social, and mental resources, these positive feelings empower us to cope effectively with life's

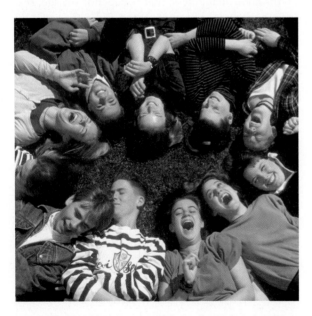

*A powerful strategy for maintaining psychosocial health is to make time for friends and activities you enjoy and that bring laughter into your life.*

challenges. While the actual emotions may be transient, their effects can be permanent and provide lifelong enrichment.[22]

## Psychosocial Health and Well-Being

In the 1970s and 1980s, a number of widely publicized studies of the health of widowed and divorced people indicated higher rates of illness and death than those of married people. Moreover, their lab tests revealed below-normal immune-system functioning. Several follow-up studies indicated unusually high rates of cancer among depressed people.[23] Are these studies conclusive evidence of the mind–body connection? Probably not, because they do not account for many other factors relevant to health. For example, some researchers suggest that people who are divorced, widowed, or depressed are more likely to drink and smoke, use drugs, eat and sleep poorly, and fail to engage in physical activity— all of which negatively affect the immune system. Another possibly relevant factor is that such people may be less tolerant of illness and more likely to report their problems.[24]

Keep in mind that the immune system changes measured in various studies of the mind–body connection are relatively small. (They are nowhere near as large as the disruptions that occur in people with AIDS, for example.) The health consequences of such minute changes are difficult to gauge because the body can tolerate a certain amount of reduced immune function without illness developing. The exact amount the body is able to tolerate and under what circumstances are still unresolved questions.[25] Thus, although there is a large body of evidence pointing to an association between emotions and physical health, there is still much to learn about this relationship. In the meantime, however, maintaining an optimistic mindset is probably sound advice.

# WHEN THINGS GO WRONG

In spite of our best efforts to remain psychosocially healthy, circumstances and events in our lives sometimes prove to be more than we can handle. Abusive relationships, stress, anxiety, loneliness, financial upheavals, and other traumatic events can sap our spirits, causing us to turn inward or act in ways different than what might be considered normal. Chemical imbalances, drug interactions, trauma, neurological disruptions, and other physical problems may also contribute to these not-so-normal behaviours. **Mental illnesses** are disorders that disrupt thinking, feeling, moods, and behaviours, and cause a varying degree of impaired functioning in daily life. Similar to a physical disease, mental illnesses can range from mild to severe and exact a heavy toll on the quality of life of the individual affected and those who come in contact with him or her. It is estimated that one in five Canadians will directly experience a mental illness at some point in his or her lifetime.[26]

# Depression

Depression is the most common emotional disorder in Canada: six percent of Canadians aged 18 and over have experienced a major depressive episode. It was estimated from the 2000/01 Canadian Community Health Survey that 9.9 percent of Canadians over the age of 12 had a possible or probable risk of depression.[27] Females have a greater risk of depression than males (12.3 vs. 7.5 percent). Individuals between 20 and 24 years of age have the greatest possible and probable risk of depression (13.3 percent), while individuals over the age of 75 have the lowest risk (5.1 percent).

There are two acknowledged forms of depression: endogenous and exogenous depression. **Endogenous depression** is of biochemical origin. Neurotransmitters (chemicals that transmit nerve impulses across synapses) in the brain responsible for mood elevation become unbalanced for unknown reasons. A decrease in these neurotransmitters gives rise to outward expressions of depression. If not treated, endogenous depression may become chronic. **Exogenous depression**, on the other hand, is usually caused by an external event such as the loss of something or someone of great value. Victims of exogenous depression can slide into chronic depression if unable to work through the grieving process necessary for overcoming event-related depression.

Similar symptoms appear in the two types of depression: lingering sadness; inability to find joy in pleasure-giving activities; loss of interest in work and reduced concentration; diminished or increased appetite; unexplainable fatigue; sleep disorders, including insomnia or early-morning awakenings; loss of sex drive; withdrawal from friends and family; feelings of hopelessness and worthlessness; and a desire to die. A depressed person may be unable to get out of bed in the morning or may find it impossible to leave the house.

A depressed person usually suffers from low self-esteem. He or she may feel alone, separated from and unable to communicate with others. After a while,

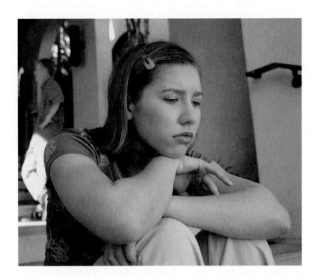

*Without appropriate treatment, depression and anxiety can become overwhelming problems that affect psychosocial well-being and physical health.*

depression becomes a vicious circle. The person feels helpless and trapped, having no way out. He or she may feel that depression is a deserved punishment for real or imagined failings. Prolonged depression may cause a person to feel utterly worthless and to view suicide as the only way out.

## Facts and Fallacies about Depression

Although depression appears to be one of the fastest-growing psychosocial health problems, the general public is uninformed and misinformed about many aspects of it. The following points may help your understanding of depression.[28]

■ *Depression is not a natural reaction to crisis and loss.* This is true. Something has happened to the mood and thinking of depressed people such that they are afflicted by pervasive pessimism, helplessness, despair, and lethargy, sometimes coupled with agitation. Individuals who are depressed may have difficulty at work and chronically negative interpersonal relationships. Symptoms may come and go, get worse, or stay stable, but won't get better without treatment. Depressed people forget what it's like to feel normal.

**Mental illnesses:** Disorders that disrupt thinking, feeling, moods, and behaviours, and cause a varying degree of impaired functioning in daily life.

**Endogenous depression:** A type of depression with a biochemical basis, such as neurotransmitter imbalances.

**Exogenous depression:** A type of depression with an external cause, such as the death of a loved one.

- *People will not snap out of depression by using a little willpower.* This is true. Telling a depressed person to snap out of it is like telling a person with diabetes to produce more insulin. Medical intervention in the form of antidepressant drugs and therapy is often necessary for recovery. Depression also tends to recur—more than half of those afflicted once will experience a recurrence. Understanding the seriousness of the disease and supporting people in their attempts to recover are important.

- *Frequent crying is not a hallmark of depression.* This is true. Some depressed people don't cry at all. In fact, biochemists theorize that crying may actually ward off depression by releasing chemicals that the body produces as a positive response to distress.

- *Depression is not "all in the mind."* This is true. In fact, depressive illnesses originate with an inherited chemical imbalance in the brain. Depression-like symptoms can also be a side-effect of certain physiological conditions (or their treatment), such as thyroid disorders, Lyme disease, diabetes, multiple sclerosis, hepatitis, mononucleosis, rheumatoid arthritis, and pancreatic cancer.

- *Only in-depth psychotherapy can cure long-term clinical depression.* This is false. No single psychotherapy method works for all cases of depression.

## Treating Depression

Depression is one of the most treatable of mental health problems;[29] various types of treatment are available including lifestyle modification (that is, engaging in regular moderate to vigorous intensity physical activity, eating well, managing stress, getting adequate sleep, and so on); talking to a physician, counsellor, psychologist, or psychiatrist; attending a support group; or taking a medication. Selecting the best treatment for a specific person involves determining his or her type and degree of depression and its possible causes. Psychotherapeutic and pharmacological modes of treatment are recommended for clinical (severe and prolonged) depression. Drugs often relieve the symptoms of depression, such as loss of sleep or appetite, while psychotherapy can improve a depressed person's social and interpersonal functioning. Treatment may be weighted toward one or the other mode depending on the specific situation. In some cases, psychotherapy alone may be the most successful treatment. The two most common psychotherapeutic therapies for depression are cognitive and interpersonal therapy.

*Cognitive therapy* aims to help an individual look at life rationally and to correct habitually pessimistic thought patterns. It focuses on the here and now rather than analyzing the past. To pull a person out of depression, cognitive therapists usually need 6 to 18 months of weekly sessions comprising reasoning and behavioural exercises. *Interpersonal therapy* is sometimes combined with cognitive therapy. It also addresses the present but differs from cognitive therapy in that its primary goal is to correct chronic human relationship problems. Interpersonal therapists focus on individuals' relationships with their families and other people.

Antidepressant drugs relieve symptoms in nearly 80 percent of people with chronic depression. In recent years, Zoloft and Prozac have become such a common part of our vocabulary that it doesn't seem at all unusual to know someone taking them. Despite how commonplace antidepressants have become, caution is warranted regarding their use. Many emergency-room visits occur when people misuse their antidepressants, in particular when they try to quit "cold turkey" or have drug interactions. There are several types of antidepressant drugs. The most commonly used are tricyclics (Tofranil); bicyclics (Effexor); seratonin selective reuptake inhibitors, or SSRIs (Prozac, Zoloft); and monoamine oxidase inhibitors (Parnate). These medications usually begin to take effect within two to four weeks, although tricyclics can take six weeks to three months to become effective.

Clinics have been established in large metropolitan areas to offer group support for depressed people. Some clinics treat all types of depressed people; others restrict themselves to specific groups, such as widows, adolescents, or families and friends of people with depression.

# Obsessive-Compulsive Disorders

An **obsessive-compulsive disorder (OCD)** is an illness in which people have obsessive thoughts or perform habitual behaviours that they cannot control. People with compulsions feel forced to engage in a repetitive behaviour, almost as if the behaviour controls them. Feeling an obsessive need for cleanliness and washing one's hands 20 times before eating, counting to a certain number while using the toilet, and checking and rechecking all the light switches in the house before leaving or going to bed are examples of compulsive behaviours. More harmful compulsive behaviours include pulling out one's hair and other forms of self-mutilation.

The causes of OCD are difficult to isolate. Some theorists believe that sufferers engage in compulsive behaviours to distract themselves from more pressing problems. Until recently, behavioural therapy, which focused on controlling and changing behaviours, was the most common treatment. However, research indicates that some of these disorders may be caused by a lack of the neurotransmitter serotonin in the limbic system (an area of the brain concerned with emotion and motivation). In 1974, a drug called clomipramine (Anafranil), which researchers believe alters the way serotonin is used in the brain, was released in Canada for prescription use. Used in conjunction with behavioural therapy, clomipramine alleviates symptoms of obsessive-compulsive disorders.

## Anxiety Disorders

Rates of anxiety disorders do not fall far behind those for depression. **Anxiety disorders**, in which people are plagued by persistent feelings of threat and anxiety about everyday problems of living, are characterized by fatigue, back pain, headaches, feelings of unreality, a sensation of weakness in the legs, and fear of losing control. Generalized anxiety disorders can last for more than six months and typically result in excessive worry about personal problems. Three major types of anxiety disorders are phobias, panic attacks, and post-traumatic stress disorder.

### Phobias

A **phobia** is a deep and persistent fear of a specific object, activity, or situation, and results in a compelling desire to avoid the source of fear. Phobias are thought to be more prevalent in women than in men. Simple phobias, such as fear of spiders, fear of flying, and fear of heights, can be treated successfully with behavioural therapy. Social phobias (fears related to interaction with others), such as fear of public speaking, fear of inadequate sexual performance, and fear of eating in public places, require more extensive therapy.

### Panic Attacks

A **panic attack** is the sudden onset of disabling terror—a form of acute anxiety that brings on an intense physical reaction. It can happen at any time: while sleeping, while sitting in traffic, or just before you deliver your class presentation. Suddenly and unexpectedly your heart starts to race, your face turns red, you can't catch your breath, you feel nauseated, you start to perspire, and you may feel like you are going to pass out or are having a heart attack. Panic attacks may have no obvious link to environmental stimuli, or they may be learned responses to environmental stimuli. Researchers believe that panic attacks are caused by some physiological change or biochemical imbalance in the brain; they are still searching for the mechanisms that trigger such attacks.

### Post-Traumatic Stress Disorder

Some victims of severe traumas such as rape, child abuse, assault, war, weather disasters (hurricanes, tornadoes, floods, forest fires), or airplane or car crashes are afflicted by **post-traumatic stress disorder (PTSD)**.

PTSD manifests itself as detachment, constricted affect, diminished interest in one or more activities, sleep disturbance, hypervigilance, guilt, memory impairment, and difficulty concentrating. It can also cause terrifying flashbacks to the sufferer's trauma.

When correctly diagnosed, anxiety disorders are treatable, usually through a combination of methods. Because undiagnosed diabetes, heart conditions, and endocrine disorders can mimic anxiety disorders, doctors recommend a thorough physical examination to rule out physical causes. If it is established that the causes are not physical, treatment usually consists of psychotherapy combined with medication.

## Seasonal Affective Disorder

**Seasonal affective disorder (SAD)**, a type of depression, affects approximately two to three percent of Canadians.[30] As much as 25 percent of the population in Canada[31] experiences a milder form of the disorder known as the *winter blues.* SAD strikes during the winter months and is associated with reduced exposure to sunlight. People with SAD suffer from irritability, apathy, carbohydrate craving and weight gain, increases in sleep time, and general sadness. Researchers believe that SAD is caused by a malfunction in the hypothalamus, the gland responsible for regulating responses to external stimuli. Stress may also play a role in SAD.

Certain factors seem to put people at risk for SAD. Women are four times more likely to suffer from SAD than men. Although SAD occurs in people of all ages, those between 20 and 40 years of age appear to be most vulnerable. Certain families also appear to be at risk. People living in cities with cold, bright winters and with an active winter culture often have lower rates of SAD than expected. Vancouver has relatively high rates of SAD due to frequent overcast skies. Some people experience a reduction in symptoms if they move south.[32]

---

**Obsessive-compulsive disorder (OCD):** A disorder characterized by obsessive thoughts or habitual behaviours that cannot be controlled.

**Anxiety disorders:** Disorders characterized by persistent feelings of threat and anxiety in coping with everyday problems.

**Phobia:** A deep and persistent fear of a specific object, activity, or situation that results in a compelling desire to avoid the source of the fear.

**Panic attack:** The sudden, rapid onset of disabling terror.

**Post-traumatic stress disorder:** A disorder characterized by terrifying flashbacks, detachment, and anxiety following a severe traumatic event.

**Seasonal affective disorder (SAD):** A type of depression that occurs in the winter months, when sunlight levels are low.

## CMHA Applauds Work of Senate Committee, Wants Recommendations to Move Forward

On May 9, 2006, the Canadian Mental Health Association (CMHA)* applauded the Senate Committee on Social Affairs, Science and Technology on the 118 recommendations it made in a report on mental health, mental illness, and addictions in Canada. This report (titled Out of the Shadows at Last) is the result of a three-year study of mental health and addiction. In the report, the Senate Committee recommends that a 5-percent tax be placed on alcoholic beverages to assist with the funding of the $5.4-billion plan to transform Canada's mental health system.

The CMHA looks forward to working with the government, its agencies, and other stakeholders across the country to make the recommendations a reality.

It should be noted that Canada is one of the only G-8 countries currently without a national strategy for mental health and mental illness. As such the CMHA, in particular, supports the Senate Committee's recommendation for a call for a strategy on mental health and mental illness for the people of Canada. The CMHA recommends that the federal government work with the provincial and territorial governments and key stakeholders in the mental health community to develop and implement a national strategy

The CMHA also strongly supports the Senate Committee's recommendation for the establishment of a Mental Health Commission that will bring together key stakeholders to improve the quality of life of those affected directly and indirectly by mental illness. Finally, the CMHA endorsed the Senate Committee's

recommendation for the creation of a Mental Health Transition Fund, which would be used to assist individuals with mental illness in obtaining affordable housing.

The complete report can be downloaded from www.parl.gc.ca/39/1/parlbus/commbus/senate/com-e/soci-e/rep-e/rep02may06-e.htm.

* The CMHA is a leading national, voluntary organization within the mental-health sector. For more than 90 years, it has existed to promote the mental health of Canadians and to serve mental-health consumers and their families and friends through education, public awareness, research, advocacy, and direct services.

There are some simple but effective therapies for SAD. The most beneficial appears to be light therapy, in which an individual is exposed to lamps that mimic sunlight. In fact, following four days of daily light exposure, 80 percent of individuals experienced relief from their symptoms. Other forms of treatment include dietary modifications (eating more foods high in complex carbohydrates), increased physical activity, stress management, sleep restriction (limiting the number of hours slept in a 24-hour period), psychotherapy, and antidepressants.

## Schizophrenia

Perhaps the most frightening of all mental disorders is **schizophrenia**, a disease that affects about one percent of the Canadian population. Schizophrenia is characterized by alterations of the senses (including auditory and visual hallucinations); the inability to sort out incoming stimuli and make appropriate responses; an altered sense of self; and radical changes

in emotions, movements, and behaviours. Individuals with this disease often cannot function in society.

For decades, researchers believed that schizophrenia was an environmentally provoked form of madness. They blamed abnormal family interactions or early-childhood traumas. Since the mid-1980s, when magnetic resonance imaging (MRI) and positron emission tomography (PET) allowed researchers to study brain function more closely, schizophrenia has been recognized as a biological brain disease. It has become evident that the brain damage involved occurs very early in life, possibly as early as in the second trimester of fetal development. However, the disease most commonly is onset in late adolescence.

Schizophrenia is treatable but not curable. Treatments usually include some combination of hospitalization, medication, and supportive psychotherapy. Supportive psychotherapy, as opposed to psychoanalysis, can help the individual acquire skills for living in society.

Even though the environmental theories of schizophrenia have been discarded in favour of biological theories, a stigma remains attached to the disease.

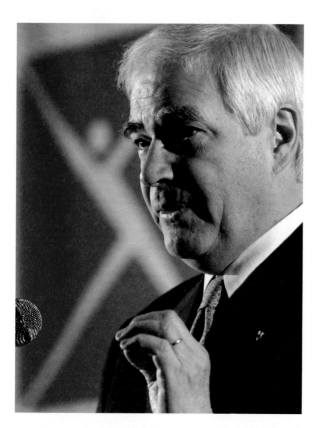

*Canadians are becoming more familiar with their psychosocial health, the risk factors for poor psychosocial health, and their treatment options partly because of people like James Bartleman, who shared his story of depression at the National Canadian Mental Health Association Conference*

Families of individuals with schizophrenia often experience anger and guilt. They often need help in the form of information, family counselling, and advice on how to meet the needs for shelter, medical care, vocational training, and social interaction of the individual with schizophrenia.

# SEX ISSUES IN PSYCHOSOCIAL HEALTH

Studies have shown that sex bias often gets in the way of correct diagnosis of psychosocial disorders. In one study, 175 mental health professionals of both sexes were asked to diagnose an individual on the basis of a summarized case history. Some of the professionals were told that the individual was male, others female. The sex of the patient made a substantial difference in the diagnosis given (though the sex of the clinician did not). When clinicians thought the case history was from a female, they were more likely to diagnose hysterical personality, a "women's disorder." When they believed the case history was from a male, the more likely diagnosis was antisocial personality, a "male disorder."

## Depression and Sex

For reasons not well understood, women have a greater probability of developing depression than men.[33] Researchers have proposed biological, psychological, and social explanations. The biological explanation rests on the observation that women appear to be at greater risk for depression when their hormone levels change significantly, as during the premenstrual period, postpartum, and the onset of menopause. Men's hormone levels appear to remain relatively stable throughout life. Researchers therefore theorized that women were inherently more at risk for depression. Yet evidence relating to this theory is either inconsistent or contrary.

Since depression is often preceded by a stressful event, some researchers theorized that women might be under more stress than men and thus more prone to depression. However, women do not report more stressful events any more frequently than men. Finally, researchers observed sex differences in coping strategies, or the response to certain events or stimuli, and thus proposed that women's strategies put them at greater risk. Results indicated that men tried to distract themselves from a depressed mood whereas women tended to focus on it. If focusing on depressed feelings intensifies these feelings, women's response style then may make them more likely than men to become clinically depressed.

## PMS: Physical or Mental Disorder?

A major controversy regarding sex bias is the inclusion of a diagnosis for premenstrual syndrome (PMS) in the American Psychiatric Association's *Diagnostic and Statistical Manual of Mental Disorders* (fourth edition; known as *DSM-IV*). The provisional diagnosis, in an appendix to DSM-IV, signals that PMS merits further study and may be included as an approved diagnosis in future editions of the DSM.

PMS is characterized by depression, irritability, and other symptoms of increased stress typically occurring just prior to menstruation and lasting for a day or two. More severe cases of PMS are known as premenstrual dysmorphic disorders (PMDD). Whereas PMS is somewhat disruptive and uncomfortable, it does not interfere with daily function; PMDD does. To be diagnosed with PMDD, a woman must have at least five symptoms of PMS for a week to ten days, at least one of which is serious enough to interfere with her ability to function at work or at home. In these more severe cases, antidepressants may be prescribed.

**Schizophrenia:** A mental illness characterized by irrational behaviours, severe alterations of the senses (hallucinations), and, often, an inability to function in society.

# SUICIDE: GIVING UP ON LIFE

There were 3,681 suicides reported in Canada in 1997 (2,914 men and 767 women)—equivalent to a rate of 12.3 per 100,000 people,[34] slightly less than the world-wide rate of 14.5 per 100,000 people reported by the World Health Organization.[35] The pressures, joys, disappointments, challenges, and changes within the college or university environment are believed to be in part responsible for these rates. However, young adults who choose not to go to post-secondary school and who search for the directions to their career and relationship goals and other life aspirations are also at risk for suicide. Experts estimate that there may actually be more cases due to the difficulty in determining the causes of suspicious deaths. Suicide is often a consequence of poor coping skills, lack of social support, lack of self-esteem, and the inability to see one's way out of a bad or negative situation. Suicide can also be viewed as an extreme form of violence—anger, rage, and hopelessness turned inward rather than outward.

University or college students are more likely than the general population to attempt suicide; suicide is the second leading cause of death in people between the ages of 15 and 24. Although women attempt suicide at four times the rate of men, more than three times as many men as women actually succeed in ending their lives. Men may be more "successful" than women because they often choose more violent measures to kill themselves (that is, firearms vs. overdose of painkillers). The suicide rate among First Nations peoples is reported to be three to eight times that of other Canadians.[36]

Risk factors for suicide include a family history of suicide, previous suicide attempts, excessive drug and alcohol use, prolonged depression, financial difficulties, serious illness in the suicide contemplator or in his or her loved ones, and loss of a loved one through death or rejection. Divorced people and former psychiatric patients have a higher risk of suicide than do others. Individuals addicted to alcohol also have a high rate of suicide.

Many of us will be touched by a suicide at some time. In most cases, the suicide does not occur unpredictably. In fact, between 75 and 80 percent of people who commit suicide give a warning of their intentions.

## Warning Signals of Suicide

Common warning signals of suicide include:

- a direct statement about committing suicide, such as "I can't take it anymore. I might as well end it all."
- an indirect statement about committing suicide, such as, "Soon this pain will be over," or, "You won't have to worry about me anymore."

- "final preparations," such as writing a will, repairing poor relationships with family or friends, giving away prized possessions, or writing revealing letters
- a preoccupation with themes of death
- a withdrawal from friends and family and from activities once found pleasurable
- change in eating habits
- change in sleeping patterns
- marked personality change, such as sadness, withdrawal, irritability, anxiety, tiredness, indecisiveness, or apathy
- frequent complaints about physical symptoms, often related to emotions, such as stomachaches, headaches, fatigue, etc.
- not tolerating praise or rewards
- changes in behaviours, such as inability to concentrate, loss of interest in classes, or a sudden and unexplained demonstration of happiness following a period of depression
- changes in personal appearance
- failure to recover from a personal loss or crisis and deepening or prolonged depression
- excessive risk taking and an "I don't care what happens to me" attitude

## Taking Action to Prevent Suicide

Many people who attempt suicide really want to live but see suicide as the only way out of an intolerable situation. Crisis counsellors and help lines may help temporarily, but the only way to prevent suicide is to get rid of conditions, situations, and substances that may precipitate attempts, including alcohol, drugs, loneliness, isolation, and access to guns. If someone you know threatens or displays warnings signs of suicide, take the following actions:

- *Monitor the warning signals.* Keep an eye on the person involved, or ensure there is someone around the person as much as possible.
- *Take any threat seriously.* Don't brush them off.
- *Do not belittle the person's feelings or say that he or she doesn't really mean it or couldn't succeed at suicide.* To some people, these comments offer the challenge of proving you wrong.
- *Let the person know how much you care about him or her.* State that you are there if he or she needs help.
- *Listen.* Try not to discredit or be shocked by what the person says to you. Empathize, sympathize, and keep the person talking. Talk about stressors and listen to responses.

# Prescribing Antidepressants for Depression in 2005: Recent Concerns and Recommendations

In 2005, a review was conducted after the safety of prescribed antidepressants (selective serotonin reuptake inhibitors [SSRIs], selective serotonin and noradrenalin reuptake inhibitors [SNRIs], and other novel antidepressants) was questioned as a first-line treatment for major depressive disorders (MDD) in adults and in children and adolescents because of the drugs' potential to cause or enhance aggression and suicide. Results from this review led to the following clinical recommendations for prescribing antidepressants:

- In adults, including the elderly, SSRIs, SNRIs, and other novel agents remain the best first-line treatments for MDD.

- In children and adolescents, only fluoxetine should be used as a first-line treatment for MDD.

- In children and adolescents, SSRIs other than fluoxetine can be used as a second-line treatment when depression is severe, chronic, and associated with other comorbid conditions or if psychosocial treatments have not worked. SNRIs and other novel agents should be used only as a third-line treatment because of their greater risk of adverse events.

- It is essential to closely monitor patients for suicidality (emerging or worsening suicidal thoughts, behaviours, and attempts), particularly in the early phases of treatment—weekly contact in the first month of antidepressant treatment is recommended. It is also critical to inform the patients and families (when appropriate) of the potential side-effects that may increase suicidality (anxiety, agitation, hypomania, and activation syndrome).

Further research is recommended; specifically to determine risks and benefits to antidepressant use in children, adolescents, and the elderly.

Source: Adapted from R. W. Lam and S. H. Kennedy, "CPA Position Statement: Prescribing Antidepressants for Depression in 2005: Recent Concerns and Recommendations," *The Canadian Journal of Psychiatry*, 49.12, 1–6, retrieved May 30, 2006, from www.canmat.org/suicidality_antidepressant/suicidality-antidepressant.html.

- *Ask the person directly, "Are you thinking of hurting or killing yourself?"*

- *Help the person think about alternatives.* Offer to go for help with the person. Call your local suicide hotline and use all available community and campus resources.

- *Make a contract to meet the person at a later time in his or her home.*

- *If the person has a plan, remove any pills or guns; get help.*

- *Remember that your relationships with others involve responsibilities.* If you need to stay with the person, take the person to a health-care facility, or provide support, give of yourself and your time.

- *Tell your friend's spouse, partner, parents, brothers and sisters, or counsellor.* Do not keep your suspicions to yourself. Don't let a suicidal friend talk you into keeping your discussions confidential. Let your friend know you must share this information with a professional. If your friend is successful in a suicide attempt, you will have to live with the consequences of your inaction. Counselling services available on campus can help you talk with your friend and suggest options for you.

## WHAT WOULD YOU DO?

If your roommate showed warning signs of suicide, what action would you take? Whom would you contact first? Where on campus might your friend get help? In your community? What if someone in your class who you hardly knew showed warning signs of suicide? What would you do?

# SEEKING PROFESSIONAL HELP

Many Canadians feel that seeking professional help for psychosocial problems is an admission of personal failure. Typically, any physical health problem, such as an abscessed tooth or prolonged severe pain, sends us to the nearest dentist or physician. On the other hand, we tend to ignore psychosocial problems until they pose a serious threat to our well-being—and even then, we

# Choosing a Therapist: Key Factors to Consider

When you are in emotional or psychological trouble, you are often in the most vulnerable of situations. The choices you make in times of desperation are often critical to your eventual health; yet, many people choose their therapists at random at their lowest emotional point. Like auto mechanics, physicians, and professors, all therapists are not created equal nor are they equally skilled at what they do. A degree or credential does not ensure compatibility with you, or even general competence. Taking some time to check out the person you are going to see and evaluating that person during your first session are important first steps in taking care of yourself. While even the most thorough check does not guarantee satisfaction, assessing the following may help make your experience a positive and fulfilling one.

1. *Does the therapist have qualities you want in a close friend?* Early in your interaction with the therapist, you should find that the therapist is someone you like, admire, and respect—someone you relate to well and would be willing to trust with your most intimate thoughts. The therapist should convey a genuine interest in you and your problems, rather than watch the clock or check his or her book to schedule your next appointment. You should enjoy sitting in the room with this person and talking. In short, you need to "connect" with your therapist.

2. *Does the therapist act professionally?* Most therapists adhere to a very basic code of ethics. They set boundaries around their relationships with clients to ensure the clients' safety, to foster a feeling of trust, and to encourage confidence in their ability to help. There are exceptions, however. Signs of unprofessional behaviour include:
   - suggestions of meetings or social interactions outside of your sessions, particularly if the therapist appears to be trying to be a personal friend or lover rather than maintaining a professional role
   - agreeing to counsel someone with whom there is a conflict of interest in the counselling situation. Former partners, business relationships, friends, and other clients should be off-limits
   - continually being late for sessions, seeming distracted in sessions, forgetting what you told them before and needing you to repeat things
   - spending too much time talking about him- or herself during the session rather than listening to you; identifying too much of what you are saying with him- or herself rather than your own situation
   - questionable billing practices, such as discrepancies in billing, billing errors to insurance companies, or seeming to want your business and the money rather than displaying a sincere desire to help
   - locking you into the therapist's own specialty; for example, a counsellor who specializes in alcoholism and adult children of alcoholics who continually tries to force you into the "adult child of alcoholic" box, even though this has little to do with your unique situation
   - continual interruptions of your session with phone calls, talking to the receptionist, or other diversions so that you do not get your full amount of time
   - never seeming to want to release you from therapy or encouraging an indefinite dependence on their help. Although the length of treatment varies with each client and his or her respective problems, one of the goals of therapy should be to get out of therapy

3. *Does the therapist work with you to set your goals, thereby empowering you to get better at your pace?* Good therapists will assess your general problem fairly early and set at least some provisional goals on which to work. These usually take the form of small steps that you can tackle each week between sessions, or things that you can do to help you think about your issues and problems. If therapy takes place only in the office, the therapist is not moving you toward recovery. A good therapist is not a detective there to solve your problem per se; his or her role is to provide insight into the things you are doing or to help you understand how your situation and personal actions contribute to your problem(s). A good therapist should serve as a catalyst for you to help yourself, rather than serving as your saviour. Good therapists help you find your answers and build on your strengths, rather than just focusing on getting rid of your weaknesses.

4. *Is the therapist willing to let you conduct an interview before committing to his or her services?* Good therapists will allow you at least one meeting (often at a minimal or reduced charge) to check out the aforementioned information and to find out about their credentials, their counselling style, their personality, and the general "fit."

Most therapy should result in at least minor improvements in six to eight weeks. If you find that you are getting nowhere, if you are repeating the same things over and over, or if you find problems with any of the above, do not be afraid to find another therapist.

Sources: "How to Choose a Therapist," CBS This Morning, July 24–26, 1996; David Meyers, *Psychology,* Chapter 16, "How to Choose a Therapist," Worth Publishing, 537–572; James W. Kalat, "Treatment of Psychologically Troubled People," in *Introduction to Psychology,* 4th edition, eds. Brooks/Cole (1996), 648–678.

may refuse to ask for the help needed. Despite this tradition, an increasing number of Canadians are turning to mental health professionals for help. Researchers believe that more people want help today because "normal" living has become more difficult. Breakdown in support systems, high expectations of the individual by society, and dysfunctional families are cited as the three major reasons more people ask for help.

You should consider seeking help under the following circumstances. Seek help if:

- you think you need help
- you experience wild mood swings
- a problem is interfering with your daily life
- your fears or feelings of guilt frequently distract you
- you begin to withdraw from others
- you have hallucinations
- you feel that life is not worth living
- you feel inadequate or worthless
- your emotional responses are inappropriate in various situations
- your daily life seems to be nothing but repeated crises
- you feel you can't "get your act together"
- you are considering suicide
- you turn to drugs or alcohol to escape your problems
- you feel out of control

# Types of Mental Health Professionals

Several types of mental health professionals, or providers, are available to help you. The most important criterion when choosing a provider is whether you feel you can work well with that person, not how many degrees he or she has.

## Psychiatrist

A **psychiatrist** is a medical doctor. After obtaining a medical doctorate, a psychiatrist spends up to 12 years studying psychosocial health and disease. As a licensed physician, a psychiatrist can prescribe medications for various mental or emotional problems and may have admitting privileges at local hospitals. Some psychiatrists are affiliated with hospitals, while others are in private practice. Psychiatric fees are normally covered by provincial or territorial health insurance.

## Psychoanalyst

A **psychoanalyst** is a psychiatrist or a psychologist with special training in psychoanalysis. Psychoanalysis is a type of therapy in which a person is helped to remember early traumas that block personal growth. Facing these traumas helps the individual to resolve the conflicts they have caused and begin to lead a more productive life.

## Psychologist

A **psychologist** usually has a Ph.D. in counselling or clinical psychology. In addition, all provinces require licensure. Psychologists are trained in various types of talk therapy. Most are trained to conduct individual and group counselling sessions. Psychologists may also be trained in certain specialties, such as family counselling, sexual counselling, or counselling related to compulsive behaviours. Psychologists may work in private practice or in publicly funded organizations. Some employee assistance programs cover a certain number of psychologist visits annually, and the extended health plan through your university or college may have some coverage for psychologists' fees.

## Clinical/Certified/Psychiatric Social Worker

A **social worker** has at least a master's degree in social work (M.S.W.) and two years of experience in a clinical setting. Some provinces require an examination for accreditation in the College of Clinical Social Work. Some social workers work in clinical settings, whereas others have private practices. Certified clinical social workers (C.S.W.) often work in private practices, and their clients are sometimes insured through employee assistance programs.

## Counsellor

Persons having a variety of academic and experiential training call themselves counsellors. The **counsellor** often has a master's degree in counselling, psychology, educational psychology, or a related human service. Professional societies recommend at least two years of graduate coursework or supervised practice as a minimal requirement. Many counsellors are trained to do individual and group counselling. They often specialize in one type of counselling, such as family, marital, relationship, children,

**Psychiatrist:** A licensed physician who specializes in treating mental and emotional disorders.

**Psychoanalyst:** A psychiatrist or psychologist with special training in psychoanalysis.

**Psychologist:** A person with a Ph.D. and training in psychology.

**Social worker:** A person with an M.S.W. degree and clinical training.

**Counsellor:** A person with a variety of academic and experiential training who deals with the treatment of emotional problems.

# Managing Your Psychosocial Health

Psychosocial health is a complex concept. Finding the best way to help yourself achieve optimal psychosocial health requires careful introspection and planned action. Remembering the following points and acting upon them whenever possible may help you along the way.

## MAKING DECISIONS FOR YOU

Psychosocial health is influenced by many factors.

- Why is being psychosocially healthy important to you? To the people close to you?

- What steps can you take to improve your mental health? What actions can you take today that will improve your emotional health? What steps could you take right now that could help you improve your social health? What could you do to improve your spiritual health?

- Finally, if you felt that you had a psychosocial problem, would you seek help? Why or why not? Who would you seek help from?

## CHECKLIST FOR CHANGE

- Consider life an opportunity for discovery and learning.
- Accept yourself as the best that you are able to be right now.
- Remember that nobody is perfect.
- Remember that the most difficult times in life occur during transitions and can be opportunities for growth even though they are painful.
- Remember that there are other perspectives than your own.
- Recognize the sources of your anxiety and act to reduce them.
- Ask for help when you need it; discuss your problems with others.
- Become sensitive to and aware of your body's signals—take care of yourself.

- Find a meaning for your life and work toward achieving your goals.
- Develop strategies to get through problem situations.
- Remain open to emotional experiences—give yourself to today rather than waiting for tomorrow.
- Even when you fail, be proud of yourself for trying.
- Keep your sense of humour—learn to laugh at yourself.
- Never quit trying to grow, to experience, to love, and to live life to its fullest.

## CRITICAL THINKING

Suppose that your roommate ended a long-term relationship last month. Ever since, your roommate no longer jogs every morning or attends religious services, and doesn't even want to attend school mixers to meet someone else. Worse yet, even minor mistakes lead your roommate to vicious self-berating.

You are concerned about your roommate's psychosocial health, but unsure of what to do. You know that your roommate has in the past said that anyone who needs therapy should be "locked up and the key thrown away." But your roommate's mood is beginning to affect you. Use the DECIDE model described in Chapter 1 to decide what you would do in this situation. Explain your decision. If the action you chose did not bring about the desired result, what would you do next? Then list some ways you can show support for a friend who shows signs of psychosocial illness.

---

drug, divorce, behavioural, or personal counselling. Remember that in Canada anyone can use the title of therapist or counsellor. Before you begin treatment, you should consider the credentials of your counsellor, your desired outcomes, and the expectations of you and your counsellor.

## Psychiatric Nurse Specialist

Although all registered nurses can work in psychiatric settings, some have chosen to continue their education and specialize in psychiatric practice. The psychiatric nurse specialist can be certified by the Registered Psychiatric Nursing Association in some provinces.

## What to Expect When You Begin Therapy

The first trip to a therapist can be extremely difficult. Most of us have misconceptions about what therapy is and about what it can do. That first visit is a verbal and mental sizing up between you and the therapist. You may not accomplish much in that first hour. If you decide that the therapist is not for you, you will at least have learned how to present your problem and what qualities you need in a therapist.

1. Before meeting a therapist, briefly explain your needs to the therapist or to the individual who you made the appointment with. Ask about the

fee. Arrive on time. Wear comfortable clothing. Expect to spend about an hour with the therapist during your first visit.

2. The therapist may want to take down your history and details about the problems that brought you to therapy. Answer as honestly as possible. Many therapists will ask how you feel about aspects of your life. Do not be embarrassed to acknowledge your feelings.

3. Therapists are not mind readers. They cannot tell what you are thinking. It is therefore critical to the success of your treatment that you have enough trust in your therapist to be open and honest.

4. Do not expect the therapist to tell you what to do or how to behave. Very few hand out behavioural prescriptions.

5. Find out if the therapist will allow you to set your own therapeutic goals and timetables. Also, find out if, later in therapy, your therapist will allow you to determine what is and what is not helping you.

6. If, after your first visit (or even after several visits), you feel you cannot work with a therapist, you must summon up the courage to say so. Do not worry about hurting the therapist's feelings. If there is a personality conflict or if you do not feel comfortable, the therapy will not be effective.

## WHAT WOULD YOU DO?

Have you ever thought about seeing a therapist? Why or why not? Did you make an appointment? If so, what made you decide to? If you didn't, did things get better quickly? Do you think you might have worked out your problem faster if you had seen a therapist?

# SUMMARY

- Psychosocial health is a complex phenomenon involving mental, emotional, social, and spiritual health.
- Many factors influence psychosocial health, including family, the environment, self-efficacy and self-esteem, and personality.
- Social bonds and social support networks contribute to the ability to cope with life's challenges.
- Common psychosocial problems include depression, obsessive-compulsive disorders, anxiety disorders (including phobias, panic attacks, and post-traumatic stress disorder), seasonal affective disorder, and schizophrenia.
- Suicide is a result of negative psychosocial reactions to life. People intending to commit suicide often give warning signs. Such people can often be helped.
- Mental health professionals include psychiatrists, psychoanalysts, psychologists, clinical/certified/ psychiatric social workers, counsellors, and psychiatric nurse specialists. Major types of therapy include behavioural, cognitive, family, and psychodynamic therapies.

# DISCUSSION QUESTIONS

1. What is psychosocial health? What indicates that you either are or aren't psychosocially healthy? Why do you think the university or college environment may provide a real challenge to your psychosocial health?

2. Discuss the factors that influence your overall level of psychosocial health. What factors can you change? Which ones may be more difficult to change?

3. What steps could you take today to improve your psychosocial health? Which steps require long-term effort?

4. What factors appear to contribute to psychosocial difficulties and illnesses? Which of the more common psychosocial illnesses is likely to affect people in your age group?

5. What are the warning signs of suicide? What would you do if you heard a stranger in the cafeteria say to no one in particular that he was going to "do the world a favour and end it all"? What if this person was a friend; how would you react then?

6. Discuss the different types of health professionals and therapies. If you felt depressed about breaking off a long-term relationship, which professional and therapy do you think would be most beneficial? Explain your answer. What services are provided by your student health centre? Are fees charged to students?

7. What psychosocial areas do you need to work on? Which are most important? Why?

## APPLICATION EXERCISE

Reread the What Do You Think? scenario at the beginning of the chapter and answer the following questions.

1. How psychosocially healthy is Marisol?

2. What factors may have contributed to Marisol's current health status?

3. What services on your campus would be available to help Marisol improve her psychosocial health?

4. As a friend, what could you do to help Marisol?

## HEALTH ON THE NET

Canadian Mental Health Association
**www.cmha.ca/bins/index.asp**

Child & Family Canada
**www.cfc-efc.ca**

University of British Columbia Mood Disorders Centre
**www.psychiatry.ubc.ca/mood/**

Canadian Network for Mood and Anxiety
**www.canmat.org/**

Health Canada
**www.hc-sc.gc.ca**

# CHAPTER 3

# MANAGING STRESS

*Toward Prevention and Control*

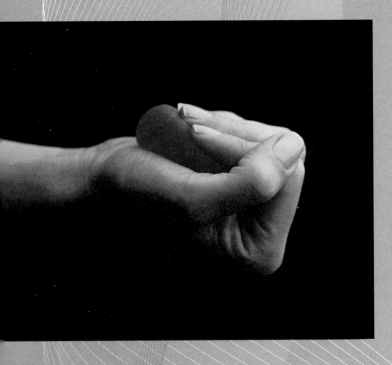

## CHAPTER OBJECTIVES

- Define stress, stressors, and stress reaction.
- Explain how stress may have direct and indirect effects on your immune system and on your overall health status.
- Explain the three phases of the general adaptation syndrome and describe what happens physiologically and psychologically when you perceive a threat.
- Discuss psychosocial, environmental, and self-imposed sources of stress.
- Examine how evolving technology and societal expectations may cause new kinds of stress.
- Examine the stressors particularly relevant to university and college students.
- Describe stress management techniques.

Rhett is taking a full load of introductory classes in his first year of post-secondary studies. He is living with his best friend from high school in a residence directly on campus and goes home one weekend each month. He is involved in several student organizations and plays intramural sports. He is doing well in his science courses, but struggling in his arts courses. Although he tries to study in his room, he finds residence life too distracting and as a result has been forced to find somewhere else to study. The library is often overcrowded and he has difficulty finding a spot. He tries to get to bed by midnight; however, the noise level in residence often keeps him awake until 1 or 2 a.m. Since being on campus, he's eaten fewer fruits and vegetables and more pasta, pizza, burgers, and fries. Unlike many of his friends who say they know what they are planning to do when they graduate, Rhett is still searching for his career path.

■ Are Rhett's experiences common for first-year university or college students? What components of first-year post-secondary studies may cause him to feel stressed? What advice would you give to him as a first-year student?

Stress: it's hard to live with it and it's almost impossible to live without it. We are bombarded by a host of subtle and not-so-subtle internal and external factors that may lead us to feel stressed from the moment we awake until we finally drift into deep sleep at the day's end. Even during our sleeping moments, noise, temperature changes, and other activities can lead to a stress response. Rarely does a day go by without someone you know talking about being under stress—from homework, financial pressures, relationship demands, or other problems. Despite our best efforts to ignore it, stress-inducing factors cannot be run from, hidden from, or wished away. For some people, these factors provide the stimulus for growth and higher levels of achievement. Yet for others, they increase the likelihood of dysfunctional or abnormal behaviours or illness.

Stress in itself is neither positive nor negative. Rather, it is our reactions to stress that can be described as positive or negative. Whether we are aware of it or not, our reactions to stress can become the habits that lead us either to health-enhancing personal growth or to debilitation in the form of migraines, substance misuse and abuse, circulatory disorders, asthma, gastrointestinal problems, and hypertension (high blood pressure). In addition, our responses to stress can lead to psychological and social problems, including dysfunctional relationships. In this chapter, we will explore why and how these reactions take place and how we may be able to control them and channel our efforts more effectively such that our health and wellness is not compromised.

## WHAT IS STRESS?

Many things that have contributed to making you who you are also influence how you respond to stressful events in your life. Stress responses—such as breaking out in a cold sweat before asking someone to go out on a date, becoming anxious around people who speak too slowly or drive too cautiously, feeling nervous when meeting new people, a racing heart rate when you are called upon to make a response in class, feeling edgy or pumped when it is time to play a game—are all unique byproducts of past experiences. Your family, friends, environmental conditions, general health status, personality, and support systems influence how you respond to a given event.

Stress means different things to different people. Often, we think of **stress** as an externally imposed factor that threatens or makes a demand on our minds and bodies. If your hard-nosed instructor tells you that you have to do a 10-page paper in the next week, that's an external stressor. However, most stress is actually self-imposed and is usually the result of an internal state of emotional tension that occurs in response to the various demands of living. Stress may manifest itself in physiological and psychological responses to the demands placed upon us, and many researchers define stress as these responses.[1] Most current definitions state that stress is the mental and physical response of our bodies to the various demands or expectations in our lives.

A **stressor** is any physical, social, or mental event or condition that causes our bodies to adjust to it. Stressors may be tangible, such as an angry parent or a disgruntled roommate, or intangible, such as the mixed emotions associated with meeting your significant other's parents for the first time. Adjustment is our attempt to cope with a given situation.[2] As we try to adjust to the various stressors in our lives, strain may develop. Strain is the wear and tear our bodies and minds sustain during the process of adjusting to or resisting a stressor.

Most of our daily activities involve situations or events that may elicit a stress response. Positive stress, or stress that presents the opportunity for personal growth and satisfaction, is called **eustress.** Getting married, starting school, beginning a career, developing new friendships, and learning a new physical skill all give rise to eustress. **Distress,** or negative stress, is caused by things such as financial problems, injury or illness, the death of a loved one, trouble at work, academic difficulties, the unexpected ending of a relationship, and not being sure of your purpose in life that result in a debilitative stress response and strain.

In most cases, we cannot prevent distress; like eustress, it is simply a part of life. However, we can learn to recognize the events that are likely to cause distress and to anticipate our reactions to them by learning to practise prestress coping skills and develop poststress management techniques. Developing these skills depends on our understanding of the major components of stress.

## The Mind–Body Connection: Physical Responses

Although much has been written about the negative effects of stress, researchers have only recently begun to untangle the complex web of physical and emotional interactions that actually cause the body to wear down over time. As a result, stress is often described generically as a "disease of prolonged arousal" that often leads to other negative health effects. Nearly all systems of the body become potential targets for this onslaught, and the long-term effects may be devastating.

Much of the initial impetus for studying the health effects of stress came from prospective observations. Specifically, researchers in the Framingham Study noted that highly stressed individuals were significantly more likely to experience cardiovascular diseases.[3] Monkeys exposed to high levels of unpredictable stressors in studies also showed significantly increased levels of disease and mortality.[4] In a study of susceptibility to cold viruses, subjects who reported recent high levels of stressors were much more likely to catch a cold after inhaling large doses of a cold virus through their nose than their counterparts who reported fewer stressors.[5] While the battle over the legitimacy of these observations continues to be waged in research labs, certain factors relating too much stress over long periods of time to selected ailments have gained credibility. What do repeated experiences of the stress response actually do to the body? Why are health and wellness experts concerned about repeated responses or reactions to stress? What are the short- and long-term health implications of the stress response?

## Stress and Impaired Immunity

Although the health effects of prolonged stress responses provide dramatic evidence of the direct and indirect impact of stress on body organs, researchers continue to seek more definitive answers about the exact physiological and psychological

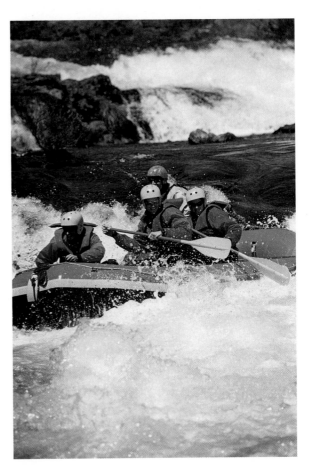

*Stress is a positive factor in life when it creates opportunities for personal growth and satisfaction rather than psychological or physiological wear and tear.*

mechanisms that lead to specific diseases. The science of **psychoneuroimmunology (PNI)** analyzes the relationship between the mind's response to stress and the functioning of the immune system.

Much of the preliminary PNI data on stress and immune functioning focused on the hypothesis that, during periods of prolonged stress, elevated levels of adrenal hormones, including cortisol, destroy or reduce the ability of the white blood cells known as *natural killer T cells*. Killer T cells aid in the immune response, and when they are suppressed the body is less effective at

**Stress:** Our mental and physical responses to the demands placed upon us.

**Stressor:** A physical, social, or mental event or condition that causes us to adjust to it.

**Eustress:** Stress perceived as "good" because it presents opportunities for personal growth.

**Distress:** Stress perceived as "bad" because it is debilitating and can have a negative effect on health and wellness.

**Psychoneuroimmunology (PNI):** Science of the interaction between the mind and the body, in particular with the immune system.

combatting illnesses. In addition to killer T suppression, many other body processes are disrupted and overall disease-fighting capacity is reduced. Although several studies have supported the hypothesis of a relationship between increased stress levels and greater risk of disease in times of grief, social disruption, poor mood, and so forth, there is much still to be learned about possible mediating factors.[6] Other studies have shown no increased risk for disease among people suffering from prolonged arousal by stressors.[7] These conflicting findings also emphasize the need to further examine the relationships of physical and mental health and wellness to stressors, stress responses, and coping mechanisms.

# THE GENERAL ADAPTATION SYNDROME

Every living organism attempts to achieve a state of balance known as **homeostasis.** In homeostasis, all physiological and psychological systems function smoothly, and equilibrium is maintained. When a stress is perceived, the mind and body adjusts with an **adaptive response,** or an attempt to restore homeostasis. This adaptive response varies in intensity and physical manifestation from person to person and from stressor to stressor. Further, this response can vary within an individual from time to time even with the same stressor.

The physiological and psychological responses to stress follow a pattern first recognized in 1936 by Hans Selye.[8] The three-stage response to stress Selye outlined is called the **general adaptation syndrome (GAS).** The phases of the GAS are alarm, resistance, and exhaustion (see Figure 3.1).

## Alarm Phase

During the alarm phase, a stressor disturbs homeostasis. The brain subconsciously perceives the stressor and prepares the body either to fight or to run away, a response sometimes called the fight or flight response. The subconscious perceptions and appraisal of the stressor stimulate the areas in the brain responsible for emotions. Emotional stimulation, in turn, starts the physical reactions that we associate with stress (see Figure 3.2). This entire process usually takes only a few seconds.

When the mind perceives a stressor (either real or imaginary), such as a potential attacker, the cerebral cortex, the region of the brain that interprets the nature of an event, is called to attention. If the cerebral cortex consciously or unconsciously perceives a threat, it triggers an instantaneous **autonomic nervous system (ANS)** response that prepares the body for action (i.e., fight or flight). The ANS is the portion of the central nervous

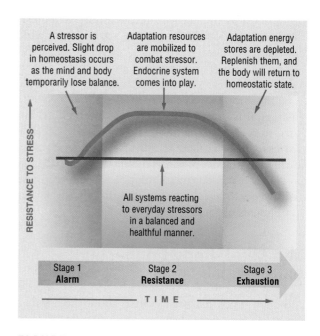

**FIGURE 3.1**
The General Adaptation Syndrome

system that regulates bodily functions that we do not normally consciously control, such as heart rate, breathing, and glandular function. When we are stressed, the rate of these bodily functions increases dramatically to give us the physical strength to protect ourselves against an attack, or to mobilize internal forces. The ANS has two branches. One branch, the **sympathetic nervous system (SNS),** energizes the body for either fight or flight by signalling the release of several stress hormones that increase heart and breathing rates, and trigger many other stress responses. The other branch, the **parasympathetic nervous system (PNS),** slows all the systems stimulated by the stress response. In other words, the PNS works in opposition to the SNS and attempts to restore homeostasis. In a healthy person, these two systems work together to maintain balance. Long-term stress can cause this balance to become strained, resulting in chronic physical and mental problems.

The response of the SNS to various stressors involves a complex series of biochemical exchanges between different parts of the body. The **hypothalamus,** a section of the brain, functions as the control centre and determines the overall reaction to stressors. When the hypothalamus perceives that extra energy is needed to fight or flee a stressor, it stimulates the adrenal glands, located near the top of the kidneys, to release the hormone **epinephrine,** also called adrenaline.

Epinephrine causes more blood to be pumped with each beat of the heart, dilates the alveoli (air sacs in the lungs) to increase oxygen intake, increases the rate of breathing, stimulates the liver to release more glucose (which fuels muscular contractions), and dilates the pupils to improve visual sensitivity. The body is then

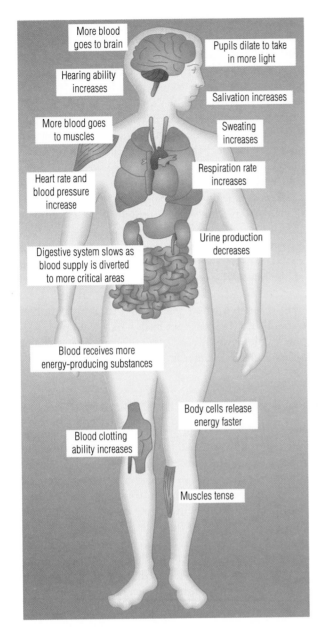

**FIGURE 3.2**
**The General Adaptation Syndrome: Alarm Phase**

available to meet energy demands. Finally, other parts of the brain and body release endorphins, the body's naturally occurring opiates, which relieve pain that may be caused by a stressor or the body's response to the stressor.

## Resistance Phase

The resistance phase of the GAS begins almost immediately after the alarm phase starts. In this phase, the body has reacted to the stressor and adjusted in a way that begins to allow the system to return to homeostasis. As the sympathetic nervous system is working to energize the body via the hormonal action of epinephrine, norepinephrine, cortisol, and other hormones, the parasympathetic nervous system is working to keep these energy levels under control and attempts to return the body to a normal level of functioning.

## Exhaustion Phase

In the exhaustion phase of the GAS, the physiological and psychological energy used to respond to a stressor (i.e., fight or flight) has been depleted. Short-term response to stress would probably not deplete all a person's energy reserves, but chronic stressors may create continuous states of alarm and resistance. When a person no longer has the adaptation energy stores for responding to a distressor, burnout and serious illness may result.

**Homeostasis:** A balanced physical and mental state in which all the body's systems function smoothly.

**Adaptive response:** Form of adjustment in which the mind and body attempt to restore homeostasis.

**General adaptation syndrome (GAS):** The pattern followed by our physiological and psychological responses to stress, consisting of the alarm, resistance, and exhaustion phases.

**Autonomic nervous system (ANS):** The portion of the central nervous system that regulates bodily functions that we do not normally consciously control.

**Sympathetic nervous system (SNS):** Branch of the ANS responsible for stress arousal.

**Parasympathetic nervous system (PNS):** Part of the ANS responsible for slowing systems stimulated by the SNS.

**Hypothalamus:** A section of the brain that controls the SNS and directs the stress response.

**Epinephrine:** Also called adrenaline, a hormone that stimulates body systems in response to stress.

**Adrenocorticotrophic hormone (ACTH):** A pituitary hormone that stimulates the adrenal glands to secrete cortisol.

**Cortisol:** Hormone released by the adrenal glands that enables the availability of stored nutrients to meet energy demands.

poised to act immediately. As epinephrine secretion increases, blood is diverted away from the digestive system, and this can cause nausea and cramping if this response occurs shortly after a meal. Further, epinephrine dries nasal and salivary tissues, producing a dry mouth.

The stress response occurring during the alarm phase also leads to longer-term reactions to stress. The hypothalamus triggers the pituitary gland, which in turn releases another powerful hormone, **adrenocorticotrophic hormone (ACTH).** ACTH signals the adrenal glands to release **cortisol,** a hormone that makes stored nutrients more readily

# SOURCES OF STRESS

Eustress and distress have many sources. These sources include psychosocial factors, such as change, pressure, inconsistent goals and behaviours, conflict, overload, and burnout; environmental stressors, such as natural and human-made disasters; and self-imposed stressors including factors related to self-concept.

## Psychosocial Sources of Stress

As you learned in the previous chapter, psychosocial health refers to the social, mental, emotional, and spiritual dimensions of health. These components combined define how we perceive our lives, relate to one another, and react to stress. Many psychosocial factors in our daily lives cause us to feel stressed. Our interactions with others, the subtle and not-so-subtle expectations we have for ourselves and others, the expectations others have for us, and the social conditions we work, play, and live in force us to adjust and readjust continually. Some of these stressors present very real threats to our mental or physical well-being; others cause us to worry about things that may never happen. Still other stressors result from otherwise good psychosocial events—being around someone you're attracted to, meeting new friends, moving to a new and better apartment, celebrating a win or successful paper or exam.

### Change

You will experience stress any time there is change, whether good or bad, in your normal daily routine. The more changes you experience and the more adjustments you must make as a result of this change, the greater the stress response may be. In 1967, Holmes and Rahe analyzed the social readjustments experienced by more than 5,000 patients, noting which events seemed to occur just before the onset of disease.[9] They determined that certain events (positive and negative) were predictive of increased risk for illness. They called their scale for predicting stress overload and the likelihood of illness the Social Readjustment Rating Scale (SRRS).[10] The SRRS has since been modified for certain groups, including university or college-aged students. Although many other factors must be considered, it is generally believed that the more stressors you have, the more likely you are to experience negative effects on your health and wellness and the more important it is to address your behaviours or situations before health problems occur. (See the Rate Yourself box.)

While Holmes and Rahe focused on such major sources of stress as a death in the family, psychologists such as Richard Lazarus have more recently focused on petty annoyances, irritations, and frustrations—collectively referred to as hassles—as sources of stress.[11] Minor hassles—losing your keys, having the grocery bag rip on the way to the door, slipping and falling in front of everyone as you walk to your seat in class, finding that you went through a whole afternoon with a big chunk of spinach stuck in your front teeth—may seem unimportant, but the cumulative effects of these minor hassles may be harmful in the long run.

### Pressure

Pressure occurs when we feel forced to speed up, intensify, or shift the direction of our behaviours to meet a higher standard of performance.[12] Pressures can be based on our personal goals and expectations or on a concern about what others may think of us. Pressure can also come from outside influences. Among the most significant and consistent of these are seemingly relentless demands from society about what we should look like and that we compete and be all that we can be. The forces that push us to attempt to shape our bodies into an image that may not even be physiologically realistic for us or to compete for the best grades, the nicest cars, the most attractive partners, and the highest paying jobs create a lot of pressure to be the personification of success.[13] Being pressured into doing something we don't want to do (for example, studying when everyone else is going to a movie or going to a party because everyone else is when you really need to be studying) can also be a source of frustration.

### Inconsistent Goals and Behaviours

For many of us, negative stress effects are magnified when there is a conflict between our goals (what we value or hope to obtain in life) and our behaviours (actions or activities that may not help us to achieve these goals). For instance, you want good grades and your family expects them, yet you party and procrastinate throughout the term resulting in

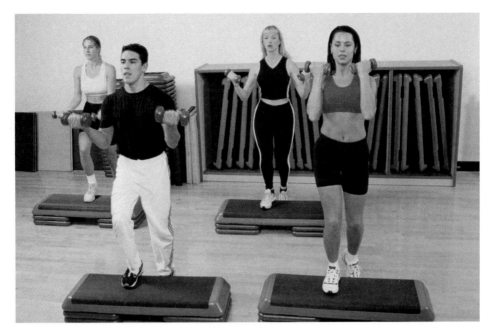

*Aerobic exercise is an effective stress management tool.*

disappointing grades. Thus, your behaviours were inconsistent with your goals and significant stress in the form of guilt and a last-minute frenzy before exams usually occurs. On the other hand, if you choose to dig in and study hard, and are committed to getting good grades, your goals and behaviours are congruent and you will not experience this kind of negative stress. Thwarted goals may lead to frustration, and frustration has been shown to be a significant disrupter of homeostasis (see Figure 3.3).

Determining whether our behaviours are consistent with the goals we want to reach is an essential component of our efforts to maintain a balance in our lives. If we consciously strive to attain our goals in a very direct manner, our chances of success are greatly improved. If we deviate from the plan, or if we act in a manner that is inconsistent with our goals, significant stress may result that makes our goals impossible, and they may then become negative sources of stress.

## Conflict

Of all life's difficulties, **conflict** is probably the most common. Conflict occurs when we are forced to make challenging decisions concerning two or more competing motives, behaviours, or impulses or when we are forced to face two incompatible demands, opportunities, needs, or goals.[14] What if your best friends choose to smoke marijuana and you don't want to but fear rejection? Such conflicts occur every day for most of us. Worrying about the alternatives, fretting, stewing, and becoming overly anxious are common responses when conflict occurs.

BEHAVIOURS          GOALS

Work ethic
Priorities
Perseverance
Commitment
Dedication
Consistency
Interpersonal interactions

Health
Grades
Love
Career success
Financial gain
Expectations/ desires
Achievement levels
Values/beliefs
Relationship satisfaction

HOMEOSTASIS

**FIGURE 3.3**

**Homeostatic Balance Requires Actions Related to Goals and Values**

**Conflict:** Simultaneous existence of incompatible demands, opportunities, needs, or goals.

# How Stressed Are You?

Each of us reacts differently to life's little challenges. Faced with a long line at the bank, most of us will get heated up for a few seconds before we shrug and move on. But for others—the one in five of us whom researchers call *hot reactors*—such incidents are an assault on good health. That's why rating your stress requires you to tally your life's stressors (Part One) and to figure out whether you are particularly susceptible to stress (Part Two). (As university or college students, you should consider your job as being a student.)

## PART ONE
### The Stress in Your Life

How often are the following stressful situations a part of your daily life?

1. Never
2. Rarely
3. Sometimes
4. Often
5. All the time

| | | | | | |
|---|---|---|---|---|---|
| I work long hours | 1 | 2 | 3 | 4 | 5 |
| There are signs my job isn't secure | 1 | 2 | 3 | 4 | 5 |
| Doing a good job goes unnoticed | 1 | 2 | 3 | 4 | 5 |
| It takes all my energy just to make it through the day | 1 | 2 | 3 | 4 | 5 |
| There are severe arguments at home | 1 | 2 | 3 | 4 | 5 |
| A family member is seriously ill | 1 | 2 | 3 | 4 | 5 |
| I'm having problems with child care | 1 | 2 | 3 | 4 | 5 |
| I don't have enough time for fun | 1 | 2 | 3 | 4 | 5 |
| I'm on a diet | 1 | 2 | 3 | 4 | 5 |
| My family and friends count on me to solve their problems | 1 | 2 | 3 | 4 | 5 |
| I'm expected to keep up a certain standard of living | 1 | 2 | 3 | 4 | 5 |
| My neighbourhood is crowded or dangerous | 1 | 2 | 3 | 4 | 5 |
| My home is a mess | 1 | 2 | 3 | 4 | 5 |
| I can't pay my bills on time | 1 | 2 | 3 | 4 | 5 |
| I'm not saving money | 1 | 2 | 3 | 4 | 5 |

**Your Total Score** _____

Below 38: You have a lower-stress life.

38 and above: You have a high-stress life.

## PART TWO
### Your Stress Susceptibility

Try to imagine how you would react in these hypothetical situations:

You've been waiting 20 minutes for a table in a crowded restaurant, and the host seats a party that arrived after you. You feel your anger rise as your face gets hot and your heart beats faster.

**True or False** _____

Your sister calls out of the blue and starts to tell you how much you mean to her. Uncomfortable, you change the subject without expressing what you feel.

**True or False** _____

You come home to find the kitchen looking like a disaster area and your partner (or roommate) lounging in front of the TV. You tense up and can't seem to shake your anger.

**True or False** _____

Faced with a public-speaking event (such as a class presentation), you get keyed up and lose sleep for a day or more, worrying about how you'll do.

**True or False** _____

On Thursday your repair shop promises to fix your car in time for a weekend trip. As the hours go by, you become increasingly worried that something will go wrong and your trip will be ruined.

**True or False** _____

Two or Fewer True: You're a Cool Reactor, someone who tends to roll with the punches when a situation is out of your control.

Three or More True: You're a Hot Reactor, someone who responds to mildly stressful situations with a "fight-or-flight" adrenaline rush that drives up blood pressure and can lead to heart rhythm disturbances, accelerated clotting, and damaged blood vessel linings. Some hot reactors can seem cool as a cucumber on the outside, but inside their bodies are silently killing them.

## WHAT YOUR SCORES MEAN

Combine the results from Parts One and Two to get your total stress rating.

**Lower-Stress Life      Cool Reactor**

Whatever your problems, stress isn't one of them. Even when stressful events do occur—and they will—your health probably won't suffer.

**Lower-Stress Life      Hot Reactor**

You're not under stress—at least for now. Though you tend to overreact to problems, you've wisely managed your life to avoid the big stressors. Before you honk at the guy who cuts you off in rush-hour traffic, remember that getting angry can destroy thousands of heart muscle cells within minutes. Robert S. Eliot, author of *From Stress to Strength*, says hot reactors have no choice but to calm themselves down with rational thought. Ponder the fact that the only thing you'll hasten by reacting is a decline in health. "You have to stop trying to change the world," Eliot advises, "and learn to change your response to it."

**High-Stress Life      Cool Reactor**

You're under stress, but only you know if it's hurting. Even if you normally thrive with a full plate of challenges, now you might be biting off more than you can chew. Note any increase in headaches, backaches, or insomnia; that's your body telling you to lighten your load. If your job is the main source of stress, think about reducing your hours. If that's not possible, find a way to make your job more enjoyable, and stress will become manageable.

**High-Stress Life      Hot Reactor**

You're in the danger zone. Make an extra effort to engage in physical activity, get enough sleep, and keep your family and friends close. Unfortunately, even being physically active and physically fit does little to protect you if your body is in perpetual stress mode. To survive, you may need to make major changes—walking away from a life-destroying job or relationship, perhaps—as well as to develop a whole new approach to life's hourly obstacles. Such effort will be rewarded, too. In one experiment, 77 percent of hot reactors were able to cool down—lower their blood pressure and cholesterol levels—by training themselves to stay calm.

Source: Reprinted by permission of the Health Publishing Group, a division of Time Publishing Ventures, Inc., from "How Stressed Are You?" *Health*, October 1994, 47. Researched by Lora Elise Ma. © 1994.

## Overload

**Overload** occurs when you experience excessive time pressure, excessive responsibility, lack of support, or excessive expectations of yourself and those around you. Have you ever felt that you had so many responsibilities that you couldn't possibly begin to fulfill them all? Have you longed for a weekend when you could just curl up and read a good book or take time out with friends and not feel guilty? These feelings typically occur when a person has been under continuous pressure for some time and as a result experiences overload. Students who are overloaded may experience anxiety about tests and assignments, poor self-concept, thoughts about dropping classes or dropping out of school, and other problems. In severe cases, in which they are unable to see any solutions to their problems, students may suffer from depression or resort to overeating or consuming alcohol or drugs.

## Burnout

People who regularly feel overload, frustration, and disappointment may eventually begin to experience **burnout,** a state of physical and mental exhaustion caused by excessive stress. People involved in the helping professions, such as teaching, social work, drug counselling, nursing, and psychology, appear to experience high levels of burnout, as do police officers, fire-fighters, and air-traffic controllers, who work in high-pressure, dangerous jobs.

## Other Forms of Psychosocial Stress

Other forms of psychosocial stress include problems with adaptation (difficulty in adapting to life's changes), frustration (the thwarting or inhibiting of natural or desired behaviours or goals), overcrowding (the presence of too many people in a space), discrimination (the unfavourable actions taken against people based on prejudices concerning race, religion, social status, gender, sex, sexual orientation, lifestyle, national origin, or physical characteristics), and socioeconomic events (inflation, unemployment, or poverty). People of different ethnic backgrounds and individuals who are homosexual may face disproportionately heavy impacts from these sources of stress.

## Environmental Stress

Environmental stress is stress that results from events occurring in our physical environment. Environmental stressors include natural disasters, such as floods, earthquakes, hurricanes, tornadoes, hail storms, and forest fires, and industrial disasters, such as chemical spills,

**Overload:** A condition in which we feel overly pressured by demands made on us.

**Burnout:** Physical and mental exhaustion caused by the continuous experience of overload.

accidents at nuclear power plants, and explosions. Often as damaging as one-time disasters are **background distressors,** such as noise, air, and water pollution or heat, humidity, cold, and wind-chills, although we may be unaware of them and their effects may not become apparent for decades. As with other distressors, our bodies respond to environmental distressors with the general adaptation syndrome. People who cannot escape background distressors may exist in a constant resistance phase, which may also contribute to the development of stress-related disorders.

# Self-Imposed Stress

## Self-Concept and Stress

How we feel about ourselves, our attitudes toward others, and our perceptions and interpretations of the stressors in our lives are part of the psychological component of stress. Also included are the defence or coping mechanisms we have learned to use in various situations that induce the stress response.

The psychological system that governs our stress responses is called the **cognitive stress system.**[15] It recognizes stressors; evaluates them on the basis of self-concept, past experiences, and emotions; and makes decisions about how to best cope with them. Our sensory organs serve as input channels for information reaching the brain. From that point on, attention to the problem, memory, reasoning, and problem solving processes are organized in various parts of the brain before we respond to the stressor. Because learning and memory involve the changing of various proteins in brain neurons, the emotions we experience during the stress response also "tickle" the memory-storage neurons and contribute to our responses. Behaviourally, we respond to the stressor in ways consistent with our memories of similar situations.

Self-esteem is closely related to the emotions engendered by past experiences. People with low self-esteem are more likely to feel helpless anger, an emotion experienced by people who have not learned to express anger in appropriate ways. People with helpless anger have usually learned that they are wrong to feel anger; therefore, instead of expressing their anger in healthy ways, they turn it inward. They "swallow" their anger in food, alcohol, or other drugs, or act in other self-destructive ways. See the Building Communication Skills box for a series of questions concerning expressing your anger effectively.

Self-esteem significantly affects various disease processes. People with low self-esteem create a self-imposed distressor that can impair the immune system's ability to combat disease. Some researchers believe that chronic distress can depress the immune system and thus increase the symptoms of such diseases as acquired immune deficiency syndrome (AIDS), herpes, multiple sclerosis, and Epstein-Barr syndrome.

## Personality Types and Hardiness

A person's personality may contribute to the kind and degree of self-imposed stress he or she experiences. The coronary-disease-prone personality was first described in 1974 by physicians Friedman and Rosenman in their book *Type A Behavior and Your Heart.*[16] Although their work is now considered controversial, it is the basis for much current research.

Friedman and Rosenman identified two stress-related personality types: Type A and Type B. Type A personalities are hard-driving, competitive, anxious, time-driven, impatient, angry, and perfectionistic. Type B personalities are relaxed and noncompetitive. According to Rosenman and Friedman, people with Type A characteristics are more prone to heart attacks than their Type B counterparts.

Researchers today believe that more needs to be discovered about Type A and Type B personalities before we can say that all Type As will have greater risks for heart disease than Type Bs. First of all, most people are not one personality type or the other all the time. Second, there are many other unexplained variables that must be explored, such as why some Type A personalities seem to thrive in stress-filled environments. Now labelled Type C personalities, these individuals appear to succeed more often than Type B personalities and have good health even while displaying Type A patterns of behaviour.

Critics of the supposed links between these personality types and risk of disease argue that attempts to explain ill health by means of personal behavioural patterns have so far been crude. For example, Ragland and Brand contend that the Type A personality may be more complex than previously described.[17] These researchers identified a "toxic core" in some Type A personalities. People with this toxic core are angry, distrustful of others, and have above-average levels of cynicism. Generally, people who are angry and hostile also have below-average levels of social support and other increased risks for ill health. It may be this toxic core rather than the hard-driving nature of the Type A personality that makes people more prone to self-imposed stress and its consequences.

**Psychological hardiness** has been identified as a characteristic that helps some people cope with the self-imposed stress associated with Type A behaviours.[18] Psychologically hardy people are characterized by control, commitment, challenge, choices, and connectedness. People with a sense of control are able to

# Expressing Anger Effectively

Expressing anger constructively is an important skill involved in learning to cope with intimate relationships, family interactions, and other stressful situations. Here are some suggestions for constructively expressing anger.

1. *Determine the reason behind your anger.* Is it due to a real event (for example, someone you trusted is spreading malicious gossip) or to a perception you have about a situation (friends are avoiding you, so you think someone may be gossiping)?

2. *Don't let your anger build.* When you become angry, take control, and decide what actions you need to take. Try not to act rashly, but don't stew for too long. If you choose to write a letter expressing your anger, sit down and write it, but don't mail the letter immediately. Put it away, wait a few days, and then reread it. Even though you may choose not to send the letter, sitting down to write it will have been beneficial.

3. *If you decide to confront a person, select an appropriate time and place for the meeting.* Try not to attack your target unexpectedly or in the presence of others: the person may become defensive. Give the person a general idea of what you want to discuss ahead of time.

4. *Stick to the main reason for your anger.* Bringing up a whole list of things that have made you angry over the last year will complicate the issue and make the other person want to create his or her own list of wrongs that you have committed. Plan in advance which issue you want to discuss. Be careful of using all inclusive statements such as "You always . . ." or "You never . . . ."

5. *Attack the problem rather than the person.* ("It made me angry that we had to leave early" versus "You made me angry because you made us leave early") Don't get into a battle over personal characteristics. Use "I" statements to communicate resentment or disappointment ("I feel angry that we had to leave the party so early"). "You" statements often put people on the defensive.

6. *Listen carefully to what the other person has to say.* Do not interrupt; give the other person a chance to speak. Listen rather than planning what you are going to say next. If the other person starts wandering from the issue, gently try to bring him or her back to the point. If the other person attacks you personally, stay in control and don't allow yourself to fight back.

7. *Treat the other person with respect.* Even though you may say the right things, your gestures and body language can reveal that you don't value what the other person has to say, that you are hostile, or that you are losing patience. Drumming your fingers, sighing, or rolling your eyes while the other person is talking can often increase friction. Remember, communication is 90 percent non-verbal.

8. *Recognize when to quit.* Sometimes even the best-laid plans go awry. No matter what you do, the problem may appear impossible to resolve. In such situations, knowing when to quit, either temporarily or permanently, is a key factor in controlling stressful anger levels. Agree to disagree. Nobody has to "win" the argument.

9. *When it's over, let it be over.* After you have done all that you can do, let go of your anger. Don't dwell in the past. Acknowledge your right to be angry, recognize it for what it was, and move on.

---

accept responsibility for their behaviours and to make changes in behaviours that they discover to be debilitating. People with a sense of commitment have good self-esteem and understand their purpose in life. These individuals choose to commit themselves to the things that matter to them. People with a sense of challenge see changes or struggles in life as stimulating opportunities for personal growth. Psychologically hardy people also make lifestyle choices that enhance their health and, finally, these individuals are connected to others in meaningful ways. This connectedness provides a level of social support that is health enhancing.

Modification of the Type A personality is possible when particular "learned" behaviours are modified. For example, some Type A people are able to reduce their hurried behaviours and become more tolerant, more patient, and better-humoured. Unfortunately, many people do not decide to modify their Type A habits until after they have become ill or suffered a heart attack or other circulatory system distress. Prevention of heart and circulatory disorders resulting from stress entails recognizing and changing dangerous behaviours before damage is done.

**Background distressors:** Environmental stressors that we may be unaware of.

**Cognitive stress system:** The psychological system that governs our emotional responses to stress.

**Psychological hardiness:** A personality characteristic characterized by control, commitment, challenge, choices, and connectedness.

# Taming Technostress

Cell phones that ring constantly; email lists that grow on your computer desktop like an out-of-control fungus; laptop computers that somehow end up in your luggage when you go on vacation; voice message systems that don't allow you to talk to a live person; and slow, slow, slow downloading of information. Can you feel your heart rate speeding up just thinking about these situations? On campuses across the country, students, faculty, and administrators are using electronic organizers, the Internet, and other forms of technology. Email, the World Wide Web, and personal digital assistants (PDAs) are no longer flashy new tools but are as commonplace as the backpack. Unfortunately, many people feel frustrated and distressed in their struggle to adapt to increasingly complex technology. As many as 85 percent of us have at least some level of discomfort around technology. If you are like millions of people today, you find that technology is often a daily terrorizer that raises your blood pressure, frustrates you, and prevents you from ever really getting away from it all. In short, you may be a victim of stressors that previous generations only dreamed (or had nightmares) about. Known as *technostress*, this problem is defined as "personal stress generated by reliance on technological devices . . . a panicky feeling when they fail, and a state of near-constant stimulation, or being perpetually 'plugged in.'" When technostress grabs you, it may interact with other forms of stress to create a synergistic, never-ending form of stimulation that keeps your stress response reverberating all day.

Part of the problem, ironically, is that technology enables us to be so productive. Because it encourages polyphasic activity, or "multitasking," people are forced to juggle multiple thoughts and actions at the same time, such as driving and talking on cell phones or checking handheld devices for appointments. People who multitask, however, are actually less efficient than those who focus on one project at a time. Moreover, there is clear evidence that multitasking contributes to auto accidents and other harmful consequences, including short-term memory loss. What is less clear is what happens to someone who is always plugged in. What are the symptoms of technology overload? It evokes typical stress responses by increasing heart rate and blood pressure and causing irritability and memory disturbances. Over time, many stressed-out people lose the ability to relax and find that they feel nervous and anxious when they are supposed to be having fun. Headaches, stomach and digestive problems, skin irritations, frequent colds, difficulty in wound healing, lack of sleep, ulcers, and other problems may result. Other red flags include gaps in your attentiveness and changes in your ability to concentrate. One study indicates that chronic stress may even thicken the waistline; increased secretions of cortisol caused even slender women to store added fat in the abdomen. Authors Michelle Weil and Larry Rosen describe *technosis*, a syndrome in which people get so immersed in technology that they risk losing their own identity. If you answer yes to questions such as, "Do you rely on preprogrammed systems to contact others?" and "Do you feel stressed if you haven't checked your email within the last couple of hours?" you may be too dependent on technology.

## TIPS FOR FIGHTING TECHNOSTRESS

- *Enjoy the natural environment.* Get away from any form of technology. Try to find a place that has few people and little noise—that usually means outdoors.
- *Become aware of what you are doing.* Log the time you spend on email, voice mail, etc. Set up a schedule to limit your use of technology. For example, spend no more than a half-hour per day answering emails.
- *Give yourself more time for everything you do.* If you are surfing the Web for resources for a term paper, start early rather than the night before the paper is due.
- *Manage the telephone—don't let it manage you.* Rather than interrupting what you're doing to answer, screen calls with an answering machine or caller ID. Get rid of call waiting, which forces you to juggle multiple calls, and subscribe to a voice mail service that takes messages when you're on the phone.
- *Set "time out" periods when you don't answer the phone, listen to the stereo, use the computer, or watch TV.* Switch off email notification systems so you aren't beeped during these periods.
- *Take regular breaks.* Even when working, get up, walk around, stretch, do deep breathing, or get a glass of water, every hour.
- *If you are working on the computer, look away from the screen and focus on something far away every 30 minutes.* Stretch your shoulders and neck periodically as you work. Play soft background music to help you relax.
- *When working on the computer, focus on one task at a time.* If you are working on a paper, close your email and instant messaging so that you can focus on your paper and not feel pressured to respond because "you've got mail" or someone has logged on to instant messaging.
- *Resist the urge to buy the newest and fastest technology.* Such purchases not only cause financial stress, but also add to stress levels with the typical glitches that occur when installing and adjusting to new technology.
- *Do not take laptops, hand-held devices, or other technological gadgets on vacation.* If you must take a cell phone for emergencies, turn it and your voice messaging system off, and use the phone only in true emergencies.

## Self-Efficacy and Control

Whether people are able to cope successfully with stressful situations often depends on their level of self-efficacy, or belief in their skills and performance abilities.[19] If people have been successful in mastering similar problems in the past, they are more likely to believe in their own effectiveness in future situations. Similarly, people who have repeatedly tried and failed may lack confidence in their abilities to deal with life's problems. In some cases, this insecurity may prevent them from trying to cope.

In addition, people who believe they lack control in a situation may become easily frustrated and give up. Those who feel they have little to no personal control over their life and what happens to them tend to have an external locus of control and a low level of self-efficacy. People who are confident their behaviours will influence the ultimate outcome of life's events tend to have an internal locus of control. People who feel that they have limited control over their lives tend to have higher levels of stress.

# STRESS AND THE POST-SECONDARY STUDENT

Stress related to university or college life is not caused only by pressure to excel academically. Post-secondary students experience numerous distressors, including changes related to being away from home for the first time, climatic differences between home and school, pressure to make friends in a new and sometimes intimidating setting, the feeling of anonymity imposed by larger classes, test-taking anxiety, and pressures related to time management.

Some students are stressed by athletic team requirements, on-campus food selection, roommates' habits, peers' expectations, new questions about personal values and beliefs, relationship problems, fraternity or sorority demands, financial worries, changed sleeping habits (including reduced sleep), or the need to be technologically savvy. For older students, worries about competing with 18-year-olds may also be distressful in addition to the pressure of determining their future career path. Technological advancements have created new pressures for students to be engaged in computer and computer-related tasks for longer time periods, which may cause mental as well as physical duress (that is, anxiety about not finding required information, sifting through the abundance of materials discovered to find credible information, and repetitive strain injuries related to overuse and poor body mechanics). Most colleges offer stress management workshops through their health centres or student counselling departments.

You should not ignore the following symptoms of stress overload. If you experience one or more of these symptoms, act promptly to reduce their impact:

- difficulty keeping up with classes or difficulty concentrating on and finishing tasks

- frequent clashes with close friends, family, or intimate partners about trivial issues such as housekeeping

- frequent mood changes or overreaction to minor problems

- lethargy caused by lack of sleep or excessive frustration

- lack of interest in social activities or tendency to avoid others

- avoidance of stressors through use of drugs or alcohol or through other extreme behaviours

- sleep disturbances, TV addiction, free-floating anxiety, or an exaggerated sense of self

- difficulty in maintaining an intimate relationship

- lack of interest in sexual relationships or inability to participate in satisfactory sexual relationships

- tendency to be intolerant of minor differences of opinion

- hunger and cravings or tendency to overeat or to eat while thinking of other things

- lack of awareness of sensory cues
- inability to listen or tendency to jump from subject to subject in conversation
- stuttering or other speech difficulties
- accident-proneness

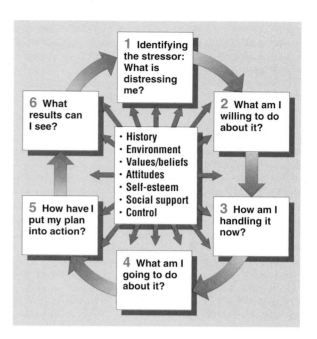

FIGURE 3.4

**A Decision-Making Model for Stress Management**

Source: Adapted from Lester A. Lefton, *Psychology,* 5th ed., 485 (Figure 13.5). © 1994 by Allyn & Bacon. Reprinted by permission.

# STRESS MANAGEMENT

Stress can be challenging or defeating depending upon how we learn to view it. The most effective way to avoid defeat is to learn a number of skills known collectively as stress management. Stress management consists primarily of finding balance in our lives. We balance rest, relaxation, physical activity, dietary intake, work, school, family, finances, and social activities. As we balance our lives, we make the choice to react constructively to our stressors. Robert Eliot, a cardiologist and stress researcher, offers two rules for people trying to cope with life's challenges: (1) "Don't sweat the small stuff," and (2) remember that "it's all small stuff."[20]

## Dealing with Stress

The first step of stress management is to examine thoroughly any problem involving stress. Figure 3.4 shows a decision-making model for managing your response to stress. As the model shows, dealing with stress involves assessing all aspects of a stressor, examining how you currently respond to the stressor and how you may be able to change your response, and evaluating various methods of coping with stress. Some stressors we cannot change, such as professors' assignments or unexpected distressors like car accidents or storm damage. Inevitably, we will take classes that bore us and for which we find no application to real life. We feel powerless when a loved one has died. The facts themselves cannot be changed; only our reactions or responses to these situations can be changed.

## Assessing Your Stressors

After recognizing a stressor, you need to assess it. Can you alter the circumstances in any way to reduce the amount of distress you are experiencing, or must you change your behaviours and reactions to the stressor to reduce your stress levels? For example, if five term papers for five different courses are due during the semester, you will probably quickly assess that you cannot alter the circumstances: your professors are unlikely to change their requirements. You can, however, alter your behaviours by working on one or two of the papers well before the due dates and spacing the others over time to avoid last-minute stress from trying to write them all in the week before they are due. Another example is if your boss is vague about directions for assignments; you cannot change the boss. You can, however, ask the boss to clarify what is expected of you—in writing, if an oral response is insufficient.

## Recognizing and Changing Your Responses

Recognizing and changing your responses to stressors requires self-reflection, practice, and emotional control. It is important to recognize your typical physical and mental responses to stress so that you can manage these responses more effectively in future situations. If your roommate is habitually messy and this causes you stress, you can choose from several responses. For example, you can express your anger by yelling, you can pick up the mess and leave a nasty note, or you can defuse the situation with humour. The first response that comes to mind is not always the best response. Stop before you react, to gain the time you need to find an appropriate response. Ask yourself, "What is to be gained from my response?" or "How will my response mediate this type of behaviour in the future?" Many people change their responses to potentially stressful events through cognitive coping strategies. These strategies help them prepare for stressors through gradual exposure to increasingly higher stress levels.

## Learning to Cope

Everyone copes with stress and their stress responses in different ways. For some people, drinking and taking drugs helps them to cope. Others choose to get help from counsellors. Still others try to get their minds off stress by engaging in physical activity or relaxation techniques. *Stress inoculation,* a newer technique, helps people prepare for stressful events ahead of time. For example, if you are petrified about speaking in front of your class, practising in front of a friend or a mirror may inoculate you and prevent you from freezing up on the day of your presentation. Some health experts compare stress inoculation to a vaccine. Stress inoculation:

- increases the predictability of stressful events
- fosters coping skills
- generates self-talking
- encourages confidence about successful outcomes
- builds a commitment to personal action and responsibility for an adaptive course of action

Regardless of how you cope with a given situation, your conscious effort to deal with it is an important step in stress management.

## Downshifting

Today's lifestyles are hectic and pressure-packed, with self-imposed stress often a result of trying to keep up. Many people are wondering if "having it all" is worth it, and as a result are taking a step back and simplifying their lives. This simplification is known as downshifting. Moving from a big city to a small town or moving from a big house to a smaller home and a host of other changes typify downshifting. Some dedicated downshifters have given up television, phones, and even computers.

Downshifting involves a fundamental alteration in values and honest introspection about what is important in life. When you consider any form of downshift or perhaps even start your career this way, it's important to move slowly and consider the following:

- *Determine your ultimate goal.* What is most important to you, and what will you need to reach that goal? What can you do without? Where do you want to live? Where do you want to work?

- *Make a short- and long-term plan for simplifying your life.* Set up your plan in doable steps, and work slowly toward each step. Begin saying no to requests for your time and determine those people and organizations to whom it is important to give your time.

- *Complete a financial inventory.* How much money will you need to do the things you want to do? Will you live alone or share costs with roommates? Do you need a car, or can you rely on active methods or public transportation? Pay off credit cards and eliminate existing debt, or consider debt consolidation. Get used to paying with cash. If you don't have the cash, don't buy. Remember, your lifestyle may be different as a student compared to when you were working or living at home.

- *Select the right career.* Look for work that you enjoy and isn't necessarily driven by salary. Can you be happy in a lower-paying job that perhaps is less stressful but still provides you with sufficient challenge and the opportunities you consider important?

- *Consider options for saving money.* Downshifting doesn't mean you renounce money; it means you choose not to let money dictate your life. It's still important to save. If you are just getting started, you need to prepare for emergencies and future plans.

- *Clear out/clean out.* A cluttered life can be distressing. Take an inventory of material items, and get rid of things you haven't worn or used the last year or so. Donate these items to appropriate charities.

# Managing Emotional Responses

Have you ever gotten all worked up about something you thought was happening only to find that your perceptions were totally wrong or that a communication problem resulted in a misinterpretation of events? This happens to most of us. We often get upset by our faulty perceptions rather than reality. For example, imagine you find out that your friends were invited to a party but you were not. You are likely to become angry as well as disappointed. Self-doubt will likely follow, and you will wonder if nobody likes you. Yet the reality may be that you were invited, but your invitation got lost or misplaced.

Stress management requires that you examine your emotional responses, including your self talk and explanatory style. With any emotional response to a distressor, you are responsible for your emotions and resulting behaviours. Learning to tell the difference between normal emotions and those based on irrational beliefs can help you to express them in a healthy and more appropriate way. Admitting your feelings and allowing them to be expressed either through communication or action is a stress management technique that can help you get through many difficult situations. Talking yourself through the situation—in a positive way—and explaining yourself to others, accepting responsibility when appropriate, and avoiding blaming others for your mistakes or setbacks are also part of managing your emotional responses and behaviours.

## Learning to Laugh and Cry

For some people, learning to express emotions freely is a difficult task. However, it is a task worth learning. Have you ever noticed that you feel better after a good laugh or cry? It wasn't your imagination. Laughter and crying stimulate the heart and temporarily rev up many body systems. Heart rate and blood pressure then decrease significantly, allowing the body to relax.

## Managing Social Interactions

The importance of your social interactions should not be underestimated in your stress management plans. Consider the nature and extent of your friendships. Do you have someone with whom you can share intimate thoughts and feelings? Is there someone you can call for help or in the case of an emergency? Do you trust your friends to be supportive? to be honest if you are doing something risky or inappropriate? Having someone to listen to you when needed and to give helpful advice is an invaluable stress management tool. It is less important to have a wide circle of acquaintances than it is to have a few really good friends. Different friends often serve different needs, so having more than one friend is usually beneficial. In university and college, friends often fulfill roles that family members did. As you continue to develop and cultivate friendships, look for individuals who:

- have values and interests that are similar to your own (as well as those with different interests that force you to grow and explore new ideas).
- are good listeners, give and share freely, are tolerant, and do not rush to judgment.

- are trustworthy and have your best interests at heart.
- are not unusually critical, negative, selfish, or only bring you down. Avoid people who enjoy "stirring things up" and always seem to be in some crisis themselves; they often precipitate rather than reduce stress responses.
- are responsible and value doing well in school but also know when and how to have fun.
- are willing to be physical-activity buddies or study partners with a mutual interest in a healthy lifestyle.
- know how to laugh, cry, engage in meaningful conversation, and feel comfortable with silence.

Just as it is important to find these characteristics in your friends, it is also important for you to bring these qualities to your friendships. Sometimes, focusing on others can help you get your problems into perspective and control.

## Making the Most of Support Groups

Support groups are an important part of stress management. Friends, family members, and co-workers can provide us with emotional and physical support. Although the ideal support group differs for each of us, you should have one or two close friends in whom you are able to confide and neighbours with whom you can trade favours. You should also take the opportunity to participate in community activities at least once a week. A healthy, committed relationship can also provide vital support.

If you do not have a close support group, you should know where to turn when the pressures of life seem overwhelming. Family members are often a steady base of support on which you can rely. Most colleges and universities have counselling services available at no cost for short-term crises. Clergy members, instructors, and residence supervisors may also be supportive resources. If university or college services are not available or if you are concerned about confidentiality, remember that most communities offer low-cost counselling through mental health clinics.

## Taking Mental Action

Stress management calls for mental action in two areas. First, positive self-esteem, which can help you cope with stressful situations, comes from learned habits. Successful stress management involves mentally developing and practising self-esteem skills. Second, because you can't always anticipate what the next distressor will be, you need to develop the mental skills necessary to manage your reactions to stresses after they have occurred. The ability to think about and react quickly to stress comes with time, practice, experience with a variety of stressful situations, and patience. Most of all, you must strive to become more aware of situations that may potentially induce stress and act quickly to deal with them. Rather than seeing stressors as adversaries, learn to view them as exercises in life.

### Changing the Way You Think

Once you realize that some of your thoughts or self-talk may be negative, irrational, or overreactive, making a conscious effort to reframe or change the way you've been thinking and focusing on more positive ways of thinking is a key element of stress management. Here are some specific actions you can take to develop these mental skills.

- *Worry constructively.* Don't waste time and energy worrying about things you can't change or things that may never happen.
- *Look at life as being fluid.* Accept change as a natural part of living and growing rather than resisting it.
- *Consider alternatives.* Remember that there is seldom only one appropriate action. Anticipating options will help you plan for change and adjust more rapidly.
- *Have moderate expectations.* Aim high, but be realistic about your circumstances and capabilities.
- *Weed out trivia.* Don't sweat the small stuff, and remember that most of it is small stuff.
- *Don't rush into action.* Think before you act.
- *Keep things in perspective.* Try not to exaggerate the importance of what has happened.
- *Focus on the positive.* Become selectively aware of the positive aspect of negative or unplanned situations. For example, if you get caught up in traffic, plan your day ahead. Or if your partner ends your relationship, think about the extra time you will have to yourself or for your friends and family.
- *See stumbling blocks as challenges rather than barriers.* Expect challenges and difficulties rather than resisting them.
- *When you think "I can't do it," break the task into smaller pieces and work on one small part at a time.* For example, if you have a paper and a laboratory report due on the same day, break each down into logical pieces and work on one piece at a time.
- *Reframe.* Rather than seeing the situation as a stumbling block, see it as a challenge and an opportunity. For example, if your date is no longer available to go out, see the unexpected evening alone as an opportunity to unwind and indulge in a bath rather than getting angry or frustrated.

## Taking Physical Action

Adopting the attitudes and behaviours necessary for effective stress management can be a satisfying accomplishment that assists in building confidence and self-esteem. Learning to use physical activity to alleviate and manage stress will complement the emotional strategies you employ in stress management.

### Physical Activity

Moderate- and vigorous-intensity physical activities play a role in stress management by increasing the levels of endorphins (mood-enhancing, pain-killing hormones) in the bloodstream. Engaging in physical activity also increases energy, reduces hostility, and improves mental alertness. Most of us have relieved stress by engaging in vigorous physical activity: joining a kick-boxing class is one example. Physical activity or exercise performed as an immediate response can help alleviate stress symptoms. However, engaging in physical activity regularly yields even more substantial benefits. Try to engage in at least 20 to 30 minutes of aerobic exercise three or four times a week. A quiet walk can also refresh your mind, calm your stress response, and replenish your adaptation energy stores. Plan walking breaks alone or with friends. In fact, walking and talking is often an effective way to manage stress. Stretch after prolonged periods of study at your desk. A short period of physical activity may provide the break you really need. For more information about physical activity, see Chapter 9.

### Relaxation

Like physical activity, relaxation can help you to cope with stressful feelings, preserve adaptation energy stores, and dissipate the excess hormones associated with the GAS. Relaxation also helps you to refocus your energies and should be practised daily until it becomes a habit. You may find that you even actually enjoy it. When you begin to feel your body respond to distress, make time to relax to give yourself added strength and to alleviate the negative physical effects of stress. As your body relaxes, your heart rate lowers, your blood pressure and metabolic rate decrease, and many other body-calming effects occur, allowing you to channel energy more effectively. See also the Your Spiritual and Emotional Health box.

# Relaxation Techniques for Stress Management

You probably experience stressful situations every day—at school, at work, at home. Stress results from a combination of many factors often beyond our control. While stress cannot be eliminated completely, you can learn how to manage your responses in a positive way. Take steps to manage your response to stressful situations by using the following simple techniques:

1. **Diaphragmatic or deep breathing:** Typically, we breathe only using the upper chest and thoracic region rather than involving the abdominal region. Diaphragmatic breathing is deep breathing that maximally expands the chest by involving the movement of the lower abdomen. This technique is commonly used in yoga exercises. The diaphragmatic breathing process occurs in three stages:
   - *Stage 1:* Assume a comfortable position. Whether sitting or lying down on your back, find the most natural position to be in. Close your eyes, unbutton your shirt or binding clothes, remove your belt, or unbutton your pants. Often it works best to fold your hands over your abdomen and get used to feeling the rise and fall of your stomach.
   - *Stage 2:* Concentrate on the act of breathing. Shut out external noise. Focus on inhaling, exhaling, and the route the air is following. Try saying to yourself, "Feel the warm air coming into your nose, warming your windpipe, and flowing into your lungs. Feel your stomach rise and fall as you inhale slowly and exhale slowly, noting the air flowing out of your nose or mouth." Repeat this action several times.
   - *Stage 3:* Visualize. The above stages seem to work best when combined with visualization. A common example is to visualize clean, fresh, invigorating air slowly entering the nose

and being exhaled as grey, stale air that has accumulated in the body. Such processes, particularly when they involve the whole body, seem to help individuals become refreshed from their experience.

2. **Progressive muscle relaxation:** Progressive muscle relaxation involves systematically contracting and relaxing each of several muscle groups; breathing deeply and concentrating on the muscles being contracted and relaxed are part of this process. Again, find a comfortable position and begin a deep breathing cycle. The difference from diaphragmatic breathing is that, as you concentrate on inhaling, you will also contract a particular muscle group (for example, the hand and fingers). Hold that position for a short period and then, as you exhale, slowly release the muscles that you have been contracting. Repeat and add more muscle groups. You might start with the hands, then move to the forearms, the entire arms, the neck, then move to the shoulders, back, buttocks, thighs, lower legs, and finish with the feet. You can add components of other relaxation techniques to this experience by saying, "My hands are getting warmer, my arm is getting warmer," and so on as you work to gain maximum control of blood flow and muscle tension in a region.

Source: Paragraph on qigong from C. Dold, "The New Yoga," *Health* (May 2004): 73–77.

## Eating Well

Is food a destressor? Do Mom's chocolate chip cookies or Grandma's apple pie really make you feel better? Whether foods can calm us and nourish our psyches is a controversial question. Much of what has been published about hyperactivity and its relation to the consumption of sweets has been shown to be scientifically invalid. High-potency stress-tabs that are supposed to provide you with resistance against stress-related ailments are nothing more than gimmicks. However, what is clear is that having a balanced, healthy dietary intake will provide you with the stamina needed to get through problems and may stress-proof you in ways that are not fully understood. It is also known that undereating, overeating, emotional eating, and an unhealthy dietary intake can create distress in the body. For more information about the benefits of sound nutrition in overall health and wellness, see Chapter 7.

## Learning Time Management

Time—everybody needs more of it, especially students trying to balance the demands of classes, social life, part-time jobs, family obligations, and time needed for relaxation and physical activity. The following tips regarding time management should become a part of your stress management program:

- *Clean off your desk.* According to Jeffrey Mayer, author of *Winning the Fight Between You and Your Desk,* most of us lose time looking for things that are lost on our desks or in our homes. Go through the things on your desk, recycle the unnecessary papers, and organize the remaining papers in "to do" piles.

- *Never handle papers more than once.* When bills and other papers come in, take care of them immediately. Write out a cheque and hold it for mailing. Get rid of the envelopes. Read your mail and file it or toss it. If you haven't looked at something in over a year, recycle it.

- *Prioritize your tasks.* Make a daily "to do" list and try to stick to it. Categorize the things you must do today, the things that you have to do but not immediately, and the things that it would be nice to do. Prioritize the Must Do Now and Have to Do Later items and put deadlines next to each. Only consider the Nice to Do items if you finish the others or if the Nice to Do list includes something fun for you. Give yourself a reward as you finish each task.

- *Avoid interruptions.* When you've got a project that requires your total concentration, schedule uninterrupted time. Unplug the phone or let your answering machine get it. Turn off the instant messaging and email software on your computer. Close your door and post a Do Not Disturb sign. Go to a quiet room in the library or student union where no one will find you. Protect your time.

- *Don't be afraid to say no.* Too often, we overcommit ourselves. It is okay to say "No, I am too busy," "No, I am not really interested," or "I would like to help out, however, I am already committed to too many projects at this time."

- *Reward yourself for being efficient.* If you've planned to take a certain amount of time to finish a task and you finish early, take some time for yourself. Have a cup of coffee or hot chocolate. Go for a walk. Read for pleasure. Differentiate between rest breaks and work breaks. Work breaks simply mean that you switch tasks for a while. Rest breaks get you away from work and let you spend time for yourself.

- *Use time to your advantage.* If you are a morning person, plan your work to take advantage of that time. If you know that by Friday afternoon you will be tired and worn out, plan to work on tasks that require minimal concentration. Take breaks when needed. Use physical activity as an energizer.

- *Become aware of your own time patterns.* For many of us, minutes and hours drift by without us even noticing them. Chart your daily schedule, hour by hour, for one week. Note the time that was wasted and the time spent in productive work or restorative pleasure. Assess how you could be more productive and make more time for yourself.

- *Remember that time is precious.* Many people learn to value their time only when they face a terminal illness. Try to value each day. Time spent not enjoying life is a tremendous waste of potential.

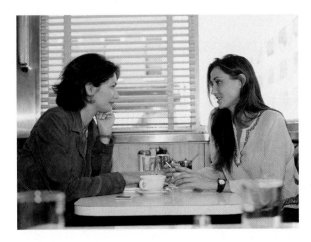

*Being able to talk comfortably to someone close to you is part of stress management.*

## Using Alternative Stress Management Techniques

The popularity of stress management as a media topic has increased the amount of advertising for various "stress fighters" such as hypnosis, massage therapies, and meditation. Some universities may provide these services through extended health coverage.

### Hypnosis

**Hypnosis** is a process that requires a person to focus on one thought, object, or voice, thereby freeing the right hemisphere to become more active. The person is then unusually responsive to suggestions. Whether self-induced or induced by another person, hypnosis can reduce certain types of stress.

### Massage

If you have ever had someone massage your stiff neck or aching feet, you know that massage is an excellent means of relaxation and a form of stress management. Massage therapists use techniques that vary from the aggressive methods typical of Swedish massage to more gentle methods such as acupressure and Esalen massage. Before selecting a massage therapist, check his or her credentials carefully. He or she should have training from a reputable program that teaches scientific principles for anatomical manipulation. Each province and territory has different requirements to become a registered massage therapist—check out the Canadian Massage Therapy Alliance website at www.cmta.ca for specific information.

**Hypnosis:** A process that allows people to become unusually responsive to suggestion.

# Managing Stress Behaviours

Stress is not something that you can run from or wish into nonexistence. To control stress, you must meet it head-on and use as many resources as you can to ensure that your coping skills are fine-tuned and ready to help you. In planning your personal strategy for stress success, you should consider the following:

## MAKING DECISIONS FOR YOU

Following a few simple guidelines may help you not only to enjoy more guilt-free time but also to become more productive during work hours.

- *Plan life, not time.* Determining what you want from life rather than what you can get done may help change the way you use time. Evaluate all your activities, even the most trivial, to determine whether they add to your life. If they don't, get rid of them.

- *Decelerate.* Rushing is part of the Canadian work ethic and mindset that says "Busy is better." It can be addictive. When rushed, ask yourself if you really need to be. What's the worst that could happen if you slow down? Tell yourself at least once a day that failure seldom results from doing a job slowly or too well. Failures happen when rushing causes a lack of attention to detail.

- *Learn to delegate and share.* The need to feel in control is powerful. If you are unusually busy, leave details to someone else. Don't be afraid to ask others to help or to share the workload and responsibilities.

- *Learn to say no.* Give priority to what is most critical to your life, your job, or your current situation. Decide what things you can do, what things you must do, and what things you want to do, and delegate the rest to someone else either permanently or until you complete some of your priority tasks. Before you take on a new responsibility, finish or drop an old one.

- *Schedule time alone.* Find time each day for quiet thinking, reading, physical activity, or other enjoyable activities.

## CHECKLIST FOR CHANGE: ASSESSING YOUR LIFE STRESSORS

- Have you assessed the major stressors in your life? Are they people, events, or specific activities?

- Have you thought about what you may be doing to elevate your stress levels? Do you often worry about things that never happen?

- Have you thought about what you could change to reduce your stress response?

- Do you have a network of friends and family members who can help you reduce your stress levels? Do you know how and where to access professional advice if needed?

- Have you thought about what changes you'd like to work on first? Have you developed a plan of action? When do you want to start?

## CHECKLIST FOR CHANGE: ASSESSING COMMUNITY STRESSORS

- Have you considered what in your environment may be perceived as stressful for you and those around you?

- Do you have control over these stressors? How could they be changed? How would changing them make a difference?

- What on your campus or in your living situation is perceived as stressful for you or your friends? What could you do to manage these stressors?

- What advice might you give to your school administrators to help them reduce unnecessary stress among students?

## CRITICAL THINKING

You just scraped by to pay your tuition bill in January, then your university announced a large tuition hike for next year. You already work a part-time job, and seem to spend all your "free time" studying. The stress you've got now is beginning to get to you, and you realize that you will have to work another five to ten hours per week just to pay your bills next year. And tuition is likely to go up in your final year as well. How can you manage your time and finances so you can complete your degree?

Use the DECIDE model described in Chapter 1 to decide what you should do. Begin with your current situation: How can you make better use of your time? Could you prioritize your week in such a way that you could find the extra time to work? Finally, even if you make enough money, you need to deal with the increased stress. What will you do to keep the stress in check?

## Meditation

Another way to relax and to manage stress is through meditation. **Meditation** generally focuses on visualization and deep breathing, allowing tension to leave the body with each exhalation. There is no "right" way to meditate. Although there are several common forms of meditation, most involve sitting quietly for 15 to 20 minutes, focusing on a particular word or symbol, controlling breathing, and getting in touch with your inner self.

**Meditation:** A relaxation technique that involves deep breathing and concentration.

# SUMMARY

- Stress is an inevitable part of our lives. Eustress refers to stress associated with positive events, distress to negative events. Psychoneuroimmunology is the science that attempts to analyze the relationship between the mind's reaction to stress and the function of the immune system. Currently, most evidence links disease susceptibility to stress.

- The alarm, resistance, and exhaustion phases of the general adaptation syndrome involve physiological responses to real and imagined stressors.

- Multiple factors contribute to stress and to the stress response. Psychosocial factors include change, pressure, inconsistent goals and behaviours, conflict, overload, and burnout. Other factors are environmental stressors, and self-imposed stress.

- University or college can be an especially stressful time. Recognizing the signs of stress is the first step in helping yourself to manage your stress.

- Managing stress begins with learning simple coping mechanisms: assessing your stressors, identifying your stress responses, changing these responses, and learning to cope. Finding out what works best for you—probably some combination of managing emotional responses, taking mental or physical action, learning time management, or using alternative stress management techniques—will help you cope better with stress in the long run.

# DISCUSSION QUESTIONS

1. Compare and contrast distress and eustress. Are both types of stress harmful?

2. Describe the alarm, resistance, and exhaustion phases of the general adaptation syndrome. During which of these phases do your perceptions and feelings about a situation often turn out to be wrong? Discuss the physiological and psychological responses that take place if you find you were wrong.

3. What are the major factors that seem to influence the nature and extent of a person's stress susceptibility? Explain how social support, self-esteem, and personality may make you more or less susceptible to stress.

4. Why are university and college students often susceptible to overload and burnout? What services are available on your campus to help you deal with excessive stress?

5. What can university and college students do to inoculate themselves or build resilience against negative stress effects? What actions can you take to manage your stressors? How can you help others to manage their stressors more effectively?

# APPLICATION EXERCISE

Reread the What Do You Think? scenario at the beginning of the chapter and answer the following questions:

1. Is it common for first-year students like Rhett to experience stress? Why or why not?

2. What should Rhett do to manage the stress he experiences as a result of his arts courses? Is there help available on your campus if you had a similar problem? Do you know how to access these services?

3. Are Rhett's experiences with residence life common? What suggestions could you make to him so that he enjoys this part of campus life and still does well academically?

4. Is it important for Rhett to know precisely what career he is headed for? Why or why not?

# HEALTH ON THE NET

Canadian Institute for Health Information
**www.cihi.ca**

Canadian Medical Association
**www.cma.ca**

Canadian Network for Mood and Anxiety Treatments
**www.canmat.org/**

Internet Mental Health
**www.mentalhealth.com/**

University of Alberta Health Centre—Students & Stress
**www.ualberta.ca/dept/health/public_html/healthinfo/stress.htm**

# CHAPTER 4

# PERSONAL SAFETY

*Reducing Violence,
Abuse, and Injury*

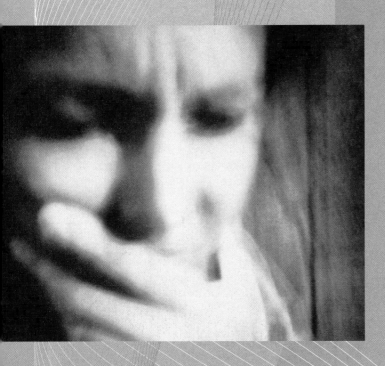

## CHAPTER OBJECTIVES

- Examine violence in Canada, including homicide, suicide, youth violence, and hate and bias crimes.

- Summarize domestic violence (abuse against women, children, men, and the elderly committed by their family members) and its causes.

- Describe sexual victimization, including sexual assault, rape, date rape, and sexual harassment, and explain why it happens.

- Identify the steps you can take to prevent personal assaults at home, on the street, or in your car.

- Examine the impact of personal injury on Canadians, and consider how to reduce the incidence of such injuries.

Freddy is wakened by the sound of loud voices. His parents are fighting again. His father is calling his mother awful names. She is shouting back. Freddy creeps to the top of the stairs. They are just below him. He hears a sickening "whack" as his father hits his mother. Then his father kicks her. There is a knock at the door. The police have been called by the neighbours. They take his father away and talk to his mother. Freddy goes back to his room, but he cannot sleep.

■ What factors in Canadian society have contributed to our growing awareness of violence in the family? What attitudes and beliefs do you encounter as you reflect on family violence? Do you feel violence in the home is increasing? Or is this a problem that has been going on for a long time?

Chances are that if you flip on the TV, you will see graphic images of violent acts and their outcomes. We live in a world caught in an epidemic of violence. The term **violence** is used to indicate a set of behaviours that produce physical, social, or emotional injuries, as well as the outcomes of these behaviours (the injuries themselves). In this chapter, we focus on those violent acts that may have particular relevance to you.

# VIOLENCE IN CANADA

Violence is a worldwide problem. Each year, more than 1.6 million people across the world lose their lives to violence.[1] Worldwide, violence is among the leading causes of death for individuals between the ages of 15 and 44 years, accounting for 14 percent of male and 7 percent of female deaths. Further, for every person who dies as a result of violence many more are injured, resulting in myriad physical, sexual, social, spiritual, and mental health problems. Violent incidents may not be as common in Canada as in some other countries, but we have had riots after sporting events and the occasional political confrontation: the 2000 melee at the Ontario provincial legislature and the 1995 standoff at Gustafson Lake in British Columbia are notable examples. We have also had police strikes with no change in the crime rate, and most cities are relatively safe to work, play, and live in. Canadians are less likely to take precautions against crime when going out than are people in other industrialized countries.[2] Yet violence exists here, in overt forms such as assault or homicide and in more subtle but nonetheless intimidating forms such as stalking. Violence can flare up between groups—as it did at Oka in 1990, between First Nations peoples and the town of Oka over disputed land—or in families, as in child, spousal, and elder abuse. In fact, the most violent group in society is the family.

The 1987 General Social Survey estimated that only 31 percent of violent crimes were reported to police. Why do victims not report violence? Stated reasons were that they felt the incident was minor, believed the police could do nothing about it, were fearful, or had dealt with it informally.[3] Although there was little change between 1988 and 1996 in the percentage of people who reported being a victim of crime, 75 percent of Canadians in 1997 reported that they thought crime had increased.[4]

In a 1995 report, the Department of Justice noted that Canada has a long history of violence toward racial or ethnic minorities. In Vancouver in 1907 a mob of whites attacked the Chinese and Japanese communities, resulting in several fatalities and damage to stores.[5] The internment of Japanese Canadians during World War II and the confiscation of their property is another example.[6] The federal government gave compensation and an apology to the Japanese-Canadian community many years later.

Vulnerable groups such as women, children, and the elderly witnessing or experiencing violence in families is of special concern. The issue of violence by men toward women and children and by adult children toward their parents is now recognized as a major social problem in Canadian society. The opening of sexual assault centres and battered women's shelters in the 1970s made this type of violence more visible for the public.

Violence relates to health through injuries and deaths that result directly from various acts of violence, as well as the subtler forms of damage caused by actual or threatened violence, such as stress, poor mental health, conduct disorders, and lack of social and emotional responsiveness. In addition to these social and emotional costs, the economic costs are very high.[7]

Although the underlying causes of violence and abuse are as varied as the individual crimes and people involved, several social, cultural, and individual factors seem to increase the likelihood. Poverty, unemployment, hopelessness, lack of education, inadequate housing, poor parental role models, cultural beliefs that objectify women and allow men to act as aggressors, lack of social support systems, discrimination, ignorance about people who are different, religious self-righteousness, breakdowns in the criminal justice system, stress, economic uncertainty, and a host of other factors may precipitate violent acts.

By learning more about the etiology of homicide, suicide, and other violent acts, you will reduce your risk of becoming a victim or perpetrator and ensure your own level of health. By taking steps to help prevent violence against others, you will safeguard the health of society.

## WHAT WOULD YOU DO?

Why do you think there is so much violent behaviour in Canada? Has violence increased or decreased in the last 10 years? Why? What actions can you take to prevent violent events from occurring? What actions could be taken on your campus? In your community?

## Homicide

There were 622 **homicides** in Canada in 2004 (73 more than in 2003), a rate of 1.95 per 100,000 people.[8] The territories have the highest rates (Yukon Territory 22.43; Nunavut 13.49; and Northwest Territories 9.34) and the Atlantic provinces the lowest rates (Prince Edward Island 0.00; Newfoundland and Labrador 0.39; New Brunswick 0.93; and Nova Scotia 1.39). Stabbing occurs most frequently (205), followed by shooting (172), beating (136), strangulation (63), fire (13), and other/not known methods (33).[9] Most victims were males (424 vs. 198), with the greatest number (103) between the ages of 18 and 24 years.[10] Similarly, a higher number of males were accused of homicide (508 vs. 58), with the highest number between the ages of 18 and 24 years (186) followed by 30 to 39 years (101). Forty youths (12–17 years), 37 male and 3 female, were accused of homicide in 2004.[11]

Despite popular fears of the violent stranger, a homicide is likely to be committed by someone known to the victim (47 percent by an acquaintance, 36 percent by a spouse).

A comparison of Western countries found that 48 percent of U.S. households owned at least one firearm. In Canada, individuals owning firearms must register them. Currently, there are about 2 million valid firearms licences issued to individuals under the Firearms Act; 1.2 million are possession only licences, 766,000 are possession and acquisition licences, and 5,570 are minor licences.[12] More than 7.1 million firearms are currently registered, with 6.89 million registered to individuals, 194,000 to businesses, and 44,500 to public agencies or museums.

## Suicide

When anger, rage, and hopelessness turn inward rather than outward, violence against the self can result. Suicide is the most extreme form of this violence. Suicide attempts may result from different causes. A suicide attempt can be "a cry for help," a signal of extreme distress and emotional pain. The physical pain of self-injury distracts the person from their never-ending emotional pain. A suicide attempt may be an explosive outburst of rage at the self; such attempts are usually fatal. Or, the suicide may be motivated by a balance of sadness, resignation, and a desire for dignity, in the case of a terminally ill person. Why some people choose suicide is unclear. Studies indicate that a combination of neurobiological,[13] psychological,[14] and social[15] factors combine to enable suicide (see Chapter 2).

What is the extent of this behaviour? According to the World Health Organization, an estimated 815,000 people killed themselves in 2000—a rate equivalent to 14.5 per 100,000 people, or roughly one suicide every 40 seconds.[16] The most recent Statistics Canada data indicate there were 3,681 suicides in Canada in 1997, equivalent to 12.3 per 100,000 people.[17] Men, on average, are more likely than women to commit suicide.[18] Specifically, men between the ages of 45 and 64 have the highest rate (25.5 per 100,000), followed closely by men between the ages of 25 and 44 (25.0 per 100,000) and men aged 20 to 24 (24.9 per 100,000). Women between ages 45 and 64 have the highest rate for females, at 7.6 per 100,000.

Suicides account for 80 percent of all firearm deaths in Canada, with the proportion of suicides involving firearms declining over the last two decades. Fewer than a quarter of the 4,000 suicides in 1995 involved a firearm, usually a rifle or shotgun. While suicides are more frequent in urban areas, the percentage involving a firearm is higher in rural areas.[19]

Those who attempt suicide are a very mixed group and may differ markedly from those who complete suicide. Most people who attempt suicide do not ultimately die from their attempt(s), though they may try frequently, and many people who die from suicide have not attempted previously.[20] We need to understand suicide more completely to respond more appropriately.

The suicide rate among Aboriginal youth is reported to be two to seven times greater than that of the population as a whole.[21] The Canadian Institute of Child Health[22] interprets these statistics as a warning that these youth need more support, recognition, respect, and hope for the future, and that society as a whole must rethink the way we work with and serve them.

**Violence:** Refers to a set of behaviours that produce injuries, as well as the outcomes of these behaviours (the injuries themselves).

**Homicide:** Death that results from intent to injure or kill.

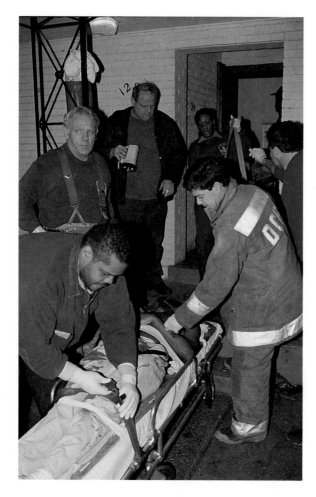

*Violence in the form of fatal stabbings, domestic beatings, and abuse of the elderly is a major cause of death and disability in Canada, and a source of fear and anxiety.*

## Youth Violence

According to the World Health Organization, violence is among the leading causes of death for people aged 15 to 44, accounting for 14 percent of all male deaths and 7 percent of all female deaths.[23] As noted previously, 103 of the 424 male homicides in Canada occurred in those between the ages of 18 and 24. Thirteen homicides occurred in males between the ages of 12 and 17. In females, 23 of the 198 homicides occurred in women between the ages of 18 and 24, and another 5 homicides in those between the ages of 12 and 17.[24] Of the 508 males accused of homicide, 186 were between the ages of 18 and 24 and 37 were between the ages of 12 and 17. In females, 14 of the 58 accused of homicide were between 18 and 24 and 3 were between the ages of 12 and 17.[25]

In 1991, 22 percent of federal statute charges were against youths. A higher proportion of youths than adults were criminally charged. In 1997–98, one in five cases (20 percent) involved violent crimes; about half were common assaults. The rate of property crime cases has dropped 25 percent since 1992, whereas the rate of violent crime has risen 4 percent. The rate of youth court cases has increased for females (by 5 percent) and decreased for males (by 12 percent) over this period.[26] Total charges against youths were double the number of charges in 1986. Does this statistic truly represent an increase in youth crime? Rather, some of the increase reflects society's increased sensitivity toward youth violence. Because of school policies of "zero tolerance" for violence, incidents that would previously have been dealt with at a school level now result in police charges and are counted in the statistics.

The youth involved are generally in their late teens (16- and 17-year-olds account for 51 percent of offenders), and the victims are generally youths between 12 and 17 years (36 percent of minor assaults), usually male (76 percent of aggravated assaults). Assaults most commonly occur in a public place (35 percent in 1997 occurred in a parking lot or on public transportation), dwellings (26 percent), or in schools (22 percent).[27]

Canada jails a high proportion of young offenders because our justice system makes little use of alternative approaches. Unlike the adult justice system, there is no parole for youth. Aboriginal youth, youth from certain racial and cultural groups, and young people from lower-income families are overrepresented in our justice system. Marginalization fosters resentment and anger, which may be vented on symbols of society, such as property. Yet it should be remembered that more than 95 percent of Canada's young people are never in trouble with the law.[28]

## The Violence of Hate

Canada has always welcomed people from other cultures—while marginalizing Aboriginal people. The degree of acceptance, however, decreases with the immigrants' physical and cultural differences from Northern European peoples. Much as we may wish otherwise, prejudice and racism have always been and continue to be a part of Canadian society.

Historically, established leaders in Canadian society (individual and institutional) have made key contributions to interracial violence, for example to the anti-Chinese riot of 1887 and the anti-Chinese and Japanese riot of 1907 in Vancouver. In both cases, the local newspapers, respectable individuals (businessmen, clergymen, politicians), and organizations played a very prominent role in at least preparing the groundwork and instigating the violence, which claimed "scores" of Chinese lives. The timing of the riots seems to have been related to white workers' alleged fears of economic competition, especially at a time of recession.[29]

## Preventing Hate and Bias Crimes

Canadian data relating to hate-motivated conduct are not collected and reported systematically by police forces on a national scale. In contrast, other jurisdictions, such as England, France, and the United States, have put in place reporting mechanisms that provide a more comprehensive national picture of the scale of hate-motivated behaviours. Others, like Australia, have created national inquiries to examine the scope of such violence throughout the country.[30]

Although the causes of intolerance remain in question, it is believed that much of it stems from a fear of change and a desire to blame others when forces such as the economy and crime seem to be out of control. What can you do to be part of the solution rather than part of the problem?

- *Support educational programs designed to foster understanding and appreciation for differences in people.* Many colleges now require diversity classes as part of their academic curriculum.

- *Examine your own attitudes and behaviours.* Are you intolerant of others? Do you engage in behaviours that demean any group of individuals? Have you thought about the reasons why you have problems with a particular group?

- *Discourage racist jokes and other forms of social or ethnic bigotry.* Do not participate in such behaviours and express your dissatisfaction with others who do. Silence condones the behaviours.

- *Vote for community leaders who respect the rights of others, value diversity, and do not have racially or ethnically motivated hidden agendas.* Vote against intolerant candidates who are attempting to control school boards and local government through planned infiltration.

- *Educate yourself.* Read, interact with, and try to understand people who appear to be different from you. Remember that you do not have to like everything about another person or group. Other people may not like everything about you, either. However, respecting people's right to be different is part of being a healthy, integrated individual.

- *Examine your own values in determining the relative worth of your friends and the others in your life.* Are you judgmental? Are you somewhat intolerant of others' differences? How do you resolve your tendencies to be judgmental and bigoted? Do you judge people on appearances? Do you take time to get to know who they are as individuals?

# Violence against Women

Canadians were shocked out of denying the existence of violence toward women by the Montreal Massacre at Concordia University in Montreal in 1989, when Marc Lepine shot and killed 14 women at the École Polytechnique because, as his writings amply explained, he hated women.

The first major empirical study on violence toward women noted that one in ten women living with a man would be abused each year.[31] This figure, initially ridiculed, is now accepted as an underestimate: more recent figures indicate that more than one woman in four (29 percent) experiences some form of domestic violence from her partner.[32] Assaults are eight times more likely in a relationship of less than two years' duration than in partnerships lasting more than 20 years.[33] Almost half (45 percent) of wife assault cases result in physical injury to the woman. The most frequent types of injuries are bruises (90 percent); cuts, scratches, and burns (33 percent); broken bones (12 percent); and fractures (11 percent).[34]

The shelter movement (begun in England in 1972 and in Canada in 1974) lobbied for zero tolerance of abuse and mandatory charging of abusers. This policy was adopted in virtually all jurisdictions in 1982, when Canada's attorney general urged police chiefs to lay charges in all cases of suspected wife abuse. The Royal Canadian Mounted Police introduced a formal policy in 1984 specifically instructing its members to lay charges in all cases where there are "reasonable and probable grounds" to believe that assault occurred. The abusive partner may be charged under the assault sections of the Criminal Code of Canada. A police charge not only highlights the criminal nature of the act, but also relieves the victim of the burden of laying charges.[35]

Discrimination and violence toward women is a global issue. On the urging of Canada, among other nations, the United Nations Convention on the Elimination of All Forms of Discrimination Against

Women adopted a resolution in 1992 accepting that states are responsible for acts of domestic violence between individuals. In December 1993, the UN passed a Declaration Against Violence Against Women.

How many times have you heard of a woman repeatedly beaten by her partner or spouse and wondered, "Why doesn't she just leave him?" There are many reasons why some women find it difficult, if not impossible, to break their ties with their abusers. Many women, particularly those with small children, are financially dependent on their partners. Others fear retaliation against themselves or their children. There are women who hope that the situation will change with time (it rarely does), and others who stay because their cultural or religious beliefs forbid divorce. Finally, there are women who still love the abusive partner and are concerned about what will happen to him if they leave.[36]

### Cycle of Violence Theory

Psychologist Lenore Walker has developed a theory known as the "cycle of violence" to explain how women (and men) can get caught in a downward spiral without knowing what is happening to them.[37] The cycle has three phases:

- *Phase One: Tension Building.* In this phase, minor battering occurs, and the woman (or man) may become more nurturant, more pleasing, and more intent on anticipating the abuser's needs in order to forestall another violent scene. The victim assumes guilt for doing something to provoke the abuser and tries hard to avoid doing it again.

- *Phase Two: Acute Battering.* At this stage, pleasing the abuser doesn't help and the victim can no longer control or predict the abuse. Usually, the abuser is trying to "teach a lesson," and will not stop until enough pain has been inflicted. When the acute attack is over, the abuser may respond with shock and denial about his or her behaviours. Usually, the abuser and victim soft-pedal the seriousness of the attacks.

- *Phase Three: Remorse/Reconciliation.* During this "honeymoon" period, the abuser may be kind, loving, and apologetic, swearing to never act violently again. The abuser may "behave" for several weeks or months, and the victim may question whether she overrated the seriousness of past abuse. Then the kind of tension that precipitated abusive incidents in the past resurfaces, the abuser loses control again, and once more beats his or her partner. Unless some form of intervention breaks this downward cycle of abuse, contrition, further abuse, denial, and contrition, it will repeat again and again, ending perhaps only when the abuser kills the victim or, less often, when the victim kills the abuser.

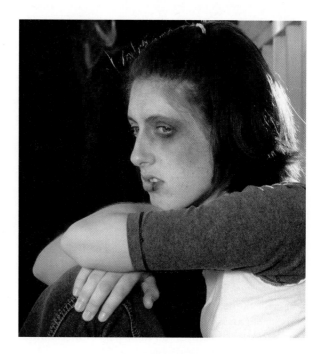

*Despite obvious physiological and psychological injury, it can be difficult for a woman to leave her abusive partner.*

It is very hard for most women who get caught in this cycle of violence (which may include forced sexual relations and psychological and economic abuse as well as physical beatings) to summon up the courage and resolution to extricate themselves. Most need effective outside intervention.

## Domestic Violence

The extent of spousal violence has only recently begun to be well documented. Statistics Canada conducted its first Violence Against Women survey in 1993. It found that 29 percent of Canadian women experienced violence at the hands of a current or past marital partner. Between 1974 and 1992, 1,435 women were killed by their husbands and 451 men were killed by their wives.[38] More recently, Statistics Canada reported rates of spousal violence by a current or previous partner in the five-year period between 1999 and 2004 to be 7 percent for women and 6 percent for men.[39] There was a significant decline in the percentage of women (8 vs. 7 percent), but the rate in men remained unchanged. A larger number of these women than men reported being beaten, choked, or threatened (23 vs. 15 percent). Women were also more likely to report more than 10 violent incidents at the hands of their partner (21 vs. 11 percent) and being injured as a result of the violence (44 vs. 18 percent). It should be pointed out that the rate of spousal violence is twice the average in those couples who are gay or lesbian (15 vs. 7 percent) and Aboriginal peoples are

## A Week without Violence

Violence can happen anywhere—at home, at school, and at work—and it can take many forms. When we think of violence, we often think of physical violence and underestimate the effect of verbal putdowns and degrading gestures. Many people endure emotional, psychological, economic, social, physical, and sexual violence in silence. Women, Aboriginal peoples, visible minorities, and individuals who are homosexual confront systemic forms of violence almost every day of their lives. This is the harsh reality of the violence that permeates our society.

Speaking about violence can help us to identify feelings of loss and anger, and to heal from them. Organized by the YWCA, the Week without Violence is a nationwide effort that encourages people to identify realistic and sustainable alternatives to violence; it occurs during the third week of October. It is believed that with active support from schools, politicians, law enforcement agencies, faith groups, and national and local community agencies we can create safer places to live, work, and play.

In 2004, more than 45,000 people and 600 schools, workplaces, and community organizations participated. For example, in Kamloops a native drumming circle of friendship was created; in Brockville a youth day focused on sports rather than violence; in Lethbridge discussions on racism and eliminating discrimination were held; and in Vancouver a mask-making workshop to empower women was hosted. For more ideas and to read more about this initiative, see www.weekwithoutviolence.ca.

Source: Adapted from YWCA of Canada, retrieved May 5, 2006, from www.weekwithoutviolence.ca.

---

3 times more likely to be victims of domestic violence (21 vs. 7 percent).

Only 27 percent of those who experience spousal abuse report the incident(s) to the police, with a greater proportion of females making the reports (37 vs. 27 percent). Approximately one-third (32 percent) of those who report their abuse to the police obtain restraining orders or protective orders against their abusers. Thirty-four percent of those who experience spousal violence seek help from a formal agency because of the violence, with more females than males seeking this help (47 vs. 20 percent).[40]

### WHAT WOULD YOU DO?

Do you know a woman who you think might be a victim of domestic violence? Can you think of a man whom you consider a likely victimizer? What about him has contributed to his current situation? Similarly, can you think of a man who you think might be a victim of domestic violence? Can you think of a woman whom you consider a likely victimizer? What about her has contributed to her current situation? In either of these situations, how could you intervene such that the anticipated violence does not occur?

### Causes of Domestic Violence

There is no single explanation for why people tend to be abusive in relationships. Although alcohol abuse is often associated with **domestic violence**, marital dissatisfaction seems to predict physical abuse better than any other variable.[41] Numerous studies also point to differences in the communication patterns between abusive relationships and nonabusive relationships.[42] While some argue that the hormone testosterone is the cause of male aggression, recent studies failed to show a strong association between physical abuse in relationships and this hormone.[43] Many experts believe that men who engage in severe violence are more likely than other men to suffer from personality disorders.[44]

The dynamics that both people bring to a relationship can result in violence and allow it to continue. Obtaining help from community support and counselling services may help determine the underlying basis of the problem and help the victim and the abuser come to a better understanding of the actions necessary to stop the cycle of abuse. The Rate Yourself box may help you determine if you are a victim (or aggressor) of abuse.

### Violence against Children

**Child abuse** is found in all societies and is almost always a highly guarded secret wherever it takes place. In countries with reliable mortality reporting, WHO

**Domestic violence:** The use of force to control and maintain power over another person in the home environment; it includes actual harm and the threat of harm.

**Child abuse:** The systematic harming of a child by a caregiver, generally a parent.

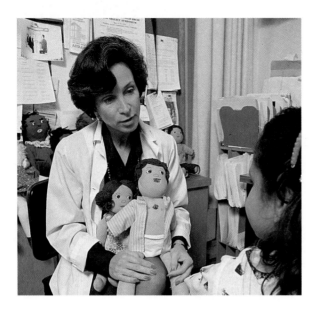

*Sympathetic and sensitive therapy can help abused children cope with the mental and physical pain inflicted on them.*

estimates that as many as 1 in 5,000 to 1 in 10,000 children under the age of five die each year from physical violence. In the same countries, every year from 1 in 1,000 to 1 in 180 children are either taken to a health-care facility or are reported to child welfare services as a consequence of abuse.

A second nation-wide study of reported child maltreatment in Canada estimated that of the estimated 217,319 investigations, 47 percent were substantiated—equivalent to an incidence rate of 21.71 per 1,000 cases of maltreatment in children.[45] It was pointed out in this report that only cases investigated by child welfare services were included, and those that were screened out or only investigated by the police were not reported. Further, it was noted that there was a change in reporting that may relate to the increase in rates of investigated and substantiated cases of maltreatment between 1998 and 2003. Of the confirmed cases of maltreatment, 15 percent involved emotional maltreatment, 28 percent of the children were exposed to domestic violence, 3 percent were sexually abused, 24 percent were physically abused, and 30 percent were neglected.

Physical violence often originates when there is a lack of parenting skills. Typically, abusive parents are unable to respond to a young child's needs and have unrealistic expectations for the stage of a child's development. Another factor is the cultural acceptance of corporal punishment and violence within a society.

Other stresses contributing to child maltreatment may include an unwanted child, an unsupported single-parent household, the absence of social support, financial pressures, and unemployment. Child maltreatment can be aggravated by substance abuse on the part of the parent or guardian. In substance-abusing families there is a strong association between physical violence, sexual abuse, and domestic violence directed at members of the family, particularly women and young children.

The perpetrators of violence or sexual abuse of children are often trusted individuals in a position of authority, usually males, and often family members.[46] Child victims of violence or sexual abuse have a high risk of becoming perpetrators of similar forms of abuse toward younger children. In later years, they may be physically violent to children in their care or to their own children. The normal reactions to harm are the expression of anger and pain. The abused child is forbidden to express anger and cannot bear to endure the pain alone. To survive, the child must repress the feelings and even the memory. The repressed emotions will gain expression in destructive acts—against others, as in criminal behaviours and even mass murder, or self-directed, as with drug and alcohol abuse.[47]

Physical violence and sexual abuse in the home is a factor contributing to the phenomenon of street children in developed and developing countries. Further abuse on the street is an everyday reality.[48]

The use of threat and power by an adult against a child breaks the deep trust of the child toward his or her protectors. That they would turn against the child is unthinkable, and so the child divorces awareness of the abuse from everyday thoughts and manages to forget the trauma. But the fear continues to influence the child's behaviours and interactions with others, often in destructive ways. Later in life, when it is safer, the memory may resurface and the person can begin to heal.

Not all child violence is physical. A child's health can be severely affected by psychological violence—assaults on personality, character, competence, independence, or general dignity as a human being. The negative consequences of this kind of victimization in close relationships can be harder to discern and therefore harder to combat. They include depression, lowered self-esteem, and a pervasive fear of doing something that will offend the abuser.

## WHAT WOULD YOU DO?

What factors in society lead to child maltreatment? What are common characteristics of children's abusers? Why are family members often the perpetrators of child abuse and child sexual abuse? What actions can be taken to prevent such behaviours? How can the cycle of the abused becoming the abuser be stopped?

# Are You a Victim of Abuse?

Ask yourself if you are being abused. Start with the following questions:

**1.** Does your partner continually criticize what you wear, what you say, how you act, and how you look? _____

**2.** Does your partner often call you insulting or degrading names? _____

**3.** Do you feel like you need to ask permission to go out and see your friends and family? _____

**4.** Do you feel that no matter what you do, everything is your fault? _____

**5.** Do you feel like you're walking on eggshells trying to avoid an argument? _____

**6.** When you're late getting home, does your partner harass you about where you were and whom you were with? _____

**7.** Is your partner so jealous that you're always being accused of having affairs? _____

**8.** Has your partner threatened to hurt you or the children if you leave? _____

**9.** Does your partner force you to have sex? _____

**10.** Has your partner threatened to hit you? _____

**11.** Has your partner ever pushed, shoved, or slapped you? _____

If you answered yes to one or more of these questions, you may be suffering abuse. The following support services are available.

## WHERE TO GO FOR SUPPORT SERVICES

- Transition house or shelter
- Police department
- Distress centre
- Sexual assault centre
- Social service agency

Telephone numbers can be found at the front of your phone book.

## DO YOU WANT TO LEARN MORE?

The National Clearinghouse on Family Violence can provide you with a list of publications that can be ordered free of charge. The Clearinghouse can also tell you about films and videos on abuse that can be borrowed through the National Film Board's regional offices.

Source: Deborah Prieur and Mary Rowles, *Taking Action: A Union Guide to Ending Violence Against Women* (BC Federation of Labour and the Women's Research Centre 1992) 14. Reprinted by permission of the BC Federation of Labour.

## Violence against Men

While women are most often the targets of violence by men, men can also be the target. In 1999 males committed 85.5 percent of violent crimes. Thirty-nine percent of violent crimes in 1999 involved males attacking other males. Men under 34 years are more likely to be perpetrators in major assaults (65 percent). In only 6 percent of reported cases did a woman commit a violent act on a man.[49] Thus, the task of overcoming violence in our society is largely a male issue. The principal reason seems to be that boys are taught—overtly or subtly—that competitiveness, power, and control are valued male attributes. Violence can be seen as an expression of frustration and stress.

## Violence against Older Adults

Violence toward older adults (elder abuse) has only recently been getting attention. The first national survey of abuse toward the elderly was done in 1989 at Ryerson University; the researchers found that 4 percent of Canadians over 65 living in private dwellings (or 98,000 seniors) reported experiencing at least one type of abuse in the last 12 months. The most prevalent types of abuse reported (listed in order of prevalence) were material abuse (such as forcing older adults to hand over money or valuable goods), chronic verbal aggression, physical abuse, and neglect.[50] The victim was more often female (67 percent), and the abuser was most frequently a spouse or a child of the victim. (See Table 4.1.) The vulnerability of this group is reflected in the lack of formal charges laid against the perpetrators, with only 13 percent of abused seniors laying charges.

Statistics Canada reports that older women are more likely than their male counterparts to be victims of family violence, with almost 40 percent of senior female victims assaulted by a family member compared to 20 percent of senior male victims.[51]

## TABLE 4.1
## Elder Abuse: The Victims and the Abusers

**Number and proportion of older adult victims of violent crime by sex of victims and relationship to accused, 2000[1]**

| Relationship of accused to victim | Total | | Female | | Male | |
|---|---|---|---|---|---|---|
| | No. | % | No. | % | No. | % |
| **Total[2]** | 3,627 | 100 | 1,792 | 100 | 1,835 | 100 |
| Unknown | 214 | 6 | 91 | 5 | 123 | 7 |
| Non-family | 2,407 | 66 | 1,052 | 59 | 1,355 | 74 |
| Family | 1,006 | 28 | 649 | 36 | 357 | 19 |
| **Total family[3]** | 1,006 | 100 | 649 | 100 | 357 | 100 |
| Spouse[4] | 312 | 31 | 236 | 36 | 76 | 21 |
| Parent[5] | 53 | 5 | 28 | 4 | 25 | 7 |
| Adult child[5] | 398 | 40 | 243 | 37 | 155 | 43 |
| Sibling[6] | 110 | 11 | 60 | 9 | 50 | 14 |
| Extended family[7] | 133 | 13 | 82 | 13 | 51 | 14 |

Percentages may not total 100 percent due to rounding.

[1] Data are not nationally representative. Based on data from 166 police departments representing 53 percent of the national volume of crime in 2000.

[2] Excludes one case where relationship between victim and accused was unknown.

[3] Excludes cases where relationship between victim and accused was unknown.

[4] Includes current and former spouses, either by legal marriage or common-law relationship.

[5] Includes a small number of cases where age or the relationship between the accused and the victim may have been miscoded.

[6] Sibling includes natural, step, half, foster, or adopted brother or sister.

[7] Extended family includes others related to the victim either by blood or by marriage, e.g., aunts, uncles, cousins, and in-laws.

Source: Number and proportion of older adult victims of violent crime by sex of victims and relationship to accused, 2000, adapted from Statistics Canada, Revised Uniform Crime Reporting Survey (UCR2), 2000.

Most (55 percent) older adult victims of family-related violence experience common assaults, while another 19 percent experience verbal aggression. The perpetrators of these assaults are most often males.

## SEXUAL VICTIMIZATION

In 1997, sexual offences reported to police represented 10 percent (30,735 sexual offences) of violent crimes. The offenders are mostly male (98 percent in 1997) and somewhat older (32 years) than the norm for all violent offenders (29 years). The 1997 rate is 25 percent lower than the peak in 1993.[52]

### WHAT WOULD YOU DO?

What factors make men likely to commit sexual assault? What might be effective in preventing such behaviours?

## Sexual Assault

**Sexual assault** can be understood in terms of a power imbalance in society "in which violence is implicit" as the base upon which sexual exploitation is built.[53] A survey of more than 6,000 post-secondary students found that 84 percent of women who had been sexually assaulted knew their attacker and that 57 percent of the rapes happened on a date.[54] Of male offenders, 19 percent were between 18 and 24 years, 32 percent were between 25 and 34 years, and 23 percent were between 35 and 44 years. Many universities coordinate "safe walk" programs, during which a person can be accompanied at night on campus from building to building or to and from the parking lots. Self-defence courses can provide some protection against attackers as well as improving self-confidence. The Skills for Behaviour Change box discusses preventing sexual assault when dating.

### Why Some Males Sexually Assault Women

Over the years, psychologists and others have proposed many theories to explain why so many males sexually victimize women. One study found that almost two-thirds of the male respondents had engaged in intercourse unwanted by the woman, primarily because of male peer pressure.[55] Peer pressure is certainly a strong factor in such behaviours, but a growing body of research suggests that sexual assault is encouraged by the normal socialization processes that males experience daily.[56]

### Social Assumptions

According to many experts, certain common assumptions in our society prevent the recognition by the perpetrator and the wider public of the true nature of sexual assault.[57] The most important of these assumptions are:[58]

- *Minimization:* It is often assumed that sexual assault of women is rare because official crime statistics show relatively few offences; however, sexual assault is the most underreported of all serious crimes.
- *Trivialization:* Incredibly enough, sexual assault of women is still often viewed as a jocular matter by many men.
- *Blaming the victim:* Many discussions of sexual violence against women display a sometimes unconscious assumption that the woman did something to provoke the attack—that she dressed too revealingly or flirted too much.
- *"Boys will be boys":* This is the assumption that men can't control themselves once they become aroused. The myth that men can't stop once they start is millennia old and typically suggests males are slaves to their sexual organs or that great physical harm can happen to the unfortunate male denied ejaculation. These notions can be countered by pointing out the following: (a) If a woman's parents walked into the room where sex was occurring, it's a sure bet that the man could stop; and (b) there has never been a documented case where a male died due to coitus interruptus.

## WHAT WOULD YOU DO?

Why do you think women are often reluctant to report sexual assault? How can we help women in this regard? Why do you think men are not aware of their sexually harassing behaviours? What can be done to increase awareness of harassing behaviours for men and women?

# PREVENTING PERSONAL ASSAULTS

After a violent act is committed against someone we know, we acknowledge the horror of the event, express sympathy for the victim, and then go on with our lives. But the brutalized person often takes a long time to recover—and sometimes complete recovery from the assault is not possible (see Table 4.2 for a summary of the most common consequences of victimization). In this section we discuss prevention of violence and abuse rather extensively because it is far better to stop a violent act than to have to recover from it.

## Self-Defence against Sexual Assault

To reduce your risk of sexual assault there are some common-sense self-defence tactics that you can learn. Self-defence is a process that includes increased awareness, learning self-defence techniques, taking reasonable precautions, and developing the self-confidence and judgment needed to determine appropriate responses to different situations.[59]

### Taking Control

Most sexual assaults by assailants unknown to the victim are planned in advance. They are frequently preceded by a casual, friendly conversation. Although many women have said that they started to feel uneasy during such a conversation, they denied the possibility of an attack to themselves until it was too late. Listen to your feelings and trust your intuition. Be assertive

**Sexual assault:** Any act in which one person is sexually intimate with another person without that other person's consent.

# Preventing Date Rape

The risk of date rapes can be reduced by following several general guidelines:

## WOMEN

- *Decide ahead of time how far you are willing to go.* Remember that it is your game, your rules, and no one should pressure or force you into going beyond your limits.

- *Think ahead of time and try to avoid "compromising" situations.* If you haven't decided to have sex, stay out of your date's bedroom, the back seat of the car, or other quiet spots away from the rest of the crowd.

- *Communicate directly.* Don't be wishy-washy. If things start to go farther than you want them to, say NO loudly and with conviction. Do not worry about hurting feelings or seeming aggressive. Be firm and stick to your words.

- *Be aware that some men, in some situations, will interpret a low-cut, sexy dress or other clothing as a come-on.* Although this is obviously wrong on their part, it is important that you do not naively assume that everyone is enlightened. Be direct and firm with anyone who seems to be assuming too much from your attire or interactions.

- *Limit your consumption of alcohol and other drugs that reduce your ability to think clearly.* Do not accept a drink from anyone. Do not leave your drink unattended.

- *Pay attention to the nonverbal and verbal cues that your date is giving you.* If he is indicating that he is interested in more, let him know you are not.

- *Be concerned about any of the following behaviours or expressions exhibited by your date:*
  - Continued suggestive or dirty language indicating disrespect for you and others.
  - Failure to listen to or to value your opinions about where to go, whom to spend time with, etc.
  - Unusual displays of jealousy or rage concerning your interactions with others.
  - Unusual roughness and forceful pushing or shoving to get you to comply with his wishes.
  - Wild anger and violent acts toward others.
  - Inability to control drinking and to display appropriate behaviours.
  - Lack of concern for your feelings; laughter or derisive comments when you say no.

## MEN

- *Take stock of your past behaviours in potentially sexual situations.* How have you behaved, what have been the outcomes of the encounters, etc.? Have you felt uncomfortable about pushing too hard to have sex with your dates in the past? Have you felt pushed yourself?

- *Know and express your sexual limits.* If you feel that you are beginning to lose control in an intimate situation, communicate your feelings and indicate why it is time to stop.

- *Understand that NO means NO—and that it is not a sign of rejection.* Respect your partner's right to say no, regardless of how far you've gone or what you thought she might have wanted. Stop NOW and do not try "another line." Think about how you'd want your sister or close female friend to be treated by another guy in a similar situation.

- *Just because you may have been intimate with the woman before doesn't mean it's okay now.* When you hear the word NO, or if the woman struggles in any way, STOP.

- *Limit alcohol and other drugs that cause you to think less clearly.* Do not accept a drink from anyone or leave your drink unattended. Do not purchase a drink for someone unless they ask for it.

- *Avoid situations likely to get you into trouble.* Until you are sure of your intentions and your date's intentions, stay out of bedrooms and avoid dark roads and the back seats of cars, or any other places away from people.

- *If you encounter a particularly aggressive woman, it is not unmanly to tell her you do not want to have sex and are not interested in being intimate in any way.* Say NO and avoid situations that may cause you to be caught in a compromising position. Forget about what she may say or what your friends will say. Remember, it is up to you whether or not you have sex.

**TABLE 4.2**

**Common Consequences of Victimization**

| Psychological | Medical |
|---|---|
| Recurrent and intrusive recollections, dreams, or flashbacks involving traumatic incidents | Death |
| Generalized anxiety, mistrust, and/or social isolation | Sexual/reproductive symptoms/consequences: chronic pelvic pain, HIV infection, urinary tract infections, premenstrual pain, fertility problems, trauma-specific pain, orgasmic difficulty |
| Difficulty in forming or maintaining nonexploitive intimate relationships | Battering-related symptoms: bruises, black eyes, fractured ribs, broken teeth, subdural haematomas, detached retinas, other head injuries |
| Chronic depression | Stress-mediated symptoms: headaches, backaches, TMJ symptoms, high blood pressure, hyperalertness, sleep disorders, gastrointestinal disorders |
| Dissociative reactions: phobic avoidance, often generalized to apparently unrelated situations; feelings of "badness," stigma, and guilt; impulsive or self-defeating behaviour | Eating disorders<br>Self-mutilation |

Source: From Marjorie Whittaker Leidig, "The Continuum of Violence against Women: Psychological and Physical Consequences," *Journal of American College Health, 40* (1992): 151. Reprinted with permission of the Helen Dwight Reid Educational Foundation. Published by Heldref Publications, 1319 Eighteenth Street NW, Washington, DC 20036-1802. © 1992.

and direct to someone who is getting out of line or threatening—this may convince the would-be rapist to back off. Stifle your tendency to be "nice," and don't fear making a scene. Let him know that you mean what you say and are prepared to defend yourself:[60]

- Speak in a strong voice and use statements like "Leave me alone" rather than questions like "Will you please leave me alone?" Avoid apologies and excuses.

- Maintain eye contact with the would-be attacker.

- Sound as if you mean what you say.

- Stand up straight, act confident, and remain alert. Walk as if you own the sidewalk.

Many rapists use certain ploys to initiate their attacks. Among the most common are:

- *Request for help.* This allows him to get close—to enter your house to use the phone, for instance.

- *Offer of help.* This can also help him gain entrance to your home: "Let me help you carry that package."

- *Guilt trip.* "Gee, no one is friendly nowadays. . . . I can't believe you won't talk with me for just a little while."

- *Authority.* Some victimized women have been fooled by the "police officer at the door" ruse. If anyone comes to your door dressed in the uniform of a police officer, firefighter, repairman, or any other individual, ask him to show you his ID before you unlock the door. You can also call the employer to get a confirmation on his ID.

If you are attacked, act immediately:

- *Don't worry about causing a scene.* Draw attention to yourself and your assailant. Scream for help.

- Report the attack to the appropriate authorities at once.

To prevent an attack from occurring:

- Always be vigilant. Even the safest cities and towns have sexual assaults. Don't be fooled by a sleepy, little-town atmosphere.

- Use campus escort services whenever possible.

- Be assertive in demanding a well-lit campus and safe-walk programs.

- Don't use the same routes all the time. Think about your movement patterns and vary them accordingly.

- Don't leave a bar alone with a friendly stranger. Stay with your friends, and let the friendly stranger come along. Don't give your address or phone number to anyone you don't know.

- Never accept a drink from another person and never leave your drink unattended. Rohypnol (often called the date rape drug) is odourless and colourless and you cannot tell if it has been put in your drink.

- Let friends or family know where you are going, what route you'll take, and when to expect your return.

- Stay close to others. Avoid shortcuts through dark or unlit paths. Don't be the last one to leave the lab or library late at night.

- Keep your windows and doors locked. Don't answer the door to strangers.

### What to Do When a Sexual Assault Occurs

If you are a sexual assault victim, it should be you who reports the attack. This gives you a sense of control. Call 911 immediately. Do not bathe, shower, douche, clean up, or touch anything the attacker may have touched. Do not throw away or launder the clothes you were wearing. They will be needed as evidence. Bring a clean change of clothes to the clinic or hospital. Contact the Rape Crisis Centre in your area and ask for advice on therapists or counselling if you need additional support.

If you want to help a sexual assault victim, the best thing you can do is to believe her. Don't ask questions that appear to implicate her in the assault. Your hindsight may find some questionable judgment on her behalf, but that doesn't mean she's to blame. Sexual assault is a violent act against someone; the victim was certainly not looking or asking for it. Encourage her to talk, and when she does, listen. Hold back on advice.

Encourage her to see a doctor immediately, as she may have medical needs but be too embarrassed to seek help on her own. Be supportive of her reporting the crime. Continue to be her friend. It may take six months to a year for emotional recovery, and you should be understanding during this time. Encourage her to seek counselling if problems persist.

## Preventing Assaults at Home

When at home, there are several precautions you can take to avoid being assaulted:[61]

- Get deadbolts and peepholes and make sure the entryway to your house is well lit and free of shrubs.

- Put a lock, solid-core door, and extension phone with a lighted dial in your bedroom.

- Get to know your neighbours and organize a neighbourhood watch.

- Don't hide your keys under a fake rock or other device. These are dead giveaways to experienced criminals.

- Don't open your door to anyone you don't know.

- Ask for identification from repairmen, police officers, fire fighters, and others and call to verify that they've sent someone out.

- Keep lights on in at least one room other than the one you're in to make it look as if you aren't home alone.

- Don't put your full name on your mailbox or in the phone book; use your initials instead.

- Use a "Beware of Dog" sign to deter assailants. Be careful of "doggy doors." Many assailants have entered a house through a pet door.

## Preventing Assaults on the Street

There are several suggestions to prevent an assault when you walk or jog:[62]

- *Walk or jog at a steady pace.* Look confident and stay alert to your surroundings.

- *Walk or jog with others.* There is safety in numbers.

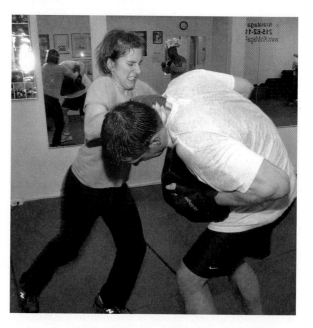

*Women who learn self-defence techniques and remember to take reasonable safety precautions lower their risk for assault.*

- *At night, avoid dark parking lots, wooded areas, and all other good hiding places for assailants.*
- *Listen for footsteps and voices.* Change the pace of your walk if you think you're being followed to see if the person behind you does likewise. If he or she does, walk down the middle of the street, staying near the streetlights. Run and yell if you feel threatened.
- *Be aware of cars that keep driving around in your area.*
- Vary your running or walking routes.

## WHAT WOULD YOU DO?

How safe are you in your own home? How about on campus? What precautions can you take to reduce your risk?

## Preventing Assaults in Your Car

Carjackings and murders of individuals driving expensive cars, rental cars, and other vehicles point out the necessity for personal actions to prevent assaults when you are in your car:[63]

- Keep your doors locked and your windows rolled up.
- Don't stop for vehicles in distress. Drive on and call for help.
- If your car breaks down, lock the doors and wait for help from the police. Do not accept assistance from strangers, particularly from individuals on isolated roads.
- If you think someone is following you, do something to attract attention. Stay in your car with locked windows and doors and drive to a fire station, police station, all-night grocery, restaurant, or other place where there are people. If you are forced to stop on a deserted road, leave your engine running and in gear. Wait until your pursuer gets out of his car, then drive away as fast as you safely can.
- Stick to well-travelled routes. Avoid dark, isolated shortcuts.
- Fill your car with gas and keep it in good running order.
- Don't put your name and address on your key ring.
- Before getting into your car, walk around it and check the back seat, floor, and undercarriage.

- On long trips, don't make it obvious you're travelling alone. Never take a map into a restaurant.
- Don't sleep in your car along the highway. This is no longer safe in many areas.
- When you stop for a traffic light, leave a car's length so that if you are approached you'll have room to pull out. If someone does approach, blow your horn and attract attention.
- If someone bumps into you, never get out of the car until a police officer arrives. Murders and carjackings have involved assailants ramming victims' cars from behind and then shooting or attacking those who got out to investigate.

# VIOLENCE AND HEALTH

If the health sector is to adequately understand and respond to violence, greater emphasis is needed on the Population Health Model now adopted by the federal government, which sees health as embracing not only medical services and personal health practices, but also the physical, social, and economic environment (see Chapter 1). Prevention of violence must be based on the creation of life conditions that reduce the occurrence of violence and lessen its effects.

Clearly, a violence-free environment is a prerequisite for health. Violence is a barrier to health and a consequence of an unhealthy environment. The Ottawa Charter for Health Promotion (an international statement on health promotion) states:

> the fundamental conditions and resources for health are peace, shelter, education, food, income, a stable ecosystem, sustainable resources, social justice and equity. Improvement in health requires a secure foundation in these basic prerequisites. [64]

## Injury Prevention

Intentional acts of violence and abuse receive more media coverage and public awareness than unintentional injuries, which kill and disable Canadians every day. Unintentional injuries—the result of falls, motor vehicle crashes, railway and pedestrian injuries, drowning and suffocation, poisoning, and fires—are the leading cause of death among Canadians up to the age of 44, and they kill more young people between the ages of 1 and 20 than all other causes of death combined. Why, then, do we not view injury as a serious population health problem? It is likely because we tend to call unintentional

# All-Terrain Vehicles: Handle with Care

All-terrain vehicles (ATVs) were introduced to Canada sometime in the early 1970s. Since then, Canada has become the biggest market per capita in the world, with approximately 2.5 million Canadians riding ATVs and approximately 850,000 owning one or more.

Along with increased use has come an increase in the number of ATV-related injuries and hospitalization. In fact, according to the Canadian Institute for Health Information, from 1996 to 2001 ATV-related hospitalizations increased 50 percent. Children and adolescents between the ages of 5 and 19 account for more than one-third of these injuries. Currently, ATV-related injuries are the third most common serious injury in the sports and recreational category after cycling and snowmobiling.

Helmets must be worn when riding an ATV, though not all riders abide by this mandatory regulation. Each province legislates the minimum age restriction for ATV use, with no restrictions in British Columbia, to age 12 and over on public property in Ontario, 14 and older in Newfoundland and Labrador, and 16 and older in the Yukon Territory and Nova Scotia. In addition to not wearing helmets, young riders are also likely to ride double and on public roads.

To reduce risk of injury, the Canadian Health Network recommends riders:

- **Buckle up**. Although ATVs don't have seatbelts, you should securely fasten the straps on your helmet and gloves.
- **Look first**. Become familiar with the terrain you are going to be driving on and know where you are going. If you plan a day-long or overnight trip, ensure that a responsible adult is aware of your plans. Take a cell phone.
- **Wear the gear.** In addition to wearing a helmet, wear wrist and eye protection. During the winter, dress for the weather.
- **Get trained.** Riders of all ages should take certification of training from a club or manufacturer. The Canada Safety council offers ATV riders' courses, including one geared for those under the age of 14.
- **Drive sober.** Do not drive an ATV under the influence of alcohol or any other drug that affects your ability to think clearly.

Further, the Canadian Paediatric Society recommends:

- children under 16 should NOT operate ATVs.
- children should never ride as passengers.
- ATVs should not be used at night.

Source: Adapted from Canadian Health Network, "All-Terrain Vehicles: Handle with Care." Retrieved on May 18, 2006, from www.canadian-health-network.ca/servelet/ContentServer?cid=1146231807156&pagename=CHN-RCS/CHNResiource/CHNResourcePagePrint.

---

injuries "accidents." This suggests the injury was due to some unavoidable circumstance over which the individual had no control. However, most injuries are predictable and preventable. Not wearing seatbelts or bicycle helmets drastically increases the risk of injury. Falls account for about 40 percent of the total injuries to Canadians, while motor vehicle crashes account for about 20 percent.

## Who Are the Victims of Unintentional Injury?

The injury rate resulting in death or hospitalization is higher for seniors than for any other age group in Canada, and is expected to grow as the population ages. The most common cause of injury among seniors is falls. More than $980 million is spent each year to cover the cost of direct medical care to treat these falls. Canadians of all ages face hazards in their everyday environment that might cause falls—ice-coated sidewalks and stairs, loose banisters, and unsafe play or work equipment.

Falls are by far the most common reason that Canadians are admitted to hospital for injury. The Canadian Institute for Health Information reports that falls account for more than 50 percent of all people admitted to hospital, 67 percent of all days spent in hospital due to trauma, and 75 percent of all people who die in hospital due to trauma.

Preventable injuries account for almost 70 percent of injury-related deaths among children and youth. Of the 3,000 people per year who die in motor vehicle crashes in Canada, 40 percent (1,200 deaths) are attributed to alcohol. Up to $25 billion is spent annually for emergency care, rehabilitation, and other costs resulting from traffic collisions.

# Dealing with Family Violence in Canada

### What Factors Contribute to Family Violence?

There is no single cause of family violence, and many people—regardless of status—may be vulnerable to abuse. Most experts believe that family violence is linked to inequalities and power imbalances in our society. Most abusers are in a position of power over their victims.

A person's vulnerability to abuse may be increased by factors such as dislocation, racism, sexism, homophobia, disability, poverty, isolation, and by lack of access to community services and support and the child welfare and criminal justice systems. For example, in the past, many children from marginalized groups in our society sent to institutions experienced abuse

### What Are the Consequences of Family Violence?

Individuals who experience—or are exposed to—family violence, can experience psychological, physiological, behavioural, academic, sexual, interpersonal, self-perceptual, or spiritual consequences, which are fatal in some cases.

### Consequences for Abusers

In some cases, abusers may have been abused—or exposed to abuse—themselves and learned that abuse is a way of exerting power and control over others. They may continue to harm others even if it destroys their relationships or has other negative consequences for their lives.

### Societal Consequences

Family violence has enormous economic costs for Canadian society. The first research study to estimate the costs of various forms of violence against women, including abuse in intimate relationships, found it costs Canadian society an estimated $4.2 billion per year in social services, education, criminal justice, labour, employment, health, and medical costs.

### Preventing and Responding to Family Violence

Victims and abusers are involved in intimate or dependent relationships, and often have strong emotional ties. Community services and supports for victims, such as shelters, are essential. All levels of government are working together to ensure that the criminal justice system responds more effectively to protect victims and hold abusers accountable via legal reform, public and professional education, research, and support for programs and services.

## DISCUSSION QUESTION

1. Besides reforming the law and enhancing its implementation, what other strategies are you aware of to prevent and respond to family violence in Canada? What interventions or programs are offered in your community? What impact do these programs have on the incidence or impact of family violence for the victims and Canadian society at large?

Source: "Family Violence: A Fact Sheet," from the Department of Justice Canada, 2002. Reproduced with the permission of the Minister of Public Works and Government Services Canada, 2003. http://canada.justice.gc.ca/en/ps/fm/familyvfs.html

## What Can Be Done?

SmartRisk suggests that each individual has the power to control the level of risk in his or her life. Smart risk-taking means that you have identified all risks beforehand and that you fully understand the consequences of your actions. Preparing for the risky activity will reduce the amount of risk you take on and enable you to make good decisions when a risky scenario presents itself. You must be prepared to choose behaviours that will reduce your likelihood of injury. Buckle up. Drive sober. Wear a bicycle helmet. Get trained. Wear the safety gear. Look first. (For more on practising smart risk, check out www.smartrisk.ca.)

# Managing Campus Safety

University and college campuses today may be healthy places for student interactions, or they may be settings for violent and aggressive interactions between students. Most campuses have initiated programs, services, and policies designed to protect students from possible violations of their personal health and safety. Answering the following questions may help you determine your college administrators' degree of interest in and commitment to a violence-free setting.

## MAKING DECISIONS FOR YOU

Setting limits on where you go, at what time, and with whom seems to be a running theme of this chapter. What types of limits do you set for yourself? Think for a moment about your next night out with friends or with your lover. What limits will you set for yourself? Will you decide ahead of time to limit your drinking? What time do you want to be home? How far will you go sexually? Will you use condoms? Decide how you will achieve your goals

## CHOICES FOR CHANGE: MAKING PERSONAL CHOICES

- Do you decide before a date to limit your sexual behaviours?
- Do you travel in groups whenever possible?
- Do you avoid being out alone at night?
- Do you avoid high-crime areas?

## CHOICES FOR CHANGE: MAKING COMMUNITY CHOICES

- Does your campus have a student health centre with a trained staff of health educators?
- Does your health centre offer workshops on prevention of sexual assault?
- Does your campus offer courses focusing on understanding human diversity?
- Does your campus offer workshops or seminars for men to help them understand their sexuality and refrain from rape and other kinds of assault against women?
- Does your campus offer workshops and information for students to help them avoid situations that put them at risk for violent sexual or other interactions?
- Does your campus offer confidential counselling or assistance to victims of sexual assault?
- Does your campus offer workshops or educational sessions dealing with suicide?
- Does your campus offer information, workshops, or services dealing with domestic violence?

- Does your campus offer information, workshops, or services dealing with child abuse and/or sexual abuse?
- Does your campus offer workshops or seminars that help males learn how to confront peers who express attitudes supportive of "overcoming" women sexually?
- Does your campus have strict substance abuse policies designed to reduce the likelihood of sexual assaults?
- Are sessions designed to negate myths and to increase understanding between the sexes offered in "safe" environments where discussions are open and positive role models encourage positive actions?
- Are services such as rides and escort services available to students after hours to prevent assaults? Do security guards patrol the campus?
- Is your campus well-lit and open in the evenings?
- Are campus health educators, counsellors, and other professionals trained to spot victimization in clients and recommend appropriate services?
- Does your campus have a code of conduct that mandates swift and prudent punishment for alcohol and other drug abuse and acts of campus violence?

## CRITICAL THINKING

Your best friend and roommate has been accused of date rape; if the charge is substantiated, he could be dismissed from school. The way your friend tells it, they had a few drinks, started making out, and eventually had intercourse. He claims that she did not try to stop him. Your friend asks you to talk to the girl; after all, she's a friend of yours from high school and you introduced them. He wants you to "find holes in her story" and see if you can get her to "forget about the whole thing." It's hard to believe your best friend is a rapist. But then it's also hard to believe she is lying.

Using the DECIDE model described in Chapter 1, decide what you will do. Reconsider the information about date rape in the chapter. Would it make a difference if she came to you to talk?

# SUMMARY

- Violence affects everyone in society—from the direct victims, to those who live in fear, to those who pay higher taxes and insurance premiums. More than half of homicides are committed by people who knew their victims. Bias and hate crimes divide people, while teaching tolerance can reduce risks.

- Sexual victimization refers to sexual assault, date rape, and sexual harassment. The possible reasons accounting for why males sexually assault females include male socialization, attitudes, sexual history and hostility, misperceptions, and situational factors. Sexual assault is not a sexual act, but a violent act.

- Prevention of violent acts begins with keeping yourself out of situations in which harm may occur. It also involves education, including understanding and accepting diversity.

# DISCUSSION QUESTIONS

1. What are common ways that violence is expressed in Canada?

2. What are the health issues of violence in society?

3. What are the causes of domestic violence? Compare spousal abuse against men and against women: What are the differences? What are the similarities?

4. What puts a child at risk for abuse? Is there anything that can be done to prevent or to decrease the amount of child abuse?

5. List the actions you can take to protect yourself from personal assault in your home, on the streets, or in your car.

6. If your friend were to tell you that she was sexually assaulted last night, what would you do? What would you suggest she do?

7. Think about a time when you did something risky. Was it a smart or foolish risk? What steps did you take to manage or limit the risk? Where did you draw the line?

# APPLICATION EXERCISE

Reread the What Do You Think? scenario at the beginning of the chapter and answer the following questions.

1. From what you have read in this chapter, do you think what Freddy has witnessed is common in Canadian society?

2. How do you think Freddy might react to the police taking his father away?

3. How might Freddy react to his mother?

4. How can Freddy break the cycle of violence and not become an abuser himself?

# HEALTH ON THE NET

Access to Justice Network
**www.acjnet.org/**

Health Canada
**www.hc-sc.gc.ca**

World Health Organization
**www.who.int/**

Child & Family Canada
**www.cfc-efc.ca/**

Canada Safety Council
**www.safety-council.org**

Alberta Centre for Injury Control & Research
**www.stop-injury.ca**

SmartRisk Canada
**www.smartrisk.ca**

Safe Communities Foundation
**www.safecommunities.ca**

CHAPTER 5

# HEALTHY RELATIONSHIPS AND SEXUALITY

*Making Commitments*

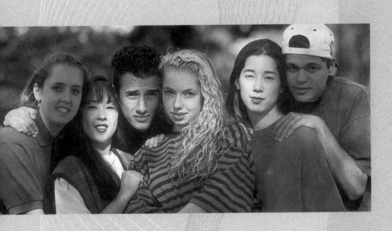

## CHAPTER OBJECTIVES

- Identify the role of communication in intimate and nonintimate relationships.

- Explain the characteristics of intimate relationships, the purposes they serve, and the type of intimacy that each of us is capable of.

- Explain the development of relationships, potential barriers to healthy relationships, and the factors important in maintaining intimate relationships.

- Describe what remaining single means for many Canadians.

- Examine child-rearing practices in Canada and the importance of a healthy family environment.

- Identify the warning signs of a failing relationship, where you can get help, and factors that ultimately lead to the relationship failing.

- Differentiate sexual and gender identity. Provide examples of each.

- Learn to develop your sexual identity.

- Describe how a person can express his or her sexuality.

- Classify sexual dysfunctions and describe each disorder.

Michael and Sara have been dating seriously for more than two years and talked about marriage. Sara has noticed that Michael often seems overly possessive of her and jealous of her time spent with others. They fight regularly about whom she does things with, potential threats to their relationship, and the like. Recently, Michael took a weekend to go hunting with the guys while Sara stayed home to get caught up on her work. When Sara's friends called her to ask her to go to a party, she decided to go. When she talked to Michael on the phone the next day, he asked her what she did the night before. Wanting to avoid a fight, she told him she stayed home to work. He responded angrily, "I tried to call you and you weren't home!"

■ What should Sara do in this situation? Why do you think she felt the need to lie? Is dishonesty in a relationship justified? Why or why not? Is Michael's jealousy a healthy, normal part of their relationship? What factors may have contributed to his jealousy? Can a relationship based on mistrust and half-truths survive? Why or why not?

Humans are social beings—we have a basic need to belong and feel loved, appreciated, and wanted. We can't live without relating to others in some way. In fact, research indicates that the ability to relate well with people, as well as give and receive love and support throughout your life, can have almost as much impact on your health as regular physical activity and good nutrition.[1] All relationships involve a degree of risk. However, only by taking these risks can we grow and truly experience all that life has to offer. By looking at our intimate and nonintimate relationships, components of sexual identity, gender roles, and sexual orientation, we will come to better understand who we are.

# COMMUNICATING: A KEY TO ESTABLISHING RELATIONSHIPS

From the moment of birth, we struggle to be understood. We flail our arms, cry, scream, smile, frown, and make sounds and gestures to attract attention, get a reaction from someone, or have someone understand what we want or need from them. By the time we enter adulthood, each of us has developed a unique way of communicating using gestures, words, expressions, and body positions. No two of us communicate in the exact same way or have the same need for connecting with others. Some are outgoing and quick to express emotions and thoughts. Others are quiet, reluctant to talk about feelings, and may prefer to spend time alone rather than with others.

Different cultures have not only different languages and dialects, but also distinct ways of expressing themselves and using body language to communicate.[2] Some cultures gesture wildly; others maintain a closed and rigid means of speaking. Some cultures are offended by apparent "fixed and dilated" staring, while others welcome a steady look in the eyes. Although people differ in the way they communicate, this doesn't mean that one sex, culture, or group is better or should be a model for the others. We have to be willing to accept differences and work to keep communication lines open and fluid. Appearing interested, actively engaged in the interaction, and open and willing to exchange ideas and thoughts is something that we typically learn with practice and hard work.

## Communicating How You Feel

Do you find it easy to express how much you care about friends and family members with hugs, kisses, and verbal expressions? If you are comfortable telling them you love them and that they mean a lot to you, chances are that you also will be able to tell them when you are feeling sad, disappointed, angry, or frustrated. However, it's important to realize that some people were not raised in affectionate families or a culture supportive of open expressions, do not readily discuss feelings or emotions, and sometimes may struggle to find the right words for expressing what they feel.

When two people begin a relationship, they bring their communication styles with them.[3] How often have you heard someone say, "We just can't communicate," or "You're sending mixed messages"? These exchanges occur regularly as people start relationships or work through communication problems in an existing relationship. Because communication is a process, our every action, word, facial expression, gesture, or body posture becomes part of our shared history and part of the evolving impression we make on others. If we are angry in our responses, others will be reluctant to interact with us. If we bring "baggage" from past bad interactions to new relationships, we may be cynical, distrustful, and guarded in our exchanges with others. If we are positive, happy, and share openly with others, they will be more likely to communicate openly with us. This ability to communicate assertively is an important skill in relationships (see Improving Communication Skills below). Assertive communicators are in touch with their feelings and values and able to directly and honestly communicate their needs or defend choices in a positive manner.

## Improving Communication Skills

Because people have such different ways of communicating, there is no recipe for how to communicate effectively in a given situation. At times, silence may be the best approach. However, there are things that each of us can do to become better communicators and to encourage and assist others in their attempts to interact with us.

### Learning Appropriate Self-Disclosure

Sharing personal information with others is called **self-disclosure.** If you are willing to share personal information with others, they will likely share personal information with you. In other words, if you want to learn more about someone, you have to be willing to share parts of your personal self with that person. Self-disclosure is not storytelling or sharing secrets; rather, it is revealing how you are reacting to the present situation and giving information about the past relevant to the other person's understanding of your current reactions.[4]

Self-disclosure can be a double-edged sword, for there is risk in divulging personal insights and feelings. If you sense that sharing feelings and personal thoughts will result in a closer relationship, you will likely take the risk. But if you believe that self-disclosure may result in rejection or alienation, you may not open up so easily. If the confidentiality of previously shared information has been violated, you may hesitate to disclose yourself in the future.

### Being a Better Listener

Listening is a vital part of interpersonal communication; it allows us to share feelings, express concerns, communicate wants and needs, and let our thoughts and opinions be known. We must do the necessary work to improve our speaking and listening skills, which will enhance our relationships, improve our grasp of information, and allow us to interpret more effectively what others say. We listen best when (1) we believe that the message is somehow important and relevant to us, (2) the speaker holds our attention through humour, dramatic effect, use of media, or other techniques, and (3) we are in the mood to listen (free of distractions and worries). When we listen effectively, we try to understand what people are thinking and feeling from their perspective. We not only hear the words, but we try to understand what is really

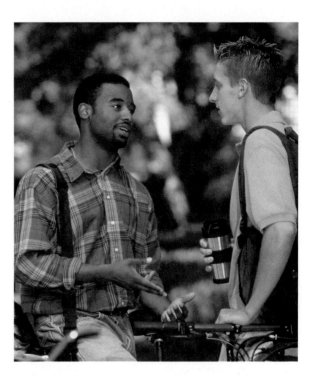

*Listening is a key component of communication.*

being said. How many times have you been caught pretending to be listening when you were not? After several moments of nodding and saying "uh-huh," your friend finally asks you a question, and you haven't a clue about what she has been saying. Sometimes this tuned-out behaviour is due to a lack of sleep, stress overload, being preoccupied, having too much to drink, or being under the influence of drugs. Other times it's because speakers are motor-mouths who talk for the sake of talking or you find them or what they are talking about boring. Some of the most common listening difficulties are things that we can work to improve.

# CHARACTERISTICS OF INTIMATE RELATIONSHIPS

There are many possible definitions of **intimate relationships.** One classic definition calls these relationships "close relationships with another person in which you offer, and are offered, validation, understanding, and a sense of being valued intellectually,

**Self-disclosure:** Sharing personal feelings or information with others.

**Intimate relationships:** "Close relationships with another person in which you offer, and are offered, validation, understanding, and a sense of being valued intellectually, emotionally, and physically."

# Learning to Really Listen

Most of us have lamented the fact that someone "never listens" and seems to monopolize the entire conversation. Although we are quick to recognize such flaws in others, we are often less likely to spot our own poor listening skills. On a daily basis, we have times when we simply "tune out." When a professor drones on about a subject we don't relate to, we begin doodling or put on a fake interested expression, even though we are thinking about dinner or what to wear to go out that night. When a friend or colleague tells the same story over and over again, we say "uh-huh"—and worry that we'll be caught when we're asked a question and don't have a clue what he or she is talking about. We grimace at the thought of certain people calling but dash for the phone when the caller ID indicates that it is someone we love to talk with. What is the difference? Why do we tune out when some people speak and tune in for others?

We gravitate toward those who seem to understand us and with whom we have fun and interesting interactions. If truth be told, most of us are only mediocre listeners.

What does it take to be an excellent listener? Practise the following skills and consciously use them on a daily basis as an important part of improving your communication.

- *Be present in the moment.* Contrary to what is often believed, good listeners don't just sit back with their mouths shut. They participate and acknowledge what the other person is saying. (Nodding, smiling, saying "yes" or "uh-huh," and asking reflective questions at appropriate times are all part of this. Take care, however, not to numbly say "uh-huh" too frequently since it can be distracting and convey insincerity.)

- *Use positive body language and voice tone.* Show that you are "with" the speaker by turning toward him or her and staying focused (wandering eyes are a sure sign that your mind is elsewhere). Avoid barrier gestures such as shaking your head "no," making negative faces, or folding your arms; smile at appropriate times and maintain appropriate eye contact (deadpan stares can be distracting). Voice tone, posture, and an attitude that conveys interest are important.

- *Show empathy and sympathy.* Watching for verbal and non-verbal clues to the other person's feelings and trying to relate can be very useful. For example, saying, "That must have been really hard for you" can encourage the speaker to talk and feel more comfortable with you as an understanding listener.

- *Ask for clarification.* If you aren't sure what the speaker means, indicate that you're not sure you understand, or paraphrase what you think you heard. This kind of feedback is invaluable in avoiding misinterpretation and lapses in overall communication. As a speaker, you may ask, "What did you think I was just saying?" but be sure to say this in a nonthreatening manner.

- *Control that deadly desire to interrupt.* Some people start nodding and gesturing before you ever get a word out of your mouth. If you are like that, squelch it, even if you have to put an inconspicuous hand over your mouth. Try taking a deep breath for two seconds, then hold your breath for another second and really listen to what is being said as you slowly exhale. Don't be so enthusiastically empathetic that you finish speakers' sentences or put words in people's mouths.

- *Avoid snap judgments based on what other people look like or are saying.* If you notice some strange mannerism, try to focus on what is being said, not how it is being said. Avoid stereotyping or labelling.

- *Resist the temptation to "set the other person straight."* Control your urge to correct errors or react defensively. Listen and hear without reacting or trying to rationalize what the speaker is trying to say.

- *Try to focus on the speaker.* Sometimes it is very tough to listen to someone who is trying to talk about a painful situation, especially if we are experiencing or have recently experienced something similar. Hold back the temptation to "tell all" and fly off into your own rendition. Give the speaker the moment and later, after he or she is done talking, you may talk about your own experience as a way of validating the feelings expressed. Don't tell him how he is feeling or how he should feel.

- *Be tenacious.* Stick with the speaker and try to stay on the topic. If they seem to wander, gently nudge them back by saying, "You were just saying. . . ." Offer your thoughts and suggestions, but remember that you should advise only up to a certain point. Clarify statements with "this is my opinion" as a reminder that it is only opinion, rather than fact.

emotionally, and physically."[5] In this context, friends, family, lovers, partners, and even people you work with or interact with at the grocery store may be included in the sphere of intimate interactions. For the purposes of this chapter, we define intimate relationships in terms of three characteristics: *behavioural interdependence, need fulfillment,* and *emotional attachment.* Each of these characteristics may be related to interactions with family, close friends, and romantic relationships.[6]

Behavioural interdependence refers to the mutual impact that people have on each other as their lives and daily activities become intertwined. What one person does may influence what the other person may want and can do. Such interdependence may become stronger over time to the point that each person would find a void in his or her life if the other person left.

Another characteristic of intimate relationships is that they fulfill psychological needs and, as such, are a means of need fulfillment. These needs may often be met only through relationships with others:

- *The need for approval and for a sense of purpose in life*—requiring the sense that what we say and do counts.
- *The need for intimacy*—requiring someone with whom we can share our feelings freely.
- *The need for social integration*—requiring someone with whom we can share our worries and concerns.
- *The need for being nurturing*—requiring someone whom we can take care of.
- *The need for being nurtured*—requiring someone who can take care of us.
- *The need for reassurance or affirmation of our own worth*—requiring someone to tell us that we matter.

In other words, rewarding, intimate relationships, partners, or friends meet each other's needs. They disclose feelings, share confidences, and discuss practical concerns; they help each other and provide reassurance. They serve as major sources of social support and reinforce our feelings that we are important and serve a purpose in life.

In addition to behavioural interdependence and need fulfillment, intimate relationships involve strong bonds of *emotional attachment,* or feelings of love and attachment. The intimacy level experienced by any two people cannot easily be judged by those outside the relationship. Although sex may often be an important part of an intimate relationship, a relationship may be very intimate without it. In fact, many satisfying and lasting intimate relationships go well beyond the need for sexual contact.

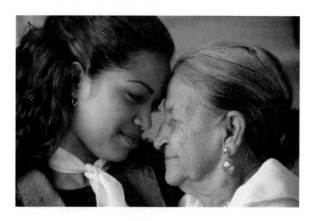

*Emotional bonding and other elements of intimate relationships are rooted in a caring, supportive family environment.*

psychologically by making ourselves unavailable emotionally. For example, after the end of a relationship, a young person may close down emotionally and carefully avoid letting her- or himself feel too much. This allows time for regrouping and healing before reaching out to people again. It also reduces the risk of a rebound romance that is often doomed to failure as a result of unresolved personal hurts and issues.

# FORMING INTIMATE RELATIONSHIPS

Throughout our lives, we go through predictable patterns of relationships. In our early years, our most significant relationships are with our families. Gradually, our relationships widen to include friends, co-workers, and acquaintances. Ultimately, most of us develop romantic or sexual relationships with significant others. Each of these relationships plays a significant role in psychological, social, spiritual, and physical health.

## Families: The Ties That Bind

Although many people consider the family the foundation of Canadian society and talk about a return to "family values" as a desirable objective, it is clear that the modern Canadian family looks quite different from families of previous generations. The *Leave It to Beaver* family type encouraged during the 1950s—Mom with her apron, staying at home, content with her role as mother and spouse; Dad with his briefcase, trying to move up the corporate ladder;

**Emotional availability,** the ability to give to and receive from others emotionally without fear of being hurt or rejected, is another characteristic of intimate relationships. At times, all of us may need to protect ourselves

**Emotional availability:** The ability to give to and receive from other people emotionally without being inhibited by fears of being hurt.

and two or three happy, well-adjusted children—is no longer the norm. More than half of today's moms work outside the home, and many children are raised by single parents, grandparents, relatives, stepparents, nannies, day-care centre workers, and other "parents."

Regardless of the form or structure of each family, all families should care for, protect, love, and socialize with one another. Whether the family is related by birth, a high level of love and regard, living arrangement, or some other factor, the family network often provides the sense of security needed to develop into healthy adults. The definition of *family* changes dramatically from culture to culture and from place to place over time.

The Vanier Institute of the Family defines family as "any combination of two or more persons bound together over time by ties of mutual consent, birth or adoption/placement and who, together, assume responsibilities for variant combinations of the following: physical maintenance and care of family members; addition of new members; socialization of children; social control of members; production, consumption and distribution of goods and services; love and affective nurturance."[7]

## Today's Family Unit

The United Nations defines seven basic types of families, including single-parent families, communal families (unrelated people living together for ideological, economic, or other reasons), extended families, and others. But most of us think of family in terms of the "family of origin" or the "nuclear family." The *family of origin* includes the people present in the household during a child's first years of life—usually parents and siblings. However, the family of origin may also include a stepparent, parents' lovers, or significant others such as grandparents, aunts, or uncles. The family of origin has a tremendous impact on the child's psychological, social, and spiritual development. The *nuclear family* consists of parents (usually, but not necessarily, married) and their offspring.

If parents are comfortable in sharing feelings, affection, and love with each other and their offspring, their children are likely to become emotionally connected adults. If the home environment provides stability and seems a safe place to be, it is likely that the children will learn to express feelings and develop intimacy skills. Sibling interactions provide a way to learn and practise interpersonal skills.[8] The family of origin and the nuclear family have the potential for encouraging significant positive interactions and growth. People can practise positive behaviours and learn the rights and wrongs of negative behaviours in a safe and nonjudgmental environment when the family itself is healthy However, if the family is psychologically or physically unhealthy, it may pose significant barriers to later relationships.

## Establishing Friendships

A Friend is one who knows you as you are,

understands where you've been,

accepts who you've become,

and still gently invites you to grow.

—*Author Unknown*

Although most of us have a fairly clear idea of the distinction between a friend and a lover, this difference is not always easy to verbalize. Some people believe that the major difference is that there is no intimate physical involvement between friends. Others have suggested that intimacy levels are much lower between friends than between lovers. But, as we have stated, people can be intimate with each other without being sexually involved. Confused? You are probably not alone. Surprisingly, there has not been a great deal of research to clarify these terms. Beyond the fact that two people participate in a relationship as equals, friendships include the following characteristics:[9]

- *Enjoyment.* Friends enjoy each other's company, although there may be temporary states of anger, disappointment, or mutual annoyance.

- *Acceptance.* Friends accept each other as they are, without trying to change the other person.

- *Trust.* Friends have mutual trust in the sense that each assumes that the other will act in his or her friend's best interests.

- *Respect.* Friends respect each other in the sense that each assumes that the other exercises good judgment in making life choices.

- *Mutual assistance.* Friends are inclined to assist and support one another. They can count on each other in times of need, trouble, or personal distress, as well as in positive times, worthy of celebration.

- *Confiding.* Friends share experiences and feelings with each other that they don't share with other people.

- *Understanding.* Friends have a sense of what is important to each other and why each person behaves as he or she does. Friends are usually not puzzled or mystified by each other's actions.

- *Spontaneity.* Friends feel free to be themselves in the relationship rather than play a role, wear a mask, or refrain from revealing their true self.

## Significant Others, Partners, Couples

Although family and friends provide necessary intimate relationships, most people choose at some point whether or not to enter into an intimate sexual relationship with another person. Most couples fit into one of four categories of significant sexual or committed relationships: married heterosexual couples, cohabiting heterosexual couples, married lesbian and gay couples, and cohabiting lesbian and gay couples. Love relationships in each of these four groups typically include all the characteristics of friendship as well as characteristics related to passion and caring:[10]

- *Fascination.* Lovers tend to pay attention to the other person even when they should be involved in other activities. They are preoccupied with the other person and want to think about, look at, talk to, or merely be with him or her.

- *Exclusiveness.* Lovers have a special relationship that usually precludes having the same relationship with a third party. The love relationship takes priority over all others.

- *Sexual desire.* Lovers want physical intimacy with their partner, desiring to touch, hold, and engage in sexual activities. However, they may choose not to act on these feelings because of religious, moral, or other practical considerations.

- *Giving the utmost.* Lovers care enough to give the utmost when the other is in need, sometimes to the point of extreme self-sacrifice.

- *Being a champion/advocate.* The depth of lovers' caring may show up as an active, unselfish championing of each other's interests and a positive attempt to ensure that the other succeeds.

For obvious reasons, the best love relationships share friendships, and the best friendships include several love components. Both relationships share common bonds of nurturance, enhancement of personal well-being, and a genuine sense of mutual regard, trust, and security.

## This Thing Called Love

What is love? Defining love is more difficult than simply listing characteristics of a loving relationship. Love has been written about and engraved on walls; it has been the theme of countless novels, poems, movies, songs, and plays. There is no one definition of *love,* and the word may mean different things to people depending on cultural values, age, sex, and situation.

Many social scientists maintain that love may be of two kinds: companionate and passionate. *Companionate* love is a secure, trusting attachment, similar to what we often feel for family members or close friends. In companionate love, two people are attracted, have much in common, care about each other's well-being, and express reciprocal liking and respect. *Passionate* love involves a state of high arousal filled with the ecstasy of being loved or the agony of being rejected.[11] The person experiencing passionate love tends to be preoccupied with his or her partner and to perceive the loved person as perfect.[12] Passionate love will not occur unless three conditions are met.[13] First, the person must live in a culture in which the concept of "falling in love" is idealized. Second, a "suitable" person to love must be present. If the culture a person is immersed in—including influence from parents, movies, books, songs, peers, and the like—projects the need to seek a particular partner with a certain level of attractiveness or belonging to a certain racial group or with a certain socioeconomic status, and none is available, the "seeker" may find it difficult to allow him- or herself to become involved. Finally, for passionate love to happen, there must be some type of physiological arousal that occurs when a person is in the presence of the object of desire. Sexual excitement is often the way this arousal is expressed.

In the "triangular theory of love," love is clarified by isolating three key ingredients:

- *Intimacy.* The emotional component, which involves feelings of closeness.

- *Passion.* The motivational component, which reflects romantic, sexual attraction.

- *Decision/commitment.* The cognitive component, which includes the decisions you make about being in love and the degree of commitment to your partner.

According to this model, the greater the intimacy, passion, and commitment, the more likely a person is to be involved in a healthy, positive love relationship (see Table 5.1).

In regard to attraction and the process of falling in love, a fairly predictable pattern is followed based on (1) *imprinting,* in which our evolutionary patterns, genetic predispositions, and past experiences trigger romantic reaction; (2) *attraction,* in which neurochemicals produce feelings of euphoria and elation; (3) *attachment,* in which endorphins— natural opiates—cause lovers to feel peaceful, secure, and calm; and (4) *production of a cuddle chemical,* in which the brain secretes the chemical oxytocin, thereby stimulating sensations during lovemaking and eliciting feelings of satisfaction and attachment.[14]

Lovers who claim to be swept away by passion may not, therefore, be far from the truth:

> A meeting of the eyes, a touch of the hands or a whiff of scent may set off a flood that starts in the brain and races along the nerves and through the blood. The familiar results—flushed skin, sweaty palms, heavy breathing—are identical to those experienced when under stress. Why? Because the love-smitten person is secreting chemical substances such as dopamine, norepinephrine, and phenylethylamine (PEA) that are chemical cousins of amphetamines.[15]

TABLE 5.1
The Triangular Theory of Love: Types of Relationships

|  | Intimacy | Passion | Decision and Commitment |
| --- | --- | --- | --- |
| Nonlove | Low | Low | Low |
| Liking | High | Low | Low |
| Infatuated love | Low | High | Low |
| Romantic love | High | High | Low |
| Empty love | Low | Low | High |
| Companionate love | High | Low | High |
| Fatuous love | Low | High | High |
| Consummate love | High | High | High |

Source: R. J. Sternberg, "The Triangular Theory of Love," *Psychological Review 93* (1986): 119–135. Copyright 1986 by the American Psychological Association. Reprinted by permission.

Although attraction may in fact be a "natural high," with PEA levels soaring, this hit of passion loses effectiveness over time as the body builds up a tolerance. Needing a continual fix of passion, many people may become attraction junkies, seeking the intoxication of love in a way similar to the drug user who seeks a chemical high.[16]

It has been speculated that PEA levels drop significantly over a three- to four-year period, relating to the "four-year itch" that shows up in the peaking fourth-year divorce rates present in more than 60 cultures. Those romances that last beyond the four-year decline of PEA are influenced by another set of chemicals known as endorphins, soothing substances that give lovers a sense of security, peace, and calm.[17]

In another theory, researchers describe the first stage as the *lust phase,* in which our biological and genetic histories converge to pique our interest and intensity of response. In the lust phase, if someone comes into our range of awareness a chemical surge can trigger our enthusiastic response. Known as *pheromones* and said to be as unique as our fingerprints, these triggers are scent-infused chemicals found in perspiration under the armpits. They trigger a unique sensory reaction in the nose and result in attraction if their producer is a match for you.[18] Following these pheromone triggers comes the *attraction phase,* often labelled the falling in love phase, and then the *attachment phase.* The two hormones most important in this last phase are oxytocin and vasopressin. Oxytocin increases the bond between lovers, is released by both sexes during orgasm, and is one of the chemicals responsible for contractions during childbirth and milk expression when breastfeeding. Scientists suspect vasopressin to be the chemical responsible for creating the desire to be monogamous with another person. The science behind this is relatively new, but the implications are interesting. The theory suggests that the more sex a couple has, the greater the bond between them.[19]

In addition to the possible chemical influences, our past experiences may significantly affect our attractions for others. Our parents' modelling of traits we believe are desirable or undesirable may play a role in drawing us to people with similar traits. Many researchers have investigated the possible link between males seeking partners similar to their mothers and females seeking partners similar to their fathers.

# GENDER ISSUES

In any relationship, understanding and communication are important ingredients for success. Sometimes it may seem that the relating styles of men and women are so different that obtaining true understanding and open communication may be next to impossible. Men's and women's social conditioning is so different that it is almost as if they are raised in two different cultures.[20] Women are brought up to feel comfortable and to share freely in their intimate relationships. As a

# Is It Love or Infatuation?

In the early stages, love and infatuation can be very similar emotions. They both produce a characteristic rush of excitement as well as a strong desire to have more of the loved one's time, energy, and contact. The primary difference is that with love, the feelings often grow deeper as you get to know the person better and come to appreciate him or her more. With infatuation or a crush, you begin to realize that Ms. or Mr. Right wasn't all you had thought. Taking the following test may help you determine whether it's the real thing or merely a case of infatuation. Respond YES or NO to the following statements:

1. I knew I was in love with the person almost immediately.
2. Even though I've known the person for a while, I still really love his/her personality.
3. I wonder sometimes if the person has changed a lot since I've known him/her because he/she acts differently around me now.
4. The more I'm with the person, the more I want to be around him/her.
5. I am less interested in the person sexually than I was in the beginning.
6. The more I know about the person, the more I want to know.
7. The more I know about the person, the less interested I am in him/her.
8. I feel really good associating with this person and being regarded as a couple.
9. I have begun to notice more things wrong with this person and spend a lot of time trying to get him/her to change.
10. Even though I have been with this person for a while, I am still as sexually interested as I was in the beginning.
11. I find that I'd just as soon do things with other people as with this person because I'd probably have more fun.
12. I am able to share my feelings with this person and trust him/her completely.
13. I really love this person but don't feel good about sharing intimate feelings with him/her yet.
14. This person brings out the best in me and genuinely seems to care about me.
15. I love this person, but I don't respect him/her the way I respect others.

## SCORING

There are no right or wrong responses to these statements. However, answering YES to the even-numbered statements may indicate that your feelings are more likely to be love-directed. In contrast, answering YES to the odd-numbered statements may indicate a tendency toward infatuation rather than love. Count the number of YES responses to the even-numbered statements and the number of YES responses to the odd-numbered statements. Look carefully at each statement. Are these things that you feel are important enough to work on? Or are your responses telling you that another person may be a better choice?

---

result, they tend to be more nurturing and less afraid to share their fears, anxieties, and emotions. It's okay if they cry, scream, or express wide emotional swings. Big boys, however, are not supposed to cry—at least according to popular beliefs. Unlike their female counterparts, they are not supposed to show emotions, and are brought up believing that being strong is often more important than close friendships. As a result, only one in ten males has a close male friend to whom he divulges his innermost thoughts.[21]

## Why the Differences?

Although there are various theories about why males and females relate the way they do, the most comprehensive analysis indicates a serious barrier to intimacy because of a basic difference in the development patterns of men and women.[22] Accordingly, men are less able to express emotions and achieve intimacy owing to the process of identity development in infancy, which is often more difficult for males than females. Males initially achieve intimacy with a female caregiver, usually a mother, at a preverbal stage. By the time they develop verbal skills, boys have physically separated from their caregiver. Thus, for males, intimacy may consist of physical proximity rather than verbal sharing. Because females do not need to separate themselves from a female caregiver, they do not separate their feelings of intimacy from their verbal constructs. As a result, women are often able to express intimacy verbally, whereas men often are not. This male/female disparity in the ability to express emotions is the single greatest difference between the sexes and the greatest threat to intimacy in many relationships. This theory has received widespread acceptance among sociologists and psychologists. The disparity in the ability to express emotions may account for common female complaints about male attitudes toward sex; emotion generates sexual feelings in women, whereas sexual feelings generate emotion in men. Sex, it seems, is one area in which men are allowed to contact deeper emotional states. In fact, sexual activity carries the major burden of emotional expression for many males and may explain the urgency with which some men approach sex.

## WHAT WOULD YOU DO?

To whom do you feel most comfortable talking about very personal issues? Do you talk with males and females about these issues, or do you tend to gravitate toward just one sex? Why do you think you do this? Similarly, who most frequently shares personal issues with you? Are males and females equally likely to open up to you, or just one sex? Why do you think they do this?

## Picking Partners: Similarities and Differences between Genders

Just as males and females may find different ways to express themselves, the process of partner selection also shows distinct patterns. In males and females, more than chemical and psychological processes influence the choice of partners.[23] One of these factors is proximity, or being in the same place at the same time. The more you see a person in your hometown, at social gatherings, or at work, the more likely an interaction will occur. Thus, if you live in Winnipeg, you'll probably end up with another Winnipegger. If you live on Prince Edward Island, you'll probably end up with another Islander.

You also pick a partner on the basis of similarities (attitudes, values, intellect, interests); the adage that "opposites attract" usually isn't true. Even though you may initially be attracted to someone extremely different from you, first flames usually die quickly and there is a subliminal hunt for common ground. If your potential partner expresses interest or liking, you may react with mutual regard, known as *reciprocity*. The more you express interest, the safer it is for someone else to return the regard, and the cycle spirals onward.

Another factor that apparently plays a significant role in selecting a partner is physical attraction. Whether such attraction is caused by a chemical reaction or a socially learned behaviour, males and females appear to have different attraction criteria. Men tend to select their mates primarily on the basis of youth and physical attractiveness. Although physical attractiveness is an important criterion for women in mate selection, they tend to place greater emphasis on partners who are somewhat older, have

good financial prospects, and are dependable and industrious. Good grooming is an almost universally desirable trait for all. If you smell or appear less than squeaky clean, you may have problems in the partner arena regardless of your sex.

# BARRIERS TO INTIMACY

Obstacles to intimacy include lack of personal identity, emotional immaturity, and a poorly developed sense of responsibility. The fear of being hurt, low self-esteem, mishandled hostility, chronic "busyness" (and its attendant lack of emotional presence), a tendency to "parentify" loved ones, and a conflict of role expectations may be equally detrimental. In addition, individual insecurities and difficulties in recognizing and expressing emotional needs can lead to an intimacy barrier. These barriers to intimacy may have many causes, including the different emotional development of men and women or an upbringing in a dysfunctional family.

## Dysfunctional Families

As noted earlier, the ability to sustain genuine intimacy is largely developed in the family of origin. Unfortunately, sharing, trust, and openness do not always occur in the family. In fact, the assumption that such intimacy existed in the family of origin may actually be unrealistic. As adults, we may discover that although we thought our family encouraged emotional intimacy, it was actually judgmental, full of expectations, controlling, and, in many ways, dysfunctional. A **dysfunctional family** is one in which the interaction between family members inhibits psychological growth rather than encouraging self-love, emotional expression, and individual growth. If you were to examine even the most pristine family under a microscope, you would likely find some type of dysfunction. No group of people who live together day in and day out can interact perfectly all the time. However, many people have begun to overuse the term dysfunctional to refer to even the smallest problems in the family unit. True dysfunctionality refers to settings where negative interactions are the norm rather than the exception. Children raised in these settings tend to face tremendous obstacles to growing up healthy. Coming to terms with past hurts may take years. However, with careful planning and introspection, support from loved ones, and counselling when needed, children from even the worst homes have proved to be remarkably resilient. Many are able to

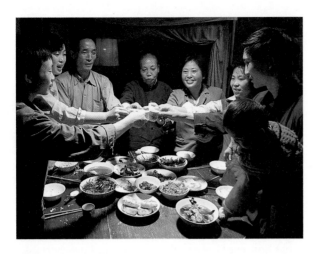

*The negative interactions in dysfunctional families that damage self-esteem and deter psychosocial growth do not exist in healthy families that encourage emotional intimacy.*

leave the past and focus on the future, developing into healthy, well-adjusted adults.[24] It is important to note that dysfunctional families are found in every social, ethnic, religious, economic, and racial group.

For more than a decade, social scientists studied the impact of the alcoholic home environment on the sexual and intimate behaviours of adult children of alcoholics (ACOAs). A number of intimacy problems have been identified as typical of ACOAs. Many ACOAs claim that they become involved in unhealthy relationships and have difficulty trusting others, problems in communicating with partners, and difficulty defining a healthy relationship.[25]

Another large group of people struggling with intimacy problems originating in the family of origin are survivors of childhood emotional, physical, or sexual abuse. Experiencing or witnessing physical, sexual, or emotional abuse as a child can have an impact on a person's intimate relationships as an adult. Domestic violence, whether directed at a child or another family member, can affect a child's ability to trust others and to maintain an intimate relationship later in life. Physical abuse may vary from spanking to violent beatings. Sexual abuse refers to any suggestive conversations, inappropriate kissing, touching, petting, oral, anal, or vaginal intercourse or any other kinds of sexual interaction between a child and an older child or adult. Emotional abuse includes name-calling and other tactics that damage a child's self-esteem.

## Jealousy in Relationships

**Jealousy** is an aversive reaction evoked by a real or imagined relationship involving your partner and another person. Contrary to what many believe,

jealousy is not a sign of intense devotion or of passionate love for the person who is the target of it. Instead, jealousy is often a sign of underlying problems that may prove to be a significant barrier to a healthy, intimate relationship. The roots of jealous feelings and behaviours may run deep and typically include:

- *Overdependence on the relationship.* People who have few social ties and rely exclusively on their significant others tend to be fearful of losing them.

- *High value on sexual exclusivity.* People who believe that sexual exclusiveness is a crucial indicator of a love relationship are more likely to become jealous. As the expectation of sexual exclusivity increases, the likelihood of becoming jealous also increases.

- *Severity of the threat.* People may feel uneasy if a person with a fantastic body, stunning good looks, and a great personality appears interested in their partner. But they may brush off the threat if they appraise the person as "unworthy" in terms of appearance or other characteristics.

- *Low self-esteem.* People who feel good about themselves are less likely to feel unworthy and to fear that someone else is going to snatch their partner away from them. The underlying question that torments people with low self-esteem is, "Why would anyone want me?" Thus, everyone other than the "beloved" becomes a threat.

- *Fear of losing control.* Some people need to feel in control of the situation. Feeling that they may be losing the attachment of or control over a partner can cause jealousy.

# COMMITTED RELATIONSHIPS

Feelings of love or sexual attraction do not always equal commitment in a relationship. There can be love—or sex—without commitment. Commitment in a relationship means that there is an intent to act over time in a way that perpetuates the well-being of the other person, you, and the relationship. A committed relationship involves tremendous diligence on the part of both partners. Over the years, partners learn about one another and constantly adjust the direction of

**Dysfunctional family:** A family in which the interaction between family members inhibits rather than enhances psychological growth.

**Jealousy:** An aversive reaction evoked by a real or imagined relationship involving a person's partner and another person.

their relationship. What separates committed from uncommitted relationships is the willingness of committed partners to dedicate themselves to acquiring and using the skills that will ensure a lasting relationship.

## Marriage

Marriage is the traditional committed relationship in many societies around the world. For many people, marriage is the ultimate expression of an intimate relationship. When two people marry in Canada, they enter into a legal agreement that includes shared financial plans, property, and responsibility in raising children. For religious people, marriage is also a sacrament that stresses the spirituality, rights, and obligations of each person.

In 2005, of the total population 48.5 percent were legally married, living common law, or legally separated; 41.8 percent were single; 4.9 percent were divorced; and 4.8 percent were widowed.[26] There were 151,334 marriages in 2005, over 5,000 more than in the previous year.[27] In the most recent year that data were available, 2003, there were 10,828 divorces.[28]

Most people believe that marriage involves **monogamy,** or exclusive sexual involvement with one partner. The lifetime pattern for many Canadians appears to be **serial monogamy,** which means that a person has a monogamous sexual relationship with one partner for the duration of a relationship before moving on to another monogamous relationship. Some people prefer to have an **open relationship,** or open marriage, in which the partners agree that each person may become sexually involved outside their relationship.

Humans are not naturally monogamous; that is, most of us are capable of being sexually or emotionally involved with more than one person at a time. Yet Canadian society frowns on involvement with an outsider when involved in a committed relationship. Many people find themselves attracted to others while in a relationship and consciously try to stop subsequent interactions. Others find themselves involved unintentionally. Still others actively seek out extra-relationship affairs. Whether by choice or chance, sexual infidelity is a common factor in many divorces and break-ups. Perhaps only those having strong self-images and a dedication to the principles of open relationships are able to maintain non-monogamy over a period of time.

As with all relationships, there are marriages that work well and bring much satisfaction to the partners, and there are marriages that are unhealthy for the people involved. A good marriage can yield much support and stability, not only for the couple, but also for those involved in the couple's life. Considerable research also indicates that married people live longer, are happier, remain mentally alert longer, and suffer fewer bouts of physical and mental ailments. However, traditional marriage does not work for everyone and is not the only path to a happy and successful committed relationship.

## Cohabitation

**Cohabitation** is defined as two unmarried people with an intimate connection who live together in the same household. The relationship can be very stable, with a high level of commitment between the partners. In the latest Canadian census data available (2001), common-law couples comprised 14 percent of all "couple families" compared to 6 percent in 1981. Married couples accounted for 70 percent of all families in 2001, down from 83 percent in 1981.[29] Between 1995 and 2001, the number of couples living common-law rose 20 percent to nearly 1.2 million couples. In contrast, the number of married couples increased by just 3 percent, growing to 6.4 million.[30] More than 40 percent of men and women aged 30 to 39 in 2001 were expected to choose a common-law union as their first union; for those aged 20 to 29, the percentage was estimated to reach 53 percent for women.[31]

The increase in common-law marriages may be partly attributed to youth's inclination to question traditional values and recognizing that marriage may not be the only legitimate basis for sexual relations. The availability of cheaper, more effective birth control has probably been another factor. Many couples also believe that living together simply because they want to may be more important than being bound by a legal document.

Although cohabitation is a viable alternative for some, many cohabitors eventually marry because of pressures from parents and friends, difficulties in obtaining insurance and tax benefits, legal issues over property, and a host of other reasons. The disadvantage of cohabitation lies in the lack of societal validation for the relationship and, in some cases, in the societal disapproval of living together without being married. Cohabiting partners do not usually experience the social incentives to stay together that they would if they were married. If they decide to separate, however, they do not experience the legal problems involved in going through a divorce. In most provinces, cohabitation that lasts more than six months is viewed as a **common-law marriage** in the eyes of the court on issues of child care and spousal support. It is not the same,

## It's a Quiet Thing: Equal Marriage Is Law

Marriage for same-sex couples is now the law in Canada. Bill C-38 was passed into law by the Canadian Senate on July 19, 2005. The following evening, Chief Justice Beverly McLaughlin gave the bill royal assent

The law was debated for more than five years in courtrooms, cabinet rooms, and living rooms across the country. The language of the debate reflected more than simply small wording changes to the marriage law, but rather how marriage is defined. Specifically, many debates were over whether individuals in same-sex unions formed families. Undoubtedly, the law indicated that such unions can and do form families.

The lack of "noise" made over this historic law (158 voted in favour and 133 against) in Canada indicates that the world simply continues, as it should.

Source: Adapted from K. Bourassa and J. Varnell, "It's a Quiet Thing: Equal Marriage Is Law: Marriage Receives Senate Approval & Royal Assent." Retrieved on May 9, 2006, from www.samesexmarriage.ca/legal/qui210705.htm.

however, as becoming legally married. Some laws treat common-law spouses the same as married spouses. For example, parents' responsibilities to their children are the same whether the parents are married to each other or not. On the other hand, some laws apply to married people and not to common-law couples, such as the one that divides matrimonial property. In still other situations, how the law treats a common-law couple depends on how long they have lived together. For example, Employment Canada considers moving to be with a spouse a valid reason to quit a job, and, for this purpose, considers a couple who have been living together for at least one year to be spouses.[32]

### Gay and Lesbian Partnerships

Most people seek intimate, committed relationships during their adult years. This is no different for homosexual couples. Lesbians and gay men are socialized like other people in our culture and place a high value on relationships. They seek the same things in their primary relationships as heterosexual partners: friendship, communication, validation, companionship, and a sense of stability. Studies of lesbian couples indicate high levels of attachment and satisfaction and a tendency toward monogamous, long-term relationships. Gay men, too, tend to form committed, long-term relationships, especially as they age.[33]

Challenges to successful homosexual relationships often stem from the discrimination they face and to difficulties dealing with social, legal, and religious doctrines. On July 19, 2005, Canada redefined the legal and social boundaries of marriage to include same-sex couples. For details, see the Health in the Media box "It's a Quiet Thing: Equal Marriage Is Law."

## SUCCESS IN COMMITTED RELATIONSHIPS

Because the traditional marriage ceremony includes the vow "till death do us part," the definition of success in a relationship tends to be based on whether a couple stays together over the years. Marriage has become the model to which relationships must conform to be considered stable or healthy. One reason for the increase in cohabitation and other alternative relationships is the need for new forms in which people can express their love and commitment to one another and still have individual needs met adequately. Success in relating to another human being may have more to do with the quality of the interaction between two people than with the number of years they live together. Many social scientists agree that the ideal in relating to another person is to develop a committed bond, the boundaries and form of which can—and

**Monogamy:** Exclusive sexual involvement with one partner.

**Serial monogamy:** Monogamous sexual relationship with one partner before moving on to another.

**Open relationship:** A relationship in which partners agree that there can be sexual involvement outside the relationship.

**Cohabitation:** Living together without being married.

**Common-law marriage:** Cohabitation lasting at least six months is treated as equivalent to marriage for some, but not all, legal purposes.

should—change to allow the maximum degree of growth over time.

## Partnering Scripts

Most parents love their children and want them to be happy. They often believe that their children will achieve happiness by living much as they have. Accordingly, children are reared with a very strong script for what is expected of them as adults. Each group in society has its own partnering script that prescribes standards regarding sex, age, social class, race, religion, physical attributes, and personality types. By adolescence, people generally know exactly what type of person they are expected to befriend or to date.

Society provides constant reinforcement for traditional couples. People who choose an "appropriate" partner usually have plenty of validation for the relationship. The love and support they feel from friends and family is genuine. It also comes with expectations of what will occur within the relationship. Decisions that the couple feels should be exclusively theirs may provoke unsolicited advice from friends and family.

As Canadian society becomes increasingly multicultural, in-group partnering is giving way to more frequent mixing of cultures and backgrounds. Nonetheless, a relationship between people of different cultural backgrounds often brings increased tension partly because of the lack of societal reinforcement. In addition to a lack of recognition to non-traditional couples, friends and family often blame the non-traditional nature of the couple if the relationship fails.

### WHAT WOULD YOU DO?

By which partnering script were you raised? Would your parents be happy if you brought a same-sex partner into your home? Or a partner of a different race, religion, or ethnicity?

### WHAT WOULD YOU DO?

What characteristics are most important to you in a potential partner? Which of these would be important to your parents or friends? If your parents or friends didn't like a potential partner, how important would their opinion be?

## The Importance of Self-Nurturance

It is often stated that you must love yourself before you can love someone else. What does this mean? Learning how you function emotionally and how to nurture yourself through all life's situations is a lifelong task. There seems to be a certain level of individual maturity that needs to be reached before a successful intimate relationship becomes possible. One can look to age of marriage and divorce rates for support. More than half of marriages between teenagers end in divorce. The divorce rate drops to 37 percent among people over 25 years of age at marriage.

Two concepts especially important to knowing yourself and maintaining a good relationship are accountability and self-nurturance. **Accountability** means that both partners see themselves as responsible for their decisions and actions. The other person is not held responsible for the positive or negative experiences in life. Each and every choice is one's own responsibility. When two people are accountable for their own emotional states, partners can be angry, sad, or frustrated without the other person taking it personally. Accountable people may even say something like, "This has nothing to do with you; I just happen to be angry right now."

**Self-nurturance** goes hand-in-hand with accountability. In order to make good choices in life, a person needs to maintain a balance of sleeping, eating, being physically active, working, relaxing, and socializing. When the balance is disrupted, as it will inevitably be, self-nurturing people are patient with themselves and try to put things back on course. When they make bad choices, as all people do, self-nurturing people learn from the experience. Learning to live in a balanced and healthy way is a lifelong process. Two people on a path of accountability and self-nurturance together have a much better chance of maintaining a satisfying relationship.

## Elements of Good Relationships

Satisfying and stable relationships share certain elements. Some of these are achieved through conscious efforts and communication; others evolve over time. People in healthy, committed relationships trust one another. Without trust, intimacy will not develop and the relationship will experience trouble and possible failure. **Trust** can be defined as the degree of confidence felt in a relationship. Trust includes three fundamental elements: predictability, dependability, and faith.

- *Predictability* means that you can predict your partner's behaviours. This sense of predictability is based on the knowledge that your partner acts in consistently positive ways.

- *Dependability* means that you can rely on your partner to give support in all situations, particularly in those in which you feel threatened with hurt or rejection.

- *Faith* means that you feel absolutely certain about your partner's intentions and behaviours.

Trust and intimacy are the foundation of healthy, committed relationships. Spouses who like and enjoy one another as people and find each other interesting frequently are happier than those who don't. Many spouses describe their partners as their best friends. Although most marriages have their share of ups and downs, successful couples are able to communicate and touch one another in an atmosphere of caring. They value a good sense of humour and exhibit communication, cooperation, and the ability to resolve conflicts constructively.

Sexual intimacy is also a major part of healthy relationships, but sex is not the major reason the relationship exists. Some couples admit to sexual dissatisfaction but feel the relationship is more important. Rather than seek an outlet in an extramarital affair, those who are dissatisfied with their sex lives adjust and spend little energy worrying about it because the relationship is satisfying in other, more important ways. Many couples report that as communication and trust increase in a long-term, committed relationship, the sexual relationship also improves.

# STAYING SINGLE

While many people choose to marry and have children, increasing numbers of young and older adults remain single. As previously noted, 41.8 percent of the population is single, 53.5 percent of which is male.[34] While many of these people seek or have sought committed relationships, in the absence of a suitable partner they find being single preferable. Singles clubs, social outings arranged by communities and churches, extended-family environments, and a large number of social services support the single lifestyle. Although some research indicates that single people live shorter lives, are less happy, more likely to be financially distressed, and more prone to illnesses than their married counterparts, other studies contradict these findings. At least one Canadian study found that it was social isolation (as measured by the social network index), not marital status, that had an impact on self-reported health.[35]

# HAVING CHILDREN

When a couple decides to raise children, their relationship changes. Resources of time, energy, and money are split many ways, and the partners no longer have each other's undivided attention. Babies and young children do not time their requests for food, sleep, and care to the convenience of adults. Therefore, individuals or couples whose basic needs for security, love, and purpose are already met make better parents. Any stresses that already exist in a relationship are further accentuated when parenting is added to the list of responsibilities. Having a child does not save a bad relationship and, in fact, may only compound problems that already exist. A child cannot and should not be expected to provide the parents with self-esteem and security.

Changing patterns in family life affect the way children are raised. In modern society, it is not always clear which partner will adjust his or her work schedule to provide the primary care of children. Remarriage creates a new family of stepparents and stepsiblings. In addition, an increasing number of individuals are choosing to have children in a family structure other than a male/female couple. Single women or lesbian couples can choose adoption or alternative (formerly "artificial") insemination as a way to create a family. Single men or gay couples can choose to adopt or obtain the services of a surrogate mother. Regardless of the structure of the family, certain factors remain important to the well-being of the unit: consistency, communication, affection, and mutual respect.

Some people become parents without a lot of forethought. Some children are born into a relationship that was supposed to last and didn't. This does not mean it is too late to do a good job of parenting. Attention, consistency, and caring can be provided by other adults if a parent cannot be physically or emotionally present for a period of time. Children are amazingly resilient and forgiving if parents show respect to them and communicate about household activities that affect their lives. Even children who grew up in a household of conflict can feel loved and respected if the parents treat them fairly. This means that parents take responsibility for any of their own conflicts and make it clear to the children that they are not the reason for the conflict.

**Accountability:** Accepting responsibility for personal decisions, choices, and actions.

**Self-nurturance:** Taking care of (i.e., nurturing) oneself as needed.

**Trust:** The degree of confidence felt in a relationship.

# Building Healthy Relationships

Couple and family therapy can often help those who experience difficulty in their relationships. All communities have a variety of services used by couples to better understand and strengthen their relationship. Below are some frequently asked questions.

### What can I do if my relationship is in trouble?

Don't put it off—get professional help *now*. Often couples are afraid to admit that there is a problem and wait too long. The distancing increases and things are said and done that are hard to take back. The right time to start improving the relationship is now, not later.

### What kind of help is there?

Many different professionals can help: clergy, medical doctors, psychologists, psychiatrists, and social workers who have taken specialized training in couple and family therapy. Most communities have a Community Information Service that lists social service agencies and therapists whose specialty is couple and family therapy. Marriage and family therapists are also listed in the telephone directory.

### What do couple and family therapists do?

By talking about your situation with a therapist, you can gain a new perspective on the issues you are dealing with. You also are helped to increase the level of communication so that the thoughts and feelings that have previously been unspoken are brought out into the open. The tension level is lowered so that old issues can be resolved.

### How do I choose a couple and family therapist?

Since you will be sharing intimate details of your relationship with your therapist, you want to make sure that there is a good match, and that you feel safe. Feel free to call several offices and get a feel for the therapist. Most therapists should be willing to have a five-minute discussion on the phone with you while you are searching for the right match.

### What kind of questions should I ask?

You are looking for two things: professional competence and personal style. For competence issues you will want to know what professional training they have, what professional associations they belong to, and if they are registered in their profession. Couple and family therapists must have at least a master's degree in relationship counselling and have been supervised for a minimum of 1,000 client hours before they can be registered. All provinces have an Association of Marriage and Family Therapists and an Association of Social Workers. They can provide you with a list of therapists in your area. You can also contact the Canadian Guidance Counsellors Association.

### How long does therapy take?

Each situation is unique. Usually the therapist will set one appointment each week for the first few weeks. Each session is generally about 50 minutes, with an average of 8 to 10 sessions. Often by that time significant changes have been made in the relationship.

### How much does therapy cost?

Costs can vary from $50 to $125 per session. Registered psychologists usually charge more than $100 per session. Public health insurance does not cover the cost of therapy unless the therapy is provided by a psychiatrist. Many employee benefit plans will cover all or portions of the cost of couple and family therapy. Check with your service provider to see what assistance you can receive.

You can expect to pay around $500 for couple therapy. Given that the cost of an uncontested divorce is about $1,300 and one that is contested can cost much more, working on the relationship may provide savings in more than one way!

### How long do I have to wait to get an appointment?

Usually you will be seen within a week or two. It depends, however, on how flexible you can be. Most therapists will have some evening hours, but these usually fill up quickly. If you require an evening appointment you might have to wait a little longer.

### Who should come to the appointment?

Whoever is involved! If it is a marital issue it is best if both partners attend. If it is a family issue, the therapist may ask the whole family to attend. This helps the therapist to see the situation in its full context and for each person involved to present how they experience the issue.

### What if my partner won't come?

The therapist may suggest some helpful strategies to lower your partner's anxiety and make it easier for him or her to attend. If, however, your partner chooses not to participate, it is still possible to proceed with only one person present.

Changes in the traditional family structure have forced society to examine alternative means of raising children. Day-care centres, extended families, and live-in babysitters are becoming important alternatives to the traditional parental unit.

# ENDING A RELATIONSHIP

## The Warning Signs

The symptoms of a troubled relationship are relatively easy to recognize. Many couples choose to ignore them, however, until the situation erupts into some type of emotional confrontation. By then, the relationship may be beyond salvaging. Breakdowns in relationships usually begin with a change in communication, however subtle. Either partner may stop listening, ceasing to be emotionally present for the other. In turn, the other feels ignored, unappreciated, or unwanted. Unresolved conflicts may increase, and unresolved anger can cause problems in sexual relations.

When a couple who previously enjoyed spending time alone together find themselves continually in the company of others, spending time apart, or preferring to stay home alone, it may be a sign that the relationship is in trouble. Of course, the need for individual privacy is not a cause for worry—it's essential to health. If, however, a partner decides to make a change in the amount and quality of time spent together without the input or understanding of the other, it may be a sign of hidden problems.

Post-secondary students, particularly those who are socially isolated and far from family and hometown friends, may be particularly vulnerable to remaining in unhealthy relationships. They may become emotionally dependent on a partner for everything from eating meals to recreational and study time; mutual obligations such as shared rental arrangements, transportation, and child care can make it tough to leave. It is also easy to mistake unwanted sexual advances for physical attraction or love. Without a network of friends and supporters with whom a student can talk, obtain validation for feelings, or share concerns, he or she may feel stuck in a relationship headed nowhere.

Honesty and verbal affection are usually very positive aspects of a relationship. In a troubled relationship, however, they can be used to cover up irresponsible or hurtful behaviours. "At least I was honest" is not an acceptable substitute for acting in a trustworthy way. The words "But I really do love you" should not be used as a licence to be inconsiderate, rude, or hurtful to a partner.

## Seeking Help: Where to Look

The first place some people look for help when there are problems in a relationship is a trusted friend. Although friends can offer needed support during trying times, few have the training and detachment necessary to resolve problems. Others find that they do not have the type of friendships that lend themselves to divulging these kinds of problems.

Most communities have private practitioners trained to counsel married or committed couples. Community mental health centres usually have trained counsellors as well. These practitioners may be psychiatrists, licensed psychologists, social workers, or counsellors with advanced degrees. These counsellors are often specially equipped to deal with the unique needs of young adults with relationship, sexual, emotional, financial, or other concerns. Most student health centres or counselling centres on campus have reduced student fees or no fees for students who need help. If you are unaware of such services, talk with your instructor and ask for his or her advice about where someone with your type of problem may get help.

## Trial Separations

Sometimes a relationship becomes so dysfunctional that even counselling cannot bring about significant change. Moving apart for a period of time may allow some preliminary healing and give both parties an opportunity to reassess themselves and their commitment to the relationship. Trial separations do not guarantee that the situation will improve, nor do they mean the relationship is ending. If both people are involved in counselling or have other support systems and mutually agree on the need for a trial separation, it may be a way to regroup and save a failing relationship.

## Why Relationships End

Although there was a gradual decrease in the number of Canadian couples experiencing divorce from the 1990s to the 2000s, the number of divorces

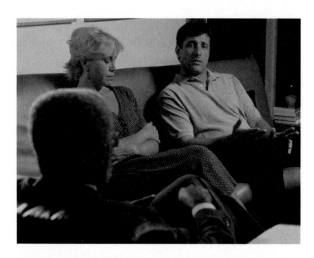

*Unresolved conflicts and frequent emotional confrontations are signs of a troubled relationship. If each partner is committed to staying together, counselling may bring about positive change.*

now remains steady. As noted previously, there were 70,828 divorces in 2003 (most recent data available).[36] The reasons for divorce and relationship breakdown are numerous. One contributing factor may be the lack of communication and cooperation between partners under the additional stress of tragedies such as the death of a child, serious illness of one partner, severe financial difficulties, and career failures. What about breakups between people who have not experienced these tragedies? These breakups arise from unmet expectations regarding marriage or relationships in general or personal roles within the relationship. Many people enter marriage with unrealistic expectations about what marriage will be like and how they and their partner will behave. Many people enter relationships looking for someone to fill the empty spots in their lives. Failure to communicate such expectations to your partner can lead to resentment and disappointment. Because many premarital expectations may be unreasonable, early exploration of these expectations is important. This exploration may take place together or within a support program.

Differences in sexual needs may also contribute to the demise of a relationship. Many partners find that their spouses desire sex at different times or in different styles and frequencies than they do. Unless sexual differences are resolved, one or both partners may begin to feel used and resent sexual activity.

The bottom line is that if couples do not grow together, they often grow apart. Without a commitment to working on their differences, many find it easier to move on, and this decision may be best for all concerned.

## Deciding to Break Up

At some point, troubled couples may feel that their relationship is not worth saving. The decision to end the relationship is usually difficult, even for couples whose relationship was over long before the decision.

For married couples, wading through divorce or dissolution proceedings may be painful as they decide child-custody issues, alimony questions, and division of property. Finding legal assistance may be difficult, because painful emotions usually affect judgment. Friends or counsellors may be able to recommend lawyers who understand the emotions that follow the ending of a relationship.

Cohabiting couples also experience difficulty in separating. Legal problems involving property, children, and alimony are often more ambiguous than in a marriage. Some couples expend much time, money, and energy working out settlements with lawyers who specialize in problems following the breakup of a common-law relationship.

Aside from legal worries, many newly separated or divorced people experience painful emotions of anger, guilt, rejection, and unworthiness. No matter how miserable the relationship, feelings of failure are not uncommon or abnormal following a divorce or breakup, and the emotional wounds take varying amounts of time to heal. Counsellors familiar with loss and grieving estimate that it takes at least a year and often longer to recover from the loss of a major relationship, whether by death or separation. With time, support from others, and community or professional help, most people do recover and establish new relationships.

## Coping with Loneliness

Some people find establishing and maintaining relationships difficult. Others find that through death, illness, or distance, their relationships disappear or grow dim with time. Loneliness, or the unfulfilled desire to engage in a close personal relationship, is a difficult emotion to experience, even for the most determined person.

The loss of an important committed relationship is usually too painful for a person to want to repeat. Reflecting on the beginning, the course, and the ending of the relationship can help you avoid the same mistakes in the future. Concentrating on the negative aspects of past behaviours of an ex-partner is a natural tendency, and may be helpful in getting in touch with emotions or in learning from the situation. It is equally important to spend time remembering what was loved in the other person and what is lovable about oneself. Intimacy, love, and commitment between people always change the lives of those involved. It is through relationships that we give and receive our greatest support and validation as worthwhile human beings. When we accept the risk and challenge of close relationships, we accept one of the greatest gifts life has to offer.

# YOUR SEXUAL IDENTITY

Although you are a sexual being from birth, you are not born knowing all about your sexuality. Learning about and becoming comfortable with your sexual self is a lifelong process. Taboos, mores, laws, and sexual myths abound and often hinder the process of learning about your sexual self. Family, friends, and the media—including print and electronic forms, music, religion, and educational institutions—provide you with information about your sexuality and how you should or should not express it. In the end, it is up to you to blend all this information with your personal experience and values to create your own sexual identity.

Your **sexual identity** is determined by a complex interaction of genetic, physiological, and environmental factors. The beginning of your sexual identity occurs at conception with the combining of chromosomes that determine your sex. Actually, it is your biological father who determines whether you will be a boy or a girl. Here's how it works. All eggs (ova) carry an X sex chromosome; sperm may carry either an X or a Y chromosome. If a sperm carrying an X chromosome fertilizes an egg, the resulting combination of sex chromosomes (XX) creates the blueprint to produce a female. If a sperm carrying a Y chromosome fertilizes an egg, the XY combination produces a male (see Figure 5.1). The genetic instructions included in the sex chromosomes lead to the differential development of male and female **gonads** at about the eighth day in utero. Once the male gonads (testes) and the female gonads (ovaries) are developed, they play a key role in all future sexual development because the gonads are responsible for the production of sex hormones. The primary sex hormones produced by females are estrogen and progesterone. In males, the hormone of primary importance is testosterone. The release of testosterone in a maturing fetus signals the development of a penis and other male genitals. If no testosterone is produced, female genitals form.

During **puberty,** sex hormones play major roles in development. Hormones released by the **pituitary gland,** called gonadotropins, stimulate the gonads (testes and ovaries) to make appropriate sex hormones. The increased production of estrogen in females and testosterone in males leads to the development of **secondary sex characteristics.** Secondary sex characteristics in males include deepening of the voice, development of facial and body hair, and genital

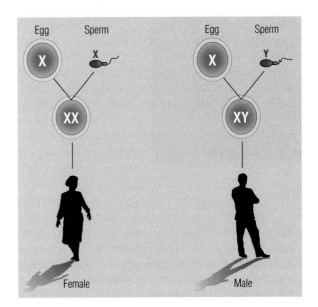

**FIGURE 5.1**
**How Sex Is Determined**

(penis and testes) development. In females, secondary sex characteristics include growth of the breasts, menarche, widening of the hips, and the development of pubic and underarm hair.

## Gender Identity and Roles

Thus far, we have described sexual identity only in terms of a person's sex. Sex simply refers to the biological condition of being male or female based on physiological and hormonal differences. **Gender,** on the other hand, refers to your sense of masculinity or femininity as defined by the society in which you live. Each of us expresses our maleness or femaleness to others on a daily basis by the **gender roles** we play.

---

**Sexual identity:** Our recognition of ourselves as sexual creatures; a composite of sex, gender, gender roles, sexual preference, body image, and sexual scripts.

**Gonads:** The reproductive organs in a male (testes) or female (ovaries).

**Puberty:** The period of sexual maturation.

**Pituitary gland:** The endocrine gland controlling the release of hormones from the gonads.

**Secondary sex characteristics:** Characteristics associated with sex developed during puberty such as vocal pitch, degree of body hair, and genital development.

**Gender:** Your sense of masculinity or femininity as defined by the society in which you live.

**Gender roles:** Expression of maleness or femaleness exhibited on a daily basis.

**Gender identity** refers to your personal sense or awareness of being masculine or feminine, a male or a female. It may sometimes be difficult for you to express your true sexual identity because you feel bound by existing gender-role stereotypes. **Gender-role stereotypes** are generalizations about how males and females should express themselves and the characteristics each possesses. Our traditional sex roles are an example of gender-role stereotyping. Men are thought to be independent, aggressive, better in math and science, logical, and in control of their emotions. Women, on the other hand, are traditionally expected to be passive, nurturing, intuitive, sensitive, and emotional. **Androgyny** is the combination of traditional masculine and feminine traits in a single person. Androgynous people do not always follow traditional sex roles but, rather, act according to the given situation. The process by which a society transmits behavioural expectations to its individual members is called **socialization.** Gender roles are shaped or socialized by our parents, peers, schools, textbooks, and many forms of media including television, advertisements, the Internet, music, and movies. Think about the current television shows or movies you watch. Do the characters play traditional gender roles?

By now you can see that defining your sexual identity is not a simple matter. Your sexual identity is made up of the unique combination of your sex, gender identity, chosen gender roles, sexual preference, and personal experiences. No other person is exactly like you, and it is up to you to take every opportunity to get to know and like yourself so that you may enjoy your life to the fullest. As the saying goes, sex is what you are born with, but sexuality is who you are.

## WHAT WOULD YOU DO?

How masculine or feminine do you feel? Why? Do you feel limited or bound by existing gender-role stereotypes? Why or why not? Do you challenge these stereotypes? In what way? What words will you use in the future?

# REPRODUCTIVE ANATOMY AND PHYSIOLOGY

An understanding of the functions of the male and female reproductive systems will help you derive pleasure and satisfaction from your sexual relationships, be sensitive to your partner's wants and needs, and be more responsible in your choices regarding your sexual health.

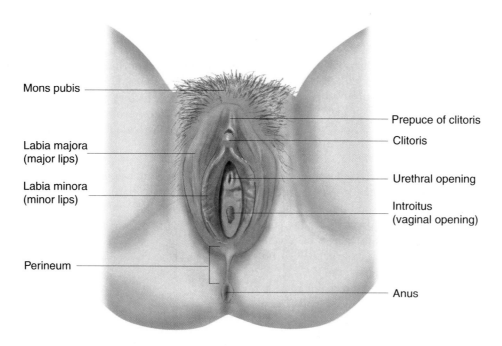

FIGURE 5.2

**External Female Genital Structures**

*Source:* R. D. McAnulty and M. M. Burnette, *Exploring Human Sexuality: Making Healthy Decisions* (Boston: Allyn & Bacon, 2001). Copyright © 2001 by Pearson Education.

# Female Reproductive Anatomy and Physiology

The female reproductive system includes two major groups of structures, the external and internal genitals (see Figures 5.2 and 5.3). The **external female genitals** include the outwardly visible structures often referred to as the vulva. The **vulva,** or external genitalia, includes the mons pubis, the labia minora and majora, the clitoris, the urethral and vaginal openings, and the vestibule of the vagina. The **mons pubis** is a pad of fatty tissue covering the pubic bone. The mons protects the pubic bone, and during puberty becomes covered with coarse hair. The **labia minora** are folds of mucous membrane and the **labia majora** are folds of skin and erectile tissue that enclose the urethral and vaginal openings. The labia minora are found just inside the labia majora.

The **clitoris** is the female sexual organ whose only known function is sexual pleasure. It is located at the upper end of the labia minora and beneath the mons pubis. Directly below the clitoris is the **urethral opening** through which urine leaves the body. Below the urethral opening is the opening of the **vagina.** In some women, the vaginal opening is covered by a thin membrane called the **hymen.** It is a myth that an intact

**Gender identity:** Your personal sense or awareness of being masculine or feminine, a male or female.

**Gender-role stereotypes:** Generalizations concerning how males and females should express themselves and the characteristics each possesses.

**Androgyny:** Combination of traditional masculine and feminine traits in a single person.

**Socialization:** Process by which a society identifies behavioural expectations to its individual members.

**External female genitals:** The mons pubis, labia majora and minora, clitoris, urethral and vaginal openings, and vestibule of the vagina and its glands.

**Vulva:** The female's external genitalia.

**Mons pubis:** Fatty tissue covering the pubic bone in females; in physically mature women, the mons is covered with coarse hair.

**Labia minora:** "Inner lips" or folds of tissue just inside the labia majora.

**Labia majora:** "Outer lips" or folds of tissue covering the female sexual organs.

**Clitoris:** A pea-sized nodule of tissue located at the top of the labia minora.

**Urethral opening:** The opening through which urine is expelled.

**Vagina:** The passage leading from the vulva to the uterus.

**Hymen:** Thin tissue covering the vaginal opening.

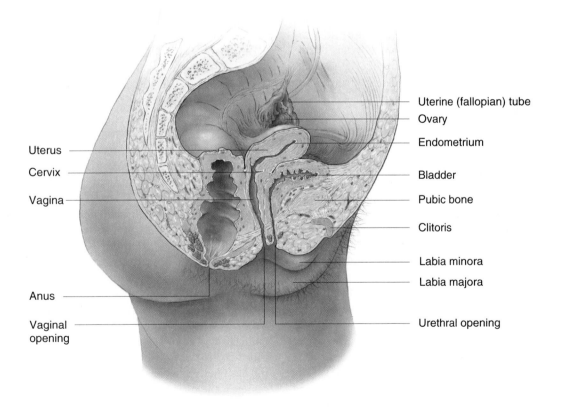

FIGURE 5.3

Side View of the Female Reproductive Organs

hymen is proof of virginity. The **perineum** is the area between the vulva and the anus. Although not technically part of the external genitalia, the tissue in this area has many nerve endings and is sensitive to touch; it can play a part in sexual excitement.

The **internal female genitals** of the reproductive system include the vagina, uterus, fallopian tubes, and ovaries. The vagina is a tubular passageway from the uterus to the outside of a female's body. This passageway allows menstrual flow to exit from the uterus during a female's monthly cycle and serves as the birth canal. The vagina also receives the penis during intercourse. The **uterus,** also known as the womb, is a hollow, muscular, pear-shaped organ. Hormones acting on the inner lining of the uterus, called the **endometrium,** either prepare the uterus for implantation and development of a fertilized egg or signal that no fertilization has taken place, in which case the endometrium deteriorates and becomes menstrual flow.

The lower end of the uterus is called the **cervix** and extends down into the vagina. The **ovaries** are almond-sized structures suspended on either side of the uterus. The ovaries produce the hormones estrogen and progesterone and are the reservoir for immature eggs. All the eggs a female will ever have are present in the ovaries at birth. Eggs mature and are released from the ovaries in response to hormone levels. Extending from the upper end of the uterus are two thin, flexible tubes called the **fallopian tubes.** The fallopian tubes are where sperm and egg meet and fertilization takes place. Following fertilization, the fallopian tubes serve as the passageway to the uterus, where the fertilized egg implants and development continues.

## The Onset of Puberty and the Menstrual Cycle

During puberty, the female reproductive system matures and secondary sex characteristics transform girls into young women. Under the direction of the endocrine system, the pituitary gland, the hypothalamus, and the ovaries secrete hormones that act as the chemical messengers among them. Working in a feedback system, hormonal levels in the bloodstream act as the trigger mechanism for release of more or different hormones (see Figure 5.4).

At the beginning of puberty in females, the **hypothalamus** receives the message to begin secreting **gonadotropin-releasing hormone (GnRH).** The release of GnRH in turn signals the **pituitary gland** to release hormones called gonadotropins. **Follicle-stimulating hormone (FSH)** and **luteinizing hormone (LH)** are two gonadotropins, and their role is to signal the gonads, in this case the ovaries, to start

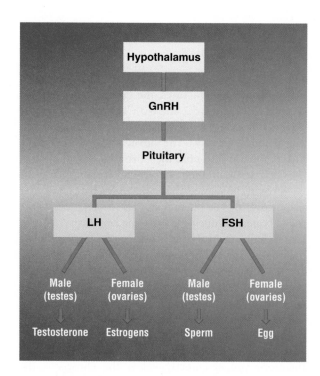

FIGURE 5.4

Hormonal Direction of the Human Reproductive System

producing **estrogens** and **progesterone.** Increased estrogen levels assist in the development of female secondary sex characteristics. In addition, estrogens are responsible for regulating the reproductive cycle. The normal age range for the onset of the first menstrual period, termed the **menarche,** is 10 to 16 years, with the average age around 12 or 13 years.

The average menstrual cycle is 28 days and divided into three phases, the proliferatory phase, the secretory phase, and the menstrual phase. During the proliferatory phase, the pituitary gland releases FSH and LH. The FSH acts on the ovaries to stimulate the maturation process of several **ovarian follicles (egg sacs).** These follicles secrete estrogens and, in response, the lining of the uterus, the endometrium, begins to grow and develop. The inner walls of the uterus become coated with a thick, spongy lining composed of blood and mucus. In the event of fertilization, the endometrial tissue will become a nesting place for the developing embryo. The increased estrogen level also signals the pituitary to slow down FSH production and to increase LH secretion. Of the several follicles developing in the ovaries, only one each month normally reaches complete maturity. Under the influence of LH, this one ovarian follicle rapidly matures, and on or about the fourteenth day of the proliferatory phase it releases an ovum into the fallopian tube—a process referred to as **ovulation.** Just prior to ovulation, the mature egg's follicle begins to increase secretion of progesterone, the first function of which is to spur the addition of further nutrients to the developing endometrium.

After ovulation, the ovarian follicle is converted into the *corpus luteum,* or yellow body, which continues to secrete estrogen and progesterone but in decreasing amounts. In addition, FSH falls back to its preproliferatory levels. Essentially, the woman's body is "waiting" to see whether fertilization will occur. During this time after ovulation, LH declines, and progesterone levels begin to rise, causing additional tissue growth in the endometrium. This phase of the cycle is called the secretory phase.

If fertilization takes place, cells surrounding the developing embryo release a hormone called **human chorionic gonadotropin (HCG).** This hormone leads to increased levels of estrogen and progesterone secretion, which maintains the endometrium while signalling the pituitary gland not to start a new menstrual cycle. If fertilization does not occur, the egg gradually disintegrates within approximately 72 hours. The corpus luteum gradually becomes nonfunctional, causing levels of progesterone and estrogen to decline. As hormonal levels decline, the endometrial lining of the uterus loses its nourishment, dies, and is sloughed off as menstrual flow. Menstruation is the third phase of the menstrual cycle.

### Menopause

Just as menarche signals the beginning of a female's potential reproductive years, **menopause**—the permanent cessation of menstruation—signals the end. Generally occurring between the ages of 40 and 60, menopause results in decreased estrogen levels, which may produce troublesome symptoms in some women. Decrease in vaginal lubrication, hot flashes, headaches, dizziness, and joint pain have been associated with menopause.

Hormones such as estrogen and progesterone have been prescribed as *hormone replacement therapy (HRT)* to relieve menopausal symptoms and reduce the risk of heart disease and osteoporosis. However, the results from some studies indicate that hormone therapy may actually do more harm than good. In particular, HRT may increase risk of breast cancer, heart attack, stroke, blood clots, and other health problems.[37] A woman needs to discuss the risks and benefits of HRT with her health-care provider and come to an informed decision. Certainly lifestyle changes such as regular physical activity and a dietary intake low in fat and adequate in calcium can also help protect postmenopausal women from heart disease and osteoporosis.

## Male Reproductive Anatomy and Physiology

The structures of the male reproductive system may be divided into external and internal genitals (see Figure 5.5). The penis and the scrotum make up the

**Perineum:** Tissue extending from the vulva to the anus.

**Internal female genitals:** The vagina, uterus, fallopian tubes, and ovaries.

**Uterus (womb):** Hollow, pear-shaped muscular organ whose function is to house the developing fetus.

**Endometrium:** Soft, spongy matter that makes up the uterine lining.

**Cervix:** Lower end of the uterus that opens into the vagina.

**Ovaries:** Almond-sized organs that house developing eggs and produce hormones.

**Fallopian tubes:** Tubes that extend from the ovaries to the uterus.

**Hypothalamus:** An area of the brain located near the pituitary gland. The hypothalamus works in conjunction with the pituitary gland to control reproductive functions.

**Gonadotropin-releasing hormone (GnRH):** Hormone that signals the pituitary gland to release gonadotropins.

**Pituitary gland:** A gland located deep within the brain; controls reproductive functions.

**Follicle-stimulating hormone (FSH):** Hormone that signals the ovaries to prepare to release eggs and to begin producing estrogens.

**Luteinizing hormone (LH):** Hormone that signals the ovaries to release an egg and to begin producing progesterone.

**Estrogens:** Hormones that control the menstrual cycle.

**Progesterone:** Hormone secreted by the ovaries; helps keep the endometrium developing in order to nourish a fertilized egg; also helps maintain pregnancy.

**Menarche:** The first menstrual period.

**Ovarian follicles (egg sacs):** Areas within the ovary in which individual eggs develop.

**Ovulation:** The point of the menstrual cycle at which a mature egg ruptures through the ovarian wall.

**Human chorionic gonadotropin (HCG):** Hormone that calls for increased levels of estrogen and progesterone secretion if fertilization has taken place.

**Menopause:** The permanent cessation of menstruation.

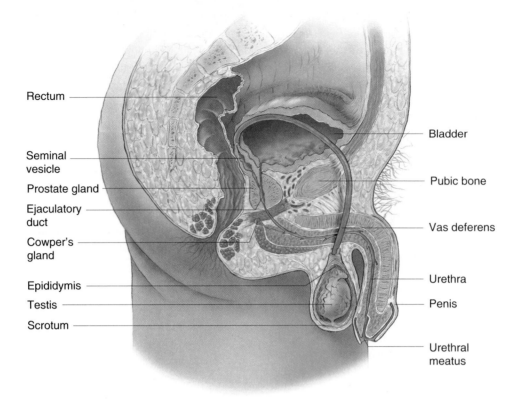

Rectum

Seminal
vesicle

Prostate gland

Ejaculatory
duct

Cowper's
gland

Epididymis

Testis

Scrotum

Bladder

Pubic bone

Vas deferens

Urethra

Penis

Urethral
meatus

FIGURE 5.5
Side View of the Male Reproductive Organs

**external male genitals.** The **internal male genitals** include the testes, epididymides, vasa deferentia, urethra, and three other structures—the seminal vesicles, the prostate gland, and the Cowper's glands—that secrete components that, with sperm, make up semen. These three structures are sometimes referred to as the **accessory glands.**

The **penis** is the organ that releases sperm during ejaculation. The urethra, which passes through the centre of the penis, acts as the passageway for semen and urine to exit the body. During sexual arousal, the spongy tissue in the penis becomes filled with blood, making it stiff, or erect. Further sexual excitement leads to **ejaculation,** a series of rapid spasmodic contractions that propel semen out of the penis.

Situated behind the penis outside the body is a sac called the **scrotum.** The scrotum protects the testes and helps control the temperature within the testes, which is vital to sperm production. The **testes** (singular: *testis*) are egg-shaped structures in which sperm are manufactured. The testes also contain cells that manufacture **testosterone,** the hormone responsible for male secondary sex characteristic development.

**Spermatogenesis** describes the development of sperm. Like the maturation of eggs in the female, this process is governed by the pituitary gland. Follicle-stimulating hormone (FSH) is secreted into the bloodstream to stimulate the testes to manufacture sperm. Immature sperm are released into a comma-shaped structure on the back of the testis called the **epididymis** (plural: *epididymides*), where they ripen and reach full maturity.

The epididymis contains coiled tubules that gradually "unwind" and straighten to become the **vas deferens.** The two *vasa deferentia,* as they are called in the plural, make up the tubular transportation system with the sole function to store and move sperm. Along the way, the **seminal vesicles** provide sperm with nutrients and other fluids that compose **semen.**

The vasa deferentia eventually connect each epididymis to the ejaculatory ducts, which pass through the **prostate gland** and empty into the urethra. The prostate gland contributes more fluids to the semen, including chemicals to aid the sperm in fertilization of an ovum, and, more importantly, a chemical that neutralizes the acid in the vagina to make its environment more conducive to sperm motility (ability to move) and potency (potential for fertilizing an ovum).

Just below the prostate gland are two pea-shaped nodules called the Cowper's glands. Their primary function is to secrete a fluid that lubricates the urethra and neutralizes any acid that may remain in the urethra after urination. Urine and semen do not come into contact with each other. During ejaculation of semen, the tube to the urinary bladder is closed off by a small valve.

### Circumcision: Risk versus Benefit

Parents must decide whether their male infant will be circumcised. Circumcision involves the surgical removal of the **foreskin,** a flap of skin covering the tip of the penis. Most circumcisions are performed for religious or cultural reasons or because of concerns about hygiene. In the uncircumcised male, oily secretions and sloughed-off dead cells (smegma) can collect under the foreskin and create an irritation or a breeding ground for infection. Removing the foreskin makes cleansing the penis easier. Today, infants can be given a local anesthetic, and circumcisions can be performed with little or no pain. This does not mean, however, that the procedure itself is without risk. All surgery involves some risk. If circumcision is performed later in life under a general anesthetic, the risk of complications is greater. Like all other elective surgical procedures, careful consideration of the risks and benefits of circumcision should be made prior to making a decision.

# EXPRESSING YOUR SEXUALITY

Finding healthy ways to express your sexuality is an important part of developing sexual maturity. Many avenues of sexual expression are available.

## Human Sexual Response

Sexual response is a physiological process that involves different stages. The biological goal of the response process is the reproduction of the species. Human psychological traits greatly influence sexual desire and response. Thus, we may find relationships with one partner vastly different from those we experience with another partner.

Sexual response generally follows a pattern, though individual differences are common. Males and females each exhibit four common stages: excitement/arousal, plateau, orgasm, and resolution. In addition, some males may experience a fifth stage, the refractory period. Regardless of the type of sexual activity (stimulation by a partner or self-stimulation), the response stages are the same.

During the first stage, *excitement/arousal,* male and female genital responses are caused by **vasocongestion,** or increased blood flow in the genital region. Increased blood flow to these organs causes them to swell. The vagina begins to lubricate in preparation for penile penetration and the penis becomes partially erect. Both sexes may exhibit a "sex flush," or light blush all over their bodies. Excitement/arousal can be generated by touching, kissing, through fantasy, viewing films or videos, or reading erotic literature.

The *plateau phase* is characterized by an intensification of the initial responses. Voluntary and involuntary muscle tensions increase. The female's nipples and the male's penis become erect. A few drops of semen, which may contain sperm, are secreted from the penis at this time.

During the *orgasmic phase,* vasocongestion and muscle tensions reach their peak, and rhythmic contractions occur through the genital regions. In females, these contractions are centred in the uterus, the outer vagina, and the anal sphincter. In males, the contractions occur in two stages. First, contractions within the prostate gland begin propelling semen through the urethra. In the second stage, the muscles of the pelvic floor, the urethra, and the anal sphincter

**External male genitals:** The penis and scrotum.

**Internal male genitals:** The testes, epididymides, vasa deferentia, ejaculatory ducts, urethra, and accessory glands.

**Accessory glands:** The seminal vesicles, prostate gland, and Cowper's glands.

**Penis:** Male sexual organ.

**Ejaculation:** The propulsion of semen from the penis.

**Scrotum:** Sac of tissue that encloses the testes.

**Testes:** Two organs, located in the scrotum, that manufacture sperm and produce hormones.

**Testosterone:** The male sex hormone manufactured in the testes.

**Spermatogenesis:** The development of sperm.

**Epididymis:** A comma-shaped structure atop the testis where sperm mature.

**Vas deferens:** A tube that transports sperm toward the penis.

**Seminal vesicles:** Storage areas for sperm where nutrient fluids are added.

**Semen:** Fluid containing sperm and nutrients that increase sperm viability and neutralize vaginal acid.

**Prostate gland:** Gland that secretes nutrients and neutralizing fluids into the semen.

**Foreskin:** Flap of skin covering the end of the penis.

**Vasocongestion:** The engorgement of the genital organs with blood.

contract. Semen usually, but not always, is ejaculated from the penis. In both sexes, spasms in other major muscle groups also occur, particularly in the buttocks and abdomen. Feet and hands may also contract, and facial features often contort.

Muscle tension and congested blood subside in the *resolution phase,* as the genital organs return to their pre-arousal states. Both sexes usually experience deep feelings of well-being, satisfaction, and profound relaxation.

As previously noted, some males experience a fifth phase—the *refractory phase.* In this phase, males experience a period of time in which their systems are incapable of subsequent arousal. This refractory period may last from a few minutes to several hours. The length of the refractory period increases with age. Following orgasm and resolution, many females are capable of being aroused and brought to orgasm again. Males and females experience the same stages in the sexual response cycle; however, the length of time spent in any one stage is variable. Thus, one partner may be in the plateau phase while the other is in the excitement or orgasmic phase. Such variations in response rates are entirely normal. Some couples believe that simultaneous orgasm is desirable for sexual satisfaction. Although simultaneous orgasm is pleasant, so are orgasms achieved at different times.

Sexual pleasure and satisfaction are possible without orgasm or intercourse. Achieving sexual maturity includes learning that sex is not a contest with a real or imaginary opponent. The sexually mature person enjoys sexual activity whether or not orgasm occurs. Expressing love and sexual feelings for another person involves many pleasurable activities, of which intercourse and orgasm may be only a part.

## WHAT WOULD YOU DO?

Why do North Americans place so much importance on the orgasmic phase of sexual response? Do you think there should be a "psychological phase" added to descriptions of the sexual response cycle? Why or why not?

## Sexual Orientation

An essential part of your sexual identity is your sexual orientation. **Sexual orientation** refers to a person's potential to respond with sexual excitement to other persons.[38] You may be primarily attracted to members of the opposite sex **(heterosexual),** the same sex **(homosexual),** or both sexes **(bisexual).**

Homosexuality refers to emotional and sexual attachment to persons of your same sex. Many homosexuals

prefer the use of *gay* and *lesbian* to describe their sexual orientations, as these terms go beyond the exclusively sexual connotation of the term *homosexual.* Although the term *gay* can be applied to men and women, the term *lesbian* is applied only to women.

Most researchers today agree that sexual orientation is best understood using a multifactorial model, which incorporates biological, psychological, and socioenvironmental factors. Biological explanations focus on research into genetics, hormones (perinatal and postpubertal), and differences in brain anatomy, while psychological and socioenvironmental studies examine parent–child interactions, sex roles, and early sexual and interpersonal interactions. Collectively, this growing body of research suggests that the origins of homosexuality, like heterosexuality, are complex. To diminish the complexity of sexual orientation to "a choice" is a clear misrepresentation of current research. Homosexuals do not "choose" their sexual orientation any more than heterosexuals do.

Irrational fear or hatred of homosexuality creates antigay prejudice and is expressed as **homophobia.** Homophobia is expressed in many subtle and not so subtle ways. Homophobic behaviours range from avoiding hugging same-sex friends to "gay bashing" (physical and verbal attacks on gays). The emergence of AIDS (acquired immune deficiency syndrome) seems to have magnified antihomosexual prejudice, as some people have erroneously assumed that homosexuality, rather than high-risk behaviours, is responsible for the epidemic.

*Bisexuality* refers to emotional attachment and sexual attraction to members of both sexes. Bisexuals may face great social stigma, as they are often ostracized by homosexuals as well as by heterosexuals. Little research has been done on this segment of the population, and many bisexuals remain hidden or closeted.

## WHAT WOULD YOU DO?

What do you think is at the root of homophobia? How does society promote or demote homophobia? What can you do to prevent homophobia?

## Developing Sexual Relationships

Perhaps the most important part of developing mature sexuality is learning to develop rewarding sexual relationships. Like all skills, developing relationships takes time, patience, and practice. Your sexual education begins with your family. You watch the significant adults in your life and pattern your behaviours after theirs. At puberty, when extrafamilial

# Online Dating Becoming Common: Love and Lies Are Alive on the Internet, Canadian Study Reveals

*By Marlene Habib—The Canadian Press*

Online dating has become so common it's being studied by experts in human behaviour and the financial stakes are growing. Sociologists Robert Brym and Rhonda Lenton call Internet use "the birth of a new society."

The study says Internet dating began about five years ago. In North America, the dating-services industry was estimated to be worth $1 billion US in 1998 and is projected to reach $1.5 billion US by 2003, says the Computer Industry Almanac. "The main important finding that's emerged from this study for us is how mainstream online dating has become," says Lenton, a professor at McMaster University in Hamilton.

Among the results: 68 percent of respondents were men, 63 percent said they had sex with someone they met online, 60 percent formed at least one long-term relationship, 27 percent met at least one partner, and three percent eventually married.

But there is a downside and some cautionary advice for those looking for real love: 18 percent of online dating users were already married or living common-law, and of that group, most were men.

As well, Lenton noted, many online daters misrepresent themselves. For instance, more than 25 percent of respondents said they had given inaccurate information in their online personal ads, with many lying about their age, marital status, and appearance.

And 26 percent of respondents said they'd been pestered after a date, while 10 percent said they'd felt frightened at least once. "We would recommend that people using online dating follow the same common-sense precautions as someone they had met at a bar," Lenton warned in an interview.

While acknowledging the pitfalls, Lenton and Brym, a professor at the University of Toronto, say online dating is booming because most experiences are positive and it's as viable a way to meet people as any other.

The convenience of connecting online appeals to a growing proportion of the population that is single, career-driven and short on time. The report offers safety tips such as using an anonymous email address, arranging a first meeting during the day in a public place, and not giving out phone numbers or addresses until trust has been established.

Judy Farrant and Mark Nesbitt are mid-40s newlyweds who met on Webpersonals and who agreed to tell their story. They said their busy lives made dating difficult. So they turned to the Internet because it was convenient and they could remain anonymous.

Farrant, a flight attendant, said she began her cybersearch in 1997. She didn't tell her two children at first "because I didn't want them to know." She met 14 men before responding to Nesbitt's ad, "which was distinctive and different from anything else I'd ever seen."

"I had become fussier, so I cut to the chase," Nesbitt said. In his online profile, he stated exactly who he was and what kind of woman he was looking for.

There is, of course, a cost for using online dating services: some companies have membership subscriptions. Webpersonals sells blocks of credits. Paul Gallucci, a Webpersonals spokesman, wouldn't say how much revenue the service generates, but added that "it's a multimillion-dollar business."

Source: The Canadian Press.

---

elements, peers, and the media become more important, you adapt some of their standards to your behaviours. Your shyness, aggressiveness or assertiveness, passiveness, and levels of comfort with your sexuality come from your personality and from what you have learned from others.

You bring not only your history to your sexual relationships, but also your peculiar chemistry. The human potential for passionate sexual love has been defined as **limerence.** The word *limerence* is derived from the name of the portion of the brain that controls sexual response, the limbic cortex. Limerence is what makes us feel sexually "turned on" by a person.

**Sexual orientation:** Attraction to and interest in members of the opposite sex, the same sex, or both sexes in emotional, social, and sexual situations.

**Heterosexual:** Refers to attraction to and preference for sexual activity with people of the opposite sex.

**Homosexual:** Refers to attraction to and preference for sexual activity with people of the same sex.

**Bisexual:** Refers to attraction to and preference for sexual activity with people of both sexes.

**Homophobia:** Irrational hatred or fear of homosexuals or homosexuality.

**Limerence:** The quality of sexual attraction based on chemistry and gratification of sexual desire.

This powerful feeling can overshadow common sense. Sexual relationships based on limerence may or may not develop into long-lasting or committed relationships. Limerence is thought to last only two years at most. Relationships based upon a love that has taken time to mature are much more likely to last. Following are some of the "symptoms" of limerence:[39]

- Intrusive thoughts about the object of desire.

- Dependence of mood on love object's actions.

- Fear of rejection, along with almost incapacitating shyness.

- Sharp sensitivity to interpret desired person's actions favourably and ability to interpret any signs from the other as hidden passion.

- Buoyant, walking-on-air feeling when reciprocation is evident.

- Intensity of feelings that leaves other concerns in the background.

- Ability to emphasize what is admirable in the love object and to avoid dwelling on the negative, or even ability to reconceptualize the negative into a positive attribute.

## WHAT WOULD YOU DO?

Do you know anyone who has used an online dating service? What precautions did they take to ensure their safety? What impact has technology made on dating in Canada? Will these changes have any impact on the psychosocial health of the Canadian public? Why or why not? What safety precautions will you take should you choose to use online dating services?

# Sexual Expression: What Are Your Options?

The range of human sexual expression is virtually infinite. What you find personally satisfying and enjoyable may not be an option for someone else. The ways you choose to meet your sexual needs today may be very different two weeks or two years from now. Knowing and accepting yourself as a sexual person with individual desires and preferences is the first step in achieving sexual satisfaction.

## Celibacy

**Celibacy** is avoidance of or abstention from sexual activities with others. A completely celibate person also does not engage in masturbation (self-stimulation), whereas a partially celibate person avoids sexual

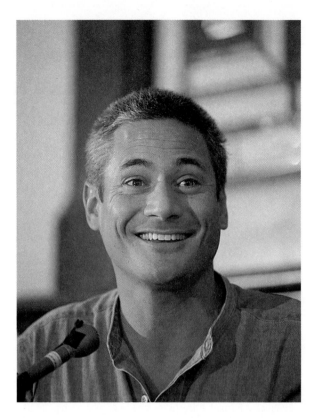

*In a society where anti-homosexual attitudes prevail, a gay person's decision to make his or her sexual preference known to the public, as Olympic diver Greg Louganis did, involves courage and a strong belief in oneself.*

activities with others but engages in autoerotic behaviours such as masturbation. Some individuals choose to be celibate for religious or moral reasons. Others may be celibate for a period of time due to illness, the break-up of a long-term relationship, or lack of an acceptable partner. For some, celibacy is a lonely, agonizing state, but others find that it can be a time for introspection, value assessment, and personal growth.

## Autoerotic Behaviours

The goal of **autoerotic behaviours** is sexual self-stimulation. Sexual fantasy and masturbation are the two most common autoerotic behaviours. **Sexual fantasies** are sexually arousing thoughts and dreams. Fantasies may reflect real-life experiences or forbidden desires or may provide the opportunity for practice of new or anticipated sexual experiences. The fact that you may fantasize about a particular sexual experience does not mean that you want to, or have to, act out that experience. Sexual fantasies are just that—fantasy. **Masturbation** is self-stimulation of the genitals. Although many people feel uncomfortable discussing masturbation, it is a common sexual practice across the life span. Masturbation is a

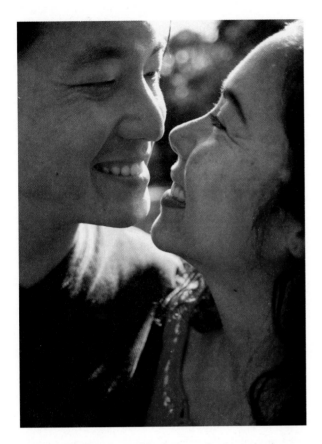

*Kissing can be a nonverbal form of sexual communication.*

natural, pleasure-seeking behaviour in infants and children. It is a valuable and important means for adolescent males and females, as well as adults, to explore their sexual feelings and responsiveness. In addition, masturbation is an important means of sexual expression for older adults whose lifelong companion has died or has a prolonged illness.

## Kissing and Erotic Touching

Kissing and erotic touching are two very common forms of nonverbal sexual communication or expression. Males and females have **erogenous zones,** or areas of the body that when touched lead to sexual arousal. Erogenous zones may include genital as well as nongenital areas, such as the earlobes, mouth, breasts, and inner thighs. Almost any area of the body can be conditioned to respond erotically to touch. Spending time with your partner exploring and learning about his or her erogenous areas is another pleasurable, safe, and satisfying means of sexual expression.

## Oral–Genital Stimulation

**Cunnilingus** is the term used for oral stimulation of a female's genitals, and **fellatio** refers to oral stimulation

of a male's genitals. Many partners find oral–genital stimulation an intensely pleasurable means of sexual expression. For some people, oral sex is not an option because of moral or religious beliefs. It is important to remember that HIV and other sexually transmitted infections (STIs) can be transmitted via unprotected oral–genital sex. Use of an appropriate barrier device is strongly recommended if either partner's disease status is in question or unknown or if either partner is not monogamous.

## Anal Intercourse

The anal area is highly sensitive to touch, and some find pleasure in the stimulation of this area. **Anal intercourse** refers to the insertion of the penis into the anus. Stimulation of the anus by mouth or with the fingers is also practised. If you do enjoy this form of sexual expression, remember to use condoms to prevent STIs. Also, anything inserted into the anus should not be directly inserted into the vagina, as bacteria commonly found there can cause infections when introduced into the vagina.

## Vaginal Intercourse

The term intercourse generally refers to **vaginal intercourse,** or insertion of the penis into the vagina. *Coitus* is another term for vaginal intercourse, the most often practised form of sexual expression. A great variety of positions can be used during coitus. Examples include the missionary position (man on top facing the woman), woman on top, side by side, or man behind (rear entry). Many partners enjoy changing and experimenting with different positions. Sexual intercourse can take on different meanings under different circumstances. It can be a hurried, unplanned event involving little communication in the back seat of a car or an erotic, sensual experience including the exchange of love and mutual emotions in a private setting. Knowledge of yourself and your

**Celibacy:** Not engaging in sexual activity.

**Autoerotic behaviours:** Sexual self-stimulation.

**Sexual fantasies:** Sexually arousing thoughts and dreams.

**Masturbation:** Self-stimulation of genitals.

**Erogenous zones:** Areas in the body that, when touched, lead to sexual arousal.

**Cunnilingus:** Oral stimulation of a female's genitals.

**Fellatio:** Oral stimulation of a male's genitals.

**Anal intercourse:** The insertion of the penis into the anus.

**Vaginal intercourse:** The insertion of the penis into the vagina.

body, along with your ability to communicate effectively with others, will play a large part in determining the enjoyment or meaning of intercourse for you and your partner. Whatever your circumstance, you should practise safe sex to avoid STIs or unwanted pregnancy.

## What Is Right for Me?

Invariably, whenever people talk about the spectrum of sexual behaviours, someone in the group will bring up the issue of normality. In *The Joy of Sex,* Alex Comfort summarizes "normality" succinctly:

> Accordingly, if you must talk about "normality," any sex behavior is normal which (1) you both enjoy, (2) hurts nobody, (3) isn't associated with anxiety, (4) doesn't cut down your scope. . . . "Normal" implies there is something which sex ought to be. That is, it ought to be a wholly satisfying link between two affectionate people, from which both emerge unanxious, rewarded, and ready for more.[40]

Many couples worry that they don't have sex often enough. Popular magazines frequently give the "average" number of times couples engage in sex every week. Such numbers are meaningless. Rather than compare yourself to these statistics, you would be wise simply to follow your own feelings. The bottom line is that you must decide what is right for you.

## Variant Sexual Behaviour

**Variant sexual behaviour** is the term used to describe sexual behaviours not engaged in by most people. The following list of variant sexual behaviours includes behaviours illegal in some provinces and territories and actions that could be harmful to others:

■ *Group sex.* Sexual activity involving more than two people. Participants in group sex run a high risk of STIs, including HIV.

■ *Transvestitism.* The wearing of clothing of the opposite sex. Most transvestites are male, heterosexual, and married.

■ *Transsexualism.* Strong identification with the opposite sex in which men or women feel "trapped in the wrong body." In some cases, transsexuals undergo sex-change operations.

■ *Fetishism.* Sexual arousal achieved by looking at or touching inanimate objects, such as underclothing or shoes.

■ *Exhibitionism.* The exposure of one's genitals to strangers in public places. Most exhibitionists are seeking a reaction of shock or fear from their victims.

■ *Voyeurism.* Observing other people for sexual gratification. Most voyeurs are men who attempt to watch women undressing or bathing. Voyeurism is illegal and an invasion of privacy.

■ *Sadomasochism.* Sexual activities in which gratification is received by inflicting pain (verbal or physical abuse) on a partner or by being the object of such infliction. A sadist is a person who receives gratification from inflicting pain, and a masochist is a person who receives gratification from experiencing pain.

■ *Pedophilia.* Sexual activity or attraction between an adult and a child. Any sexual activity involving a minor, including creating, possessing, or selling of child pornography, is illegal.

■ *Autoerotic asphyxiation.* The practice of reducing or eliminating oxygen to the brain, usually by tying a cord around one's neck, while masturbating. Tragically, some individuals accidentally hang themselves in the process.

### WHAT WOULD YOU DO?

How does our society decide what sexual behaviours are normal and which are variant? Are some sexual behaviours that we consider normal looked upon as abnormal or perverse in other countries or cultures? Why are some individuals willing to try various sexual behaviours while others are not?

# DIFFICULTIES THAT CAN HINDER SEXUAL FUNCTIONING

Research indicates that problems that hinder sexual functioning are quite common in this country. The label given to the various problems that can interfere with sexual pleasure is **sexual dysfunction.** You should not be embarrassed if you experience a sexual dysfunction at some point in your life. The sexual part of yourself does not come with a lifetime warranty. You can have breakdowns involving your sexual function just as you can have breakdowns in any of your other body systems. Sexual dysfunctions can be divided into four major classes: sexual desire disorders, sexual arousal disorders, orgasm disorders, and sexual pain disorders. In most cases, sexual dysfunctions can be treated successfully if both partners are willing to work together to solve the problem.

## Sexual Desire Disorders

The most frequent reason people seek a sex therapist is **ISD, or inhibited sexual desire.**[41] ISD is the lack of a sexual appetite or simply a lack of interest and pleasure in sexual activity. In some instances, it can result from stress or boredom with sex. **Sexual aversion disorder** is another type of desire dysfunction, characterized by sexual phobias (unreasonable fears) and anxiety about sexual contact. The psychological stress of a punitive upbringing, rigid religious background, or a history of physical or sexual abuse may be a source of these desire disorders.

## Sexual Arousal Disorders

The most common disorder in this category is **erectile dysfunction.** Erectile dysfunction, or *impotence*, refers to difficulty in achieving or maintaining a penile erection sufficient for intercourse. At some time in his life, every man experiences impotence. Causes are varied and include underlying diseases, such as diabetes or prostate problems, reactions to some medications (for example, medication for high blood pressure), depression, fatigue, stress, alcohol, performance anxiety, and guilt over real or imaginary problems (such as when a man compares himself to his partner's past lovers). Impotence generally becomes more of a problem as men age, affecting one in four men over the age of 65.[42]

Chronic impotence (impotence lasting more than three months) should be treated by a physician. A complete medical examination and history are necessary to rule out physical causes. Viagra (sildenafil citrate), Levitra, and Cialis are used as treatments for erectile dysfunction. Taken by mouth one hour before sexual activity, Viagra is reported to manage erectile dysfunction successfully in 60 to 80 percent of cases.[43] The medication is not, however, without risk. The most commonly reported side effects include headache, flushing, stomach ache, urinary tract infection, diarrhea, dizziness, rash, and mild and temporary visual changes.[44] There have been several deaths among Viagra users, prompting more caution in prescribing it to patients with known cardiovascular disease and those taking commonly prescribed short- and long-acting nitrates, such as nitroglycerin. Impotence due to psychological factors can be treated with psychotherapy. Such treatment is effective in 90 percent of cases.

## Orgasm Disorders

Up to 50 percent of the male population are affected by premature ejaculation at some time in their lives. **Premature ejaculation** is ejaculation that occurs prior to or very soon after the insertion of the penis into the vagina. Another orgasm disorder in males is **retarded ejaculation,** or the inability to ejaculate once the penis is erect. Treatment for premature ejaculation involves a physical examination to rule out organic causes. If the cause of the problem is not physiological, therapy is available to help a man learn how to control the timing of his ejaculation. Fatigue, stress, performance pressure, and alcohol can be contributing factors to these orgasmic disorders in men.

When a woman is unable to achieve orgasm with her partner, she often blames herself and fakes orgasm to preserve her partner's ego. Research has reported that up to 66 percent of women have faked an orgasm at one time or another.[45] Until recently, our society dictated that women were not supposed to enjoy sex but were to engage in it only to fulfill their "marital duty." The Kinsey reports in the 1950s and Masters and Johnson's findings in the 1960s and 1970s raised questions about these female sexual myths. We recognize today that women enjoy sexual activity as much as men. In the past, women who did not experience orgasm were called *frigid*. This term is no longer used because it implies that the woman is at fault. Instead, the term **preorgasmic** is used, since many women can be taught to become orgasmic.

For women whose sexual pleasure is hampered, therapy is available. A physical examination to rule out organic causes is generally the first step. Masturbation is usually a primary focus in teaching a woman to become orgasmic. Through masturbation, a woman can learn how her body responds sexually to various types of touch. Once a woman has become orgasmic through masturbation, she must learn to communicate her needs to her partner. The investment of time and caring by both partners is usually worth the effort, for 70 percent of preorgasmic women can be helped.

**Variant sexual behaviour:** A sexual behaviour not engaged in by most people.

**Sexual dysfunction:** Problems associated with achieving sexual satisfaction.

**Inhibited sexual desire (ISD):** Lack of sexual appetite or simply a lack of interest and pleasure in sexual activity.

**Sexual aversion disorder:** Type of desire dysfunction characterized by sexual phobias and anxiety about sexual contact.

**Erectile dysfunction:** Also known as impotence; difficulty in achieving or maintaining a penile erection sufficient for intercourse.

**Premature ejaculation:** Ejaculation that occurs prior to or almost immediately following penile penetration.

**Retarded ejaculation:** The inability to ejaculate once the penis is erect.

**Preorgasmic:** In women, the state of never having experienced an orgasm.

# Building Better Relationships

After reading this chapter, it should be apparent that relationships involve complex interactions between individuals. To build strong relationships, you must carefully assess the values you put on friendships, significant others, and other forms of interpersonal interactions. Healthy relationships involve developing intimacy in several dimensions. It may be helpful for you to take a personal inventory of your relationships to assess how healthy they are.

## MAKING DECISIONS FOR YOU

Think about the most important relationship in your life. Why is this relationship important to your overall health and well-being? Are there any behaviours that you could change to strengthen this relationship? To make such a change, begin by listing the reasons why the change is important. Who will benefit from this change? What steps will you take to make this change occur? What will you do to make sure that you keep up with or maintain this behaviour change?

## CHECKLIST FOR CHANGE: MAKING PERSONAL CHOICES

■ What relationships are most important to you right now?

■ How have these relationships affected your relationships with others? Are you giving enough time to your other relationships?

■ Have you thought about how good your relationships are from an emotional perspective? A psychological perspective? A physical perspective? A spiritual perspective? Which of these factors is the most important to you? Why?

■ What would an ideal set of relationships look like for you? How many close interactions would you want to make time for? What would be the nature and extent of these relationships?

■ Do you feel comfortable with yourself sexually? Are you satisfied with your current choice(s) of sexual expression?

■ What do you expect in a long-term, committed relationship? What would you be willing to accept in terms of behaviours from your committed partner? What do you expect of yourself?

■ What do you think are the three most important attributes of a friend? Do you display these attributes with your friends?

■ Do you feel limited or bound by gender-role stereotypes? Which ones?

■ Have you considered your values or beliefs about what is most important to you in a prospective lifelong partner? Are you asking for the same attributes that you would be able to give to a partner?

## CHECKLIST FOR CHANGE: MAKING COMMUNITY CHOICES

■ Do you make a habit of putting yourself in the other person's shoes when discussing how your actions may have made that person feel or how that person may be feeling in general?

■ Do you take time to listen to your friends? Your parents? Your acquaintances? Do you find yourself thinking about your own problems, thoughts, or issues when someone is trying to tell you about his or her problems?

■ Do you reach out to friends having problems in their relationships?

■ Are you supportive of couples having problems in their relationship without being judgmental or taking sides?

■ Do you try to work through your problems with others, or do you run from, avoid, or get angry rather than try to talk through your difficulties?

■ Are you supportive of counselling services and other campus and community services that offer help for people who have troubled relationships?

■ Do you listen carefully to what your legislators propose in the way of family and individual policies and programs that may unfairly harm others?

## CRITICAL THINKING

After leading what you consider a normal sexual life, which has included several intimate sexual relationships, you meet that special person. When you first started dating you learned that this person was a practising member of an Eastern religion, but you never really gave much thought to what that meant to your relationship. Now, several months later, as you want to become intimate, you realize that this religion does not accept intercourse before marriage.

You feel sexually frustrated. But at the same time, you are sincerely in love and believe that this relationship could lead to marriage. Using the DECIDE model in Chapter 1, think about what the two of you could do to satisfy physical and emotional feelings.

## Sexual Pain Disorders

Two common disorders in this category are dyspareunia and vaginismus. **Dyspareunia** is pain experienced by a female during intercourse. This pain may be caused by endometriosis, uterine tumours, chlamydia, gonorrhea, or urinary tract infections. Damage to tissues during childbirth and insufficient lubrication during intercourse may also cause pain or discomfort. Dyspareunia can also be psychological in origin. As with other problems, dyspareunia can be treated with good results. The first step in treatment is a thorough pelvic examination to rule out physical disease. Diseases or disorders can usually be cured with medication or surgery. Vaginal lubricants can be purchased to help with inadequate lubrication. Psychologically caused dyspareunia is much more difficult to treat.

**Vaginismus** is the involuntary contraction of vaginal muscles, making penile insertion painful or impossible. Most cases of vaginismus are related to fear of intercourse or to unresolved sexual conflicts. Treatment of vaginismus involves teaching a woman to achieve orgasm through nonvaginal stimulation. Becoming orgasmic is important because research has indicated that treatment for vaginismus is more successful in orgasmic women. The woman and her partner are then taught methods for dilating the vagina, either with fingers or a vibrator. As dilation is achieved, the woman is taught to relax in order to allow penetration. Cure rates are close to 100 percent.

## Drugs and Sex

Because psychoactive drugs affect our entire physiology, they also affect our sexual behaviours. Promises of increased pleasure make drugs very tempting to those seeking greater sexual satisfaction. Too often, however, drugs become central to sexual activities and damage the relationship. Alcohol is notorious for reducing inhibitions and giving increased feelings of well-being and desirability. At the same time, alcohol inhibits sexual response; thus, the mind may be willing, but not the body. Perhaps the greatest danger associated with use of drugs during sex is the tendency to blame the drug for negative or irresponsible behaviours: "I can't help what I did last night because I was stoned" is a response that demonstrates sexual immaturity. A sexually mature person carefully examines risks and benefits and makes decisions accordingly. If drugs are necessary to increase erotic feelings, it is likely that the partners are being dishonest about their feelings for each other. Good sex should not be dependent on chemical substances.

### WHAT WOULD YOU DO?

Why do we find it so difficult to discuss sexual dysfunction in our society? Do you think it is more difficult for men to talk about dysfunction? Why or why not? Have you ever used alcohol or some other drug to enhance your sexual performance? If you were experiencing sexual dysfunction, what would you tell your partner?

**Dyspareunia:** Pain experienced by women during intercourse.

**Vaginismus:** A state in which the vaginal muscles contract so forcefully that penetration cannot be accomplished.

# SUMMARY

- Communication is an important factor of any relationship. It is important not only to express yourself effectively, but also to listen effectively.

- Intimate relationships have several different characteristics that play significant roles in determining how happy, healthy, and well adjusted you are as you interact with others.

- Men and women often relate differently in intimate relationships. Understanding these differences and learning how to deal with them is an important aspect of healthy relationships.

- Success in committed relationships requires understanding the roles that partnering scripts play, the importance of self-nurturance, the elements of a good relationship, and the ability to confront couple issues.

- Today's family structure may look different from that of previous generations, but love, trust, and commitment continue to be the cornerstones of successful child rearing.

- Sexual identity is determined by a complex interaction of genetic, physiological, and environmental factors. Sex, gender, gender roles, and gender-role stereotypes are all blended into our sexual identity.
- The major components of the female sexual anatomy include the mons pubis, labia minora and majora, clitoris, urethral and vaginal openings, vagina, cervix, fallopian tubes, and ovaries. The major components of the male sexual anatomy are the penis, scrotum, testes, epididymides, vasa deferentia, ejaculatory ducts, and urethra.
- Sexuality can be expressed in many ways. Physiologically, males and females experience four phases of sexual response: excitement/arousal, plateau, orgasm, and resolution. In addition, men experience a fifth phase known as the refractory period. Sexual orientation refers to a person's preference for emotional, social, and sexual attractions. Sexual activities include celibacy, autoerotic behaviours, kissing and erotic touch, oral–genital stimulation, anal intercourse, and vaginal intercourse. Numerous variant sexual behaviours also exist.
- There are many strategies for building better relationships. Taking a careful look at your own behaviours, those things you may need to change, and those things that you are willing to do to help develop a relationship are all important ingredients of success.

# DISCUSSION QUESTIONS

1. What is the role of communication in nonintimate and intimate relationships? How can you become a better listener? Speaker?
2. What are behavioural interdependence, need fulfillment, and emotional attachment, and why is each of these important in subsequent relationship development?
3. What are the common types of intimate relationships? Which of these do you think is most important to you right now? Why?
4. Why are your relationships with your family important? Explain how your family unit was similar to or different from the family unit of the early 1900s. Who made up your family of origin? Your nuclear family?
5. How can you tell the difference between a love relationship and one that is based primarily on attraction? What common characteristics do love relationships share?
6. What can serve as barriers to intimacy? Are there actions you can take to reduce or remove these barriers?
7. What are the common elements of good relationships?
8. What actions can you take to improve your own interpersonal relationships?
9. What are the functions of the various hormones during puberty? What physical changes are brought about by menopause?
10. What are "normal" sexual behaviours? Is sexual orientation primarily determined by biological or environmental factors? Do men and women differ in sexual response?
11. Do drugs and alcohol enhance sexual performance? What risks are involved in such experimentation?

# APPLICATION EXERCISE

Reread the What Do You Think? scenario at the beginning of the chapter and answer the following questions.

1. From what you have read in this chapter, what problems do Michael and Sara have in their relationship?
2. Why do you think people are often forced to tell lies or half-truths in their relationships with others?

3. Are there times when it is okay to be dishonest or to not tell the truth, or should you always be totally honest and truthful about your actions?

4. Do you believe that you should tell your partner about all of your sexual interactions? Why or why not?

## HEALTH ON THE NET

Canadian Paediatric Society
**www.cps.ca/english/index.htm**

Child & Family Canada
**www.cfc-efc.ca/**

Family Service Canada
**www.familyservicecanada.org/**

British Columbia Council for Families
**www.bccf.bc.ca**

Sex Information and Education Council of Canada
**www.sieccan.org**

Sexuality and U
**http://sexualityandu.ca/**

CHAPTER 6

# BIRTH CONTROL, PREGNANCY, AND CHILDBIRTH

*Managing Your Fertility*

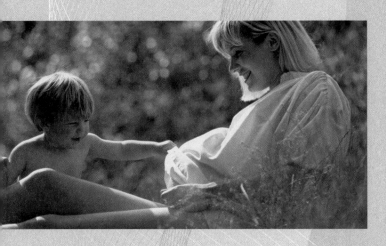

## CHAPTER OBJECTIVES

- List permanent and reversible contraceptive methods, discuss their effectiveness in preventing pregnancy and sexually transmitted infections, and describe how these methods are used.

- Summarize the legal decisions surrounding abortion and the various types of abortion procedures used today.

- Discuss emotional health, maternal health, financial evaluation, and contingency planning in terms of your life's goals as aspects that you should consider before becoming a parent.

- Explain the importance of prenatal care and the process of pregnancy.

- Describe the basic stages of childbirth as well as complications that can arise during labour and delivery.

- Review the primary causes of and possible solutions to infertility.

Kari and Dave have been dating for several months. After a wonderful evening together, they go back to Dave's place with the intention of having sex. When they arrive at Dave's, Kari discovers that Dave does not have any condoms. He thought that Kari was taking the birth control pill. Rather than spoil the evening, Kari and Dave have unprotected sex. The next day, they have an argument over who exactly was responsible for the birth control.

■ What mistakes were made in this relationship? When should a couple talk about this responsibility as well as preventing sexually transmitted infections? Who is responsible for providing birth control? What were the risks involved in engaging in unprotected sex? What were the alternatives?

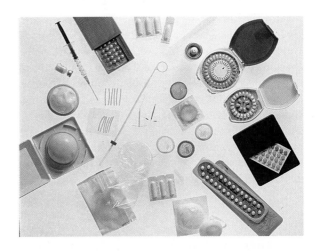

*For couples who want to avoid pregnancy, a wide variety of contraceptives are available, including male and female condoms, IUDs, cervical caps, diaphragms, and different types of pills.*

# MANAGING YOUR FERTILITY

**Fertility** is a mixed blessing for some women. The ability to participate in the miracle of birth is an incredible experience for many. Yet the responsibility for controlling one's fertility can also seem overwhelming. Today, we not only understand the intimate details of reproduction but also possess technologies designed to control or enhance our fertility. Along with information and technological advance comes choice, and choice goes hand-in-hand with responsibility. Choosing if and when to have children is one of our most important decisions. A woman and her partner have much to consider before planning or risking a pregnancy. Children, whether planned or unplanned, change people's lives. They require a lifelong personal commitment of love and nurturing.

Before you plan or risk a pregnancy, you have the responsibility to make certain you are physically, emotionally, and financially prepared to care for another human being. One measure of maturity is the ability to discuss reproduction, birth control, and sexually transmitted infection (STI) protection with your sexual partner before succumbing to sexual urges. If you cannot discuss birth control or STI protection then you may not be mature enough to engage in sex. Men often assume that their partners are taking care of birth control. Women often feel that if they bring up the subject, it implies that they are "easy" or "loose." You will find embarrassment-free discussion a lot easier if you understand human reproduction and contraception and honestly consider your attitudes toward these matters before you get into compromising situations.

**Conception** refers to the fertilization of an ovum by a sperm. The sperm enters the ovum. Its tail breaks off, and a protective chemical barrier secreted by the ovum surrounds the sperm and prevents other sperm from entering. A viable egg, a viable sperm, and possible access to the egg by the sperm are necessary conditions for conception.

**Contraception** refers to methods of preventing conception. Society has and continues to search for a simple, infallible, and risk-free method of preventing pregnancy. Our present methods of contraception fall into two categories: *reversible methods,* such as the pill, condoms, and abstinence; and *permanent methods,* such as vasectomy (for men) and tubal ligation (for women).

## Reversible Contraception
### Abstinence and "Outercourse"

Strictly defined, abstinence means not engaging in intercourse. Traditionally, individuals could still engage in such forms of sexual intimacy as massage, kissing, and solitary masturbation and consider themselves abstainers. However, many people today have broadened the definition of abstinence to include all forms of sexual contact, even those that do not culminate in sexual intercourse.

**Fertility:** A person's ability to reproduce.

**Conception:** The fertilization of an ovum by a sperm.

**Contraception:** Methods of preventing conception.

Couples who go a step farther than massage and kissing and engage in such activities as oral–genital sex and mutual masturbation are sometimes said to be engaging in "outercourse." Like abstinence, outercourse can be 100-percent effective for birth control as long as the male does not ejaculate near the vaginal opening. Unlike abstinence, however, there is still a risk of STIs when engaging in outercourse. Oral–genital contact can result in transmission of an STI, although the risk can be reduced by using a condom on the penis or a dental dam on the vaginal opening.

## Condoms

The **condom** is a strong sheath of latex rubber or other material designed to fit over an erect penis (Figure 6.1). The condom catches the ejaculate, thereby preventing sperm migration toward the egg. The condom is the only temporary means of birth control available for men and the only barrier that effectively prevents the spread of STIs, including HIV. Regardless of your preferred method of birth control, you should always use a condom. Condoms come in a wide variety of styles: coloured, ribbed for "extra sensation," lubricated, nonlubricated, and with or without reservoirs at the tip. All may be purchased with or without spermicide in pharmacies, in some schools, and in some public washrooms. Some health clinics, including those on many college and university campuses, provide condoms free of charge. A new condom must be used for each act of intercourse or oral sex.

Condoms help prevent the spread of some STIs, including genital herpes and HIV. They may also slow or reduce the development of cervical abnormalities in women that can lead to cancer. The theoretical **perfect-use effectiveness rate** for condoms is 98 percent, meaning that *when they are used correctly and consistently,* 2 women out of 100 will become pregnant in one year. In reality, however, their effectiveness, or **typical-use rate,** is only 85 percent (15 out of every 100 women who use condoms will become pregnant in one year) because they are so often used incorrectly or inconsistently. The unintended pregnancies or failure rates of contraceptives are shown in Table 6.1 according to typical and perfect-use rates. Condoms should always be used for vaginal, anal, and oral sex. They must be rolled on the erect penis before the penis touches the vagina, leaving about a one-centimetre space at the tip to collect ejaculated semen. The condom should be held at the base of the penis after ejaculation for removal to avoid spilling any semen. For greatest efficacy, they should be used with a spermicide containing nonoxynol-9.

Another reason why condoms are not as effective in real life as in theory is that they can break during intercourse, especially if they are old or poorly stored. They must be stored in a cool place (not in a wallet or hip pocket) and should be inspected before use for small tears.

Some people claim that a condom ruins the spontaneity of sex. Stopping to put it on breaks the mood for them. Others report that the condom decreases sensation. These perceived inconveniences also contribute to improper use. Couples who learn to put the condom on together as part of foreplay are generally more successful with this form of birth control and STI protection.[1]

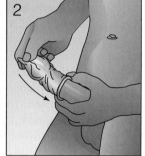
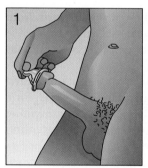
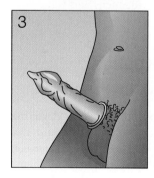
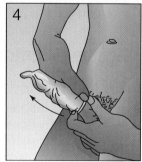

### FIGURE 6.1
#### How to Use a Condom

The condom should be rolled over the erect penis as soon as it is erect (even during outercourse). A small space (about 1 cm) should be left at the end of the condom to collect the semen after ejaculation. Hold the tip of the condom, and unroll it all the way to the base of the penis. Hold the base of the condom before withdrawal to avoid spilling any semen.

**Condom:** A sheath of thin latex or other material designed to fit over an erect penis to catch semen upon ejaculation.

**Perfect-use effectiveness rate:** The percentage rate of women who will become pregnant in one year when the contraceptive method is used correctly and consistently.

**Typical-use effectiveness rate:** The percentage of women who will become pregnant in one year when the contraceptive method is used incorrectly or inconsistently.

## TABLE 6.1

### Contraceptive Effectiveness and STI Prevention: Number of Unintended Pregnancies per 100 during First Year of Use

| Method | Typical Use | Perfect Use |
|---|---|---|
| Continuous abstinence* | 0.00 | 0.00 |
| Outercourse† | N/A | N/A |
| Norplant implant | 0.05 | 0.05 |
| *Sterilization* | | |
| Men | 0.15 | 0.1 |
| Women | 0.5 | 0.5 |
| Depo-Provera injection | 0.3 | 0.3 |
| *IUD (intrauterine device)* | | |
| ParaGard (copper T380A) | 0.8 | 0.6 |
| Mirena | 0.1 | 0.1 |
| Oral contraceptives (The Pill) | 8.0 | 0.3 |
| Male condom† | 15.0 | 2.0 |
| *Sponge* | | |
| Women who have not given birth | 16.0 | 9.0 |
| Women who have given birth | 32.0 | 20.0 |
| Ortho Evra (The Patch) | 8.0 | 0.3 |
| NuvaRing | 8.0 | 0.3 |
| Withdrawal | 27.0 | 4.0 |
| Diaphragm† | 20.0 | 6.0 |
| *Cervical cap†* | | |
| Women who have not given birth | 16.0 | 9.0 |
| Women who have given birth | 32.0 | 26.0 |
| Female condom† | 21.0 | 5.0 |
| *Periodic abstinence* | 25.0 | |
| Postovulation method | | 1.0 |
| Symptothermal method | | 2.0 |
| Cervical mucus (ovulation) method | | 3.0 |
| Calendar method | | 9.0 |
| Fertility awareness methods | N/A | N/A |
| Spermicide† | 26.0 | 6.0 |
| No method | 85.0 | 85.0 |

*Emergency contraception*

Emergency contraception pills: Treatment initiated within 72 hours after unprotected intercourse reduces the risk of pregnancy by 75–89% (with no protection against STIs). Emergency IUD insertion: Treatment initiated within seven days after unprotected intercourse reduces the risk of pregnancy by more than 99 percent (with no protection against STIs).

Notes: "Typical Use" refers to failure rates for men and women whose use is not consistent or always correct.
"Perfect Use" refers to failure rates for those whose use is consistent and always correct.
N/A means that effectiveness rates are not available.
*indicates complete protection from STIs
†indicates limited protection from STIs

Source: R. Hatcher et al., "Contraceptive Effectiveness Rates," *Contraceptive Technology,* 18th ed. (New York: Ardent Media, 2004). Reprinted by permission of Ardent Media.

# Talking with Your Partner About Using Condoms

Knowing what's best for our health and doing something about it can be two different things. Bringing up the subject of condoms can be hard—especially the first time. Here are some suggestions:

1. Think about what you want to say ahead of time. Sort out your feelings about using condoms before you talk with your partner.

2. Choose a time to talk before that first intimate moment. Getting things straight before you engage in sexual activity means you'll both be prepared and relaxed.

3. Decide how you want to start the conversation. You might say, "I need to talk with you about something that's important to both of us," or, "I've been hearing a lot lately about safer sex. Have you ever tried condoms?" or, "I feel kind of embarrassed, but I care too much about you and myself not to talk about this."

4. Remember, starting to talk is the hardest part. Don't be surprised if your partner responds with, "I'm glad you brought it up. I was worried too," or, "I like sharing the responsibility of sex. I appreciate a woman who's willing to let me."

5. Once you've agreed to use condoms, do something positive and fun. Go to the store together. Buy lots of different brands and colours. Plan a special day when you can experiment. Just talking about how you will use all those condoms can be a turn-on.

## Oral Contraceptives

**Oral contraceptive pills** were first marketed in Canada in 1961 and quickly became the most widely used reversible method of fertility control. Most oral contraceptives work through the combined effects of synthetic estrogen and progesterone. Because the levels of estrogen in the pill are higher than those produced by the body, the pituitary gland is not signalled to produce follicle-stimulating hormone (FSH), without which ova will not develop in the ovaries. Further, progesterone in the pill prevents growth of the uterine lining and thickens the cervical mucus, forming a barrier against sperm.

Pills are meant to be taken in a cycle. At the end of each three-week cycle, the user discontinues the drug or takes a placebo pill for one week. The resultant drop in hormones causes the uterine lining to disintegrate, and the user will have a menstrual period, usually within one to three days. The same cycle is repeated every 28 days. Menstrual flow is generally lighter than in a non–pill user because the hormones in the pill prevent thick endometrial build-up.

Today's pill is different from the one introduced more than three decades ago. The original pill contained large amounts of estrogen, which caused certain risks for the user, whereas the current pill contains the minimal amount of estrogen necessary to prevent pregnancy.

Because the chemicals in oral contraceptives change the way the body metabolizes certain nutrients, all women using the pill should check with their prescribing practitioners regarding dietary supplements. The nutrients of concern include vitamin C and the B-complex vitamins—B2, B6, and B12. A nutritious diet that includes whole grains, fresh fruits and vegetables, lean meats, fish and poultry, and nonfat dairy products is advised. Oral contraceptives can interact negatively with other drugs. Some antibiotics diminish the pill's effectiveness, as can the 24-hour flu or diarrhea. A backup contraceptive should be used for the rest of the pill pack if these circumstances occur. Women in doubt should check with their prescribing practitioners, their pharmacists, or other knowledgeable health professionals. You can learn more about health methods and contraceptive choice in the Skills for Behaviour Change box.

Although return of fertility may be delayed after discontinuing the pill, it is not known to cause infertility. Women who had irregular menstrual cycles before going on the pill are more likely to have problems conceiving, regardless of pill use.

The perfect-use effectiveness rate of oral contraceptives is 99.7 percent, making them one of the most effective reversible methods of fertility control. Using the pill is convenient and does not interfere with sexual activity. It may lessen menstrual difficulties, such as cramps and premenstrual syndrome (PMS). Women using oral contraceptives have lower risks for developing endometrial and ovarian cancers. They are also less likely than nonusers to develop fibrocystic

# Choosing a Contraceptive

Part of sexual maturity is taking responsibility for your personal health regarding contraceptives and STI protection. Aside from simply worrying about contraceptive effectiveness and convenience, you need to consider the effects that your birth control method may have on your health now and in the future. Here are some things to keep in mind when you decide on your contraceptive method:

1. Talk to your medical professional about your and your family's medical history. Is there anything that would discourage the use of one method or another? Some contraceptive methods may have serious side effects according to your medical history (for example, if there is a history of high blood pressure in your family, you may choose not to use oral contraceptives).

2. Learn about the potential side effects. If you find yourself experiencing the side effects of a contraceptive, you should talk to your doctor immediately. Your doctor may suggest switching to a different contraceptive or may simply assure you that the "side effects" don't appear related to contraceptive use.

3. Devise a method to ensure that you can't miss using it. If you take the pill, take it at the same time every day. Associating it with a certain time or event (for instance, taking a morning shower) will reinforce your memory. If you use condoms, you might keep some in your sport coat pocket so they will

be there when you need them. Or you might keep your diaphragm packed in your overnight bag.

4. Learn how to talk to your partner about your choice of contraception and STI protection. Decisions about contraceptives should be made as a couple, taking each person's health and desires into account.

5. Learn about drug interactions with your birth control method. While we will discuss this in more detail in Chapter 10, it is important to know what medications may interact with your method of birth control. For example, interactions may occur between alcohol and contraceptive pills or between antibiotics and contraceptive pills. Specifically, alcohol and antibiotics may diminish the effectiveness of birth control pills in some women. Ask your doctor about drug interactions if you receive a prescription drug. If there is a potential for diminished effectiveness of your contraceptive, ask when you can resume normal sexual relations without taking added precautions.

---

breast disease. In addition, pill users have lower incidences of ectopic pregnancies, ovarian cysts, pelvic inflammatory disease, and iron deficiency anemia.[2] Possible serious health problems associated with the pill include the tendency for pill users' blood to form clots and an increased risk for high blood pressure in a few women. Clotting can lead to strokes or heart attacks. The risk is low for most healthy, non-smoking women under 35; it increases with age and, especially, with cigarette smoking.

Although the perfect-use rate of oral contraceptives is 99.7 percent, the typical-use effectiveness is only 92 percent. The typical-use rate may relate to the fact that the pill must be taken every day. If a woman misses taking one pill, she is advised to use an alternative form of contraception for the remainder of that cycle. The cost of the pill may also be a problem for some women. Finally, some younger teenagers report that the requirement to have a complete gynecological examination in order to get a prescription for the pill is an obstacle. Fully 69 percent of female teenagers think that this requirement frightens their peers away from use of the pill.[3] Educating young women about what goes on in a gynecological exam may ease their anxiety, along with confirmation that their examination and prescription remains confidential.

## Progestin-Only Pills

Progestin-only pills (or minipills) contain small doses of progesterone. Women who feel uncertain about using estrogen pills, who suffer from side effects related to estrogen, or who are nursing may want to take these pills rather than combination pills. There is still some question about the specific ways progestin-only pills work. Current thought is that they change the composition of the cervical mucus, thus impeding sperm travel. They may also inhibit ovulation in some women. The effectiveness rate of progestin-only pills is 96 percent, which is lower than that of estrogen-containing pills. Also, their use usually leads to irregular menstrual bleeding.

## Birth Control Patch (Evra)

Health Canada recently approved a new form of birth control in a dermal patch that may be applied to the skin. Since January 2003, Canadian women have been able to obtain the patch by prescription and use it in

**Oral contraceptive pills:** Pills taken daily for three weeks of the menstrual cycle that prevent ovulation by regulating hormones.

place of birth control pills or injections. The patch contains the hormones progestin and estrogen, two ingredients also found in birth control pills. It works like a smoking cessation patch, releasing medication through the skin into the bloodstream. The patch can be worn on the buttocks, upper outer arm, abdomen, back, or stomach. A new patch is applied every week for three weeks each month. During the fourth week, no patch is worn to allow for menstruation. If a patch falls off at any time you must replace it within a 24-hour period to maintain your normal birth control cycle.

While the patch will not protect you from STIs, it may be an alternative worth considering for those who frequently forget to take birth control pills and who do not like injections. The patch has similar effectiveness rates as the pill: perfect use is 99.7 percent and typical use is 92 percent. A small percentage of women may find that they are not able to use the patch because it irritates the skin.

### Depo-Provera

**Depo-Provera** is a long-acting synthetic injected intramuscularly every three months. Although used in other countries for years, the Health Protection Branch did not approve it for use in Canada until 1997. Researchers believe that the drug prevents ovulation. Depo-Provera encourages sexual spontaneity because the user does not have to remember to take a pill or insert a device. Its effectiveness in preventing pregnancy is greater than 99 percent. Its use may prevent menstrual blood loss, iron deficiency anemia, premenstrual tension, and endometriosis. The main disadvantage is irregular bleeding, which can be troublesome at first, but within a year most women are amenorrheic (have no menstrual cycles). Weight gain (an average of 2.5 kg in the first year) is common. A report from Planned Parenthood indicates some other disadvantages, such as fatigue, mood disturbances, loss of libido, and increased risk of osteoporosis and diabetes. Dizziness, nervousness, and headache are other possible side effects. Unlike other methods of contraception, this method cannot be stopped immediately if problems arise. Fertility may not return right away after Depo-Provera use is discontinued.

### NuvaRing

Introduced in 2002, this effective contraceptive offers protection for four weeks at a time when used as prescribed. **NuvaRing** is a soft flexible ring about 5 cm in diameter that the user inserts into the vagina and leaves in place for three weeks. The user removes it for one week during her menstrual period. Once the ring is inserted, it continuously releases estrogen and progestin.

Advantages to NuvaRing include protection against pregnancy for one month; no pill to take daily; no requirement to be fitted by a clinician; no requirement to use spermicide; and the quick return of the ability to become pregnant when no longer in use. Possible side effects include increased vaginal discharge and vaginal irritation or infection. Oil-based vaginal medicine to treat yeast infections cannot be used when the ring is in place, and a diaphragm or cervical cap cannot be used as a backup method.

## Emergency Contraceptive Pills

**Emergency contraceptive pills** can be used when a condom breaks, after a sexual assault, or any time unprotected sexual intercourse occurs. Although often referred to as "the morning-after pill," they can be taken up to three days after unprotected intercourse to reduce the risk of pregnancy by 75 percent. It is not clear how emergency contraceptive pills prevent pregnancy, but it seems that they prevent ovulation rather than implantation of a fertilized egg. The most common emergency contraceptive pill prescribed is a combination of estrogen and progesterone. Nausea, vomiting, menstrual irregularities, breast tenderness, headaches, abdominal pain and cramps, and dizziness are the most likely side effects of these drugs.

Preven was approved by Health Canada in November 1999. It contains two hormones that stop or delay ovulation and may prevent a fertilized egg from implanting in the uterus. Two pills are to be taken within 24 hours of intercourse and another two 12 or more hours after that. This drug is intended for a woman who uses a method that fails or a woman who has experienced non-consensual sex. It is not "the abortion pill." Side effects are as listed above.

## Foams, Suppositories, Jellies, and Creams

Like condoms, these contraceptive preparations are available without a prescription. Chemically, they are referred to as **spermicides**—substances designed to kill sperm.

Jellies and creams are packaged in tubes, and foams are available in aerosol cans. They must be inserted far enough into the vagina to cover the cervix, providing both a chemical barrier that kills sperm and a physical barrier that stops sperm from continuing toward an egg (Figure 6.2).

Suppositories are waxy capsules placed deep in the vagina that melt once they are inside. They must be inserted 10 to 20 minutes before intercourse to have time to melt, but no longer than one hour prior to

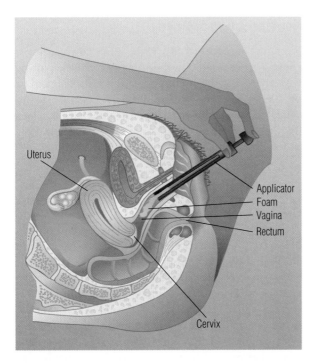

### FIGURE 6.2

The Proper Method of Applying Spermicide within the Vagina

intercourse or they lose their effectiveness. Additional contraceptive chemicals must be applied for each subsequent act of intercourse. Jellies, creams, suppositories, and foam do not require a prescription. When used in conjunction with a condom, their effectiveness rate is nearly 98 percent. They help prevent the spread of certain sexually transmitted infections. Jellies and creams are designed to be used with a diaphragm. Used alone, their effectiveness rate is only 79 percent. Foam, which is designed to be used alone, also has an effectiveness rate of 79 percent.

## Contraceptive Film

This product is available in Canada but is not widely distributed. It is a translucent square that is inserted to cover the cervix, close to the time of intercourse. Some women prefer it since it is less messy than jellies or foam. It does not have to be removed, because it dissolves.

## Female Condoms

The **female condom** is a single-use, soft, loose-fitting polyurethane sheath. It is designed as one unit, with two diaphragm-like rings. One ring, which lies inside the sheath, serves as an insertion mechanism and internal anchor. The other ring, which remains outside

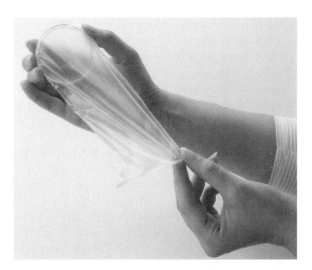

*The female condom.*

the vagina once the device is inserted, protects the labia and the base of the penis from infection. Tests conducted by the manufacturers found that it was 87.6 percent effective. Many women like the female condom because it gives them more control over their reproduction than the male condom.

## Diaphragm with Spermicidal Jelly or Cream

Invented in the mid-nineteenth century, the **diaphragm** was the first widely used birth control method for women. Before that, most women had to rely on their male partners to use a condom or to withdraw before ejaculation. The diaphragm is a soft, shallow cup made of thin latex rubber. Its flexible, rubber-coated ring is designed to fit snugly behind the pubic bone in front of the cervix and over the back of the cervix on the other side. Diaphragms are manufactured in different sizes and must be fitted to the woman by a trained practitioner. The practitioner should also be certain that the user knows how to

**Depo-Provera:** An injectable method of birth control that lasts for three months.

**NuvaRing:** A soft, flexible ring inserted into the vagina that releases hormones that prevent pregnancy.

**Emergency contraceptive pills:** Drugs taken up to three days after intercourse to reduce the risk of pregnancy.

**Spermicides:** Substances designed to kill sperm.

**Female condom:** A single-use polyurethane sheath for internal use by women.

**Diaphragm:** A latex, saucer-shaped device designed to cover the cervix and block access to the uterus; should be used with spermicide.

insert her diaphragm correctly before she leaves the practitioner's office.

Diaphragms must be used with spermicidal cream or jelly. The spermicide is applied to the inside of the diaphragm before insertion. The jelly or cream is held in place by the diaphragm, creating a physical and chemical barrier against sperm. Additional spermicide must be applied before each subsequent act of intercourse, and the diaphragm must be left in place for six to eight hours after intercourse to allow the chemical to kill any sperm remaining in the vagina (see Figure 6.3).

The typical-use effectiveness rate of the diaphragm is only 82 percent; perfect-use effectiveness is 94 percent. Further, using the diaphragm during the menstrual period or leaving the diaphragm in place beyond the recommended time increases the risk of developing **toxic shock syndrome (TSS).** This condition results from the multiplication of a type of bacteria that spreads to the bloodstream and causes sudden high fever, rash, nausea, vomiting, diarrhea, and a sudden drop in blood pressure. If not treated, TSS can be fatal. The diaphragm (as well as tampons left in place too long) creates conditions conducive to the growth of these bacteria. To reduce the risk of TSS, women should wash their hands carefully with soap and water before inserting or removing the diaphragm.

Another problem with the diaphragm is that it can put undue pressure on the urethra, blocking urinary flow and predisposing the user to bladder infections. A further disadvantage is that inserting the device can be awkward, especially if the woman is rushed. When inserted incorrectly, the effectiveness rate of the diaphragm decreases.

## Contraceptive Sponge

First manufactured in 1983, the contraceptive sponge increased in popularity among young women during the 1980s and early 1990s. Plagued by problems with reliability, allergic reactions, and other serious concerns, the original sponge was discontinued. In Canada, a new sponge is available called Protectaid.

## Cervical Cap

**Cervical caps** are one of the oldest methods used to prevent pregnancy. Early caps were made from beeswax, silver, or copper. The modern cervical cap has been available in Europe for several years and has been approved for use in Canada by the Health Protection Branch since 1982. The cervical cap is a small cup made of latex designed to fit snugly over the entire cervix. It must be fitted by a practitioner and is designed for use with contraceptive jelly or cream. It is somewhat more difficult to insert than a diaphragm because of its smaller size.

The cap keeps sperm out of the uterus. It is held in place by suction created during application. Insertion may take place anywhere up to two days prior to intercourse, and the device must be left in place for six to eight hours after intercourse. The maximum length of time the cap can be left on the cervix is 48 hours. If removed and cleaned, it can be reinserted immediately.

The effectiveness rate of the cap differs according to whether or not a woman has had a baby previously. Perfect-use rates for women who have not previously had a baby are 91 percent, while typical-use rates are

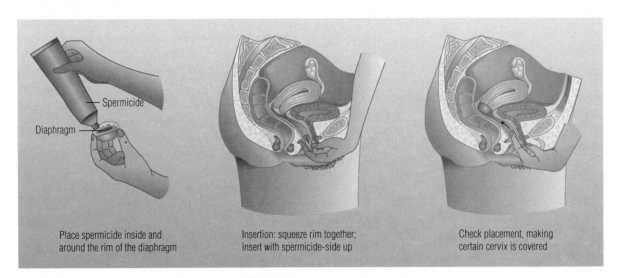

Place spermicide inside and around the rim of the diaphragm

Insertion: squeeze rim together; insert with spermicide-side up

Check placement, making certain cervix is covered

FIGURE 6.3

**The Proper Use and Placement of a Diaphragm**

84 percent. Perfect-use and typical-use effectiveness are only 74 and 68 percent respectively for women who have had a baby. Some women report unpleasant vaginal odours after use. Because the device can become dislodged during intercourse, placement must be checked frequently. It cannot be used during the menstrual period or for longer than 48 hours because of the risk of toxic shock syndrome.

### Intrauterine Device

Widespread use of **intrauterine devices (IUDs)** for contraception began in the mid-1960s, when these devices were advertised as less risky and more convenient than the pill. The devices fell out of favour in the mid-1970s following negative publicity about the Dalkon Shield, a device associated with pelvic inflammatory disease and sterility. The manufacturer stopped making Dalkon Shields in 1975. We are not certain how IUDs work, despite the fact that women have been using them since 1909. Although it was once thought that IUDs act by preventing implantation of a fertilized egg, most experts now believe that they interfere with the sperm's fertilization of the egg.

A physician must fit and insert the IUD. For insertion, the device is folded and placed into a long, thin plastic applicator. The practitioner measures the depth of the uterus with a special instrument and then uses these measurements to place the IUD accurately. When in place, the arms of the T open out across the top of the uterus. One or two strings extend from the IUD into the vagina so the user can check to make sure that her IUD is in place. The device is removed by a practitioner when desired.

Although IUDs have a perfect-use rate greater than 99 percent, the discomfort and cost of insertion may be a disadvantage. When in place, the device can cause heavy menstrual flow and severe cramps. There is also risk of uterine perforation. Women using IUDs have a higher risk of ectopic pregnancy, pelvic inflammatory disease, infertility, and tubal infections. If a pregnancy occurs while the IUD is in place, the chance of miscarriage ranges from 25 to 50 percent. Removal of the device as soon as the pregnancy is known is advised. Doctors often offer therapeutic abortion to women who become pregnant while using an IUD because of the serious risks (including premature delivery, infection, and congenital abnormalities) associated with continuing the pregnancy.

### Withdrawal

This not very effective method of birth control is most commonly used by people who have not taken the time to consider alternatives. The **withdrawal** method involves withdrawing the penis from the vagina just prior to ejaculation. Because there can be up to half a million sperm in the drop of fluid at the tip of the penis before ejaculation, this method is unreliable. Timing withdrawal is also difficult; males concentrating on accurate timing may not be able to relax and enjoy intercourse. The typical-use effectiveness rate for the withdrawal method is 73 percent; perfect-use effectiveness is 94 percent.

## Oral Contraceptives for Men?

The development of an oral contraceptive for men has been slow. Evidently, the mechanisms involved in the manufacture and release of sperm are not as easy to manipulate as the female ovulatory and uterine cycles. Some oral contraceptives for men have been tested, but they produced unpleasant side effects such as diminished sex drive and impotence. At the present time, research into the development of new male contraceptives is being carried on in various countries. One compound undergoing research is *gossypol*, a substance derived from the cotton plant. Chinese and Canadian researchers have found that gossypol inhibits sperm production, causing infertility. Difficulties in reversing the effects of the drug are presenting problems, as are concerns over long-term health consequences and possible genetic effects.

Other researchers are investigating the possibility of using ultrasound as a male contraceptive. In this method, a high-frequency sound machine is placed in contact with the scrotum. The device emits sound waves that slow sperm production, thereby lowering sperm counts. In some cases, sperm counts have remained lowered for up to two years after the procedure. Reduced sperm count, as opposed to total destruction of sperm, may suffice as a contraceptive measure because a minimum number of sperm are needed for fertilization. Before this method can be made available, the risks for testicular cancer and genetic damage must be thoroughly explored.

**Toxic shock syndrome (TSS):** A potentially life-threatening disease that occurs when specific bacterial toxins are allowed to multiply unchecked in wounds or through improper use of tampons or diaphragms.

**Cervical cap:** A small cup made of latex that is designed to fit snugly over the entire cervix.

**Intrauterine device (IUD):** A T-shaped device that is implanted in the uterus to prevent pregnancy.

**Withdrawal:** A method of contraception that involves withdrawing the penis from the vagina before ejaculation.

# Fertility Awareness Methods (FAM)

Methods of fertility control that rely upon the alteration of sexual behaviours are called **fertility awareness methods (FAM).** These methods include observing female "fertile periods" by examining cervical mucus or keeping track of internal temperature and then abstaining from sexual intercourse (penis–vagina contact) during these fertile times.

Although the "rhythm method" is often the object of ridicule because of its low effectiveness rates, it is the only method of birth control available to women belonging to religious denominations that forbid the use of oral contraceptives, barrier methods, and sterilization. Our present reproductive knowledge enables women and their partners to use natural methods of birth control better with fewer risks of pregnancy, although these methods remain less effective than others.

Fertility awareness methods of birth control rely upon basic physiology. A released ovum can survive for up to 48 hours after ovulation. Sperm can live for as long as five days in the vagina. Natural methods of birth control teach women to recognize their fertile times. Changes in cervical mucus prior to and during ovulation and a rise in basal body temperature are two indicators frequently used in natural contraceptive techniques. Another method involves charting a woman's menstrual cycle and ovulation times on a calendar. Any combination of these methods may be used to determine fertile times more accurately.

## Cervical Mucus Method

The **cervical mucus method** requires women to examine the consistency and colour of their normal vaginal secretions. Before ovulation, vaginal mucus becomes gelatinous and stringy, and normal vaginal secretions may increase. Sexual activity involving penis–vagina contact must be avoided while this "fertile mucus" is present and for several days after.

## Body Temperature Method

The **body temperature method** relies on the fact that the female's basal body temperature rises between 0.4 and 0.8 degrees after ovulation. For this method to be effective, the woman must chart her temperature for several months to learn to recognize her body's temperature fluctuations. Abstinence from intercourse and any other penis–vagina contact must be observed preceding the temperature rise and until several days after the temperature rise was first noted.

## Calendar Method

The **calendar method** requires women to record the exact number of days in their menstrual cycle. Since few women menstruate with complete regularity, a record of the menstrual cycle must be kept for 12 months, during which some other method of birth control must be used. The first day of a woman's period is counted as day one. To determine the first fertile unsafe day of the cycle, she subtracts 18 from the number of days in the shortest cycle. To determine the last unsafe day of the cycle, she subtracts 11 from the number of days in the longest cycle. This method assumes that ovulation occurs during the midpoint of the cycle (see Figure 6.4). The couple must abstain from penis–vagina contact during the fertile time.

Women interested in fertility awareness methods of birth control are advised to take supervised classes. The risks of an unwanted pregnancy are great for the untrained woman. Reading a book or watching a film on the subject or talking to the proprietor of the local health food store will not likely provide the necessary training to ensure maximum effectiveness. Incidentally, information on these methods can also be helpful to couples who are trying to conceive.

# Permanent Contraception

**Sterilization,** permanent fertility control achieved through surgical procedures, has become a popular method of contraception for women and men. Although some of the newer surgical techniques make reversal of sterilization theoretically possible, anyone considering sterilization should assume that the operation is not reversible. Before becoming sterilized, people should think through such possibilities as divorce and remarriage or a future improvement in their financial status that may make them want a larger family.

## Female Sterilization

One method of sterilization in females is called **tubal ligation.** It is achieved through a surgical procedure that involves tying the fallopian tubes closed or cutting them and cauterizing (burning) the edges to seal the tubes so that access by sperm is blocked. The operation is usually done in a hospital on an outpatient basis. First, the abdomen is inflated with carbon dioxide gas through a small incision in the navel. The surgeon then inserts a *laparoscope* into another incision just above the pubic bone. This specially designed instrument has a fibre-optic light source that enables the physician to see the fallopian tubes clearly. Once located, the tubes are cut and tied or cauterized.

Ovarian and uterine functions are not affected by a tubal ligation. The woman's menstrual cycle continues,

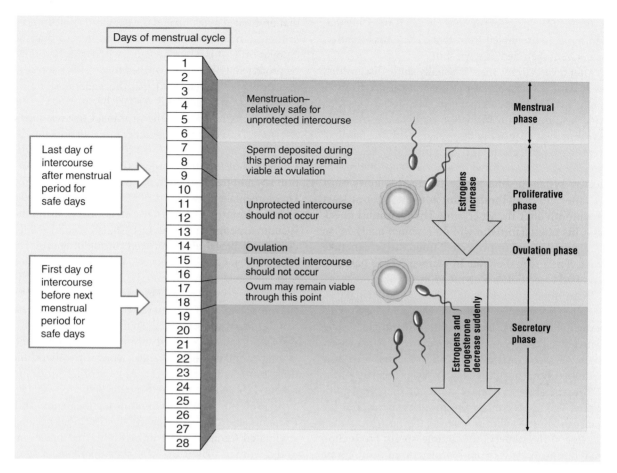

Days of menstrual cycle

| 1 |
| 2 |
| 3 | Menstruation– relatively safe for unprotected intercourse | Menstrual phase |
| 4 |
| 5 |
| 6 |
| 7 | Sperm deposited during this period may remain viable at ovulation |
| 8 |
| 9 |
| 10 | Unprotected intercourse should not occur | Proliferative phase |
| 11 |
| 12 |
| 13 |
| 14 | Ovulation | Ovulation phase |
| 15 | Unprotected intercourse should not occur |
| 16 |
| 17 | Ovum may remain viable through this point |
| 18 |
| 19 |
| 20 | Secretory phase |
| 21 |
| 22 |
| 23 |
| 24 |
| 25 |
| 26 |
| 27 |
| 28 |

Last day of intercourse after menstrual period for safe days

First day of intercourse before next menstrual period for safe days

Estrogens increase

Estrogens and progesterone decrease suddenly

FIGURE 6.4

**The Fertility Cycle**

and released eggs simply disintegrate and are absorbed by the lymphatic system. As soon as her incision is healed, the woman may resume sexual intercourse with no fear of pregnancy.

As with any kind of surgery, there are risks. Some patients are given general anesthesia, which presents a small risk; others receive local anesthesia. The procedure itself usually takes less than an hour, and the patient is generally allowed to return home within a short time after waking up. Women considering a tubal ligation should thoroughly discuss all the risks with their physician before the operation.

A **hysterectomy,** or removal of the uterus, is a method of sterilization requiring major surgery. It is usually done only when the patient's uterus is diseased or damaged.

## Male Sterilization

Sterilization in men is less complicated than in women. The procedure, called a **vasectomy,** is usually done on an outpatient basis using a local anesthetic. The surgeon makes an incision on each side of the

**Fertility awareness methods (FAM):** Include several types of birth control that require alteration of sexual behaviours rather than chemical or physical intervention.

**Cervical mucus method:** A birth control method that relies upon observation of changes in cervical mucus to determine when the woman is fertile so the couple can abstain from intercourse during those times.

**Body temperature method:** A birth control method that requires a woman to monitor her body temperature for the rise that signals ovulation and to abstain from intercourse around this time.

**Calendar method:** A birth control method that requires mapping the woman's menstrual cycle on a calendar to determine presumed fertile times and abstaining from intercourse and any other penis–vagina contact during those times.

**Sterilization:** Permanent fertility control achieved through surgical procedures.

**Tubal ligation:** Sterilization of the female that involves cutting and tying off of the fallopian tubes.

**Hysterectomy:** The removal of the uterus.

**Vasectomy:** Sterilization of the male that involves the cutting, cauterizing, and tying off of the vasa deferentia.

scrotum. The vas deferens on each side is then located, and a piece is removed from each. The ends are often cauterized, then tied or sewn shut.

After a vasectomy, there is usually some discomfort, local pain, swelling, and discolouration for about a week. In a small percentage of cases, more serious complications occur: formation of a blood clot in the scrotum (which usually disappears without medical treatment), infection, and inflammatory reactions. Because sperm are stored in other areas of the reproductive system besides the vas deferens, couples must use alternative methods of birth control for at least one month after the vasectomy. The man must check with his physician (who will do a semen analysis) to determine when unprotected intercourse can take place. The pregnancy rate in women whose partners have had vasectomies is about 15 in 10,000.

Many men are reluctant to consider sterilization because they fear the operation will affect their sexual performance. Such fears are unfounded and can be alleviated by talking to men who have already had a vasectomy. A vasectomy in no way affects sexual response. Because sperm constitute only a small percentage of the semen, the amount of ejaculate is not changed significantly. The testes continue to produce sperm, but the sperm are prevented from entering the ejaculatory duct because of the surgery. After a time, sperm production may diminish. Any sperm manufactured disintegrate and are absorbed into the lymphatic system.

Although a vasectomy should be considered a permanent procedure, surgical reversal is sometimes successful in restoring fertility. Improvements in microsurgery techniques have resulted in annual pregnancy rates of between 40 and 60 percent for women whose partners have had reversals. The two major factors influencing the success rate of reversal are the doctor's expertise and the time elapsed since the vasectomy.

## WHAT WOULD YOU DO?

Do you feel comfortable discussing birth control with your partner? Why or why not? What are the most important factors you and your partner considered when selecting a method of birth control? Have you discussed with your partner what you would do if you became pregnant? Why or why not?

# ABORTION

The law on **abortion** has seen a number of changes in Canada and much activity federally and provincially. In 1869, two years after Confederation, a law was enacted

that prohibited abortion and the penalty was life imprisonment. Those who oppose abortion believe that the embryo or fetus is a human being with rights that must be protected. Others have worked to get easier access to abortion for women. In 1967, the Federal Standing Committee on Health and Welfare began considering proposed amendments to the Criminal Code relating to abortion. Dr. Henry Morgentaler, an abortion activist and physician, appeared "on behalf of the Humanist Fellowship of Montreal, urging the repeal of the abortion law and freedom of choice on abortion."[4] In 1969, Dr. Morgentaler closed his general practice and opened a clinic in Montreal to specialize in abortion, using the vacuum aspiration method. In 1970, 1971, and 1973, 13 charges of illegal abortion were brought against Dr. Morgentaler. On November 13, 1973, a jury acquitted him. The next year, however, he was convicted by the Quebec Court of Appeal. Dr. Morgentaler appealed to the Supreme Court of Canada but in 1975 the appeal was dismissed and he served ten months in jail. In 1983, Dr. Morgentaler opened clinics in Toronto and Winnipeg and was again charged, along with other clinic doctors and the head nurse. Appeal procedures and renewed charges continued through 1986.

In 1988 the Supreme Court of Canada ruled that Canada's abortion law was unconstitutional because it violated Canada's Charter of Rights and Freedoms and a woman's right to "life, liberty and security of the person."[5] In an attempt to recriminalize abortion, Bill C-43 was introduced in Parliament. This bill, which sought to prohibit abortion unless a physician deemed it necessary for the mother's physical, mental, or psychological health, was defeated by the Senate in 1991. Harassment and threats of violence by antiabortion protesters have caused some physicians to stop performing abortions. On May 8, 1992, a firebomb destroyed the Morgentaler clinic in Toronto. On November 8, 1992, in Vancouver, abortion provider Dr. Garson Romalis was shot and seriously wounded at his home.

Another focus of debate is who will pay for abortions. Abortions conducted in hospitals are covered by public health insurance. Clinics, though, may be fully covered, partly covered, or not covered at all.[6] In 1995, the federal government ruled that if the provinces accept that abortion is medically necessary, they must pay the full cost of abortions or lose money from federal transfer payments under the Canada Health Act.[7]

In 2003, there were 103,768 (or 15.2 per 1,000 women aged 15–44) abortions performed in a hospital or clinic in Canada.[8] The highest rate of abortions occurs in the Northwest Territories, with 24.5 per 1,000 women, followed by Quebec (19.7), the Yukon (17.7), and British Columbia (17.2). The lowest rate of abortions occurs on

**Abortion:** The medical means of terminating a pregnancy.

# Contraceptive Comfort and Confidence Scale

These questions will help you assess whether the method of contraception you are using now or may consider using in the future will be effective for you. Answering yes to any of these questions predicts potential problems. Most individuals will have a few yes answers. If you have more than a few yes responses, however, you may want to talk to a health-care provider, counsellor, partner, or friend to decide whether to use this method or how to use it so that it will really be effective. In general, the more yes answers you have, the less likely you are to use this method consistently and correctly with every act of intercourse.

Method of contraception you use now or are considering:
_____

Length of time you used this method in the past:
_____

| Answer yes or no to the following questions: | Yes | No |
|---|---|---|
| 1. Have I ever had problems using this method? | ❑ | ❑ |
| 2. Have I ever become pregnant while using this method? | ❑ | ❑ |
| 3. Am I afraid of using this method? | ❑ | ❑ |
| 4. Would I really rather not use this method? | ❑ | ❑ |
| 5. Will I have trouble remembering to use this method? | ❑ | ❑ |
| 6. Will I have trouble using this method correctly and consistently? | ❑ | ❑ |
| 7. Do I still have unanswered questions about this method? | ❑ | ❑ |
| 8. Does this method make menstrual periods longer or more painful? | ❑ | ❑ |
| 9. Does this method cost more than I can afford? | ❑ | ❑ |
| 10. Could this method cause serious complications? | ❑ | ❑ |
| 11. Am I opposed to this method because of any religious or moral beliefs? | ❑ | ❑ |
| 12. Is my partner opposed to this method? | ❑ | ❑ |
| 13. Am I using this method without my partner's knowledge? | ❑ | ❑ |
| 14. Will using this method embarrass my partner? | ❑ | ❑ |
| 15. Will using this method embarrass me? | ❑ | ❑ |
| 16. Will I enjoy intercourse less because of this method? | ❑ | ❑ |
| 17. If this method interrupts lovemaking, will I avoid using it? | ❑ | ❑ |
| 18. Has a nurse or doctor ever told me not to use this method? | ❑ | ❑ |
| 19. Is there anything about my personality that could lead me to use this method incorrectly? | ❑ | ❑ |
| 20. Am I at risk of being exposed to HIV (the human immunodeficiency virus) or other sexually transmitted infections (STIs) if I use this method? | ❑ | ❑ |

Total number of yes answers: _____

## MAKE IT HAPPEN!

**Making a Change:** In order to change your behaviours, you need to develop a plan. Follow these steps and complete your Behaviour Change Contract to take action.

1. Evaluate your behaviours, and identify patterns. What can you change now? What can you change in the near future?

2. Select one pattern of behaviour that you want to change.

3. Fill out a behaviour change contract. It should include your long-term goal for change, your short-term goals, the rewards you'll give yourself for reaching these goals, potential obstacles along the way, and strategies for overcoming these obstacles. For each goal, list the small steps and specific actions that you will take.

4. Chart your progress in a journal. At the end of a week, consider how successful you were in following your plan. What helped you be successful? What made change more difficult? What will you do differently next week?

5. Revise your plan as needed: Are the short-term goals attainable? Are the rewards satisfying?

**Example:** Marissa had been using a diaphragm as her form of birth control. When she completed the self-assessment, she discovered that there were several aspects of it that made her uncomfortable. The questions to which she answered "yes" showed that she sometimes forgot to bring her diaphragm when she planned to see her boyfriend, Ben, and she disliked using it because it interrupted her sexual activity. She also was embarrassed to use it because she didn't like inserting it in front of Ben. She decided she should investigate other birth control options and discuss them with Ben. Her first step was to visit her student health centre and, based on her likes and dislikes, to choose one or two alternatives to the diaphragm. Among the options suggested to her were the contraceptive patch (Ortho Evra) and the vaginal ring (NuvaRing), both of which she would not have to remember to use and would not interrupt sexual activity. Marissa's next step was to talk to Ben about his likes and dislikes and then to make a final decision based on her confidence in the method, its convenience, and its cost.

Source: From R. A. Hatcher et al., *Contraceptive Technology*, 17th ed. (New York: Ardent Media, 1998), 238. Reprinted by permission of Ardent Media.

Prince Edward Island (4.7), in New Brunswick (5.9), and in Newfoundland and Labrador (7.9). Women between the ages of 20 and 24 have the highest rate of abortions, with 30.5 per 1,000 women. The next highest rate is found in 18- and 19-year-olds, at 28.1 per 1,000 women.[9]

Even the best birth control methods can fail. Pregnancies can occur despite due diligence. Women may be raped. When an unwanted pregnancy occurs, the decision whether to terminate, to carry to term and keep the baby, or to carry to term and give the baby up for adoption must be made. This is a personal decision each woman must make according to her personal beliefs, values, and resources after carefully considering the alternatives.

## Methods of Abortion

The type of abortion procedure used is determined by how many weeks pregnant the woman is. Pregnancy length is calculated from the first day of a woman's last menstrual period. If performed during the first trimester of pregnancy, abortion presents a relatively low risk to the mother. The most commonly used method of first-trimester abortion is **vacuum aspiration.** The procedure is usually performed with a local anesthetic. The cervix is dilated with instruments or by placing *laminaria,* a sterile seaweed product, in the cervical canal. The laminaria is left in place for a few hours or overnight and slowly dilates the cervix. After it is removed, a long tube is inserted into the uterus through the cervix. Gentle suction is then used to remove the fetal tissue from the uterine walls.

Pregnancies that progress into the second trimester can be terminated through **dilation and evacuation (D&E),** a procedure that combines vacuum aspiration with a technique called **dilation and curettage (D&C).** For this procedure, the cervix is dilated with laminaria for one to two days and a combination of instruments and vacuum aspiration is used to empty the uterus (see Figure 6.5). Second-trimester abortions are frequently done under general anesthetic. Both procedures can be performed on an outpatient basis (usually in the physician's office) with or without pain medication. Generally, the woman is given a mild tranquillizer to help her relax. Both procedures may cause moderate to severe uterine cramping and blood loss.

The **hysterotomy,** or surgical removal of the fetus from the uterus, may be used during emergencies or when the mother's life may be in danger and when other types of abortions are deemed too dangerous.

The risks associated with abortions include infection, incomplete abortion (when parts of the placenta remain in the uterus), missed abortion (when the

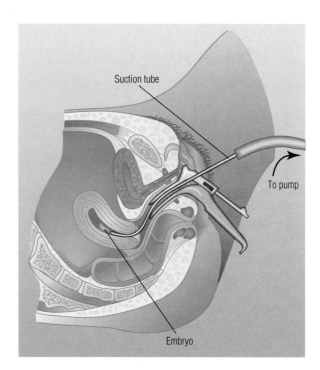

**FIGURE 6.5**
**Vacuum Aspiration Abortion**

fetus is not actually removed), excessive bleeding, and cervical and uterine trauma. Follow-up and attention to dangerous signs decrease the chances of any long-term problems.

The mortality rate for first-trimester abortions is 0.8 per 100,000 women. The rate for second-trimester abortions is higher, at 4.3 per 100,000 women. This higher rate is due to the increased risk of uterine perforation, bleeding, infection, and incomplete abortion due to the fact that the uterine wall becomes thinner as the pregnancy progresses.

Two other methods used in second-trimester abortions, though less commonly than the D&E method, are prostaglandin or saline **induction abortions.** In these methods, prostaglandin hormones or a saline solution is injected into the uterus. The injected solution kills the fetus and causes labour contractions to begin. After 24 to 48 hours the fetus and placenta are expelled from the uterus.

### WHAT WOULD YOU DO?

If you or your partner unexpectedly became pregnant, would you choose to terminate the pregnancy? What factors would you consider in making your decision? Why? How might an abortion affect your relationship? If you were married, would your decision be different? Why?

# Decision Making about Unplanned Pregnancy

Making decisions about unexpected health issues is often difficult, including those around an unplanned pregnancy. For many women, an unplanned pregnancy can be one of the first times that they have to deal with a decision about their health and the course of their life.

If you experience an unplanned pregnancy you have three options:

- continue the pregnancy and raise the child
- continue the pregnancy and place the child for adoption
- end the pregnancy with an abortion

You may reflect on many aspects of your life when considering these options. Unplanned pregnancy can happen at different stages of a woman's life. Often the decision is about what is best at this time; at another point in your life the decision might be different.

You may:

- think about your personal beliefs, values, and practices and those of others in your life
- assess your existing relationships (partners, family, friends) and the support that these relationships need and can provide
- evaluate financial and social realities
- consider your living conditions and life circumstances
- examine your feelings about becoming a mother and about parenting
- explore spiritual, religious, and cultural beliefs
- consider the reactions of others to your decision

As with any decision, you need to come to grips with making a decision and living with that decision. It is very common for women to have a variety of emotional reactions to an unplanned pregnancy. Dealing with your feelings is an important part of making a decision you can live with. Each woman is unique and the time and effort needed to make a decision will be different for each one.

## WHOM TO TALK TO

Weighing the pros and cons of such a personal decision can feel reassuring, stressful, and challenging. You may wish to seek advice before making this decision. Whom a woman chooses to talk to varies; each of us has individual needs for privacy and for emotional, physical, economic, and spiritual support. You may look for people to help you in the decision-making process who are:

- knowledgeable (able to provide information or referrals)
- non-judgmental
- able to provide support whatever the decision
- someone you feel comfortable talking to

Some women only want to talk to health-care providers; others want to include a partner or family member, a friend, or a clergy person. Whomever you talk to, you should never feel coerced or forced to make a decision that is not your own.

Source: www.womenshealthmatters.ca. Brought to you by Sunnybrook and Women's Health Sciences Centre.

# PLANNING A PREGNANCY

The technological ability to control your fertility gives you choices not available when your parents were born. The loosening of social restrictions in the areas of marriage and parenting also affords single men and women the opportunity to become parents. Regardless of your marital status, the preparation to become a parent involves similar considerations and decisions. If you are in the process of deciding whether to have children, you need to take the time to evaluate your emotions, finances, and health.

**Vacuum aspiration:** The use of gentle suction to remove fetal tissue from the uterus.

**Dilation and evacuation (D&E):** An abortion technique that combines vacuum aspiration with dilation and curettage; fetal tissue is sucked and scraped out of the uterus.

**Dilation and curettage (D&C):** An abortion technique in which the cervix is dilated with laminaria for one to two days and the uterine walls are scraped clean.

**Hysterotomy:** The surgical removal of the fetus from the uterus.

**Induction abortion:** A type of abortion in which chemicals are injected into the uterus through the uterine wall; labour begins and the woman delivers a dead fetus.

## Emotional Health

First and foremost, consider why you want to have a child: To fulfill an inner need to carry on the family? Out of loneliness? Any other reasons? Can you care for this new human being in a loving and nurturing manner? Are you ready to make the sacrifices necessary to bear and raise a child? You can prepare yourself for this change in your life in several ways. Reading about pregnancy and parenthood, taking classes, talking to parents of children of all ages, and joining a support group are helpful forms of preparation. If you choose to adopt, you will find many support groups available to you as well.

## Maternal Health

Before becoming pregnant, a woman should have a thorough medical examination. **Preconception care** should include assessment of possible pregnancy complications. Medical problems such as diabetes and high blood pressure should be discussed, as should any genetic disorders that run in either family. Additional suggestions for a healthy pregnancy include:

- engage in regular physical activity
- eat a healthy diet, following Canada's Food Guide to Healthy Eating
- maintain a normal weight
- do not smoke, drink alcohol, or use other illicit drugs
- reduce or eliminate caffeine intake
- avoid exposure to X-rays and environmental chemicals such as lawn and garden chemicals
- prior to becoming pregnant, have your annual dental X-rays and your regular checkup

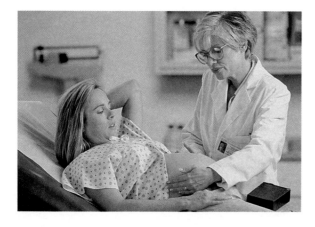

*Good prenatal care involves regular medical checkups by a practitioner with whom the mother feels she can communicate freely.*

## Paternal Health

It is common wisdom that mothers-to-be should steer clear of toxic chemicals that can cause birth defects. Even women trying to conceive are cautioned to avoid toxic environments and to eat a nourishing diet, to stop smoking and drinking alcohol, and to avoid most medications. Now similar precautions are made for fathers-to-be. New research suggests that a man's exposure to chemicals influences not only his ability to father a child but also the future health of his child.

Fathers-to-be have been overlooked in the past for several reasons. Researchers assumed that the genetic damage leading to birth defects and other health problems always occurred while a child was in the mother's womb or was caused by random errors of nature. Scientists have recently discovered that how sperm look has little to do with how they act. Misshapen sperm can penetrate an egg, and they do not necessarily carry defective genetic goods. Moreover, sperm that look healthy and swim well can be the true genetic culprits. DNA fluorescent markers have identified normal-looking yet genetically flawed sperm that carry too many or too few chromosomes. Fathers contribute the extra chromosome 21 in about 6 percent of children with Down syndrome, which causes learning disabilities; the extra X chromosome in 50 percent of boys with Klinefelter's syndrome, which causes abnormal sexual development; and the shortened chromosome 15 in about 85 percent of children with Prader-Willi syndrome, a disorder characterized by physical and learning disabilities and obesity.

Although some birth defects are caused by the random errors of nature, it now appears that some disorders can be traced to sperm damaged by chemicals. Sperm are naturally vulnerable to toxic assault and genetic damage. Many drugs and ingested chemicals can readily invade the testes from the bloodstream; others ambush sperm after they leave the testes and pass through the epididymides, where they mature and are stored. By one route or another, half of 100 chemicals studied so far (including by-products of cigarette smoke) apparently harm sperm. Some researchers believe that vitamin C is nature's way of protecting sex cells from damage. Poor dietary intake, exposure to toxic chemicals, cigarette smoking, and not enough foods rich in vitamin C are probably the biggest culprits in sperm damage.[10]

## Financial Evaluation

You also need to evaluate your finances. Both partners should find out about their employers' policies concerning parental leave, including length of leave available and conditions for returning to work.

# The Impact of a Reduced Fertility Rate on Women's Health

Total fertility rates (number of children each woman bears, on average) have decreased worldwide and in particular in Canada over the past 40 years. In fact, the Canadian fertility rate dropped from 3.90 children per woman in 1960 to 1.49 in 2000. Although there have been improvements in maternal and reproductive health over this time period, such as decreases in mortality and other pregnancy complications, little is known about the impact of reduced fertility, delayed fertility, and births to unmarried women.

Data from the General Social Survey Cycle 10—The Family (1995) were used to examine:

■ the relationship between family size and specific determinants of health,

■ the distribution of family and work attitudes by age and education, and

■ the relationship between attitude and intention to have one or more children in the future.

The results indicated that total fertility rates had decreased over the last 40 years, with considerable variation according to geographic location and socio-demographic subgroup. Further results indicated that the relationships between family size and selected determinants of health (marital status, education, employment, home ownership, and self-perceived health) were different for men and women. Specifically, a woman with one child was four times more likely to be "coupled" than a childless woman. Women with two children were as likely to be "coupled" as a woman with one child. Men were five times more likely to be married than their childless counterparts regardless of the number of children. In regard to education, women with two or more children were more likely to have not completed high school compared to their childless counterparts. A similar, but less strong relationship was noted in men. For employment, there was a negative relationship between number of children and employment status (that is, the more

children, the less likely women were to be employed outside the home). In men, this relationship existed only with five or more children (that is, a man was less likely to be employed outside the home if he had five or more children). In regard to home ownership, there was a direct, positive relationship regardless of the number of children in men and only with two children in women. No clear relationships existed with self-perceived health and number of children in either women or men. In the analysis of the associations between attitude and intention to have one or more children in the future, similarities were found among men and women, though differences existed by age group and level of education. Specifically, women who intended to have one or more children in the future were older, had a higher level of education, were employed, and believed that having a child and home were an important part of their happiness. In men, the intention to have one or more children in the future was related to their age, a better than high school education, not being employed full time, the belief that a child is important to happiness, and the belief that what a women really wants is a home and children.

Source: Adapted from J. Payne, Public Health Agency of Canada (PHAC), "The Impact of a Reduced Fertility Rate on Women's Health," retrieved May 16, 2006, from www.phac-aspc.gc.ca/publicat/whsrrssf/chap_10_e.html.

---

Raising a child exacts a tremendous strain on most families' finances. Expenses during the first year of life average to at least $10,000. The expense of raising a child from birth to 18 years of age is currently estimated to be more than $166,000—not including the cost of post-secondary education!

Parents should decide if either is willing to put their career on hold and spend the formative years raising their child(ren). The financial implications of this decision should be considered as well. Alternatively, the cost and availability of quality child care should be considered. Prospective parents should realistically assess how much family assistance they can expect with a new baby, as well as the availability and cost of nonfamily child care.

## Contingency Planning

A final consideration is how to provide financially and practically for your child should something happen to you and your partner. If both of you were to die while the child is young, do you have relatives or close friends who would raise the child? If you have more than one child, would they have to be split up or could they be kept together? What sort of financial situation would your child(ren) be in? Unpleasant though it may be to think about, this sort of contingency planning is extremely important.

**Preconception care:** Medical care received prior to becoming pregnant that helps a woman assess and address potential maternal health.

# PREGNANCY

## Prenatal Care

A successful pregnancy requires the mother's ability to take care of herself and her unborn child. It is essential to have regular medical checkups, beginning as soon as possible (certainly within the first three months). Early detection of fetal abnormalities and identification of high-risk mothers and infants are the major purposes of prenatal care. On the first visit, the practitioner should obtain a complete medical history of the mother and her family and note any hereditary conditions that could put a woman or her fetus at risk.

Regular checkups to measure weight gain and blood pressure and monitor the size and position of the fetus should continue throughout the pregnancy. This early care reduces infant mortality and low birthweight. Experts recommend obstetrical visits once a month to 28 weeks, biweekly to 36 weeks, and weekly to 40 weeks.

Additional concerns include the mother's physical condition, her level of nutrition, her confidence in her ability to give birth, her use of drugs and medications, and the availability of a skilled practitioner who can oversee the pregnancy and delivery. A woman planning a pregnancy also needs a support system (spouse or partner, family, friends, community groups) willing to give her and her child the love and emotional support needed during and after her pregnancy. In most areas prenatal classes are available, including some for pregnant teens.

## Choosing a Practitioner

A woman should carefully choose a practitioner who will attend her pregnancy and delivery, although in some localities physicians and specialists may be in short supply. If possible, this choice should be made before she becomes pregnant. Recommendations from friends satisfied with the care they received during pregnancy may be a good starting point. The woman's family physician may also be able to recommend a specialist. The pregnant woman needs to find a practitioner she can trust with her own life and that of the baby and with whom she can communicate freely.

When choosing a practitioner, parents should ask a number of questions concerning credentials and professional qualifications. Besides this information, a pregnant woman must ask questions specific to her condition. Prospective parents should also inquire about the practitioner's experience in handling various complications, commitment to being at the mother's side during delivery, and beliefs and practices concerning the use of anesthesia, fetal monitoring, induced labour, and forceps delivery. What are the practitioner's attitudes toward circumcision and alternative birthing procedures? The practitioner's approach to physical activity, nutrition, and medication during pregnancy should be similar to the woman's own. Finally, the parents must learn under what circumstances the practitioner would perform a caesarean section.

Two types of physicians can attend pregnancies and deliveries. The *obstetrician-gynecologist* (ob-gyn) is an M.D. who specializes in obstetrics (pregnancy and birth) and gynecology (care of women's reproductive organs). These practitioners are trained to handle all types of pregnancy- and delivery-related emergencies. A *family practitioner* is a licensed M.D. who provides comprehensive care for people of all ages. The majority of family practitioners have obstetrical experience but will refer a patient to a specialist if necessary. Unlike the ob-gyn, the family practitioner can serve as the baby's physician after attending the birth.

*Midwives* are also experienced practitioners who can attend pregnancies and deliveries. Most midwives work in private practice or in conjunction with physicians. Those who work with physicians have access to traditional medical facilities to which they can turn in an emergency.

## Alcohol and Drugs

A woman should avoid all drugs during pregnancy unless prescribed by a doctor—and then she should ask whether the medication is really necessary and whether there are safer alternatives. Always tell a physician, dentist, or other practitioner if you are

**TABLE 6.2**

Teratogenic Effects of Drugs

| Drug | Effect |
| --- | --- |
| Alcohol | Cognitive disabilities; growth retardation; increased spontaneous abortion |
| Amphetamines | Suspected nervous system damage |
| Aspirin | Newborn bleeding |
| Cocaine | Uncontrolled jerking motions; paralysis; depressed interactive behaviour; poor organizational response to environmental stimuli |
| Opioids | Immediate withdrawal in newborns; permanent learning disabilities |
| Tetracycline | Tooth discolouration |
| Sulfa drugs | Facial and skeletal abnormalities |
| Barbiturates | Congenital malformations |
| Streptomycin | Deafness |
| Accutane | Small or absent ears; small jaw; heart defects |
| Valium | Possible congenital anomalies |

Source: Mike Samuels, M.D., and Nancy Samuels, *The Well Pregnancy Book* (New York: Summit Books, 1986) 131. Copyright 1986. Reprinted by permission of the Elaine Markson Literary Agency and Mike Samuels, M.D., and Nancy Samuels.

pregnant or think you might be pregnant. Even common over-the-counter medications such as Aspirin and beverages such as coffee and tea can damage a developing fetus. The fetus is particularly susceptible to the **teratogenic** (birth-defect-causing) effects of some chemical substances during the first three months of pregnancy. The fetus can also develop an addiction to or tolerance for drugs that the mother is using.

Of particular concern to medical professionals is the use of tobacco and alcohol during pregnancy. Women who drink heavily may have normal first babies and then subsequently deliver children with a fetal alcohol spectrum disorder. **Fetal alcohol spectrum disorder (FSAD)** describes a number of disorders related to alcohol consumption during pregnancy including fetal alcohol syndrome, fetal alcohol effects, partial fetal alcohol effects, alcohol-related neurodevelopmental disorders, and neurobehavioural disorder–alcohol exposed. FSAD manifests in lifelong developmental and cognitive disabilities in children. The exact amount of alcohol necessary to cause FASD is not known, but researchers doubt that any level of alcohol consumption is safe. Therefore, total abstinence from alcohol during pregnancy—and when trying to get pregnant—is recommended.

Table 6.2 provides a list of teratogenic effects of alcohol and other drugs ingested by the mother.

Cigarette smoking during pregnancy has more predictable effects than alcohol. Studies indicate a 25 to 50 percent higher rate of fetal and infant deaths among women who smoke during pregnancy than among those who do not.[11] Women who smoke more than 10 to 15 cigarettes a day during pregnancy have higher rates of miscarriage, stillbirth, premature births, and low-birthweight babies than nonsmokers. Fetal research on the effects of "secondhand" or side-stream smoke (inhaling smoke produced by others) is inconclusive, but babies whose parents smoke can be twice as susceptible to pneumonia, bronchitis, and related illnesses as other babies.

**Teratogenic:** Causing birth defects; may refer to drugs, environmental chemicals, X-rays, or diseases.

**Fetal alcohol spectrum disorders (FASD):** A number of disorders related to alcohol consumption during pregnancy—including fetal alcohol syndrome, fetal alcohol effects, partial fetal alcohol effects, alcohol-related neurodevelopmental disorders, and neurobehavioural disorder–alcohol exposed—that result in lifelong developmental and cognitive disabilities in children.

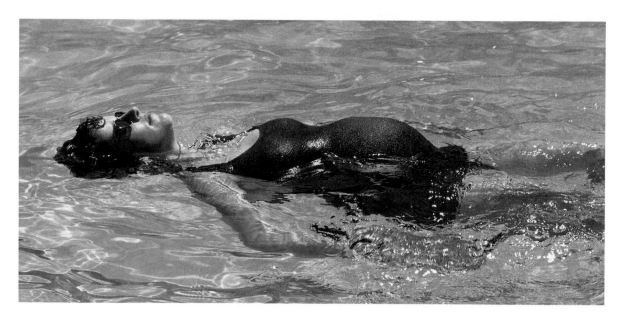

*Doctor-approved physical activity during pregnancy helps the mother control her weight and contributes to easier deliveries and healthier babies.*

## X-Rays

X-rays present a clear danger to the fetus. Although most diagnostic tests produce minimal amounts of radiation, even low levels may cause birth defects or other problems, particularly if several low-dose X-rays occur over a short time period. Pregnant women are advised to avoid X-rays unless absolutely necessary.

## Nutrition and Physical Activity

Pregnant women have additional needs for protein, calories, and certain vitamins and minerals, so their dietary intake should be carefully monitored by a qualified practitioner. Special attention should be paid to getting enough folic acid (found in dark leafy greens and in fortified cereals), iron (dried fruits, meats, legumes, liver, egg yolks), calcium (nonfat or lowfat dairy products, some canned fish), and fluids. Vitamin supplements can alleviate some deficiencies, but there is no true substitute for a well-balanced dietary intake. Babies born to mothers whose nutrition has been poor run high risks of substandard mental and physical development (see Table 6.3).

Weight gain during pregnancy helps nourish a growing baby. For a woman of normal weight before pregnancy, the recommended weight gain during pregnancy ranges from 11 to 16 kilograms (25–35 pounds); a woman carrying twins needs to gain about 16 to 20 kilograms (35–45 pounds). Usually the mother can expect to gain about 5 kilograms (10 pounds) during the first 20 weeks and about 0.5 kilograms (1 pound) per week during the rest of the pregnancy.

Of the total number of kilograms gained during pregnancy, about 3 to 4 are the baby's weight. The baby's birth weight is important, since a low weight can mean health problems during labour and the baby's first few months. Eating right and gaining enough weight helps reduce the chances of having a low-birthweight baby. If a woman gains an appropriate amount of weight while pregnant, chances are that her baby will gain weight properly, too. Pregnancy is not a time to think about losing weight—doing so may endanger the baby.[12]

As in all other stages of life, physical activity is an important factor in weight control during pregnancy as well as in overall maternal health. Regular, moderate-intensity physical activity of 45 minutes, three days per week has been associated in one study with heavier-birthweight babies, fewer surgical births, and shorter hospital stays after birth.[13] Pregnant women should consult with their physicians before starting any new physical activities.

## Other Factors

A pregnant woman should avoid exposure to toxic chemicals, heavy metals, pesticides, gases, and other hazardous compounds. She should not clean cat-litter boxes because cat feces can contain organisms that cause a disease called toxoplasmosis. If a pregnant woman contracts this disease, her baby may be stillborn or have cognitive disabilities or other birth defects.

Before becoming pregnant, a woman should be tested to determine if she has had rubella (German

**TABLE 6.3**
**Nutrient Deficiency Effects**

| Nutrient | Deficiency Effect |
| --- | --- |
| Overall caloric intake | Low infant birthweight |
| Protein | Reduced infant head circumference, low infant birthweight |
| Folic acid | Miscarriage and neural tube defects |
| Vitamin D | Decreased infant bone density |
| Calcium | Decreased infant bone density |
| Iron | Low infant birthweight and premature birth |
| Iodine | Varying degrees of mental and physical disabilities |
| Zinc | Congenital malformations |

Source: Reprinted by permission from Linda Kelly Debruyne and Sharon Rady Rolfes, *Life Cycle Nutrition: Conception through Adolescence.* Copyright 1989 by West Publishing Company. All rights reserved.

measles). If she has not had the disease, she should get immunized for it and wait the recommended length of time before becoming pregnant. A rubella infection can kill the fetus or cause blindness or hearing disorders in the infant. If a woman has ever had genital herpes, she should inform her physician. The physician may want to deliver the baby by caesarean section, especially if the woman has active lesions. Contact with an active herpes infection during birth can be fatal to the infant.

## A Woman's Reproductive Years

More than half of the average Canadian woman's expected life span is spent between menarche (first menses) and menopause (last menses), a period of approximately 40 years. During this 40-year period, she must make many decisions about her reproductive health. Deciding if and when to have children, as well as how to prevent pregnancy when necessary, are long-term concerns.[14]

Today, a pregnant woman over 35 has plenty of company. While births to women in their 20s are declining, the rate of first births to women between the ages of 30 and 39 has doubled in the past decade, and births to women over 39 have increased by more than 50 percent. Many women who wait until their 30s to consider having a child find themselves wondering, "Am I too old to have a baby?" Researchers believe that there is a decline in the quality and viability of eggs produced after age 35, which has resulted in an increase in the number of

women struggling with fertility issues and a concomitant increase in the use of fertility clinics. Statistically, the chances of having a miscarriage or a baby with birth defects do rise after the age of 35. **Down syndrome,** a condition characterized by mild to severe cognitive disabilities and a variety of physical abnormalities, is the most common birth defect found in babies born to older mothers. The incidence of Down syndrome in babies born to mothers aged 20 is 1 in 10,000 births; it rises to 1 in 365 births when the mother is 35, to 1 in 109 when she is 40, and to 1 in 32 when she is 45. Women who choose to delay motherhood until their late 30s also worry about their physical ability to carry and deliver their babies. For these women concerned about their ability to carry and deliver babies, comprehensive and regular physical activity will help to maintain good posture and promote a successful delivery.

## Pregnancy Testing

A woman may suspect she is pregnant before she has a pregnancy test. A typical sign is a missed menstrual period, yet this is not always an accurate indicator. A woman can miss her period for a variety of reasons: stress, excessive physical activity without an adequate dietary intake, or emotional upset. Confirmation of a pregnancy should be obtained from a pregnancy test scheduled in a medical office or birth control clinic.

**Down syndrome:** A condition characterized by cognitive disabilities and a variety of physical abnormalities.

## Researchers Develop Exercise Guidelines for Pregnancy

*by Marlene Habib—The Canadian Press*

Super-fit Beth Sweeney began worrying about how much exercise she should be doing when she learned she was expecting.

Sweeney, a 30-year-old fitness instructor in the resort town of Grand Bend, Ont., didn't want to take chances with her first pregnancy. So she enrolled in a study at the University of Western Ontario in London assessing how much exercise extremely fit pregnant women should be doing.

The study, by Michelle Mottola of Western and Larry Wolfe of Queen's University in Kingston, Ont., aimed to develop exercise guidelines for pregnant women like aerobics instructors, military personnel, police officers and firefighters who are intense exercisers.

Early findings from the study indicated that super-active pregnant women can continue their regimens with proper monitoring.

Sweeney's body fat, blood pressure, weight and blood-sugar levels were recorded 16 weeks into her pregnancy. She was also given a 45-minute treadmill test to determine her maximum heart rate and fitness level.

Sweeney then continued exercising with the intensity she was used to throughout much of her pregnancy, measuring her heart rate while instructing or doing other exercise to ensure it wasn't beyond the safe level determined by Mottola.

Sweeney felt so good that she was scheduled to teach an aerobics class the day she gave birth—nine days earlier than expected. She returned to lead aerobics classes in Grand Bend just five weeks postpartum.

The study by Mottola and Wolfe breaks new ground for exercising mums-to-be. Currently, there are only national guidelines for mild to moderate physical activity.

Avid exercisers like Sweeney aren't covered under these guidelines. She's among the five fit women who have been followed through their pregnancies so far by Mottola. The researcher plans to recruit a few dozen more to monitor their energy changes and other fitness aspects before the first phase ends. "We're finding a lot of really active women cut back on their activity when they don't have to," Mottola said in a telephone interview. The Canadian Forces Personnel Support Agency is funding the study. It hopes the findings will help women taken off active duty when they become pregnant keep in shape so they can return to work after maternity leave.

General safety considerations for physically active pregnant women.

- Avoid prolonged or strenuous exertion during the first trimester.
- Avoid isometric exercise or straining while holding your breath.
- Maintain adequate nutrition and hydration—drink liquids before, during, and after physical activity.
- Limit physical activity in warm or humid environments.
- Avoid exercise while lying on your back past the fourth month of pregnancy.
- Avoid activities which involve physical contact or danger of falling.
- Periodic rest periods may help to minimize possible low oxygen or temperature stress to the fetus.
- Know the reasons to stop physical activity and consult a qualified physician immediately if they occur.

Source: The Canadian Press.

Women who wish to know immediately whether or not they are pregnant can purchase home pregnancy test kits. These kits, sold over the counter in drugstores, are about 85 to 95 percent reliable. A positive test is based on the secretion of **human chorionic gonadotropin (HCG)** found in the woman's urine. Home test kits come equipped with a small sample of red blood cells coated with HCG antibodies, to which the user adds a small amount of urine. If the concentration of HCG is great enough, it will clump together with the HCG antibodies, indicating that the user is pregnant.

There are some problems with the accuracy of these home tests. If taken too early in the pregnancy, they may show a false negative. Other causes of false negatives are unclean test tubes, ingestion of certain drugs, and vaginal or urinary infections. Accuracy also depends on the quality of the test itself and the user's ability to perform it and interpret the results. Blood tests administered and analyzed by a medical laboratory give more accurate results.

## The Process of Pregnancy

Pregnancy begins the moment a sperm fertilizes an ovum in the fallopian tubes (see Figure 6.6). From there, the single cell multiplies, becoming a

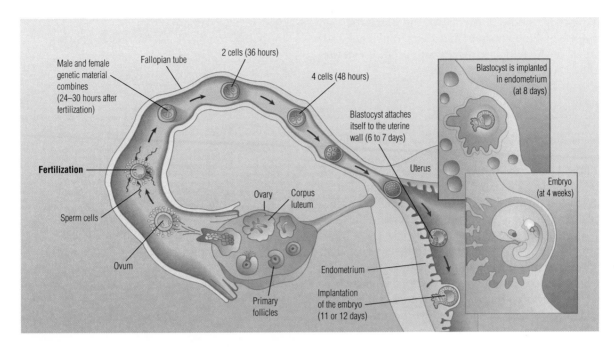

**FIGURE 6.6**
Fertilization

sphere-shaped cluster of cells as it travels toward the uterus, a journey that may last three to four days. Upon arrival, the embryo burrows into the thick, spongy endometrium and is nourished from this carefully prepared lining.

## Early Signs of Pregnancy

The first sign of pregnancy is usually a missed menstrual period (although some women "spot" in early pregnancy, and such spotting may be mistaken for a period). Other signs of pregnancy include:

- Breast tenderness
- Extreme fatigue
- Sleeplessness
- Emotional upset
- Nausea
- Vomiting (especially in the morning)

A pregnancy typically lasts 40 weeks. The due date is calculated from the expectant mother's last menstrual period. Pregnancy is typically divided into three phases, or **trimesters,** of approximately three months each.

## The First Trimester

During the first trimester, there are few noticeable changes in the maternal body. The expectant mother may urinate more frequently and experience morning sickness, swollen breasts, or undue fatigue. These symptoms may not be frequent or severe, so she may not realize she is pregnant at this time unless she has a pregnancy test.

During the first two months after conception, the **embryo** differentiates and develops its various organ systems, beginning with the nervous and circulatory systems. At the start of the third month, the embryo is called a **fetus,** indicating that all organ systems are in place. For the rest of the pregnancy, growth and refinement occur in each major body system so that they can function independently, yet in coordination, at birth.

## The Second Trimester

At the beginning of the second trimester, physical changes in the mother become more visible. Her breasts swell and her waistline thickens. During this time, the fetus makes greater demands upon

**Human chorionic gonadotropin (HCG):** Hormone detectable in blood or urine samples of a woman within the first few weeks of pregnancy.

**Trimester:** A three-month segment of pregnancy; used to describe specific developmental changes in the embryo or fetus.

**Embryo:** The fertilized egg from conception until the end of two months' development.

**Fetus:** The name given the developing baby from the third month of pregnancy until birth.

the mother's body. In particular, the **placenta,** the network of blood vessels that carry nutrients and oxygen to the fetus and fetal waste products to the mother, becomes well established.

## The Third Trimester

This is the period of greatest fetal growth. The fetus gains most of its weight during these last three months. During the third trimester, the fetus must get large amounts of calcium, iron, and nitrogen from the food the mother eats. Approximately 85 percent of the calcium and iron the mother digests goes into the fetal bloodstream. Although the fetus may live if it is born during the seventh month, it needs the layer of fat it acquires during the eighth month and time for the organs (especially the respiratory and digestive organs) to develop to their full potential. Babies born prematurely usually require intensive medical care.

# Prenatal Testing and Screening

Modern technology has enabled medical practitioners to detect health defects in a fetus as early as the fourteenth to eighteenth weeks of pregnancy. One common testing procedure, **amniocentesis,** which is strongly recommended for women over the age of 35, involves inserting a long needle through the mother's abdominal and uterine walls into the **amniotic sac,** the protective pouch surrounding the baby (see Figure 6.7). The needle draws out 15–20 mL of fluid, which is analyzed for genetic information about the baby. This test can reveal the presence of 40 genetic abnormalities, including Down syndrome, Tay-Sachs disease (a fatal disorder of the nervous system common among Jewish people of Eastern European descent), and sickle-cell anemia (a debilitating blood disorder found primarily among individuals of African descent). Amniocentesis can also reveal the sex of the child, a fact many parents choose not to know until the birth. Although widely used, amniocentesis is not without risk. Chances of fetal damage and miscarriage as a result of testing are 1 in 400.

Another procedure, *ultrasound* (or *sonography*), uses high-frequency sound waves to determine the size and position of the fetus. Ultrasound can also detect defects in the central nervous system and digestive system of the fetus. Knowing the position of the fetus assists practitioners in performing amniocentesis and in delivering the child.

A third procedure, *chorionic villus sampling (CVS),* involves snipping tissue from the developing fetal sac. CVS can be used at 10 to 12 weeks of pregnancy, and the test results are available in 12 to 48 hours. This test

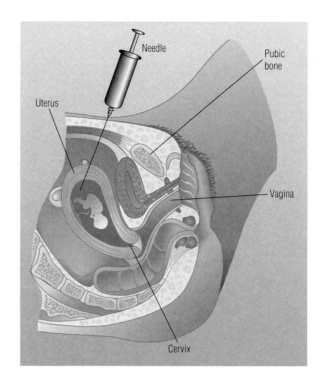

### FIGURE 6.7

## Amniocentisis

The process of amniocentesis can detect certain congenital problems as well as the sex of the fetus.

is an attractive option for couples at high risk for having a baby with Down syndrome or a debilitating hereditary disease.

If any of these tests reveals a serious birth defect, parents are advised to undergo genetic counselling. In the case of a chromosomal abnormality such as Down syndrome, the parents are usually offered counselling regarding their options.

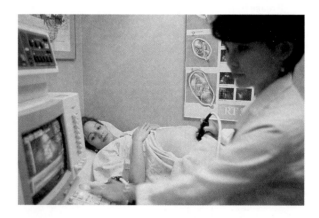

*Ultrasound testing can reveal defects in the developing fetus, and, as the time of delivery nears, it can provide useful information about the size and position of the unborn child.*

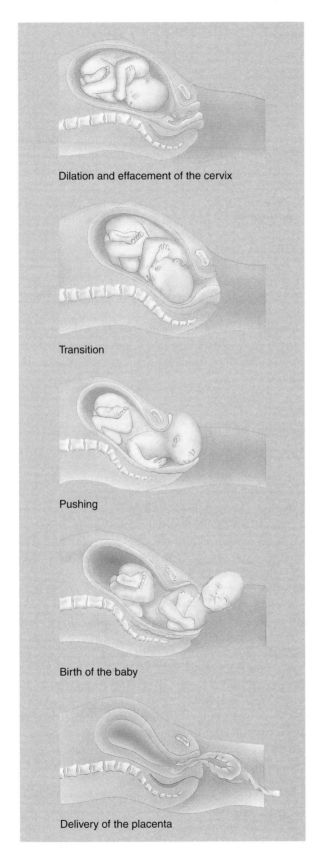

Dilation and effacement of the cervix

Transition

Pushing

Birth of the baby

Delivery of the placenta

FIGURE 6.8
**The Birth Process**

# CHILDBIRTH

## Where to Have Your Baby

Today's prospective mothers have many delivery options. These range from the traditional hospital birth to home birth. When considering birthing alternatives, parental values are important. Many couples, for instance, feel that the modern medical establishment has dehumanized the birth process; thus they choose to deliver at home or at a *birthing centre,* a homelike setting outside a hospital where women can give birth and receive postdelivery care from a team of professional practitioners, including physicians and registered nurses.

## Labour and Delivery

The birth process has three stages. The exact mechanisms that signal the mother's body that the baby is ready to be born are unknown. During the few weeks preceding delivery, the baby normally shifts and turns to a head-down position, and the cervix begins to dilate (open up). The junction of the pubic bones also loosens to permit expansion of the pelvic girdle during birth (see Figure 6.8).

In the first stage of labour, the amniotic sac breaks, causing a rush of fluid from the vagina (commonly

**Placenta:** The network of blood vessels that carries nutrients to the developing infant and carries wastes away; it connects to the umbilical cord.

**Amniocentesis:** A medical test in which a small amount of fluid is drawn from the amniotic sac; it tests for Down syndrome and other genetic diseases.

**Amniotic sac:** The protective pouch surrounding the baby.

referred to as "breaking of the waters"). Contractions in the abdomen and lower back also signal the beginning of labour. Early contractions push the baby downward, putting pressure on the cervix and thereby causing it to dilate further. The first stage of labour may last from a couple of hours to more than a day for a first birth, and is usually much shorter during subsequent births.

The end of the first stage of labour, called **transition,** is the part of the process when the cervix becomes fully dilated and the baby's head begins to move into the vagina, or the birth canal. Contractions usually come quickly during transition. Transition usually lasts 30 minutes or less.

The second stage of labour follows transition when the cervix has become fully dilated. Contractions become rhythmic, stronger, and more painful as the uterus works to push the baby through the birth canal. The second stage of labour (called the *expulsion stage*) may last between one and four hours and concludes when the infant is finally pushed out of the mother's body. In some cases, the attending practitioner will do an **episiotomy,** a straight incision in the mother's **perineum,** to prevent the baby's head from causing tearing of vaginal tissues and to speed the baby's exit from the vagina. Sometimes women can avoid an episiotomy by engaging in regular physical activity and obtaining a healthy dietary intake throughout pregnancy, by trying different birth positions, or by having an attendant massage the perineal tissue. However, the skin's natural elasticity and the baby's size are limiting factors.

After delivery, the attending practitioner cleans the baby's mucus-filled breathing passages, and the baby takes its first breath, generally accompanied by a loud wail. (The traditional "slap" on the baby's buttocks, often romanticized in old movies, is no longer a common practice because of the trauma associated with it.) In the meantime, the mother continues into the third stage of labour, during which the placenta, or afterbirth, is expelled from the womb. This stage is usually completed within 30 minutes after delivery. The umbilical cord is then tied and severed. The stump of cord attached to the baby's navel dries up and drops off within a few days.

## Prenatal Education

In terms of facilities and professionals, expectant parents in Canada can receive a variety of services for prenatal education in the community where they live. Most prenatal programs include instruction in a range of comfort measures as well as preparation in breathing.

## Drugs in the Delivery Room

Because painkilling drugs given to the mother during labour can cause sluggish responses in the newborn, many women choose drug-free labours and deliveries. Drug-free labour involves the use of physical activity, massage, and controlled rhythmic breathing to control pain. Many women who choose "natural" childbirth mistakenly believe that the activities taught in their classes will make their labour and delivery painless. When it comes time to give birth, they may feel inadequate because they experience the normal pain associated with childbirth. Pain is to be expected, and if it becomes too intense, the mother can be given painkilling medication.

A discussion with the attending practitioner before the birth of the baby will alert the mother to the practitioner's feelings about the use of painkilling drugs during delivery. Many experts believe that women should be offered the option of drugs before and during delivery. To refuse to give a mother medicine to ease the pain is considered poor medical practice by some authorities.

## Breast-Feeding and the Postpartum Period

Although the new mother's milk will not begin to flow for two or more days, her breasts secrete a yellowish substance called *colostrum*. Because this fluid contains vital antibodies to help fight infection, it is wise to allow the newborn baby to suckle. As a result of recent scientific findings, it is strongly recommended that full-term newborns be breast-fed. This recommendation does not mean that breast milk is the only adequate method of nourishing a baby. Prepared formulas can also provide nourishment that allows a baby to grow and thrive.

There are many advantages to breast-feeding. Breast milk is perfectly suited to a baby's nutritional needs. Breast-fed babies have fewer illnesses and a much lower hospitalization rate because breast milk contains maternal antibodies and immunological cells that stimulate the infant's immune system. When breast-fed babies do get sick, they recover more quickly. They are also less likely to become obese than babies fed formulas, and they have fewer allergies.

When deciding whether to breast- or bottle-feed, mothers need to consider their own desires and preferences. Both feeding methods can supply the physical and emotional closeness so essential to the parent–child relationship.

The *postpartum period* typically lasts four to six weeks after delivery. During this time, the mother's reproductive organs revert to a nonpregnant state.

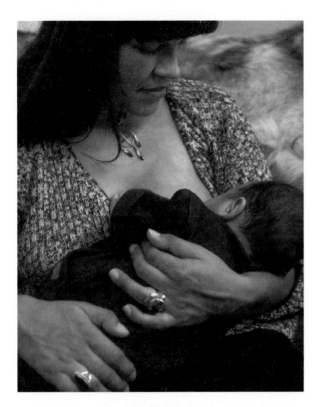

*Breast-feeding enhances the development of intimate bonds between mother and child.*

Many women experience energy depletion, anxiety, mood swings, and depression during this period. This experience, known as **postpartum depression,** appears to be a normal end-product of the birth process. For most women, the symptoms gradually disappear as their bodies return to normal. For others, the symptoms, coupled with the stresses of managing a new family, can cause more severe depression that lasts for several months.

## WHAT WOULD YOU DO?

What do you think are the advantages and disadvantages of breast-feeding? How does society view breast-feeding? Why? Are we effective in enabling women to breast-feed? Why or why not? What will you do to increase awareness and to make it easier for women to breast-feed in your community?

## Complications

Problems and complications can occur during labour and delivery even following a successful pregnancy. Such possibilities should be discussed with the practitioner prior to labour so the mother understands what medical procedures may be necessary for her safety and for that of her child.

### Caesarean Section (C-Section)

If labour lasts too long, if a baby is presenting wrong (about to exit the uterus anything but head first), or if the baby is in duress, a **caesarean section (C-section)** may be necessary. This surgical procedure involves making an incision across the mother's abdomen and through the uterus to remove the baby. This operation is also performed in cases in which labour is extremely difficult, maternal blood pressure falls rapidly, the placenta separates from the uterus too soon, the mother has diabetes, or other problems occur.

A caesarean section can be traumatic for the mother if she is not prepared. Risks to the mother are the same as for any major abdominal surgery, and recovery from birth takes considerably longer. Although a caesarean section may be necessary in certain cases, some physicians and critics feel that the option has been used too frequently in this country. The 1986 National Conference on Aspects of Caesarean Birth recommended guidelines to deal with rising caesarean rates. Overall rates of caesarean section subsequently dropped from 20 percent in 1987 to 15 percent in 1993. The guidelines dealt with three scenarios: breech presentation, prolonged labour, and previous caesarean section. The adage was formerly "Once a caesarean, always a caesarean." Now, however, surgical techniques allow many women who had a caesarean section to deliver subsequent children vaginally. Repeat caesareans decreased from 39 percent in the mid-1980s to 34 percent in 1993.[15]

### Miscarriage

One in ten pregnancies does not end in delivery. Loss of the fetus before it is viable is called a **miscarriage** (also referred to as *spontaneous abortion*). An estimated

**Transition:** The process during which the cervix becomes nearly fully dilated and the head of the fetus begins to move into the birth canal.

**Episiotomy:** A straight incision in the mother's perineum.

**Perineum:** The area between the vulva and the anus.

**Postpartum depression:** The experience of energy depletion, anxiety, mood swings, and depression that women may feel during the postpartum period.

**Caesarean section (C-section):** A surgical procedure in which a baby is removed through an incision made in the mother's abdominal and uterine walls.

**Miscarriage:** Loss of the fetus before it is viable; also called spontaneous abortion.

70 to 90 percent of women who miscarry eventually become pregnant again.

Reasons for miscarriage vary. In some cases, the fertilized egg has failed to divide correctly. In others, genetic abnormalities, maternal illness, or infections are responsible. Maternal hormonal imbalance may also cause a miscarriage, as may a weak cervix or toxic chemicals in the environment. In most cases, the cause is not known.

A blood incompatibility between mother and father can cause **Rh factor** problems, and sometimes miscarriage. Rh is a blood protein. Rh problems occur when the mother is Rh-negative and the fetus is Rh-positive. During a first birth, some of the baby's blood passes into the mother's bloodstream. An Rh-negative mother may manufacture antibodies to destroy the Rh-positive blood introduced into her bloodstream at the time of birth. Her first baby will be unaffected, but subsequent babies with positive Rh factor will be at risk for a severe anemia called *hemolytic disease* because the mother's Rh antibodies will attack the fetus's red blood cells.

Medical advances now offer prevention and treatment for this condition. The mother and fetus can be tested, and if Rh incompatibility is found, intrauterine transfusions can be given or an early delivery by caesarean section can be done, depending upon the individual case. Prevention of the problem is preferable to treatment. All women with Rh-negative blood should be injected with a medication called RhoGAM within 72 hours of any birth, miscarriage, or abortion. This injection will prevent them from developing the Rh antibodies.

Another cause of miscarriage is **ectopic pregnancy,** or implantation of a fertilized egg outside the uterus. A fertilized egg may implant itself in the fallopian tube or, occasionally, in the pelvic cavity. Because these structures are not capable of expanding and nourishing a developing fetus, the pregnancy cannot continue. Such pregnancies are surgically terminated. Most often, the affected fallopian tube is also removed.

Ectopic pregnancy is generally accompanied by pain in the lower abdomen or an aching feeling in the shoulders as the blood flows toward the diaphragm. If bleeding is significant, blood pressure drops and the woman can go into shock. If an ectopic pregnancy goes undiagnosed and untreated, the fallopian tube ruptures, and the woman is then at significant risk of hemorrhage, peritonitis (infection in the abdomen), and death.

The incidence of ectopic pregnancy has escalated and no one really understands why. We do know that ectopic pregnancy is a potential side effect of pelvic inflammatory disease (PID), which has become increasingly common in recent years, because the scarring or blockage of the fallopian tubes characteristic of this disease prevents the fertilized egg from passing to the uterus. About 50 percent of women who have had an ectopic pregnancy conceive again although they are at a higher risk of having another.

**Stillbirth** is one of the most traumatic events a couple can face. A stillborn baby is one that is born dead, often for no apparent reason. The grief experienced following a stillbirth is usually devastating and can last for years. In many cases, no amount of reassurance from the attending physician, relatives, or friends can assuage the grief or guilt. In Canada, 8,934 (or a rate of 1.1 per 1,000 live births) were stillbirths in 2003.[16] The highest rates of stillbirth occur in women ages 25 to 29 (2.1) and 30 to 34 (2.0).

## Sudden Infant Death Syndrome

The sudden death of an infant under one year of age for no apparent reason is called *sudden infant death syndrome (SIDS)*. SIDS is the leading cause of death for Canadian infants between 28 days and one year of age. The overall rate of SIDS has decreased from 1.2 per 1,000 live births in 1980 to 0.5 per 1,000 live births in 1996.[17] SIDS, also referred to as crib death, is not a disease itself but rather is designated the cause of death after all other possibilities are ruled out. A SIDS death is sudden and silent; the death occurs quickly, often associated with sleep and with no signs of suffering.

Because SIDS is a diagnosis of exclusion, doctors do not know what causes it. However, several risk factors have been identified: [18]

- risk is greater in males
- risk is greater in infants 2 to 4 months
- risk is greater in infants from families of lower socioeconomic status
- risk is greater when infants sleep on their front vs. back; there may also be an increased risk when infants sleep on their sides
- risk is greater with maternal smoking during pregnancy
- risk is greater when the infant is exposed to second-hand smoke in the home
- risk is greater if the infant's head is covered during sleep
- risk is greater with overheating
- risk may be greater when the infant shares a bed with his or her parents
- breast-feeding appears to provide a protective factor from SIDS

Because the death of an infant—whether a result of a known cause or not—is a disruption of the natural order, it is traumatic for parents, family, and friends. The lack of a discernible cause, the suddenness of the tragedy, and the involvement of the legal system make a SIDS death especially difficult, leaving a great sense of loss and a need for understanding. Some communities have support groups to help parents and other family members through this grieving process. On a more positive note, infant mortality rates have been declining over the past 35 years.[19] In 1995, the infant mortality rate was 6.2 per 1,000 compared to 27.3 per 1,000 in 1960.

# INFERTILITY

An estimated one in six Canadian couples experiences **infertility,** or difficulties in conceiving. The reasons for this phenomenon include the trend toward delaying childbirth (as a woman gets older, she is less likely to conceive), the use of IUDs, and the rise in the incidence of pelvic inflammatory disease.

## Causes in Women

As noted, one cause of infertility in women is **pelvic inflammatory disease (PID),** a serious infection that scars the fallopian tubes and blocks sperm migration. Women often develop PID as a result of a gonorrhea or chlamydia infection that progresses to the fallopian tubes and the ovaries. The risk of infertility after one bout of PID is 12 percent. After two bouts, it doubles to nearly 25 percent, and following three bouts, it increases to more than 50 percent.[20]

**Endometriosis** is a major cause of infertility. In this disorder, parts of the endometrial lining of the uterus implant themselves outside the uterus—in the fallopian tubes, lungs, intestines, outer uterine walls, ovarian walls, or on the ligaments that support the uterus. The disorder can be treated surgically or with hormonal preparations. Success rates vary. Approximately 35 percent of women diagnosed with endometriosis are infertile.

## Causes in Men

Among men, the single largest fertility problem is **low sperm count.** Although only one viable sperm is needed for fertilization, research indicates the other sperm in the ejaculate aid in the fertilization process. There are normally 60 to 80 million sperm per millilitre of semen. When the count drops below 20 million, fertility declines. Low sperm count may be attributable to environmental factors such as exposure of the scrotum to intense heat or cold, radiation, or altitude,

or even to wearing excessively tight underwear or outerwear. The mumps virus damages the cells that make sperm. Varicose veins above one or both testicles can also render men infertile. Male infertility problems account for around 40 percent of infertility cases.

## Treatment

For the couple desperately wishing to conceive, the road to parenthood may be long and frustrating. Fortunately, medical treatment can identify the cause of infertility in about 90 percent of affected couples. The chances of becoming pregnant range from 30 to 70 percent, depending on the specific cause of the infertility. The countless tests and the invasion of privacy that characterize some couples' efforts to conceive can put stress on an otherwise strong, healthy relationship. Before starting fertility tests, the wise couple will reassess their priorities. Some will choose to undergo counselling to help clarify their feelings about the fertility process. A good physician or fertility team will take the time to ascertain the couple's level of motivation.

Fertility work-ups for men include a sperm count, a test for sperm motility, and analysis of any disease processes present. Women are thoroughly examined by an obstetrician/gynecologist for the composition of cervical mucus, extent of tubal scarring, and evidence of endometriosis. Complete fertility work-ups may take four to five months and can be unsettling. In some cases, surgery can correct structural problems such as tubal scarring. In others, administering hormones can improve the health of ova and sperm. Sometimes pregnancy can be achieved by collecting the male's sperm from several ejaculations and inseminating the female at a later time.

---

**Rh factor:** A blood protein related to the production of antibodies. If an Rh-negative mother is pregnant with an Rh-positive fetus, the mother will manufacture antibodies that can kill the fetus, causing miscarriage.

**Ectopic pregnancy:** Implantation of a fertilized egg outside the uterus, usually in a fallopian tube; a medical emergency that can end in death from hemorrhage for the mother.

**Stillbirth:** The birth of a dead baby.

**Infertility:** Difficulties in conceiving.

**Pelvic inflammatory disease (PID):** An infection that scars the fallopian tubes and consequently blocks sperm migration, causing infertility.

**Endometriosis:** A disorder in which uterine lining tissue establishes itself outside the uterus.

**Low sperm count:** A sperm count below 60 million sperm per millilitre of semen.

When all surgical and hormonal methods fail, the couple still has some options. **Fertility drugs** such as Clomid and Pergonal stimulate ovulation in women. Ninety percent of women who use these drugs will begin to ovulate, and half will conceive. Fertility drugs are associated with a number of side effects including headaches, irritability, restlessness, depression, fatigue, edema (fluid retention), abnormal uterine bleeding, breast tenderness, vasomotor flushes (hot flashes), and visual difficulties. Women using fertility drugs are also at increased risk of multiple ovarian cysts (fluid-filled growths) and liver damage. The drugs sometimes trigger the release of more than one egg. Thus a woman treated with one of these drugs has a 1 in 10 chance of having multiple births. Most such births are twins, but triplets and even quadruplets are not uncommon.

**Alternative insemination** of a woman with her partner's sperm is another treatment option. If this procedure fails, the couple may choose insemination by an anonymous donor through a "sperm bank." Many men sell their sperm to such banks. The sperm are classified according to the physical characteristics of the donor (for example, blonde hair, blue eyes), and then frozen for future use. Sperm can survive in this frozen state for up to five years. The woman being inseminated usually chooses sperm from a man whose physical characteristics resemble those of her partner or match her own personal preferences. In the last few years, concern has been expressed about the possibility of transmitting the AIDS virus through alternative insemination. As a result, donors are routinely screened for the disease before they donate.

**In vitro fertilization,** often referred to as "test tube" fertilization, involves collecting a viable ovum from the prospective mother and transferring it to a nutrient medium in a laboratory, where it is fertilized with sperm from the woman's partner or a donor. After a few days, the embryo is transplanted into the mother's uterus, where, it is hoped, it will develop normally.

In **gamete intrafallopian transfer (GIFT),** the egg is "harvested" from the woman's ovary and placed in the fallopian tube with her partner's or a donor's sperm. Less expensive and time-consuming than in vitro fertilization, GIFT mimics nature by allowing the egg to be fertilized in the fallopian tube and to migrate to the uterus according to the normal timetable. The success rate for this procedure is approximately 20 percent.

In **nonsurgical embryo transfer,** a donor egg is fertilized by the man's sperm and then implanted in the woman's uterus. This procedure may also be used in cases involving the transfer of an already-fertilized ovum into the uterus of another woman.

**Embryo transfer** is another treatment for infertility. In this procedure, an ovum from a donor's body is artificially inseminated by the man's sperm, allowed to stay in the donor's body for a time, and then transplanted into the woman's body. Some laboratories are experimenting with **embryo freezing,** in which a fertilized embryo is suspended in a solution of liquid nitrogen. When desired, it is gradually thawed and implanted into the prospective mother. The first birth of a frozen embryo in the United States was reported in June 1986. In the future, this technique may make it possible for young couples to produce an embryo and save it for later implantation when they are ready to have a child, thus reducing the risks of fertilization of older eggs.

## Surrogate Motherhood

Between 60 and 70 percent of infertile couples are able to conceive after treatment. The rest decide to live without children, adopt, or attempt surrogate motherhood. In this option, the couple hires a woman to be alternatively inseminated by the husband. The surrogate then carries the baby to term and surrenders it at birth to the couple. Surrogate mothers are reportedly paid about $10,000 for their services and reimbursed for applicable medical expenses. Legal and medical expenses can run as high as $30,000 for the infertile couple. Couples considering surrogate motherhood are advised to consult a lawyer regarding contracts between the involved parties.

### WHAT WOULD YOU DO?

What option would you most likely select if you found that you and your partner had fertility problems? Why? Do you think cloning or embryo freezing is ethical? Why or why not?

**Fertility drugs:** Hormones that stimulate ovulation in women not ovulating; often responsible for multiple births.

**Alternative insemination:** Fertilization accomplished by depositing a partner's or a donor's semen into a woman's vagina via a thin tube; almost always done in a doctor's office.

**In vitro fertilization:** Fertilization of an egg in a nutrient medium and subsequent transfer back to the mother's body.

**Gamete intrafallopian transfer (GIFT):** An egg is harvested from the female partner's ovary and placed with the male partner's sperm in her fallopian tube, where it is fertilized and then migrates to the uterus for implantation.

**Nonsurgical embryo transfer:** In vitro fertilization of a donor egg by the male partner's (or donor's) sperm and subsequent transfer to the female partner's or another woman's uterus.

**Embryo transfer:** Alternative insemination of a donor with male partner's sperm; after a time, the embryo is transferred from the donor to the female partner's body.

**Embryo freezing:** The freezing of an embryo for later implantation.

# SUMMARY

- Only latex condoms, when used correctly for vaginal, oral, and anal sex, are effective in preventing sexually transmitted infections.

- To prevent pregnancy, contraceptive methods include abstinence, outercourse, oral contraceptives, condoms, foams, jellies, suppositories, creams, the female condom, the diaphragm, the cervical cap, intra-uterine devices, withdrawal, Norplant, Preven, Depo-Provera, film, and the sponge. Fertility awareness methods rely on altering sexual practices to avoid pregnancy. Sterilization is permanent contraception.

- Abortion is currently legal through the second trimester. Abortion methods include vacuum aspiration, dilation and evacuation (D&E), dilation and curettage (D&C), hysterotomy, and induction abortion.

- Parenting is a demanding job requiring careful planning. Emotional health, maternal health, financial evaluation, and contingency planning should be considered prior to conception.

- Prenatal care includes a complete physical exam within the first trimester and avoidance of alcohol, drugs, cigarettes, X-rays, and chemicals having teratogenic effects. Full-term pregnancy covers three trimesters, or 40 weeks.

- Childbirth occurs in three stages. Parents should jointly make decisions about labour early in the pregnancy to be better prepared when it occurs. Complications of pregnancy and childbirth include miscarriage, ectopic pregnancy, stillbirth, and the necessity for caesarean section.

- Infertility in women may be caused by pelvic inflammatory disease or endometriosis. In men, it may be caused by low sperm count. Treatment may include alternative insemination, in vitro fertilization, gamete intrafallopian transfer, nonsurgical embryo transfer, and embryo transfer. Surrogate motherhood involves hiring a fertile woman to be alternatively inseminated by the male partner.

# DISCUSSION QUESTIONS

1. Draw up a list of the most effective contraceptive methods. What are the pros and cons for their use? What medical conditions could keep you from using them?

2. Outline the varied methods of abortion.

3. What are some of the most important decisions that your parents made concerning raising you? Would you raise your child differently? The same?

4. Describe the growth of the fetus through the three trimesters. What medical checkups or tests should be done during each trimester?

5. List the varied decisions that parents face when thinking about childbirth. Consider where to have the child and whether to use painkilling drugs during delivery. How does the first-time parent decide what to do?

6. If you and your spouse were having difficulty getting pregnant, what would your options be? If you proved infertile, what would your options be then? What would you do?

# APPLICATION EXERCISE

Reread the What Do You Think? scenario at the beginning of the chapter and answer the following questions:

1. What concerns you most about Kari and Dave's relationship? Is it realistic that two people can date for several months and never discuss sex? What would you have done differently from Kari and Dave? Why?

2. If you could tell incoming first-year students three personal rules about using birth control and protection from sexually transmitted infections, what would they be?

# HEALTH ON THE NET

Canadian Paediatric Society
**www.cps.ca/**

Canadian Association of Family Resource Programs
**www.frp.ca/**

Planned Parenthood
**www.plannedparenthood.org**

Canadian Federation for Sexual Health
**www.cfsh.ca**

IVF (In Vitro Fertilization) Canada & the Life Program
**www.ivfcanada.com**

Infertility Network
**www.familyhelper.net/iy/in.html**

The Society of Obstetricians and Gynaecologists of Canada
**http://sogc.medical.org/**

Women's Health Matters
**www.womenshealthmatters.ca**

# CHAPTER 7

# NUTRITION

*Eating for*
*Optimum Health*

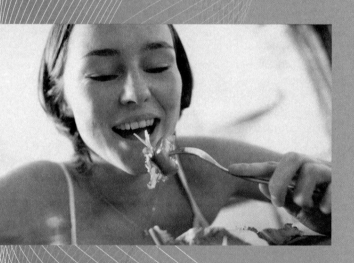

## CHAPTER OBJECTIVES

- Summarize the history of Canada's Food Guide to Healthy Eating and the objectives that guided the development of each version.

- Explain how the Food Guide can be used to obtain a healthy dietary intake and to maintain a healthy body weight.

- Identify the major essential nutrients (water, proteins, carbohydrates, fats, vitamins, and minerals) and indicate what purpose each serves in maintaining overall health.

- Define the different types of vegetarianism and discuss possible health benefits and risks.

- Describe the unique problems that university students may have when trying to eat healthy and the actions they can take to ensure they follow the Food Guide. Specifically, discuss eating healthy on a budget, fast food, and eating at a dormitory.

- Explain some of the food-safety concerns consumers should be aware of, including food irradiation, food-borne illnesses, food allergies, and organic foods.

Jeff is a first-year student living in the dormitory of a small college. His parents opted for the food service meal plan in the hope that Jeff would eat at least one good meal per day. This particular food service has the same sorts of choices for students each day (burgers and fries, pizza, stir fry, pasta and sauce, soup and sandwiches); foods are often overcooked, there are few fresh fruits or vegetables, and beverages offered include sodas, iced tea, milk, and various watered-down juices. Although Jeff eats at the food service most of the time, he supplements his dietary intake with fast food and ice cream snacks. He is gaining weight and is worried about some of the recent news stories on TV discussing high-fat diets and diets lacking certain nutrients. He decides he'd better do something about his eating habits, but when he goes to the cafeteria at school, he is not sure what to choose.

■ Why do some people find their dietary choices relatively easy, while others have huge problems adjusting their daily food intake? What factors contribute to students' attitudes and behaviours in regard to their food choices? Do you think Jeff should change his eating habits? Why or why not? Do you have friends who have similar problems? Where on your campus could they go for help?

Today, we face dietary choices and nutritional challenges that our grandparents never dreamed of—exotic foreign foods; dietary supplements; artificial sweeteners; no-fat, low-fat, and artificial-fat alternatives; and cholesterol-free, high-protein, high-carbohydrate, and low-calorie products. Thousands of alternatives bombard us daily. Caught in the crossfire of advertised claims by the food industry and advice provided by health and nutrition experts, most of us find it difficult to make wise dietary choices. The ability to sift through the untruths, half-truths, and scientific realities and select a dietary plan that meets your individual needs is an essential health-promoting skill—particularly when you are living away from home for the first time. Past patterns of eating influence your current dietary attitudes and behaviours more than you realize. Understanding the reasons behind your nutritional choices may help you change negative dietary patterns and enhance positive behaviours.

# HEALTHY EATING

Eating is one activity that most of us take for granted. We assume that we will have sufficient food to get us through the day, and rarely are forced to eat things that we do not like for the sake of staying alive. In fact, although we have all undoubtedly experienced **hunger** before mealtime, few of us have ever experienced the type of hunger that continues for days and threatens our survival. Most of us eat because of **appetite**, a learned psychological desire to consume certain foods whether or not we are hungry. Our appetite is triggered by smell, taste, time of day, special occasions, or proximity to favourite foods such as freshly baked bread. If our appetite is stimulated, we may want to eat something because it looks or smells good, even though we are not actually hungry. Finding the right balance between eating to maintain body functions (eating to live) and eating to satisfy our appetite (living to eat) is a problem for many of us, as evidenced by the rising levels of overweight and obesity in our population.

Many factors influence when we eat, what we eat, why we eat, and how much we eat. As mentioned, sensory stimulation, such as smelling, seeing, and tasting foods, can entice us to eat. Social pressures, including family traditions, social events that involve eating, and busy work schedules, can also influence our dietary intake. Although our ancestors typically sat down to three complete meals per day, they also laboured heavily in the fields or at other work and burned the calories they consumed. Today, eating three large meals combined with an inactive lifestyle is the perfect recipe for weight gain—and, in particular, fat gain.

Cultural factors also play a role in how we eat. People from Middle Eastern cultures tend to eat more rice, fruits, and vegetables and Japanese people eat more seafood than the typical Canadian. Typically, each culture has healthy and not-so-healthy eating habits. The Spiritual and Emotional Health box provides suggestions for incorporating culture-specific foods.

**Nutrition** is the science that investigates the relationship between physiological function and the elements of the foods we eat. With the abundance of food available in our society, the vast number of choices, and our easy access to almost every **nutrient** (proteins, carbohydrates, fats, vitamins, minerals, and water) 24 hours a day, Canadians should have few nutritional problems. However, nutritionists believe that our "diet of affluence" is responsible for many of our diseases and disabilities. This country's history as a land of agricultural abundance accounts for the traditional Canadian diet: high in fats and calories and weighted toward red meats, potatoes, and rich desserts. More recent trends indicated that Canadians

# Blending Spirituality and Cultural Practices with Healthy Eating

Spirituality and culture permeate all aspects of life, including food preparation and eating customs. While certain dishes may be closely linked to a culture's tradition and spirit, they may not represent a very healthy food choice. (For example, many cultures restrict or emphasize certain foods or food groups due to long-held religious beliefs.) Thus, it is important to learn to choose healthier dishes and limit the less healthy items from each culture. Remember that all foods can fit into a healthy dietary intake, some in smaller amounts.

## MAKING THE FOOD GUIDE WORK FOR YOU

Some people are overwhelmed by their first glance at the Food Guide. They think they have to consume a lot of food to obtain the recommended number of servings. But when you consider breakfast, lunch, dinner, and snacks in between, it is really quite easy to get all the servings that are recommended, particularly when you understand what constitutes a serving size.

Although everyone is different, it is generally recommended that you try to consume foods from at least two different food groups at each snack or meal, preferably three, and that you consume grain products throughout the day. As such, you might consider starting the day with a breakfast of a bowl of cereal with low-fat milk, toast, and juice, or a bowl of cereal with low-fat milk, a piece of fruit, and a half bagel or English muffin. Keep in mind that you should consider the amount of fibre and fat in the chosen grain product. Many people are duped into thinking that granola is a health food, regardless of fat content, or that bran muffins are better than bagels or bread. Sometimes these products are loaded with fat, sugar, and calories. Read the labels on packaged products and opt for reduced-fat, whole-grain products with 2 to 3 grams of fibre per serving when trying to meet the Canada's Food Guide to Healthy Eating requirements.

---

are changing to a white-meat diet with less fats and more fruits and vegetables.

Despite these dietary improvements, heart disease, certain types of cancer, hypertension (high blood pressure), cirrhosis of the liver, tooth decay, and obesity continue to be major health problems. Why do so many of us have nutritional problems? Much of our preoccupation with food and our tendency to eat too much of certain foods stems from our early eating habits.

### WHAT WOULD YOU DO?

Think about your eating habits. What is your ideal meal? Do you think of the meat on your plate first? Do you think of what you will have for dessert? Would you be happy with a veggie-laden salad and some wheat bread for your evening meal, or would you prefer a hot, meat-and-potatoes dining experience? Why do you think you feel the way you do? How did your family eat when you were growing up? Is everyone in your family of origin still eating the same way they did when they were young? Why or why not? How can you change your food choices and eating habits to better match the Food Guide?

## Responsible Eating

Canadians consume more calories per person per day than many other people in the world. A **calorie** is a unit of measure that indicates the amount of energy we obtain from a particular food. Calories are eaten in the form of *proteins, fats,* and *carbohydrates,* three of the basic nutrients necessary for life. Three other nutrients also necessary for life—*water, vitamins,* and *minerals*—do not contribute calories to our dietary intake.

Excess calorie consumption is a major factor in gaining weight. However, it is not just the quantity of food we eat that causes weight problems and associated diseases: it is also the relative proportion of

---

**Hunger:** The feeling associated with the physiological need to eat.

**Appetite:** The desire to eat; normally accompanies hunger, but is more psychological than physiological.

**Nutrition:** The science that investigates the relationship between physiological function and the essential elements of foods we eat.

**Nutrients:** The constituents of food that sustain us physiologically: water, proteins, carbohydrates, fibre, fats, vitamins, and minerals.

**Calorie:** A unit of measure that indicates the amount of energy we obtain from a particular food.

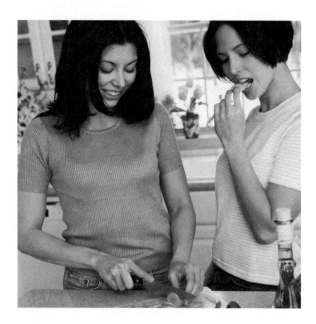

*It takes knowledge, resources, and planning to make healthy food choices, whether you are eating out, in the dining hall, or cooking your meals at home.*

nutrients consumed and, perhaps more importantly, our lack of physical activity. Canadian adults obtain their dietary energy from proteins (16–18 percent), carbohydrates (50–56 percent), and fats (29–31 percent), close to the recommended levels for their specific age/sex groups.[1] It is the high concentration of fats in the Canadian diet— particularly saturated fats (largely animal fats) and trans fats (produced when polyunsaturated oils are hydrogenated)—that appears to most increase our risk for various chronic diseases, including heart disease. High concentrations of highly processed sugars seem to increase the risk for other diseases, particularly tooth decay. Over the years, several agencies have worked to modify the average Canadian's dietary intake through a series of dietary goals and guidelines.

## Canada's Food Guide to Healthy Eating

In July 1942, the Official Food Rules, Canada's first food guide, was introduced.[2] The Official Food Rules attempted to promote healthy eating, prevent nutritional deficiencies, and improve the health of Canadians while recognizing the impact of wartime food rationing. Although the food guide has been transformed many times—and is currently in transition—it has never wavered from its original purpose of guiding food selection and promoting the health of Canadians. In addition to new looks and formats, the title of Canada's food guide has changed over time: from Canada's Official Food Rules (1942), to Canada's Food Rules (1944, 1949), to Canada's Food Guide (1961, 1977, 1982), and finally to Canada's Food Guide to Healthy Eating (1992), which is commonly referred to as the Food Guide. As mentioned, the most recent Food Guide is currently under review and is expected to be available to the public in the fall of 2006.[3]

Since 1992 and the introduction of the latest version of the Food Guide, research has advanced the understanding of the relationship between dietary intake and health.[4] As such, it was necessary to review the Food Guide and ensure that it (1) promotes a pattern of eating that meets nutrient needs, (2) promotes health, and (3) minimizes the risk of nutrition-related chronic disease. This review confirmed that the Food Guide is a useful and valid tool from a scientific and an educational perspective. However, challenges were identified related to the understanding and application of the Food Guide by individual Canadians. As such, Health Canada is revising Canada's Food Guide to Healthy Eating with the following guiding principles:[5]

- the Food Guide will promote a pattern of eating that will meet nutrient needs, promote health, and minimize the risk of nutrition-related chronic disease;
- revisions to the Food Guide will be based on the most up-to-date evidence;
- the Food Guide will be linked to public health priorities and initiatives;
- the development of messages for the Food Guide will be based on the premise that they need to be easily understood and implemented by the public; and
- the process to revise the Food Guide will be conducted in an open and transparent manner.

Further, the newest version of the Food Guide is intended to help Canadians 2 years of age and older to make food choices that promote health. Specifically, the objectives of the new Food Guide are to:[6]

- describe a pattern of eating sufficient to meet nutrient needs;
- describe a pattern of eating that reduces risk of nutrition-related health problems;
- describe a pattern of eating that supports the achievement and maintenance of a healthy body weight;
- describe a pattern of eating that reflects the diversity of foods available to Canadians;

# Vitamin D: Many Canadians May Not Be Getting Enough

A May 25, 2006, news release from the Dietitians of Canada, the national professional association of dietitians, suggested that many Canadians may not be getting enough Vitamin D.

### Why is there concern about vitamin D?

In addition to playing a vital role in bone health for people of all ages, vitamin D may have a positive effect on some types of cancers, in particular colorectal cancer, and other immune-related diseases.

We normally obtain vitamin D in one of two ways: (1) from the sun via UVB radiation absorbed through our skin, and (2) through our dietary intake, most often from fortified cows' milk.

### Who is at greatest risk for inadequate vitamin D?

All Canadians—and anyone else who lives above 37° latitude—may be at risk in the winter months when there is insufficient UVB radiation from the sun, partly because of the reduced daylight hours and because of the level of the solstice. Other groups particularly at risk include:

- **The elderly**—because they have a reduced production of vitamin D in their bodies as a result of the aging process. Other contributing factors include limited exposure to the sunlight because the elderly are more likely to be housebound and an inadequate dietary intake.

- **Individuals with dark skin**—because the darker one's skin, the lower the production of vitamin D.

- **Exclusively breast-fed infants**—because the vitamin D content of breast milk is not sufficient.

- **Individuals who wear clothing covering the majority of their body**—because there is no exposed skin to absorb vitamin D from the sun and its UVB radiation.

- **Individuals with poor dietary intakes of vitamin D.**

### Can diet alone provide enough vitamin D?

As mentioned previously, most of the vitamin D obtained via dietary intake comes from fortified cows' milk. Other dietary sources include fatty fish, such as salmon and sardines, infant formulas, meal replacements, and nutritional supplements.

The dietary reference intakes (DRIs), the new dietary standard for Canada and the United States, recommend that adults up to the age of 50 years obtain 200 IU each day, those between the ages of 51 and 70 require 400 IU per day, and individuals over 71 years need 600 IU per day. Further, the Osteoporosis Society of Canada recommends that adults over the age of 50 and at risk for osteoporosis obtain 800 IU of vitamin D or the equivalent of 750 mL of milk (around three glasses) per day.

### Are vitamin D supplements recommended, and if so how much should one take?

Health Canada and the Canadian Paediatric Society currently recommend that exclusively breast-fed infants receive a daily supplement of 400 IU vitamin D per day.

If children and adults are able to have regular, brief, unprotected daily exposure to the sun and follow Canada's Food Guide to Healthy Eating, they should obtain sufficient vitamin D. However, adults over 50 years of age at risk of osteoporosis may need to supplement. These individuals should consult their physician and have their dietary intake evaluated by a registered dietitian. A blanket recommendation should not be made for everyone.

## STUDY QUESTIONS

**1.** How much vitamin D do you need?

**2.** Where do you get your vitamin D from?

**3.** What can you do to ensure an adequate intake of vitamin D?

**4.** Are vitamin D supplements an essential part of healthy living? Why or why not?

Source: Adapted from Dietitians of Canada News Releases, May 25, 2006, "Vitamin D—Many Canadians May Not Be Getting Enough." Retrieved on May 25, 2006, from www.dietitians.ca/news/media.

- support Canadians' awareness and understanding of what constitutes a pattern of healthy eating; and

- emphasize that healthy eating and regular physical activity are important for health.

Finally, the revision addresses challenges identified during the review of the Food Guide.

Figure 7.1 shows Canada's Food Guide to Healthy Eating (1992), including recommended foods. On the second page of the Food Guide are examples of one serving from each of the major food groups.

## WHAT WOULD YOU DO?

Do you use the Food Guide? Why or why not? Examine the current version of the Food Guide (Figure 7.1). Which food groups are you most likely to eat the recommended amounts of during a typical day? Which ones are you most likely to skimp on? Why? What are some simple changes that you could make right now to help you meet the recommendations in the Food Guide?

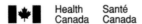

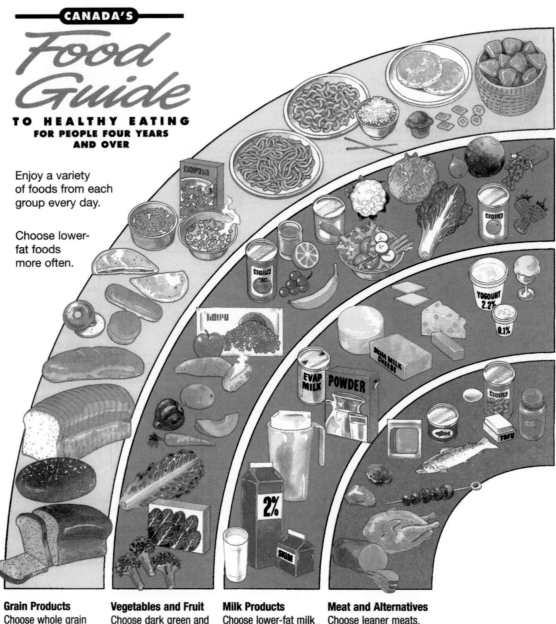

**Enjoy a variety of foods from each group every day.**

**Choose lower-fat foods more often.**

**Grain Products**
Choose whole grain and enriched products more often.

**Vegetables and Fruit**
Choose dark green and orange vegetables and orange fruit more often.

**Milk Products**
Choose lower-fat milk products more often.

**Meat and Alternatives**
Choose leaner meats, poultry and fish, as well as dried peas, beans and lentils more often.

Canada

FIGURE 7.1

Canada's Food Guide to Healthy Eating

Source: Canada's Food Guide to Healthy Eating, www.hc-sc.gc.ca/hpfb-dgsa/onpp-bppn/
food_guide_rainbow_e.htnl, Health Canada, 1992. Reproduced with the permission of the Minister
of Public Works and Government Services Canada, 2007.

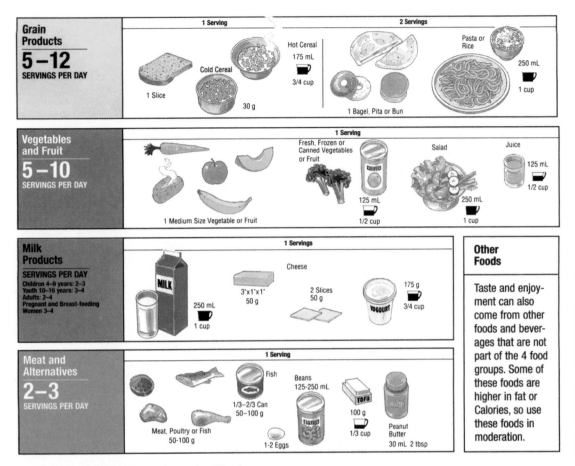

**Grain Products**
**5–12**
SERVINGS PER DAY

1 Serving
1 Slice
Cold Cereal
30 g
Hot Cereal
175 mL
3/4 cup

2 Servings
Pasta or Rice
250 mL
1 cup
1 Bagel, Pita or Bun

**Vegetables and Fruit**
**5–10**
SERVINGS PER DAY

1 Serving
1 Medium Size Vegetable or Fruit
Fresh, Frozen or Canned Vegetables or Fruit
125 mL
1/2 cup
Salad
250 mL
1 cup
Juice
125 mL
1/2 cup

**Milk Products**
SERVINGS PER DAY
Children 4–9 years: 2–3
Youth 10–16 years: 3–4
Adults: 2–4
Pregnant and Breast-feeding Women 3–4

1 Servings
MILK
250 mL
1 cup
Cheese
3"x1"x1"
50 g
2 Slices
50 g
175 g
3/4 cup

**Other Foods**

Taste and enjoyment can also come from other foods and beverages that are not part of the 4 food groups. Some of these foods are higher in fat or Calories, so use these foods in moderation.

**Meat and Alternatives**
**2–3**
SERVINGS PER DAY

1 Serving
Meat, Poultry or Fish
50-100 g
1-2 Eggs
Fish
1/3–2/3 Can
50–100 g
Beans
125-250 mL
TOFU
100 g
1/3 cup
Peanut Butter
30 mL  2 tbsp

### Different People Need Different Amounts of Food

The amount of food you need every day from the 4 food groups and other foods depends on your age, body size, activity level, whether you are male or female and if you are pregnant or breast-feeding. That's why the Food Guide gives a lower and higher number of servings for each food group. For example, young children can choose the lower number of servings, while male teenagers can go to the higher number. Most other people can choose servings somewhere in between.

Consult *Canada's Physical Activity Guide to Healthy Active Living* to help you build physical activity into your daily life.

*Enjoy eating well, being active and feeling good about yourself. That's* VITALIT

FIGURE 7.1 (continued)
Canada's Food Guide to Healthy Eating

# The Digestive Process

Food provides the chemicals we need for physical activity and body maintenance. Because our bodies cannot synthesize or produce certain essential nutrients, we must obtain them from the foods we eat. Nutrients are the elements of food that physiologically sustain us, and include water, protein, carbohydrates, fibre, fats, vitamins, and minerals. Before foods can be utilized, the digestive system must break them down into smaller, more usable forms. The process by which foods are broken down and either absorbed or excreted by the body is known as the **digestive process.**

**Digestive process:** The process by which foods are broken down and absorbed or excreted by the body.

Even before you take your first bite, your body has already begun a series of complex digestive responses. Your mouth prepares for the food by increasing saliva production. **Saliva** contains mostly water, which aids in chewing and swallowing, but it also contains important enzymes that begin the process of food breakdown. One such enzyme, amylase, begins to break down carbohydrates. From the mouth, the food passes down the **esophagus**, a 23- to 25-centimetre tube that connects the mouth to the stomach. A series of contractions and relaxations by the muscles lining the esophagus gently moves food to the next digestive organ, the **stomach**. Here food mixes with enzymes and stomach acids. Hydrochloric acid begins to work in combination with pepsin, another enzyme, to break down proteins. In most people, the stomach secretes enough mucus to protect the stomach lining from these harsh digestive juices. In others, there are problems with the lining that result in ulcers or other gastric problems.

Further digestive activity takes place in the **small intestine**, an eight-metre-long coiled tube containing three sections: the *duodenum,* the *jejunum,* and the *ileum*. Each section secretes digestive enzymes that, when combined with enzymes from the liver and the pancreas, further contribute to the breakdown of proteins, fats, and carbohydrates. Once broken down, these nutrients are absorbed into the bloodstream to supply body cells with energy. The liver is the major organ that determines whether nutrients are stored, sent to cells or organs, or excreted. Solid wastes consisting of fibre, water, and salts are dumped into the large intestine, where most of the water and salts are reabsorbed into the system and the fibre is passed out through the anus. The entire digestive process takes approximately 24 hours (see Figure 7.2).

# OBTAINING ESSENTIAL NUTRIENTS

## Water

If you were to go on a survival trip, which would you take with you—food or water? You may be surprised to learn that you could survive much longer without food than without water. Even in severe conditions, the average person can go for weeks without certain vitamins and minerals before experiencing serious deficiency symptoms. However, **dehydration** (abnormal depletion of body fluids) can cause serious problems within a matter of hours and death after a few days.

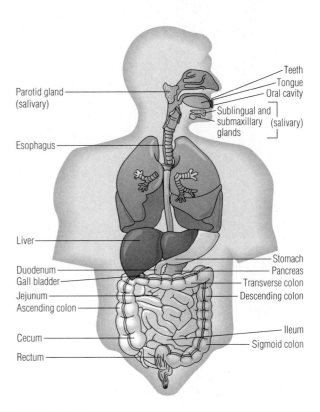

**FIGURE 7.2**
**The Digestive System**

Just what function does water serve in the body? Between 50 and 60 percent of our total body weight is water. The water in our system bathes cells, aids in fluid and electrolyte balance, maintains pH balance, and transports molecules and cells throughout the body. Water is the major component of blood, which carries oxygen and nutrients to the tissues and is responsible for maintaining cells in working order.

How much water do you need? Most experts believe that six to eight glasses of water per day are necessary. Because of high concentrations of water in most foods we consume, the actual number of glasses needed each day is somewhat less than this for the average person. Individual needs vary drastically according to dietary factors, age, size, environmental temperature and humidity levels, physical activity, and the effectiveness of the individual's system. It is not unusual for athletes to lose 1 to 2 litres of fluid per hour in hot, humid weather if they are exercising at a high intensity. To maintain hydration levels, athletes should weigh themselves before and after their workouts and drink one litre of fluid for every kilogram of weight lost. Thirst is not a good indicator of the body's need for fluids. In fact, if you wait until you are thirsty to replenish your fluids, you have waited too long. The best method of ensuring the body is adequately hydrated is to monitor the colour

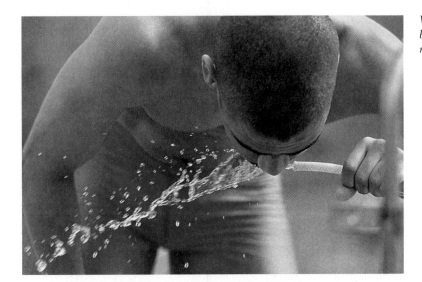

*While you may not be conscious of your body's need for water, it is actually our most necessary nutrient.*

of your urine. If it is a pale yellow, the body is sufficiently hydrated; if it is a darker yellow, the body needs fluids.

Is bottled water better than tap water? In some cases, when you buy "spring" or bottled water you are actually purchasing chlorinated water from another area of the country, and the water may not be any better than your city's tap water. Some of the better bottled waters go through a process to remove chemicals. Is it worth the extra cost? Some experts think not. If you are concerned about your drinking water, have it tested.

Are sports drinks necessary? Not likely as often as they are consumed. Most sports drinks are absorbed as well as water, and some are absorbed better than juice. In terms of hydration, it is important to note that people are likely to drink more fluid when it is flavoured. The intent of sports drinks is to replenish electrolytes lost through sweating. They are also used to replenish glycogen or energy stores. Thus, when your sweating is profuse for 60 minutes or longer, a sports drink may be necessary. However, for your physical activity of shorter durations or that's without much sweating, a sports drink is not needed; water can adequately meet your needs.

## Proteins

Next to water, proteins are the most abundant substances in the human body. **Proteins** are major components of nearly every cell and are often referred to as "building blocks" because of their role in the development and repair of bone, muscle, skin, and blood cells. Proteins are also the key elements of the antibodies that protect us from disease, of enzymes that control chemical activities in the body, and of hormones that regulate bodily functions. Moreover, proteins aid in the transport of iron, oxygen, and nutrients to all the body's cells. Normally proteins are not a source of energy, but will be broken down to supply energy if carbohydrates and fat are not available. Proteins provide 4 calories of energy per gram of intake. In short, an adequate protein dietary intake is vital to many body functions and to your survival.

Most Canadians consume more protein than needed. In particular, they consume too much protein in the form of high-fat animal flesh and dairy products, which are associated with higher blood cholesterol levels.[7] The recommended protein intake for the average person is 0.8 gram per kilogram of body weight per day, equivalent to about 12 to 20 percent of total energy intake.[8] The excess is stored, like other extra calories, as fat.

Proteins are made up of smaller molecules known as **amino acids**. Amino acids are composed of chains

**Saliva:** Fluid secreted by the salivary glands; enzymes in the fluid aid in the breakdown of certain foods for digestion.

**Esophagus:** Tube that transports food from the mouth to the stomach.

**Stomach:** Large muscular organ that temporarily stores, mixes, and digests foods.

**Small intestine:** Muscular, coiled digestive organ; consists of the duodenum, jejunum, and ileum.

**Dehydration:** Abnormal depletion of body fluids; a result of lack of water.

**Proteins:** An essential constituent of nearly all body cells, necessary for the development and repair of bone, muscle, skin, and blood, and key elements of antibodies, enzymes, and hormones.

**Amino acids:** The building blocks of protein.

that link together like beads on a necklace in differing combinations. More than 22 different types of amino acids are found in animal tissue, and humans cannot synthesize all of them. The eight amino acids that the adult body cannot make in adequate amounts are referred to as **essential amino acids.** They must be obtained from foods.

**Complete (high-quality) proteins** are found in foods that naturally contain the eight essential amino acids together. If we consume a food deficient in some of the essential amino acids, the total amount of protein that can be synthesized by the other amino acids is limited by the missing amino acid(s). It is important to remember that even though essential amino acids are present in a food does not guarantee that they will be synthesized. Quality of protein depends on the presence of amino acids in digestible form and in amounts proportional to body requirements.

The most common sources of dietary protein in Canada are meats, poultry, seafood, dairy products, eggs, soy products, legumes, whole grains, and nuts. In addition to providing high-quality proteins, some of these sources of protein (meats, poultry, high-fat dairy products, and eggs) also contain high levels of saturated fat and cholesterol. Selecting leaner cuts of meat, removing the fat and skin from chicken, and choosing low-fat dairy products enables you to get high-quality proteins without excess fat or cholesterol.

What about plant sources of protein? Proteins from plant sources are often **incomplete proteins** in that they are missing one or two essential amino acids. Nevertheless, it is relatively easy for the non–meat eater to combine plant foods effectively and eat complementary sources of plant protein (see Figure 7.3). An excellent example of this mutual supplementation process is eating peanut butter on whole-grain bread. Although each of these foods is deficient in essential amino acids, eating them together provides high-quality protein.

Plant sources of protein fall into three general categories: legumes (beans, peas, peanuts, and soy products), grains (whole grains, corn, and pasta products), and nuts and seeds. Certain vegetables, such as leafy green vegetables and broccoli, also contribute valuable plant proteins. Mixing two or more foods from each of these categories at the same meal will provide all the essential amino acids necessary to ensure adequate protein absorption. People not interested in obtaining all their protein from plants can combine incomplete plant proteins with complete low-fat animal proteins such as chicken, seafood, turkey, and lean cuts of pork or beef. Low-fat cottage cheese, skim milk, egg whites, and nonfat dry milk all provide high-quality proteins, few calories, and little dietary fat. However, it is important to note that low-fat products come at a cost: there is less calcium in

Selecting from two or more of these columns will help you use a process known as *mutual supplementation*, combining two protein-rich foods to form *complementary* proteins with all of the essential amino acids. These combinations make complete proteins and help avoid possible protein deficiencies.

| Grains | Legumes | Seeds and Nuts | Vegetables |
|---|---|---|---|
| Barley | Dried | Sesame | Leafy |
| Bulgar | beans | seeds | greens |
| Cornmeal | Dried | Sunflower | Broccoli |
| Oats | lentils | seeds | Others |
| Rice | Dried peas | Walnuts | |
| Whole-grain | Peanuts | Cashews | |
| breads | Soy | Other nuts | |
| Enriched | products | Nut berries | |
| pasta | | | |

FIGURE 7.3

**Complementary Proteins**

Source: Adapted by permission from page 205 of *Nutrition Concepts and Controversies,* 6th ed., by Eva Hamilton, Eleanor Whitney, and Frances Sizer. Copyright 1994 by West Publishing Company. All rights reserved.

low-fat dairy products, and egg whites do not provide the lecithin that the whole egg with the yolk gives.

# Carbohydrates

Although the importance of proteins in the body cannot be underestimated, it is **carbohydrates** that supply us with the energy needed to sustain normal daily activity. Carbohydrates provide 4 calories of energy per gram. Long maligned by weight-conscious people, carbohydrates can actually be metabolized more quickly and efficiently than proteins. Carbohydrates are a quick source of energy for the body, easily converted to glucose, the fuel for the body's cells. In fact, carbohydrates are the preferred fuel for red blood cells and nerve cells—including those in the brain.[9] These foods also play an important role in the functioning of the internal organs, the nervous system, and the muscles. They are the best source of energy for endurance athletes because they provide an immediate and a time-released energy source as they are digested easily and then consistently metabolized in the bloodstream.

There are two major types of carbohydrates: **simple carbohydrates,** which are mostly sugars, including those found in fruits, and **complex carbohydrates,** which are found in grains, cereals, dark green leafy vegetables, yellow fruits and vegetables (carrots, yams), *cruciferous* vegetables (such as broccoli, cabbage, and cauliflower), and certain root vegetables, such as potatoes. Most of us do not get enough complex carbohydrates in our daily dietary intake.

Most Canadians typically consume large amounts of simple sugars. The most common form is *glucose*. Eventually, the human body converts all simple sugars to glucose to provide energy to cells. In its natural form, glucose is sweet and is obtained from substances such as corn syrup, honey, molasses, vegetables, and fruits. *Fructose* is another simple sugar found in fruits and berries. Glucose and fructose are classified as **monosaccharides** because they contain only one molecule of sugar.

**Disaccharides** are combinations of two monosaccharides or two molecules of sugar. Perhaps the best-known disaccharide is common granulated table sugar (known as sucrose), which is made of fructose and glucose. Lactose, found in milk and milk products, is another disaccharide, formed by the combination of glucose and galactose (another simple sugar). Disaccharides must be broken down into simple sugars before they can be used by the body.

Controlling the amount of sugar you consume can be difficult because sugar, like sodium, is often present in food products where you might not expect to find it. Such diverse items as ketchup, Russian dressing, Coffee-Mate, and Shake'n'Bake derive 30 to 65 percent of their calories from sugar. Thus, reading nutrition labels carefully before purchasing food products is a must.

**Polysaccharides** are complex carbohydrates formed from the combination of long chains of saccharides. Like disaccharides, they must be broken down into simple sugars before they can be utilized by the body. There are two major forms of complex carbohydrates: *starches* and **fibre.**

Starches make up the majority of the complex carbohydrates. We obtain dietary starches from flours, breads, pasta, potatoes, and related foods. They are stored in the muscles and liver in a polysaccharide form called **glycogen.** When the body requires a sudden burst of energy, it breaks down glycogen into glucose. While we often think of starches as an alternative to fats, starches aren't better for some people, particularly those individuals who are insulin-resistant.

## Carbohydrates and Athletic Performance

In the last decade, carbohydrates have become the "health foods" of many people involved in athletic competition. Many fitness enthusiasts consume concentrated sugary foods or drinks before or during athletic activity, thinking that the sugars will provide

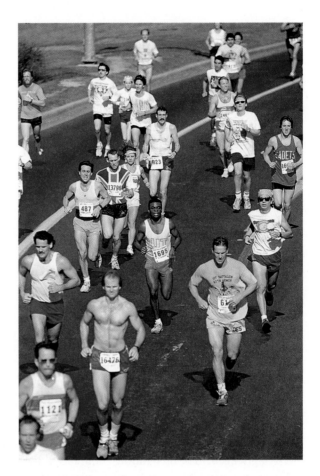

*Carb-loading before an endurance event is a training strategy used by many athletes to build energy reserves for the last few kilometres.*

**Essential amino acids:** Eight of the basic nitrogen-containing building blocks of protein that we obtain from foods.

**Complete (high-quality) proteins:** Proteins that contain all eight essential amino acids.

**Incomplete proteins:** Proteins lacking in one or more of the essential amino acids.

**Carbohydrates:** Basic nutrients that supply the body with the energy needed to sustain normal activity.

**Simple carbohydrates:** A major type of carbohydrate that provides short-term energy.

**Complex carbohydrates:** A major type of carbohydrate that provides sustained energy.

**Monosaccharide:** A simple carbohydrate that contains only one molecule of sugar.

**Disaccharide:** A combination of two monosaccharides.

**Polysaccharide:** A complex carbohydrate formed by the combination of long chains of saccharides.

**Fibre:** Cellulose, a major form of complex carbohydrates.

**Glycogen:** The polysaccharide form in which glucose is stored in the liver.

extra energy. However, in some situations, they may actually be counterproductive.[10] One possible problem involves the gastrointestinal tract. If your intestines react to physical activity (or the nervousness before competition) by moving material through the small intestine more rapidly than usual, undigested disaccharides or unabsorbed monosaccharides will reach the colon, which can result in a very inopportune bout of diarrhea.[11]

Consuming large amounts of sugar during exercise can also have a negative effect on hydration. Concentrations exceeding 24 grams of sugar per 250 mL of fluid can delay stomach emptying and hence absorption of water. Some fruit juices, fruit drinks, and other sugar-sweetened beverages have more than this amount of sugar. If you use these products, you should dilute them with ice cubes or water.

Marathon runners and other people who require reserves of energy for demanding tasks often attempt to increase stores of glycogen in the body by a process known as *carbohydrate loading*. This process involves modifying the nature of workouts and dietary intake, usually during the week or so before competition. The athletes train very hard early in the week while eating small amounts of carbohydrates. Right before competition, they dramatically increase their intake of carbohydrates to force the body to store increased levels of glycogen, to be used during endurance activities (such as the last kilometre or so of a marathon).

### The Myth of Sugar and Hyperactivity

Contrary to early media and teacher reports the day after Halloween, extensive research done during the last two decades indicates that sugars *do not* cause hyperactivity.[12] In well-controlled dietary studies, consuming sugar has not been shown to have negative effects on motor activity, spontaneous behaviours, performance in psychological tests, learning, memory, attention span, or problem-solving ability.

### Carbohydrates and Weight Loss

Throughout the 1990s and the low-fat diet craze, a plate of pasta was viewed as a healthy alternative to those who were trying to cut down on high-fat meats. More recently, carbohydrates have once again captured national (and international) attention of would-be-dieters. This time, dieters dramatically reduce the amount of carbohydrates they consume when following regimens such as the Atkins Diet, Protein Power, The Zone, the South Beach Diet, and other similar low-carbohydrate diet plans. Since carbohydrates are our preferred fuel source, our body must find another source of energy when we do not

eat enough. As a result, the body will break down stored fat in a process called *ketosis*.[13] Ketosis produces a fuel called ketones and is an important process that ensures sufficient energy is provided to the brain. When inadequate carbohydrate intake continues for an extended period of time, excessive ketones are produced resulting in acidic blood and a condition called *ketoacidosis*. Ketoacidosis interferes with basic body functions resulting in the loss of lean body mass and damage to many of the body's tissues.[14] Thus, although it appears that a low-carbohydrate dietary intake may be successful in reducing body fat (at least in the short term), the long-term negative health effects have serious implications.

> ## WHAT WOULD YOU DO?
>
> How can the Food Guide be used to ensure that you eat enough proteins, carbohydrates, and fats? How can you use the Food Guide to help maintain your weight?

## Fibre

Fibre, often referred to as "bulk" or "roughage," is the indigestible portion of plant foods that helps move foods through the digestive system and softens stools by absorbing water. *Insoluble fibre,* which is found in bran, whole-grain breads and cereals, and most fruits and vegetables, is associated with gastrointestinal benefits and reduces the risk for several forms of cancer. *Soluble fibre* appears to be a factor in lowering blood cholesterol levels, thereby reducing risk for cardiovascular disease. Major sources of soluble fibre include oat bran, dried beans (such as kidney, garbanzo, pinto, and navy beans), and some fruits and vegetables.

The best way to increase dietary fibre intake is to eat more complex carbohydrates, such as whole grains, fruits, vegetables, dried peas and beans, nuts, and seeds. As with most nutritional advice, however, too much of a good thing can pose problems. Sudden increases in dietary fibre may cause flatulence (intestinal gas), cramping, or a bloated feeling. Consuming plenty of water or other liquids may reduce such side effects and is important because fibre absorbs water in the colon prior to excretion. If insufficient water is present, constipation and significant discomfort may result.

### Fibre and Your Health

A few years ago, fibre was thought to be the remedy for just about everything. Much of this hope was exaggerated. However, current research supports the following benefits of fibre:[15]

- *Protection against colorectal cancer.* Several studies reported that fibre-rich diets, particularly those including insoluble fibre, prevent the development of precancerous growths. This protection may be a result of food moving through the colon faster (thereby reducing the colon's contact time with cancer-causing substances), or because insoluble fibre reduces bile acids and some bacterial enzymes that may promote cancer.

- *Protection against breast cancer.* Research into the effects of fibre on breast-cancer risks is very inconclusive. However, some studies indicate that wheat bran (rich in insoluble fibre) reduces blood-estrogen levels, which may reduce risk for breast cancer. Another theory suggests that people who eat more fibre have proportionally less fat in their diets and that this is what reduces overall risk.

- *Protection against constipation.* Insoluble fibre, consumed with adequate fluids, is the safest, most effective way to prevent or treat constipation. The fibre acts like a sponge, absorbing moisture and producing softer, bulkier stools easily passed. Fibre also helps produce gas, which, in turn, may initiate a bowel movement.

- *Protection against diverticulosis.* About half of Canadians over 60 suffer from *diverticulosis*, a condition in which tiny bulges or pouches form on the large intestinal wall. These bulges become irritated and cause chronic pain if under strain from constipation. Insoluble fibre helps to reduce constipation and pain. This condition is rare in those under 30.

- *Protection against heart disease.* Many studies indicate that soluble fibre (as in oat bran, barley, and fruit pectin) helps reduce blood cholesterol, primarily by lowering LDL ("bad") cholesterol. Whether this reduction is a direct effect or occurs instead through the displacement of fat calories by a high-fibre dietary intake remains in question.

- *Protection against diabetes.* Some studies have suggested that soluble fibre improves control of blood sugar and can reduce the need for insulin or medication in people with diabetes. Soluble fibre seems to delay the emptying of the stomach and slow the absorption of glucose by the intestine. Whether fibre protects against diabetes or not, it is clear that it does play a role in controlling blood glucose levels.

- *Protection against obesity.* Because most high-fibre foods are high in carbohydrates and low in fat, they help control caloric intake. Many take longer to chew, which slows you down at the table and helps you feel full sooner.

The adequate intake for fibre is 25 grams per day for women and 38 grams per day for men—or an amount equivalent to 14 grams of fibre for every 1,000 calories consumed.[16] To do this, the following steps are recommended:[17]

- Select breads and cereals made with whole grains such as wheat, oats, barley, and rye.

- Choose foods with at least 2 or 3 grams of fibre per serving.

- Choose fresh fruits and vegetables whenever possible. When appropriate, eat the peel or skin of fresh fruits and vegetables (for example, on potatoes, pears, apples, and kiwi fruit)

- Eat legumes frequently—every day, if possible. Canned or fresh beans, peas, and lentils are excellent sources of complex carbohydrates, fibre, vitamins, and minerals.

- Drink plenty of fluids.

## Fats

**Fats** (or *lipids*), another group of basic nutrients, are perhaps the most misunderstood of the body's required energy sources. Most of us do not realize that fats play a vital role in the maintenance of healthy skin and hair, insulation of the body organs against shock, maintenance of body temperature, and the proper functioning of the cells themselves. Fats make our foods taste better and carry the fat-soluble vitamins A, D, E, and K to the cells. They also provide a concentrated form of energy in the absence of sufficient amounts of carbohydrates. In fact, fats provide more than twice the energy than carbohydrates at 9 calories per gram. If fats perform all these functions, why are we constantly urged to reduce our intake?

Although moderate consumption of fats is essential to health maintenance, overconsumption can be dangerous. The most common form of fat circulating in the blood is the **triglyceride,** which makes up about 95 percent of total body fat. When we consume too many calories, the excess is converted into triglycerides in the liver, which are stored in all-too-obvious places on our bodies. The remaining five percent of body fat is composed of substances such as **cholesterol,** which can accumulate on the inner walls of arteries, causing a narrowing of the channel through which blood

**Fats:** Basic nutrients composed of carbon and hydrogen atoms; needed for the proper functioning of cells, insulation of body organs against shock, maintenance of body temperature, and healthy skin and hair.

**Triglyceride:** The most common form of fat in the body; excess calories are converted into triglycerides and stored as body fat.

**Cholesterol:** A form of fat circulating in the blood that can accumulate on the inner walls of arteries.

flows. This buildup, called plaque, is a major cause of *atherosclerosis* (discussed in detail in Chapter 12).

Fat cells consist of chains of carbon and hydrogen atoms. Those not able to hold any more hydrogen in their chemical structure are labelled **saturated fats.** They generally come from animal sources, such as meats and dairy products, and are solid at room temperature. **Unsaturated fats,** which come from plants and include most vegetable oils, are generally liquid at room temperature and have room for additional hydrogen atoms in their chemical structure. The terms *monounsaturated fat* (MUFA) and *polyunsaturated fat* (PUFA) refer to the relative number of hydrogen atoms missing. Peanut and olive oils are high in monounsaturated fats, whereas corn, sunflower, and safflower oils are high in polyunsaturated fats.

Controversy continues to swirl about which type of unsaturated fat is most beneficial. Today many researchers believe that PUFAs may decrease beneficial HDL levels while reducing LDL levels. PUFAs come in two forms: omega-3 fatty acids and omega-6 fatty acids. MUFAs, such as olive oil, seem to lower LDL levels and increase HDL levels and thus are currently the preferred—or least harmful—fat. MUFAs are also resistant to oxidation, a process that leads to cell and tissue damage. For a breakdown of the types of fats found in common vegetable oils, see Figure 7.4.

## Reducing Fat in Your Diet

Finding the best ways to reduce fat from your dietary intake is largely dependent on you, your lifestyle, and determining what works for you. The following basic guidelines are a good place to start:

- *Know what you are putting in your mouth.* Read food labels. Remember that no more than 10 percent of your total calories should come from saturated fat, and no more than 30 percent should come from all forms of fat.

- Choose fat-free or low-fat versions of foods whenever possible.

- Use olive oil for baking, stir frying, and sautéing. Studies using animal subjects indicate that this oil doesn't raise cholesterol or promote the growth of tumours.

- Whenever possible, use liquid, diet, or whipped margarine: these forms have far less trans-fatty acids than solid fat.

- Choose lean meats, seafood, or poultry. Remove skin. Broil or bake whenever possible. In general, the more well-done the meat, the fewer the calories. Drain off fat after cooking. Cut off visible fat before serving.

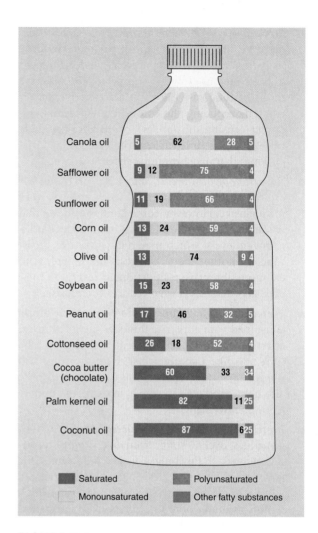

FIGURE 7.4

Percentages of Saturated, Polyunsaturated, and Monounsaturated Fats in Common Vegetable Oils

- Choose fewer cold cuts, bacon, sausage, hot dogs, and organ meats. Be careful of products claiming to be "95 percent fat-free" as they may still have high levels of fat.

- Select nonfat dairy products whenever possible. Part-skim-milk cheeses such as mozzarella, farmer's, lappi, and ricotta are good choices.

- When cooking, use substitutes for butter, margarine, oils, sour cream, mayonnaise, and salad dressings. Chicken broths, wine, vinegar, and low-calorie dressings make good flavourings and cooking ingredients.

- Remember to think of your food intake as an average over a day or a couple of days. If you have a high-fat breakfast or lunch, have a low-fat dinner to balance it.

For more specific ways to reduce fat in your dietary intake, see the Skills for Behaviour Change box.

# How to Reduce Fat in Your Dietary Intake

The small choices you make in your daily food consumption can add up to a tremendous difference in the amount of fat you eat over time. Trimming just 5 mL each day can cut more than two kilograms of fat from your dietary intake in one year—without removing great-tasting foods or causing noticeable changes. Consider the following:

1. "Butter" your toast, muffins, or bagels with "fruit-only" jams instead of sugary jellies and jams, butter, margarine, or other high-calorie spreads.

| | | |
|---|---|---|
| ■ 15 mL sugarless jam | 8 calories | 0 g fat |
| ■ 15 mL butter or margarine | 108 calories | 12 g fat |
| ■ **Savings** | **90 calories** | **12 g fat** |

2. Sauté or stir fry meat and vegetables in chicken broth or wine (most of which burns off during cooking) rather than oil.

| | | |
|---|---|---|
| ■ 15 mL oil | 240 calories | 27 g fat |
| ■ wine or broth | 0 calories | 0 g fat |
| ■ **Savings** | **240 calories** | **27 g fat** |

3. Remove the skin from chicken before cooking.

| | | |
|---|---|---|
| ■ 100 g breast | 193 calories | 8 g fat |
| ■ 100 g skinless breast | 142 calories | 3 g fat |
| ■ **Savings** | **51 calories** | **5 g fat** |

4. Use low-calorie, low-fat salad dressings on your sandwiches instead of mayonnaise.

| | | |
|---|---|---|
| ■ 15 mL mayonnaise | 100 calories | 11 g fat |
| ■ 15 mL low-cal dressing | 7 calories | 0 g fat |
| ■ **Savings** | **93 calories** | **11 g fat** |

5. Choose nonfat frozen yogurt instead of ice cream.

| | | |
|---|---|---|
| ■ 125 mL ice cream | 400 calories | 25 g fat |
| ■ 125 mL nonfat yogurt | 120 calories | 0 g fat |
| ■ **Savings** | **280 calories** | **25 g fat** |

6. For a skinny version of cream cheese that only tastes fattening, mix in a blender three parts low-fat cottage cheese with one part nonfat yogurt and use as a delicious dip, spread, or topping.

| | | |
|---|---|---|
| ■ 30 mL cream cheese | 99 calories | 10 g fat |
| ■ 30 mL mock cream cheese | 20 calories | 0 g fat |
| ■ **Savings** | **79 calories** | **10 g fat** |

7. For a warming meal minus a lot of fat and calories, eat broth-based rather than cream-based soups.

| | | |
|---|---|---|
| ■ 250 mL cream of chicken soup | 191 calories | 15 g fat |
| ■ 250 mL chicken noodle soup | 75 calories | 2 g fat |
| ■ **Savings** | **116 calories** | **13 g fat** |

8. Substitute seafood for meat at least once a week.

| | | |
|---|---|---|
| ■ 85 g top round beef | 162 calories | 5 g fat |
| ■ 85 g cod | 70 calories | 0.5 g fat |
| ■ **Savings** | **92 calories** | **4.5 g fat** |

9. Substitute two egg whites for one whole egg in recipes or omelettes.

| | | |
|---|---|---|
| ■ 1 whole egg | 79 calories | 6 g fat |
| ■ 2 egg whites | 32 calories | 0 g fat |
| ■ **Savings** | **47 calories** | **6 g fat** |

10. Load up on protein without excess fat by selecting meatless entrées such as lentil soup or vegetarian chili.

| | | |
|---|---|---|
| ■ 270 g beef chili | 256 calories | 6 g fat |
| ■ 270 g lentil soup | 164 calories | 1 g fat |
| ■ **Savings** | **92 calories** | **5 g fat** |

## GENERAL ADVICE

Become a fat sleuth. Read food labels carefully and select products that contain no more than three grams of fat for every 100 calories, which will keep your fat calories to a maximum of 30 percent of total calories.

List the small changes that you can make this week to reduce fat from your dietary intake:

1.

2.

3.

4.

5.

What other things can you do to help reduce your overall fat consumption?

Source: Adapted by permission of the author from Evelyn Tribole, "24 Ways to Trim Fat," *Shape*, July 1990, 92–93.

## Trans-Fatty Acids: Still Bad?

Since the mid-1960s, Canadians have decreased their intake of butter by almost two-thirds and substituted margarine, which became known as the "better butter" after reports labelled unsaturated fats as the "heart-healthy" alternative. But a widely publicized study in

**Saturated fats:** Fats that are unable to hold any more hydrogen in their chemical structure; derived mostly from animal sources; solid at room temperature.

**Unsaturated fats:** Fats that do have room for more hydrogen in their chemical structure; derived mostly from plants; liquid at room temperature.

1990 questioned the benefits of margarine; it indicated that margarine contains fats that raise blood cholesterol at least as much as the saturated fat in butter.[18] The culprits? **Trans-fatty acids** (fatty acids having unusual shapes) are produced when polyunsaturated oils are *hydrogenated,* a process in which hydrogen is added to unsaturated fats to make them more solid and resistant to chemical change.[19] Besides raising cholesterol levels, trans-fatty acids have been implicated in the development of certain types of cancer, increased risk for diseases such as Alzheimer's, and inflammatory processes that increase the risk of cardiovascular disease.[20]

Keep in mind that *trans* fatty acids, even MUFAs, alter blood cholesterol the same way as some saturated fats; they raise LDLs and lower HDLs. The bottom line? Moderation in all fat intake is the best rule of thumb. Probably the best advice is to continue to reduce overall fat in your dietary intake to less than 30 percent of total calories. Whenever possible, opt for other condiments on your bread, such as jams, fat-free cream cheeses, garlic, or other toppings. Some experts advocate using low-fat salad dressings as toppings for bread and pasta, or using olive oil in moderation to add a bit of flavour. If you have high cholesterol, reducing all types of fat and cholesterol in your dietary intake is sound advice.

# Vitamins

**Vitamins** are potent, essential, organic compounds that promote growth and help maintain life and health. Every minute of every day, vitamins help maintain your nerves and skin, produce blood cells, build bones and teeth, heal wounds, and convert food energy to body energy. And they do all of this without adding any calories to your diet.

Age, heat, and other environmental conditions can destroy vitamins in food. Vitamins are classified as either *fat-soluble,* meaning that they are absorbed through the intestinal tract with the help of fats, or *water-soluble,* meaning that they are easily dissolved in water. Vitamins A, D, E, and K are fat-soluble; B-complex vitamins and vitamin C are water-soluble. Fat-soluble vitamins tend to be stored in the body, and toxic accumulations in the liver may cause cirrhosis-like symptoms. Water-soluble vitamins are generally excreted and cause few toxicity problems (see Table 7.1).

Despite all media suggestions to the contrary, few Canadians suffer from true vitamin deficiencies if they consume the recommended number of servings from each of the food groups at least part of the time. Nevertheless, Canadians continue to purchase and consume large quantities of vitamin supplements. For the most part, vitamin supplements are unnecessary and in certain instances may even be harmful. Overuse of vitamin supplements can lead to a toxic condition known as **hypervitaminosis.**

## Dietary Reference Intake vs. Recommended Nutrient Intake

Scientists in Canada and the United States have been working together to develop new, common recommendations for nutrient intake. Canada previously used Recommended Nutrient Intake (RNI) while the U.S. utilized the Recommended Dietary Allowance (RDA), with slight variations between the two. The new recommendations, called Dietary Reference Intakes (DRIs), are based on the amount of water, proteins, carbohydrates, fibre, fats, vitamins, and minerals we need to avoid deficiencies and reduce our risk for chronic diseases while attempting to avoid overconsumption. [21]

---

**WHAT WOULD YOU DO?**

Of all of the nutrients discussed in this section, which one do you worry most about not getting enough of? Why? Are there any nutrients you consume too much of? What actions do you plan to make sure your daily dietary intake is adequate?

---

# Minerals

**Minerals** are the inorganic, indestructible elements that aid physiological processes within the body. Without minerals, vitamins could not be absorbed. Minerals are readily excreted and usually are not toxic. **Macrominerals** are minerals that the body needs in fairly large amounts: sodium, calcium, phosphorus, magnesium, potassium, sulphur, and chloride. **Trace minerals** include iron, zinc, manganese, copper, iodine, and cobalt, so-called because only trace

---

**Trans-fatty acids:** Fatty acids produced when polyunsaturated oils are hydrogenated to make them more solid.

**Vitamins:** Essential organic compounds that promote growth and reproduction and help maintain life and health.

**Hypervitaminosis:** A toxic condition caused by overuse of vitamin supplements.

**Minerals:** Inorganic, indestructible elements that aid physiological processes.

**Macrominerals:** Minerals that the body needs in fairly large amounts.

**Trace minerals:** Minerals that the body needs in only very small amounts.

TABLE 7.1

Dietary Reference Intakes (DRIs): Estimated Average Requirements for Groups

| Life Stage Group | CHO (g/d) | Protein (g/d)[a] | Vit A (µg/d)[b] | Vit C (mg/d) | Vit E (mg/d)[c] | Thiamin (mg/d) | Riboflavin (mg/d) | Niacin (mg/d)[d] | Vit B6 (mg/d) | Folate (µg/d)[e] | Vit B12 (µg/d) | Copper (µg/d) | Iodine (µg/d) | Iron (mg/d) | Magnesium (mg/d) | Molybdenum (µg/d) | Phosphorus (mg/d) | Selenium (µg/d) | Zinc (mg/d) |
|---|---|---|---|---|---|---|---|---|---|---|---|---|---|---|---|---|---|---|---|
| **Infants** | | | | | | | | | | | | | | | | | | | |
| 7–12 mo | | 9 | | | | | | | | | | | | 6.9 | | | | | 2.5 |
| **Children** | | | | | | | | | | | | | | | | | | | |
| 1–3 y | 100 | 11 | 210 | 13 | 5 | 0.4 | 0.4 | 5 | 0.4 | 120 | 0.7 | 260 | 65 | 3.0 | 65 | 13 | 380 | 17 | 2.5 |
| 4–8 y | 100 | 15 | 275 | 22 | 6 | 0.5 | 0.5 | 6 | 0.5 | 160 | 1.0 | 340 | 65 | 4.1 | 110 | 17 | 405 | 23 | 4.0 |
| **Males** | | | | | | | | | | | | | | | | | | | |
| 9–13 y | 100 | 27 | 445 | 39 | 9 | 0.7 | 0.8 | 9 | 0.8 | 250 | 1.5 | 540 | 73 | 5.9 | 200 | 26 | 1055 | 35 | 7.0 |
| 14–18 y | 100 | 44 | 630 | 63 | 12 | 1.0 | 1.1 | 12 | 1.1 | 330 | 2.0 | 685 | 95 | 7.7 | 340 | 33 | 1055 | 45 | 8.5 |
| 19–30 y | 100 | 46 | 625 | 75 | 12 | 1.0 | 1.1 | 12 | 1.1 | 320 | 2.0 | 700 | 95 | 6 | 330 | 34 | 580 | 45 | 9.4 |
| 31–50 y | 100 | 46 | 625 | 75 | 12 | 1.0 | 1.1 | 12 | 1.1 | 320 | 2.0 | 700 | 95 | 6 | 350 | 34 | 580 | 45 | 9.4 |
| 51–70 y | 100 | 46 | 625 | 75 | 12 | 1.0 | 1.1 | 12 | 1.4 | 320 | 2.0 | 700 | 95 | 6 | 350 | 34 | 580 | 45 | 9.4 |
| >70 y | 100 | 46 | 625 | 75 | 12 | 1.0 | 1.1 | 12 | 1.4 | 320 | 2.0 | 700 | 95 | 6 | 350 | 34 | 580 | 45 | 9.4 |
| **Females** | | | | | | | | | | | | | | | | | | | |
| 9–13 y | 100 | 28 | 420 | 39 | 9 | 0.7 | 0.8 | 9 | 0.8 | 250 | 1.5 | 540 | 73 | 5.7 | 200 | 26 | 1055 | 35 | 7.0 |
| 14–18 y | 100 | 38 | 485 | 56 | 12 | 0.9 | 0.9 | 11 | 1.0 | 330 | 2.0 | 685 | 95 | 7.9 | 300 | 33 | 1055 | 45 | 7.3 |
| 19–30 y | 100 | 38 | 500 | 60 | 12 | 0.9 | 0.9 | 11 | 1.1 | 320 | 2.0 | 700 | 95 | 8.1 | 255 | 34 | 580 | 45 | 6.8 |

*continued*

TABLE 7.1 (continued)

## Dietary Reference Intakes (DRIs): Estimated Average Requirements for Groups

| Life Stage Group | CHO (g/d)[a] | Protein (g/d)[a] | Vit A (µg/d)[b] | Vit C (mg/d) | Vit E (mg/d)[c] | Thiamin (mg/d) | Riboflavin (mg/d) | Niacin (mg/d)[d] | Vit B6 (mg/d) | Folate (µg/d)[e] | Vit B12 (µg/d) | Copper (µg/d) | Iodine (µg/d) | Iron (mg/d) | Magnesium (mg/d) | Molybdenum (µg/d) | Phosphorus (mg/d) | Selenium (µg/d) | Zinc (mg/d) |
|---|---|---|---|---|---|---|---|---|---|---|---|---|---|---|---|---|---|---|---|
| **Females (continued)** | | | | | | | | | | | | | | | | | | | |
| 31–50 y | 100 | 38 | 500 | 60 | 12 | 0.9 | 0.9 | 11 | 1.1 | 320 | 2.0 | 700 | 95 | 8.1 | 265 | 34 | 580 | 45 | 6.8 |
| 51–70 y | 100 | 38 | 500 | 60 | 12 | 0.9 | 0.9 | 11 | 1.3 | 320 | 2.0 | 700 | 95 | 5 | 265 | 34 | 580 | 45 | 6.8 |
| >70 y | 100 | 38 | 500 | 60 | 12 | 0.9 | 0.9 | 11 | 1.3 | 320 | 2.0 | 700 | 95 | 5 | 265 | 34 | 580 | 45 | 6.8 |
| **Pregnancy** | | | | | | | | | | | | | | | | | | | |
| 14–18 y | 135 | 50 | 530 | 66 | 12 | 1.2 | 1.2 | 14 | 1.6 | 520 | 2.2 | 785 | 160 | 23 | 335 | 40 | 1055 | 49 | 10.5 |
| 19–30 y | 135 | 50 | 550 | 70 | 12 | 1.2 | 1.2 | 14 | 1.6 | 520 | 2.2 | 800 | 160 | 22 | 290 | 40 | 580 | 49 | 9.5 |
| 31–50 y | 135 | 50 | 550 | 70 | 12 | 1.2 | 1.2 | 14 | 1.6 | 520 | 2.2 | 800 | 160 | 22 | 300 | 40 | 580 | 49 | 9.5 |
| **Lactation** | | | | | | | | | | | | | | | | | | | |
| 14–18 y | 160 | 60 | 885 | 96 | 16 | 1.2 | 1.3 | 13 | 1.7 | 450 | 2.4 | 985 | 209 | 7 | 300 | 35 | 1055 | 59 | 10.9 |
| 19–30 y | 160 | 60 | 900 | 100 | 16 | 1.2 | 1.3 | 13 | 1.7 | 450 | 2.4 | 1000 | 209 | 6.5 | 255 | 36 | 580 | 59 | 10.4 |
| 31–50 y | 160 | 60 | 900 | 100 | 16 | 1.2 | 1.3 | 13 | 1.7 | 450 | 2.4 | 1000 | 209 | 6.5 | 265 | 36 | 580 | 59 | 10.4 |

Notes: This table presents Estimated Average Requirements (EARs), which serve two purposes: for assessing adequacy of population intakes, and as the basis for calculating Recommended Dietary Allowances (RDAs) for individuals for those nutrients. EARs have not been established for vitamin D, vitamin K, pantothenic acid, biotin, choline, chromium, fluoride, manganese, or other nutrients not yet evaluated via the DRI process.

[a] For individual at reference weight.

[b] As retinol activity equivalents (RAEs), 1 RAE = 1 µg retinol, 12 µg β-carotene, 24 µg α-carotene, 24 µg β-cryptoxanthin. The RAE for dietary provitamin A carotenoids is two-fold greater than retinol equivalents (RE), whereas the RAE for preformed vitamin A is the same as RE.

[c] As α-tocopherol, α-Tocopherol includes RRR-α-tocopherol, the only form of a α-tocopherol that occurs naturally in foods, and the 2R-stereoisomeric forms of α-tocopherol (RRR-β RSR-β RRS-β and RRS-α-tocopherol) that occur in fortified foods and supplements. It does not include the 2S-stereoisomeric forms of α-tocopherol (SRR-β SSR-β SRS-β SSS-β and SSS-α-tocopherol), also found in fortified foods and supplements.

[d] As niacin equivalents (NE), 1 mg of niacin = 60 mg of tryptophan.

[e] As dietary folate equivalents (DFE),1 DFE = 1 µg food folate = 0.6 µg of folic acid from fortified food or as a supplement consumed with food = 0.5 µg of a supplement taken on an empty stomach.

Source: Reprinted with permission from the National Academies Press, Copyright 2005, National Academy of Sciences.

amounts of these minerals are needed. Serious problems may result if excesses or deficiencies occur. Specific types of minerals are listed in Table 7.1. Although minerals are necessary for body function, there are limits on the amounts of each that we should consume.

## Sodium

Sodium is necessary for the regulation of blood and body fluids, for the successful transmission of nerve impulses, for heart activity, and for certain metabolic functions. However, we consume much more sodium every day than we need. It is estimated that the average adult who does not sweat profusely needs only 1,500 mg of sodium per day,[22] yet the average Canadian consumes at least 12 times this amount. The most common source of sodium for Canadians is table salt. The remainder of dietary sodium comes from the water we drink and from highly processed foods infused with sodium to enhance flavour. Pickles, salty snack foods, processed cheeses, many breads and bakery products, and smoked meats and sausages often contain several hundred milligrams of sodium per serving. Many fast-food entrées and convenience entrées have 500 to 1,000 mg of sodium per serving. Soft drinks are also likely culprits for added sodium.

Many experts believe that there is a link between excessive sodium intake and hypertension (high blood pressure). Although this theory is controversial, many organizations recommend that Canadians cut back on sodium consumption to reduce their risk for cardiovascular diseases. Sodium has also been linked to stomach cancer.

## Calcium

The issue of calcium consumption has gained national attention with the rising incidence of osteoporosis (see Chapter 14) among the elderly, particularly among older women. Although calcium plays a vital role in building strong bones and teeth, contracting muscles, clotting blood, transmitting nerve impulses, regulating heartbeat, and balancing fluid within cells, most Canadians between ages 19 and 50 do not consume the recommended 1,000 mg of calcium per day.[23] Older Canadians (>50 years) are advised to consume 1,200 mg of calcium per day.[24]

Increasing Your Dietary Calcium Intake Because calcium intake is so important throughout your life for a strong bone structure, it is critical that you consume the minimum required each day. More than half our calcium intake usually comes from milk, one of the best sources of dietary calcium. Although many green, leafy vegetables are good sources of calcium, some contain oxalic acid, which makes their calcium harder to absorb. Spinach, chard, and beet greens are not particularly good sources of calcium, whereas broccoli, cauliflower, and many peas and beans offer good supplies (pinto beans and soybeans are among the best). Many nuts, particularly almonds, brazil nuts, and hazelnuts, and seeds such as sunflower and sesame contain good amounts of calcium. Molasses is fairly high in calcium. Some fruits—such as citrus fruits, figs, raisins, and dried apricots—have moderate amounts.

Of interest to those who drink carbonated soft drinks is the fact that the added phosphoric acid (phosphate) in these drinks can cause you to excrete calcium, which may result in calcium being pulled out of your bones. Calcium and phosphorus imbalances may lead to kidney stones and other calcification problems, as well as to increased atherosclerotic plaque.[25]

We also know that sunlight increases the manufacture of vitamin D in the body, and is therefore like having an extra calcium source, because vitamin D improves absorption of calcium. (See also the Focus on Canada box earlier in this chapter.) Stress, on the other hand, tends to contribute to calcium depletion. It is generally best to consume calcium throughout the day in foods containing protein, vitamin D, and vitamin C for optimum absorption. Experts differ on which type of supplemental calcium is most readily and efficiently absorbed, although bone meal, aspartate, or citrate salts of calcium are among those most often recommended. The best way to obtain calcium, like all the other nutrients, is to consume it as part of a balanced, varied dietary intake.

## Iron

Although it is found in every cell of all living things, many individuals have difficulty getting enough iron in their daily dietary intake. Females aged 19 to 50 need 18 mg per day, and males aged 19 to 50 need about 8 mg per day.[26] After the age of 50 (postmenopausal for women), men and women each require about 8 mg of iron per day.[27] Pregnant women require 27 mg of iron per day.[28] Iron deficiencies can lead to **anemia,** a problem resulting from the body's inability to produce hemoglobin, the bright red, oxygen-carrying component of the blood. When this occurs, body cells receive less oxygen, and carbon dioxide wastes are removed less efficiently, causing a person to feel tired and run down. Women are more

**Anemia:** Iron-deficiency disease that results from the body's inability to produce hemoglobin.

likely than men to suffer from iron deficiency problems, partly because they typically eat less than men, therefore their diets contain less iron, and because of blood loss from menstrual flows. Another problem with iron deficiency is that the immune system becomes less effective, which can lead to increased risk of illness. A less common problem, iron toxicity, is caused by too much iron in the blood.

## Sex Differences in Nutritional Needs

Men and women differ in body size, body composition, and overall metabolic rates. They therefore have differing needs for most nutrients throughout the life cycle (see Tables 7.1 and 7.2) and face unique difficulties in keeping on track with their dietary goals. Some of these differences have already been discussed.

However, there are some dietary factors that need further consideration. One factor is that women have a lower ratio of lean body mass to adipose (fatty) tissue at all ages, particularly after puberty. Also, after puberty, metabolism is higher in men, meaning that they will burn more calories than women doing the same things.

**Different Cycles, Different Needs** In addition to the above differences, women have many more "landmark" times in their lives when their nutritional needs vary significantly. From menarche to menopause, women undergo cyclical physiological changes that can have dramatic effects on metabolism, nutritional needs, and efforts to stick to a nutritional plan. For example, during pregnancy and lactation, nutritional requirements increase substantially for women. Those unable to follow the dietary recommendations of their doctors may find themselves

TABLE 7.2

Dietary Reference Intakes (DRIs): Recommended Macronutrient Intakes for Individuals

| Life Stage Group | Total Water[a] (L/d) | Carbohydrate (g/d) | Total Fibre (g/d) | Fat (g/d) | Linoleic Acid (g/d) | α-Linolenic Acid (g/d) | Protein[b] (g/d) |
|---|---|---|---|---|---|---|---|
| Infants | | | | | | | |
| 0–6 mo | 0.7* | 60* | ND | 31* | 4.4* | 0.5* | 9.1* |
| 7–12 mo | 0.8* | 95* | ND | 30* | 4.6* | 0.5* | 11.0 |
| Children | | | | | | | |
| 1–3 y | 1.3* | 130 | 19* | ND | 7* | 0.7* | 13 |
| 4–8 y | 1.7* | 130 | 25* | ND | 10* | 0.9* | 19 |
| Males | | | | | | | |
| 9–13 y | 2.4* | 130 | 31* | ND | 12* | 1.2* | 34 |
| 14–18 y | 3.3* | 130 | 38* | ND | 16* | 1.6* | 52 |
| 19–30 y | 3.7* | 130 | 38* | ND | 17* | 1.6* | 56 |
| 31–50 y | 3.7* | 130 | 38* | ND | 17* | 1.6* | 56 |
| 51–70 y | 3.7* | 130 | 30* | ND | 14* | 1.6* | 56 |
| > 70 y | 3.7* | 130 | 30* | ND | 14* | 1.6* | 56 |
| Females | | | | | | | |
| 9–13 y | 2.1* | 130 | 26* | ND | 10* | 1.0* | 34 |
| 14–18 y | 2.3* | 130 | 26* | ND | 11* | 1.1* | 46 |

TABLE 7.2 (continued)

Dietary Reference Intakes (DRIs): Recommended Macronutrient Intakes for Individuals

| Life Stage Group | Total Water[a] (L/d) | Carbohydrate (g/d) | Total Fibre (g/d) | Fat (g/d) | Linoleic Acid (g/d) | α-Linolenic Acid (g/d) | Protein[b] (g/d) |
|---|---|---|---|---|---|---|---|
| Females (continued) | | | | | | | |
| 19–30 y | 2.7* | 130 | 25* | ND | 12* | 1.1* | 46 |
| 31–50 y | 2.7* | 130 | 25* | ND | 12* | 1.1* | 46 |
| 51–70 y | 2.7* | 130 | 21* | ND | 11* | 1.1* | 46 |
| > 70 y | 2.7* | 130 | 21* | ND | 11* | 1.1* | 46 |
| Pregnancy | | | | | | | |
| 14–18 y | 3.0* | 175 | 28* | ND | 13* | 1.4* | 71 |
| 19–30 y | 3.0* | 175 | 28* | ND | 13* | 1.4* | 71 |
| 31–50 y | 3.0* | 175 | 28* | ND | 13* | 1.4* | 71 |
| Lactation | | | | | | | |
| 14–18 y | 3.8* | 210 | 29* | ND | 13* | 1.3* | 71 |
| 19–30 y | 3.8* | 210 | 29* | ND | 13* | 1.3* | 71 |
| 31–50 y | 3.8* | 210 | 29* | ND | 13* | 1.3* | 71 |

Bold indicates Recommended Dietary Allowances (RDAs).

* indicates Adequate Intakes (AIs).

[a] Total Water includes all water contained in food, beverages, and drinking water.

[b] Based on 0.8 g/kg body weight for the reference body weight.

Source: Reprinted with permission from the National Academies Press, Copyright 2005, National Academy of Sciences.

gaining more weight during pregnancy and retaining it afterward. During the menstrual cycle, many women report significant food cravings that may cause them to overeat. With the advent of menopause, nutritional needs again change rather dramatically. With the hormone estrogen depleted, the body needs more calcium to reduce losses in bone mineral density. Women must pay closer attention to their physical activity habits and to obtaining sufficient calcium in their dietary intake or run the risk of developing osteoporosis.

## Changing the Meat and Potatoes Man

Although men do not have the same cyclical patterns and dietary needs as women, they often have dietary excesses or habits resistant to change. Consider the following:

- Men who eat red meat as a main dish five or more times a week have four times the risk of colorectal cancer than men who eat red meat less than once a month.

- Heavy-red-meat-eaters are more than twice as likely to get prostate cancer and nearly five times as likely to get colorectal cancer (as noted above).

- For every three servings of fruits or vegetables consumed per day men can expect a 22 percent lower risk of stroke.

- High fruit and vegetable dietary intakes may lower the risk of lung cancer in smokers, from 20 times the risk of nonsmokers to "only" 10 times the risk. They may also protect against oral, throat, pancreas, and bladder cancers, all of which are more common in smokers.

- While obesity seems to be a factor in cancer of the esophagus, an increasingly common malignancy among men, consumption of fruits and vegetables can help protect against it.

# VEGETARIANISM

For aesthetic, animal rights, economic, personal, health, cultural, or religious reasons, some people choose specialized diets. Approximately four percent of Canadians claim to be some form of **vegetarian**.[29] Vegetarianism can provide a superb alternative to the typical high-fat, high-calorie, meat-based cuisine. However, without proper information and careful food selection, vegetarians can have dietary problems.

The term *vegetarian* means different things to different people. Strict vegetarians, or *vegans*, avoid all foods of animal origin, including dairy products and eggs. The few people who fall into this category must carefully plan their dietary intake to ensure that they get the necessary nutrients. Far more common are people who are *lacto-vegetarians*. These people eat dairy products but avoid flesh foods; as a result their diet is often low in fat and cholesterol, but only if they consume skim milk and other low-fat or nonfat dairy products. *Ovo-vegetarians* add eggs to their diet, while *lacto-ovo-vegetarians* eat dairy products and eggs. *Pesco-vegetarians* eat seafood, dairy products, and eggs, while *semi-vegetarians* eat chicken, seafood, dairy products, and eggs. Some people in the semi-vegetarian category prefer to call themselves *non–red meat eaters*.

Generally, people who follow a balanced vegetarian diet weigh less, have better cholesterol levels, fewer problems with irregular bowel movements (constipation and diarrhea), and a lower risk of heart disease than nonvegetarians. Some preliminary evidence suggests that vegetarians may also have a reduced risk for colorectal and breast cancer. Whether these lower risks are due to the vegetarian diet per se or to some combination of lifestyle variables remains unclear.

The modern vegetarian is usually extremely adept at combining the right types of foods to ensure proper nutrient intake. People who eat dairy products and small amounts of chicken or seafood are seldom nutrient-deficient; in fact, while vegans typically get 50 to 60 grams of protein per day, lacto-ovo-vegetarians normally consume between 70 and 90 grams per day, well beyond the DRIs. Vegan diets may be deficient in vitamins B2 (riboflavin), B12, and D. Riboflavin is found mainly in meat, eggs, and dairy products; broccoli, asparagus, almonds, and fortified cereals are also good sources. Vitamins B12 and D are found only in dairy products and fortified products such as soy milk. Vegans are also at risk for calcium, iron, zinc, and other mineral deficiencies, but these nutrients can be obtained from supplements. Strict vegans have to pay much more attention to what they eat than the average person, but by eating complementary combinations of plant products they can obtain an adequate amount of essential amino acids.

# EATING WELL AS A UNIVERSITY OR COLLEGE STUDENT

Post-secondary students often face unique challenges when trying to obtain a healthy dietary intake. Some students live in dorms and eat at university or college food services where food choices are limited. Further, most of these students do not have their own cooking or refrigeration facilities. Others live in crowded apartments where everyone forages in the refrigerator for everyone else's food. Most students have time constraints that make buying and preparing food and eating well a difficult task. In addition, many lack the financial resources needed to buy many foods that their parents purchased

**Vegetarian:** A term with a variety of meanings: vegans avoid all foods of animal origin; lacto-vegetarians avoid flesh foods but eat dairy products; ovo-vegetarians avoid flesh foods but eat eggs; lacto-ovo-vegetarians avoid flesh foods but eat dairy products and eggs; pesco-vegetarians avoid meat but eat seafood, dairy products, and eggs; semi-vegetarians eat chicken, seafood, dairy products, and eggs.

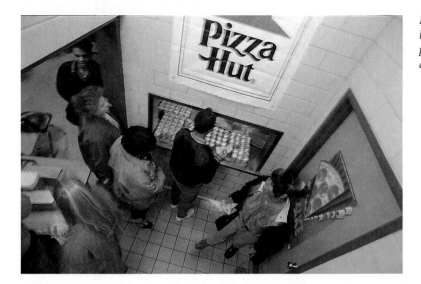

*Maintaining a healthy dietary intake can be a challenge for post-secondary students, particularly with fast-food chains on most campuses.*

while they lived at home. What's a student to do? While we can't come in and guard your refrigerator to make sure your roommates don't eat your food, we can offer some suggestions for choices that may make your eating attitudes and behaviours healthier.

## Fast Foods: Eating on the Run

If your campus is like many others across the country, you've probably noticed a distinct move toward fast-food restaurants in your student union building so that it now resembles the food courts found in most major shopping malls. These new eating centres fit students' needs for a fast bite of food at a relatively reasonable price between classes and bring in needed dollars to your school. Most of us know that many fast foods are high in fat and sodium—so is it possible to eat well and consume these fast foods?

Not all fast foods are created equal and not all of them are bad for you. Keep in mind, as well, that all foods can fit; some simply in lesser quantities than others. On a positive note, many fast-food places are offering several excellent choices for the discriminating eater. The key word is *discriminating*. It is possible to eat well at fast food chains if you follow these suggestions and those found in the Skills for Behaviour Change box:

- Ask for nutritional analyses of items on the menu so that you can make informed choices.

- Order it "your way"—avoid mayonnaise or sauces and other add-ons. Some places even have fat-free or reduced fat mayonnaise, so ask.

- Order single, small burgers rather than large, high-calorie, bacon- or cheese-topped choices. Put on your own ketchup and keep portions small.

- Order salads, and be careful how much dressing you put on. Many people think they are being health-smart by eating salad, only to smother it with calorie- and fat-rich dressings. Try the vinegar and oil or low-fat alternative dressings. Limit high-fat add-ons such as bacon bits.

- When ordering a chicken sandwich, order the skinless broiled version rather than the deep-fried kind.

- Check to see what type of oil is used to cook fries if you must have them. Avoid lard-based or other saturated-fat products.

- Order whole-wheat buns and bread and ask them to hold the butter or margarine.

- Limit fried foods in general, including hot apple pies and other crust-based fried foods.

- Opt to eat at spots where foods tend to be broiled rather than fried.

## When Funds Are Short

Balancing the need for adequate nutrition with the many other activities that are part of college or university life can become a difficult task. However, if you take the time to plan a healthy dietary intake, you may find that you are eating better, enjoying eating more, and actually saving money. Understanding the terminology used by the food industry may also help you eat healthier. The Building Communication Skills box reviews some of these pertinent terms. Figure 7.5 shows an example of a Nutrition Facts label.

In addition, you can take these steps to help ensure a quality diet:

- Buy fruits and vegetables in season for their lower cost, higher nutrient quality, and greater variety. Out-of-season, flash-frozen varieties are available at

# What's Good on the Menu?

While some restaurants offer hints for health-conscious diners, you're on your own most of the time. To help you order wisely, here are lighter options and high-fat pitfalls. "Best" choices contain fewer than 30 grams of fat, a generous meal's worth for an active, medium-size woman. "Worst" choices have up to 100 grams of fat.

## FAST FOOD

**Best**    Grilled chicken sandwich; roast beef sandwich; single hamburger; salad with light vinaigrette

**Worst**    Bacon burger; double cheeseburger; french fries; onion rings

**Tips**    Order sandwiches without mayo or special sauce. Limit deep-fried items like fish fillets, chicken nuggets, and french fries.

## ITALIAN

**Best**    Pasta with red or white clam sauce; spaghetti with marinara or tomato-and-meat sauce

**Worst**    Eggplant parmigiana; fettuccine alfredo; fried calamari; lasagna

**Tips**    Stick with plain bread instead of garlic bread made with butter or oil. Ask for the server's help in avoiding cream- or egg-based sauces. Try vegetarian pizza–without extra cheese.

## MEXICAN

**Best**    Bean burrito (no cheese); chicken fajitas

**Worst**    Beef chimichanga; chile relleno; quesadilla; refried beans

**Tips**    Choose soft tortillas (not fried) with fresh salsa. Special-order grilled shrimp, fish, or chicken. Ask for beans made without lard or fat and for cheeses and sour cream provided on the side. Ask for low-fat or no-fat varieties.

## CHINESE

**Best**    Hot-and-sour soup; stir-fried vegetables; shrimp with garlic sauce; Szechuan shrimp; wonton soup

**Worst**    Crispy chicken; kung pao chicken; moo shu pork; sweet-and-sour pork

**Tips**    Share a stir-fry; help yourself to steamed rice. Ask for vegetables steamed or stirfried with less oil. Order moo shu vegetables instead of pork. Limit fried rice, breaded dishes, egg rolls, spring rolls, and items loaded with nuts. Limit high-sodium sauces.

## JAPANESE

**Best**    Steamed rice and vegetables; tofu as a substitute for meat; broiled or steamed chicken and fish

**Worst**    Fried rice dishes; miso (very high in sodium); tempura

**Tips**    Limit soy sauces. Use caution in eating sashimi and sushi (raw fish) dishes to reduce risk of bacteria or parasites.

## THAI

**Best**    Clear broth soups; stir-fried chicken and vegetables; grilled meats

**Worst**    Coconut milk; peanut sauces; deep-fried dishes

**Tips**    Limit coconut-based curries. Ask for steamed, not fried, rice.

## BREAKFAST

**Best**    Hot or cold cereal with 1 percent or skim milk; pancakes or French toast with syrup; scrambled eggs with hash browns and plain toast

**Worst**    Belgian waffle with sausage; sausage and eggs with biscuits and gravy; ham-and-cheese omelette with hash browns and toast

**Tips**    Ask for whole-grain cereal or shredded wheat with 1 percent or skim milk or whole wheat toast without butter or margarine. Order omelettes without cheese, and fried eggs without bacon or sausage.

## SANDWICHES

**Best**    Ham and Swiss cheese; roast beef; turkey

**Worst**    Tuna salad; Reuben; submarine

**Tips**    Ask for mustard; hold the mayo and cheese. See if turkey-ham is available.

## SEAFOOD

**Best**    Broiled bass, halibut, or snapper; grilled scallops; steamed crab or lobster

**Worst**    Fried seafood platter; blackened catfish

**Tips**    Order fish broiled, baked, grilled, or steamed–not pan-fried or sautéed. Ask for fresh lemon instead of tartar sauce. Limit creamy and buttery sauces.

Sources: American Dietetic Association, 2002, www.eatright.org; *Health* 10 (November/December 1996): 79.

# Understanding Nutrition Claims

Nutritional labelling regulations became mandatory for packaged foods distributed from larger businesses on December 12, 2005. Smaller businesses have until December 12, 2007 to follow the regulations. These new regulations require labels on most pre-packaged foods to carry a Nutrition Facts table that lists calories and 13 key nutrients in a specified amount of food (that is, a usual serving). The regulations were introduced in 2003, with many food distributors adapting their food labels to meet the regulations prior to the mandatory date.

In addition to the labelling regulations, Health Canada updated the requirements of more than 40 nutrient content claims and decided to allow only certain health claims (re: the diet–health relationships) on food labels or in advertisements. It is up to the manufacturer whether to include a nutrition content or diet–health claim on the label or in the advertisement of the food. Often the claims are made—and done so attractively—because they positively influence consumers.

### Examples of Nutrient Content Claims:

**Source of fibre**–the food must contain at least 2 grams of dietary fibre in the amount of food specified as a serving in the Nutrition Facts table.

**Low fat**–the food contains no more than 3 grams of fat in the amount of food specified as a serving in the Nutrition Facts table.

**Cholesterol-free**–the food has a negligible amount of cholesterol (less than 2 mg) in the amount of food specified as a serving in the Nutrition Facts table. The food must also be low in saturated and trans fat.

**Sodium-free**–the food contains less than 5 mg of sodium in the amount of food specified as a serving in the Nutrition Facts table.

**Reduced in calories**–the food has at least 25 percent fewer calories than the food it is compared to.

**Light**–in regard to the nutritional characteristics of a product, "light" is allowed on foods reduced in fat or reduced in calories. "Light" may also be used to describe sensory characteristics associated with a particular food—so long as that characteristic is clearly identified with the claim (for example, light tasting, light coloured).

### What Do the Words in Nutrient Content Claims Mean?

**Free**–none or hardly any

**Low**–a small amount

**Reduced**–at least 25 percent less than in a similar product

**Light**–allowed only on labels reduced in fat or reduced in calories. If used in reference to the characteristic of the food, the characteristic must accompany the claim.

**Source**–contains a useful amount

**High or good source**–contains a high amount

**Very high or excellent source**–contains a very high amount

### What Are Health Claims?

Only the following diet–health claims can be made:

1. A healthy diet low in saturated and trans fat may reduce the risk of heart disease.

2. A healthy diet with adequate calcium and vitamin D, and regular physical activity, helps to achieve strong bones and may reduce the risk of osteoporosis.

3. A healthy diet rich in a variety of vegetables and fruit may help reduce the risk of some types of cancer.

4. A healthy diet containing foods high in potassium and low in sodium may reduce the risk of high blood pressure, a risk factor for stroke and heart disease.

Source: Adapted from Health Canada: Food and Nutrition, "Interactive Nutrition Label: Get the Facts." Retrieved on May 25, 2006, from www.hc-sc.gc.ca.

a reasonable price and are a high-nutrient-quality choice for fruits and vegetables.

- Use coupons and specials to get price reductions.

- Shop whenever possible at discount warehouse food chains; capitalize on volume discounts and no-frills products.

- Plan ahead to get the most for your dollar and limit extra trips to the store. Make a list and stick to it.

- Purchase meats and other products in volume, freezing portions for future needs. Or purchase small amounts of meats and other expensive proteins and combine them with beans and plant

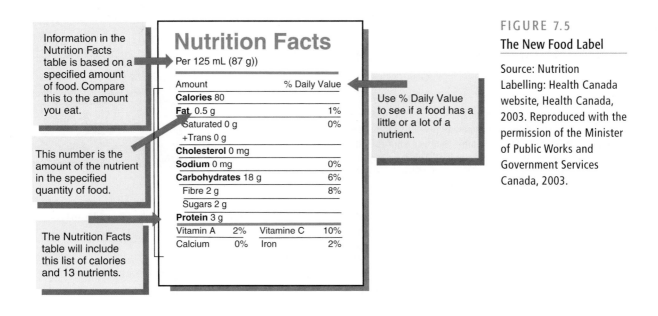

**FIGURE 7.5**

**The New Food Label**

Source: Nutrition Labelling: Health Canada website, Health Canada, 2003. Reproduced with the permission of the Minister of Public Works and Government Services Canada, 2003.

proteins for lower total cost, lower calories, and lower fat.

- Cook large meals and freeze smaller portions for later use.

- If you find that you have no money for food, check with the local food bank or social service department. Assistance may be available.

## Healthy Eating in the Dormitory

Some university or college food services have responded positively to new guidelines for low-fat, high-carbohydrate eating. Many offer vegetarian entrées, choices among broiled, baked, or fried foods, skim milks, nonfat yogurts, and full-service salad and pasta bars. Unfortunately, many others have not changed and offer limited choices for students, providing only high- and higher-fat choices.

If you find that you are in a health-conscious food service or dormitory, the guidelines and tips provided throughout this chapter should serve you well (see also Table 7.3). If you are in a food service or dormitory that has a long way to go, there are some possible actions you might take to help them change their food choices and cooking practices:

- Ask if anyone has ever done a food analysis of menu items at the food service or dorm. If they have, find out what happened to the information obtained. If not, find out what you can do to get one done. Your student health service, health class, nutrition department, or local hospital may be a good resource.

- Once you've identified the nutrient content of these meals, take your findings to the student newspaper and the student government and find someone willing to push for food service reform.

- If you are dissatisfied with cafeteria foods, make your complaints known in writing to the director of student services or the food service administrator. Be sure to include recommendations for improvements.

- Find out what is being done on other campuses in your province and throughout the country. Competition among universities and colleges often goes beyond the sports playing field. You may spur someone to action.

- Use the suggestion box provided in the cafeteria. If there isn't one, try to get one.

- Be positive in your approach. More support is gained from providing suggestions for change rather than criticism of current practice.

### WHAT WOULD YOU DO?

What problems cause you the most difficulty when you try to eat better? Are these problems that you have noted in your family, too, or are they unique to your current situation as a student? What actions can you take that would help improve your current eating attitudes and behaviours?

**TABLE 7.3**

**Eating Well in the Dining Hall**

Choose lean meats, grilled chicken, seafood, or vegetable dishes. Avoid fried chicken, fatty cuts of red meat, or dishes smothered in creamy or oily sauce.

Hit the salad bar and load up on leafy greens, beans, tuna, or tofu. Choose items such as avocado or nuts for a little "good" fat, and go easy on the dressing.

Get creative: Choose items such as a baked potato with salsa, or add a grilled chicken breast to your salad. Toast some bread, and top it with veggies, hummus, or grilled chicken or tuna.

When choosing foods from a made-to-order food station, ask the preparer to hold the butter or oil, mayonnaise, sour cream, or cheese or cream-based sauce. Do ask for extra servings of veggies and lean meats.

Limit going back for seconds and consuming large portions. Many colleges and universities limit the number of visits you make each day to the dining hall; don't view this as a reason to overeat.

If there is something you'd like but you don't see it in your dining hall, or you are vegetarian and feel like your food choices are limited, speak to your food services manager and provide suggestions.

Limit high-calorie, low-nutrient rich foods such as sugary cereals, soft-serve ice cream, waffles, and other sweet treats. Choose fruit or low-fat yogurt to satisfy your sweet tooth.

# FOOD SAFETY: INCREASING CONCERNS

## Irradiation

As we become increasingly worried that the food we put in our mouths may be contaminated with potentially harmful bacteria, insects, worms, or other not-so-nice substances, the food industry has come under fire. To convince us that our products are safe for consumption, some manufacturers have come up with "new and improved" ways of protecting our foods. One of these methods, food irradiation, has become the subject of much controversy. What is food irradiation? Should you buy irradiated foods?

**Food irradiation** involves treating foods with gamma radiation from radioactive cobalt or some other source of X-rays. When foods are irradiated they are exposed to low doses of radiation (ionizing energy), which breaks chemical bonds of harmful bacteria in the DNA, destroys pathogens, and keeps them from replication. These rays pass through the food without leaving any radioactive residue.[30]

Irradiation lengthens food products' shelf life and prevents microorganism and insect contamination. Because this results in less waste, the food industry can make higher profits while charging consumers lower prices. It is also claimed that irradiation will reduce the need to use many of the toxic chemicals currently used to preserve foods and prevent contamination from external contaminants. The following foods have already received approval for irradiation by Health Canada: onions, potatoes, wheat flour, whole wheat flour, whole or ground spices, and dehydrated seasoning preparations.

## Food-borne Illness

Most of us have experienced the characteristic symptoms of diarrhea, nausea, cramping, and vomiting that prompt us to say, "It must be something I ate." The number of cases of food poisoning in Canada has been growing (there are 10,000 reported cases per year; for every reported case there are many more unreported cases). Symptoms of food-borne illness vary according to the type of organism and the amount of contaminant eaten. These symptoms may appear as early as a half hour after eating the food, or take several days or weeks to develop. In most people, they come on five to eight hours after eating and last only a day or two. In others, such as the very old and very young and those with a compromised immune system, food-borne illness can be life-threatening.

**Food irradiation:** Treating foods with gamma radiation from radioactive cobalt, cesium, or some other source of X-rays to kill microorganisms.

Several factors may be contributing to the increase in food-borne illnesses. One factor is the move away from a traditional meat-and-potato dietary intake to "heart-healthy" eating—increased consumption of fruits, vegetables, and grains—because it has spurred demand for fresh foods not in season most of the year.[31] This means that we must import fresh fruits and vegetables, thus putting ourselves at risk for ingesting exotic pathogens. Although we are told when we travel to developing countries to "boil it, peel it, or don't eat it," we bring these foods into our kitchens and eat them, often without even washing them.[32] Food can become contaminated by being watered with contaminated water, fertilized with "organic" fertilizers (animal manure), or not subjected to the same rigorous pesticide regulations as Canadian-raised produce. To give you an idea of the implications, studies have shown that *Escherichia coli* (a lethal bacterial pathogen) can survive in cow manure for up to 70 days and multiply in foods grown with manure unless heat or additives such as salt or preservatives are used to kill them.[33] There are essentially no regulations that prohibit farmers from using animal manure to fertilize crops.

Other key factors associated with the increasing spread of food-borne diseases include inadvertent introduction of pathogens into new geographic regions and insufficient education about food safety.[34]

Part of the responsibility for preventing food-borne illness lies with consumers: more than 30 percent of such illnesses result from unsafe handling of food at home. The following are actions you can take to minimize your risk:[35]

- When shopping, pick up your packaged and canned foods first and frozen foods and perishables such as dairy products, meat, poultry, and seafood at the end. Try to put these foods in separate plastic bags so that drippings don't run onto and contaminate other foods.

- Check for cleanliness at the salad bar and meat and seafood counters. For instance, cooked shrimp lying on the same bed of ice as raw seafood can easily be contaminated.

- When shopping for seafood, buy from markets that get their supplies from approved sources; stay clear of vendors who sell shellfish from roadside stands or the back of trucks. If you're planning to harvest your own shellfish, check the safety of the water in the area.

- Remember that most cuts of meat, seafood, and poultry should be kept in the refrigerator no more than one or two days. They shouldn't be in the grocery store meat counter beyond their dated shelf life, either. Check the shelf life of all products before buying. If expiration dates are close, freeze or eat immediately.

- Leftovers should be eaten within three days.

- Use a thermometer to ensure that meats are completely cooked. Remember that the rarer the steak, the greater the number of bacteria swarming on the plate. Beef and lamb should be cooked to at least 60°C, pork to 66°C, and poultry to 74°C. Don't eat poultry that is pink inside.

- Fish is done when the thickest part becomes opaque and the fish flakes easily when poked with a fork.

- Cooked food should never be left standing on the stove or table for more than two hours. Disease-causing bacteria grow in temperatures between 5°C and 60°C. Keep hot foods hot and cold foods cold.

*Learning to shop carefully for fresh, high-quality foods can help ensure that your food is safe and help you to attain nutritional health.*

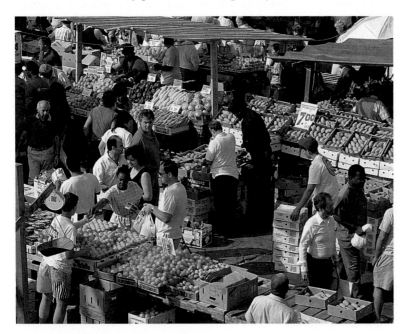

## Health Canada Comments on a Recent Study Relating to the Safety of Aspartame*

**HEALTH IN THE MEDIA**

*In June 2005, the* European Journal of Oncology *published the results of a study on the safety of aspartame conducted by the European Ramazzini Foundation of Oncology and Environmental Science. After reviewing this paper, the scientists from Health Canada reported no need to change the existing restrictions on aspartame use as outlined in the current Food and Drug Regulations. A similar report (that is, that no changes needed to be made to the previously established acceptable daily intake of aspartame) was made by the European Safety Authority.*

Nonetheless, the scientists from Health Canada are currently analyzing the data obtained from the Ramazzini Foundation to provide further support that no changes to current restrictions need to be made. Should any conclusive evidence be found that links aspartame consumption to adverse health effects, Health Canada will take appropriate action.

Source: Adapted from Health Canada: Food and Nutrition, "Health Canada Comments on the Recent Study Relating to the Safety of Aspartame." Retrieved on May 25, 2006, from www.hc-sc.gc.ca/fn-an/securit/facts-faits/aspartame/aspartame_statement_e.htm.

*Aspartame is a non-nutritive sweetener currently permitted for use in Canada (and in many other countries) as a sweetener in foods and as a tabletop sweetener. Health Canada provided approval for aspartame in 1981.

- Never thaw frozen foods at room temperature. Put in the refrigerator for a day to thaw, or thaw in cold water, changing the water every 30 minutes.

- Wash your hands with soap and water between courses when preparing food, particularly after handling meat, seafood, or poultry. Wash the countertop and all utensils thoroughly and with a bacteria-killing cleanser before using them for other foods.

## Food Allergies

Up to 8 percent of children, and a smaller proportion of adults, are allergic to at least one food. True **food allergies** occur when the body overreacts to normally harmless proteins, perceiving them as allergens. The body then produces antibodies that activate immune cells known as *histamines,* triggering a variety of allergic symptoms. Such allergic reactions vary tremendously and may range from a case of hives or a body rash to swelling of certain body parts (especially the lips), to pain, itchiness, diarrhea, nausea, or vomiting. In more severe cases, irregularities in breathing and heartbeat are experienced, along with blood pressure fluctuations, shock, and, if untreated, death. Symptoms may occur within minutes or over a two- to three-hour period.

The most common culprits are soybeans, legumes (including peanuts), nuts, shellfish, eggs, wheat, and milk. People are often allergic to a whole family of foods; this is called cross-reactivity. Unlike many other allergies, food allergies do not appear to be inherited. Individuals breast-fed as infants seem to have fewer food allergies. If you think you have a food allergy, get tested by a trained allergist.

Some common reactions to food that may imitate allergies but do not involve the immune system are listed below.[36]

- **Food intolerance,** which occurs in people who lack certain digestive enzymes and suffer adverse effects when they consume substances they are intolerant to because their bodies have difficulty breaking them down. One of the most common examples is lactose intolerance, experienced by people who do not have the digestive enzymes needed to break down the lactose in milk.

- Reactions to food additives, such as sulphites and MSG.

**Food allergies:** Overreaction by the body to normally harmless proteins perceived as allergens. In response, the body produces antibodies, triggering allergic symptoms.

**Food intolerance:** Adverse effects resulting when people who lack the digestive chemicals needed to break down certain substances eat those substances.

# Managing Your Nutrition

Let's face it. Eating for health is not easy. It takes knowledge, careful thought and analysis, and the ability to put it all together and make the best decisions for your lifestyle and personal goals within your budgetary limits. But by paying attention, reading, seeking help from reputable, trained professionals, and planning ahead, you can increase your nutritional health. The following recommendations will help you improve your nutritional status:

## MAKING DECISIONS FOR YOU

1. List the four biggest things about your current dietary intake that you want to change.

2. Prioritize the items in the above list. Determine when you want to accomplish each item and outline a plan of action for accomplishing each goal.

3. List the little actions that you can take that may make a difference in your overall plan. List the big changes that you can make to accomplish your overall goals.

4. On the basis of your past history of trying to change these behaviours, what techniques do you think may be most likely to work for you? Indicate what you will use from these past tries and what you will do differently.

## CHECKLIST FOR CHANGE: MAKING PERSONAL CHOICES

■ *Eat lower on the food chain.* Try to substitute fruits, vegetables, nuts, or grains for animal products at least once a day.

■ *Eat seasonal foods whenever possible.* By eating foods at the peak of harvest, you are most apt to avoid nutrient losses incurred by storage, freezing, canning, and so on—and are likely to be obtaining a lower-cost option.

■ *Eat lean.* The evidence against high-fat foods mounts daily. Pay attention to labels, assess your food intake, and balance high-fat with low-fat choices. Choose leaner cuts of meat and bake, grill, boil, or broil whenever possible.

■ *Eat more colour.* Generally, the more vibrant the colours in the fruit or vegetable, the more nutrients are available. In particular eat more dark greens and oranges. Try a new fruit or vegetable each week.

■ *Increase your consumption of fruits and vegetables.* Use the real thing instead of juices and get more for your money.

■ *Combine foods for optimum nutrition.* Identify the best ways to combine grains, beans, fruits, vegetables, nuts, and other foods. You will then be able to optimize dietary returns. Ask your instructor or your local public health service for advice.

■ *Practise responsible consumer safety.* Avoid unnecessary chemicals and buy, prepare, and store foods prudently to avoid food-borne illness.

■ *Eat in moderation.* Learn to separate true hunger feelings from the food cravings that come from boredom. Recognize when your body is signalling that it is getting full, and stop eating. Moderate your caloric consumption and reduce your consumption of sugars and other dietary "extras."

■ *Keep your systems functioning well.* Even the best plans are doomed to fail if life problems are dragging your systems down, particularly your digestive system.

■ *Keep dietary foods in balance.* Consume appropriate amounts of water, proteins, carbohydrates, fibre, fats, vitamins, and minerals.

■ Pay attention to changing nutrient needs. Various factors in your life, such as pregnancy or illness, may require adjustments to your nutritional intake. Prepare for these changes and remain informed about reputable sources of information concerning nutrient benefits and risks.

## CHECKLIST FOR CHANGE: MAKING COMMUNITY CHOICES

■ *Evaluate the types of eating establishments available on your campus.* If you don't have the options you think you should, take action. Involve your student newspaper and student organizations, talk with food service representatives, involve your student health service, and solicit the support of key campus representatives.

■ *Assess your elected officials' priorities regarding nutrition as it pertains to the elderly, pregnant women, and the homeless.* Are they supporting actions to help ensure adequate nutrition for high-risk groups? If not, why not? Write letters asking for clarification of their positions. Seek alternative candidates if these individuals do not represent your views.

■ *If you patronize certain food establishments, review the food choices.* Tell them when they are doing a good job and request other options.

■ *Find out about government-subsidized foods.* Who is eligible for these programs? What is their purpose? What are their limitations? Strengths? Be informed about these programs. Support or refute them on the basis of sound information rather than on emotional reactions.

■ *Be informed about key nutritional concepts.* Speak up when you see information that is false or misleading. Demand accuracy in reported claims. Give advice only when you have taken the time to read and study the issues. Read reliable nutritional sources. When in doubt, seek help from professors or experts in the community.

## CRITICAL THINKING

Bill and Sarah have been married for almost six months. Sarah enjoys cooking large meals, many of them featuring fried foods. Bill, on the other hand, is more used to eating dishes built around rice, fruits, and vegetables. He is concerned about their eating habits, especially the higher fat and cholesterol content, but he doesn't want to say anything that would affect their otherwise perfect marriage. Using the DECIDE model described in Chapter 1, decide how Bill can open up a discussion about better eating without hurting Sarah's feelings.

- Reactions to substances occurring naturally in some foods, such as tyramine in cheese, phenylethylamine in chocolate, caffeine in coffee, and some compounds in alcohol.

- Unknown reactions in people who have adverse symptoms that they attribute to foods and that may actually go away when treated as allergies but for which there is no physiological basis.

## Organic Foods

Due to mounting concerns about food safety, many people refuse to buy processed foods and mass-produced agricultural products. Instead, they purchase foods that are **organically grown**—foods reported to be pesticide- and chemical-free. Less than a decade ago, buying organic foods meant going to a specialty store and paying premium prices for produce that was likely wilted, wormy, and smaller than its nonorganic alternative. Further, there was no guarantee that these products were really grown in an organic environment. People who bought these foods did so out of the desire to eat healthier produce and to avoid chemicals they were increasingly told caused cancer, immune system problems, and a host of other ailments.

Enter the organics of the twenty-first century—larger, more attractive, and fresher looking but still carrying a hefty price tag. Another difficulty is in ensuring that what you buy as organic does not have "second-hand" pesticides or chemicals on it. Currently, Canadian farms can be certified as organic so long as they do not use chemicals themselves. However, there are no controls on what chemicals the neighbouring farms use. Thus, even though a farm may be certified organic, its produce may obtain second-hand chemicals in a way similar to a non-smoker being exposed to second-hand smoke.

Is buying organic really better for you? Perhaps if we could put a group of people in a pristine environment and ensure that they never ate, drank, or were exposed to chemicals, we could test this hypothesis. In real life, however, it is almost impossible to assess the health impact of organic versus inorganic produce. Nevertheless, the market for organics has increased each year.

**Organically grown:** Foods grown without pesticides or chemicals.

## SUMMARY

- Recognizing that we eat for more reasons than survival is the first step toward changing our health. Canada's Food Guide to Healthy Eating provides easy to follow guidelines for healthy eating.

- The major nutrients essential for life and health include water, proteins, carbohydrates, fibre, fats, vitamins, and minerals. DRIs serve as guides to adequate intakes of specific nutrients.

- Vegetarianism can provide a healthy alternative for those wishing to reduce fat and cholesterol from their dietary intake.

- University and college students face unique challenges in eating well. Using the knowledge in this chapter, you can learn to make better choices when funds are short, at fast-food restaurants, and in the dorm.

- Food irradiation, food-borne illnesses, food allergies, and other food-safety and health concerns are becoming increasingly important to health-wise consumers. Recognition of potential risks and active steps taken to prevent problems are part of a sound nutritional plan.

## DISCUSSION QUESTIONS

1. What are several factors that influence the dietary patterns and behaviours of the typical university or college student? What factors have the greatest influences on your eating attitudes and behaviours? Why is it important that you know about your dietary influences as you think about changing your eating attitudes and behaviours?

2. What are the four major food groups in Canada's Food Guide to Healthy Eating? How many servings do you need of each? What groups might you find it difficult to get enough servings from? What food group do you get too many servings from? What can you do to increase or decrease your intake of selected food groups? What can you do to remember the four groups?

3. What are the major types of nutrients that you need to obtain from the foods you eat? What happens if you fail to get enough of one or more of these nutrients?

4. Distinguish between the different types of vegetarianism. Which types are most likely to lead to nutrient deficiencies? What can be done to ensure that even the strictest vegetarian obtains enough of each nutrient?

5. What are the major problems that many post-secondary students face when trying to eat well? List five actions that you and your classmates could take immediately to improve your eating.

6. What are the potential benefits and risks of food irradiation? Why is it being used? What are the major risks for food-borne illnesses and what can you do to protect yourself at school? At home? How are food illnesses and food allergies different?

## APPLICATION EXERCISE

Reread the What Do You Think? scenario at the beginning of the chapter and answer the following questions.

1. Critique Jeff's eating habits. What suggestions could you make to help him? How could you make these suggestions in a way that won't offend him?

2. Is there anything Jeff can do to improve his eating situation? Do you think that his dorm food is really that unhealthy or does he need more knowledge and motivation to make better choices?

## HEALTH ON THE NET

Heart & Stroke Foundation of Canada
**www.heartandstroke.ca**

Canadian Council of Food and Nutrition
**www.ccfn.ca/**

Dietitians of Canada
**www.dietitians.ca**

Health Canada: Food and Nutrition
**www.hc-sc.gc.ca/fn-an/index_e.html**

American Council on Science and Health
**www.acsh.org**

CHAPTER 8

# MANAGING YOUR WEIGHT

*Finding a Healthy Balance*

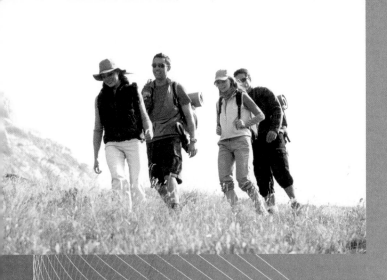

## CHAPTER OBJECTIVES

- Describe how healthy weight is determined using weight and body fat.

- Describe the major techniques used to estimate body fat.

- Describe the factors that place people at risk of developing obesity.

- Explain the roles of physical activity, dieting, dietary intake, and other factors in weight maintenance.

- Explain the health risks associated with the three major eating disorders.

- Discuss the safety and efficiency of popular fad diets.

Ray, aged 20, is desperately trying to lose the "frosh 15"—that is, the 7 kilograms (or 15 pounds) he put on during his first year at university. During that year, he spent much of his time studying, made little time for physical activity, and often rewarded his hard work with food-related breaks with his friends. Because he wants to lose the extra weight fast and be buff for spring break, Ray goes on a crash diet and begins an intense running and weightlifting program. After three weeks on the diet, his friends tell him how great he is starting to look. Bolstered by their support, Ray decides to cut his already low food intake even more, increase his exercise, and start taking a fat-loss supplement.

■ What risks are associated with Ray's plan for rapid weight loss? Is his thinking typical of people you know on similar "fast" weight loss plans? What are his motivations for losing weight, and how do the opinions of others appear to influence him? As a friend, what could you do to ensure that Ray doesn't harm himself during his quest to lose weight?

Millions of Canadians are concerned about their body weight and shape. In spite of being part of a generation of health and physical fitness buffs who exercise, forsake high-fat foods, and mesmerize ourselves with self-help diet and fitness books, by all accounts we are not doing any better in our quest for health and fitness. In fact, almost half of us are at a weight (BMI > 25.0) that may put our health at risk.[1]

What are these Canadians doing to shed their excess weight? Many opt for nutritionally balanced diets that include sufficient physical activity to burn the calories they consume. Others elect to get help from weight-loss gurus, trained professionals, or weight-loss franchises. Still others purchase questionable products and services that claim to help people "shed unsightly pounds fast and effortlessly." Some are starving themselves in pursuit of the perfect body. Finally, there is a group that has given up because they have already tried a number of different diets and not achieved their desired results.

In fact, in spite of good intentions, few people get beyond the first few days of a weight-loss effort. Those who do continue on their weight-loss programs and take off a significant amount of weight tend to gain it back. Follow-up studies of people on controlled diets indicate that at least half of the weight lost is regained within two to four years.[2]

This chapter focuses on the obsession with body weight and shape and explores the reasons why so many of us seem to be trapped in overweight bodies from which we can't escape. It is designed to help you better understand what overweight and obesity really mean and why weight maintenance is essential to your overall health. Finally, this chapter shows you how to develop strategies for maintaining your weight, losing weight, and gaining weight.

# BODY IMAGE

Most of us think of the obsession with thinness as a phenomenon of recent years. Beginning with super-model Twiggy in the 1960s and continuing with supermodel Kate Moss in the 1990s, the thin look seems to dominate fashion ads. And not only that: television, movies, the Internet, and magazines constantly project images of lean, fit bodies. We have been led to believe that if we are thin, with shapely curves or well-defined muscles, we will be more desirable.

But the thin look has been around for a long time. Anorexia nervosa, an eating disorder characterized by an obsession with thinness, an intense fear of weight gain, and the belief that one is fat though reality is the reverse, has been defined as a psychiatric disorder since 1873. During the Victorian era, corsets were used to achieve unrealistically tiny waists. By the 1920s, it was common knowledge that obesity was linked to poor health. Today, beautiful female models and underweight beauty pageant contestants in size 4 clothes exemplify desirability and success, delivering the subtle message that thin is in. In addition, we are bombarded with warnings that being obese increases our risk of heart disease, certain types of cancer, arthritis, gallbladder disease, diabetes, poor emotional health, and a host of other problems that decrease our life expectancy. What's a body to do?

In response to our irrational and emotional quests to be thin, a multibillion-dollar diet industry has developed, purveying liquid diets, freeze-dried foods, nonfat and low-fat foods, artificial sweeteners, diet books by the hundreds, and a host of weight-loss clinics. We are offered devices that are supposed to "melt away," "burn away," and "jiggle away" fat, and pills that claim to "burn fat" while you eat whatever you like and avoid physical activity. While some advertised claims are valid, others are designed to make big profits at your expense.

How do you find a safe, effective means of maintaining your weight or losing those extra kilograms?

A good way to start is by gathering accurate information about weight-loss products and services, learning what triggers you to eat, and analyzing your lifestyle to determine your problem areas. Developing the skills to set rational weight maintenance or weight-loss goals and taking advantage of social and community supports are also part of the process.

# REDEFINING OBESITY: WEIGHT VERSUS FAT CONTENT

Confusion exists in understanding the difference between overweight and obesity (see Figure 8.1). Whereas *overweight* refers to a weight greater than expected for a specific height (and is usually assessed using height–weight charts or calculating BMI), **obesity** refers to an excessive accumulation of body fat such that the individual is at increased risk of developing health problems. A person can be overweight and not overfat. For example, a male weightlifter may be 30 to 40 percent overweight because of his lean body mass according to the height–weight charts and his BMI classification. Similarly, a person can be overfat without being overweight. A 40-year-old woman who prides herself on weighing the same 60 kilograms that she did in high school may be shocked to learn that her body contains more than 40 percent fat compared with the 15 percent fat of her high school days. Thus, weight by itself is not a valid indicator of obesity or fatness.

Physical health risks associated with an excessive accumulation of fat (that is, obesity) include, but should not be limited to, an increased chance of developing atherosclerosis, coronary artery disease, hypertension, colon cancer, postmenopausal breast cancer, type 2 diabetes, gallbladder disease, and osteoarthritis.[3] Excessive fatness may also contribute to a poor body image and reduced self-esteem. Although sources vary slightly, most agree that a level of body fat that exceeds 20 percent of total body mass for a man puts him at risk of health problems. A woman would be considered obese if her body fat exceeded 30 percent of her total body mass. Table 8.1 provides general ratings for adults aged 18 to 30 in terms of overall percentages of body fat.

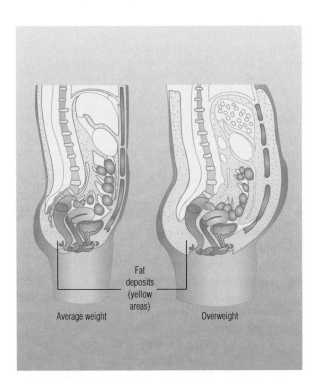

FIGURE 8.1

The figure compares a person with an average level of body fat to a person with excess body fat. Note the fat deposits under the skin and around the internal organs.

Average weight

Overweight

Fat deposits (yellow areas)

TABLE 8.1

General Ratings of Body Fat Percentages by Age and Sex

| Rating | Males (ages 18–30) (%) | Females (ages 18–30) (%) |
|---|---|---|
| Athletic* | 6–10 | 10–15 |
| Good | 11–14 | 16–19 |
| Acceptable | 15–17 | 20–24 |
| Overfat | 18–19 | 25–29 |
| Obese | 20 or over | 30 or over |

*The ratings in the Athletic category are general guidelines for athletes, such as gymnasts and long-distance runners, whose need for a "competitive edge" in selected sports may compel them to try to lose as much weight as possible. However, for the average person, such low body fat may put him or her at health risk.

**Obesity:** An excessive accumulation of body fat at which risk for health problems, such as heart disease, some types of cancers, and type 2 diabetes, is increased.

# Nutrition: Findings from the Canadian Community Health Survey Measured Obesity

Information on the prevalence of obesity (based on BMI) in adults gathered from the 2004 Canadian Community Health Survey (CCHS) was released in July 2005. Unique to this survey was that the height and weight data collected to calculate body mass index (BMI) (that is, weight in kilograms divided by height in metres squared) was measured rather than self-reported. Typically when data on height and weight is self-reported, people overestimate their height and underestimate their weight. The result of these over- and underestimates is an underestimation of BMI. Thus, the data reported in previous surveys may have underestimated the prevalence of overweight and obesity in the Canadian population.

Results from the CCHS indicate that 23.1 percent of adult Canadians (ages 18 or older) were classified as obese (BMI > 30). Further, 36.1 percent of Canadian adults were considered overweight (BMI > 25 < 30). All together, more than half (59.1 percent) of the Canadian population is overweight or obese. Of significant concern is the percentage of the population that meet the criteria for Class II (BMI 35.0 to 39.99) and Class III (BMI 40 or greater) obesity; that is, 5.1 percent and 2.7 percent, respectively.

A significantly greater number of males (42.0%) are classified as overweight than females (30.2%). Although, there is no significant difference in the estimates of males (22.9%) and females for obesity (23.2%) when the three classes are combined, there are a greater percentage of females (3.8 vs. 1.6%) in the Class III category.

Obesity rates were greatest among the 45- to 54-year-olds and lowest in the 18- to 24-year-olds (29.9 vs. 10.7%). Overweight was greatest in the 65- to 74-year-olds and lowest in the 18- to 24-year-olds (52.7 vs. 27.0%).

In regard to provincial data, the highest rates of obesity were found in Newfoundland and Labrador (33.3%), New Brunswick (30.8%), and Saskatchewan (30.4%), while the lowest rate was found in British Columbia (18.2%).

## STUDY QUESTIONS:

1. Why do think the rate of overweight and obesity has increased in the Canadian population?

2. What effect will the rise in overweight and obesity have on Canada's Health System?

Source: Adapted from Statistics Canada, 2005, Nutrition: Findings from the Canadian Community Health Survey, Measured Obesity, Adult Obesity in Canada: Measured Height and Weight, Catalogue No. 82-620-MWE2005001. Retrieved on December 9, 2005, from www.statcan.ca/english/research/82-620-MIE/2005001/articles/adults/aobesity.htm.

Why the difference between men and women? Much of it may be attributed to the normal structure of the female body and to sex hormones. It is important to think of body composition in terms of lean body mass and body fat. Lean body mass is made up of the structural and functional elements in cells, body water, muscle, bones, and other body organs such as the heart, liver, and kidneys. Body fat is composed of two types: essential fat and storage fat. Essential fat is necessary for normal physiological functioning, such as nerve conduction. Essential fat makes up approximately 3 to 7 percent of total body weight in men and approximately 10 to 15 percent of total body weight in women. Storage fat, which serves to insulate, pad, and protect the body from cold and trauma, makes up the remainder of our fat. It accounts for only a small percentage of total body weight for very lean people and between 5 and 25 percent of body weight of most Canadian adults. Female bodybuilders, who are among the leanest of female athletes, may have body fat percentages ranging from 8 to 13 percent, nearly all of which is essential fat.

There is a level of body fat below which we should not go. A minimal amount is necessary for insulating the body, for cushioning between parts of the body and vital organs, and for maintaining body functions. Although tremendous variation exists, it is generally suggested that in men this lower limit is approximately 3 to 4 percent and for women 8 percent.

Excessively low body fat in females may lead to amenorrhea, a disruption of the normal menstrual cycle. The critical level of body fat necessary to maintain normal menstrual flow is believed to be between 8 and 13 percent, but there are numerous exceptions to this rule and many additional factors that affect the menstrual cycle. Under extreme circumstances, such as starvation diets and certain diseases, the body often uses all available fat reserves and begins to break down muscle tissue in a last-ditch effort to obtain nourishment.

Too much fat and too little fat are both potentially harmful in that they each may elevate risk for developing health problems. The key is to find a level at which you are not at risk for health problems and at which you are comfortable with your appearance.

## Assessing Your Body Content

An accurate assessment of total body fat requires a different type of measurement than the traditional height–weight charts or calculations of BMI. How do you decide which techniques available for calculating your total body fat are the best for you? If you are interested in obtaining the most accurate measure before and after a program of diet and exercise, you may find the expense of some of the more sophisticated measures worth the investment. If you simply want a general idea of how much body fat you have, inexpensive skinfold measurements may be all that you need. On the other hand, if you know, based on the bulges around your middle or the size and fit of your jeans, that you are obese, perhaps the exact amount of fat that you have does not matter as much as the fact that you need to take action.

Assessments of body composition generally attempt to quantify body weight into its basic components.[4] In assessments of the health-related components of physical fitness, estimates of body fat are considered most important.

### Dual-Energy X-Ray Absorptiometry

**Dual-energy X-ray absorptiometry (DXA)** measures bone mineral content, lean, and fat tissue.[5] This technique requires a low radiation exposure from a low-energy and high-energy photon beam. Based on appropriate computer algorithms and the amount of absorption of the photon beams by the atoms in bone mineral and soft tissues, an estimate of bone mineral, fat-free soft tissue, and fat tissue is made. Some consider DXA to be the most accurate assessment of body composition.

### Hydrostatic Weighing

**Hydrostatic weighing** was previously considered the gold standard for measuring body composition. This method measures the amount of water a person displaces when completely submerged. Because fat tissue has a lower density than muscle or bone tissue, a relatively accurate indication of actual body fat can be computed using a person's underwater and out-of-water weights.

### Air Displacement Plethysmography

Based on the same premises as hydrostatic weighing, a new technique called **air displacement plethysmography (ADP)** has become popular in recent years to

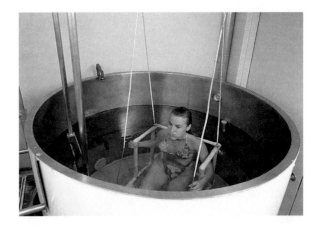

*Hydrostatic weighing is one technique used to estimate body fat.*

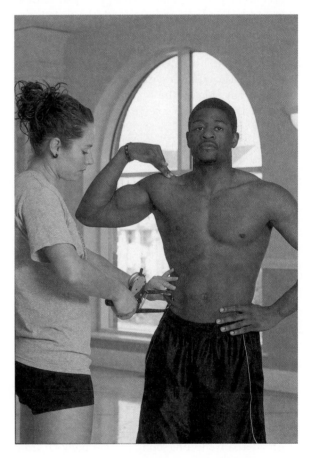

*In the hands of a trained professional, skinfold calipers can be used to provide an accurate measure of body fat for people who are not overly fat.*

**Dual-energy X-ray absorptiometry (DXA):** A method of body composition assessment where estimates are made of bone mineral content, lean, and fat mass.

**Hydrostatic weighing:** A method of determining body fat by measuring the amount of water displaced when a person is completely submerged.

**Air displacement plethysmography (ADP):** A method used to determine body fat from estimates of total body volume.

measure body composition. Similar to underwater weighing, it measures total body volume from which an estimate of body fat can be made. The major assumption of hydrostatic weighing and ADP is that the density of fat and fat-free mass (all components of the body except fat) is constant. Thus, with estimates of total body volume (either in water or air) and recognizing that density = mass ÷ volume, an estimate of fat can be determined.[6]

## Skinfold Measurements

Perhaps the most commonly used method to estimate body fat is **skinfold measurements.** In this procedure, a person grabs (that is, pinches) folds of skin and the underlying tissue with the thumb and index finger. A specially calibrated instrument called a skinfold caliper is then applied to the double fold of skin and the underlying tissue (that is, subcutaneous fat). The eight sites most commonly measured on the right side of the body include the triceps (back of the arm), biceps (front of the arm), subscapular (on the back), iliac crest (on the side of the body—near the "love handles"), supraspinale (along the front of the body over the hip), abdominal (next to the umbilicus—belly button), front thigh (middle of the upper leg), and medial calf (middle, inside of the lower leg). Once these sites are measured, special formulas can be used to predict total body fat. In the hands of trained technicians, this procedure can be fairly accurate. However, the fatter a person is, the more prone this technique is to error. For chronically obese people, difficulties in assessment are magnified because of problems distinguishing between flaccid muscles and fat. Also, most skinfold calipers do not expand far enough to obtain measurements from the moderately obese (20 to 40 percent overfat) or the morbidly obese (more than 50 percent overfat). Additional errors in skinfold assessments may occur as a result of failure to account for certain age, sex, and ethnic differences in the calculations.

An alternative to predicting percent body fat from skinfold measurements is to simply total them. A "sum of skinfolds" also allows for comparison of "before" and "after" measurements. A loss in total sum of skinfolds indicates a loss of total body fat. Similarly, a gain in sum of skinfolds indicates a gain in total body fat.

## Waist Circumference

A common method of assessing abdominal body fat is the **waist circumference**. A simple measuring tape is used to take the girth, or circumference, measurement at the narrowest point of the waist. A waist circumference greater than 102 cm in men and 88 cm in women[7] may indicate increased risk of heart disease, hypertension, and hyperlipidemia.[8]

## Bioelectrical Impedance Analysis

Another method of determining body fat levels, **bioelectrical impedance analysis (BIA),** involves sending a weak electric current through the subject's body. The rationale for this technique is based on the greater electrolyte and water content of lean versus fat tissue.[9] The amount of resistance to the current, along with the person's age, sex, and other physical characteristics, is then fed into a computer that uses special formulas to determine the total amount of lean and fat tissue. This technique has increased in use in recent years likely because of its convenience, low cost, noninvasiveness, and rapidly determined estimate of body fat. It is important for the body to be normally hydrated when using BIA because even small fluctuations in body water content result in an inaccurate assessment of body composition. Even with adequate hydration and nutritional status, significant error can result in body composition estimates from BIA.

Although all these methods can be useful, they can also be inaccurate and even harmful unless the testers are skillful and well trained. Before agreeing to any procedure, be sure you are aware of the expense, potential for accuracy, risks, and training of the tester.

---

### WHAT WOULD YOU DO?

Why is it important to consider your percentage of body fat rather than only weight when determining how fat you really are? Which of the above tests would you feel comfortable taking? Would any make you feel uncomfortable?

---

# DETERMINING THE RIGHT WEIGHT FOR YOU

The answer to whether you are overweight or obese is somewhat subjective and depends on your body structure and how your weight is distributed. Traditionally, people have compared their weight with data from some form of standard height-and-weight chart. These charts usually give the "ideal" weight for males and

TABLE 8.2

Health Risk Classification for Adults* According to BMI

| BMI | Weight Classification | Risk of Developing a Health Problem |
|---|---|---|
| 30.0 | Obese | High |
| 30.1 – 34.9 | Obese Class I | High |
| 35.0 – 39.9 | Obese Class II | Very high |
| > 40.0 | Obese Class III | Extremely high |

*These cut-off values and weight and health classifications are not applicable to growing children and adolescents.

females of given height and frame size. If you are above your ideal weight, you would be classified as overweight.

Another common method used to determine weight status in adults is based on calculating **body mass index (BMI).** Table 8.2 shows the classification for health risk according to BMI for men and women.[10] BMI is obtained by dividing your weight (in kilograms) by your height (in metres) squared. Weight should be taken without shoes or clothing, and height should be measured without shoes. In general, a BMI range of 18.5 to 24.9 is considered normal weight. BMI values above 25.0 have been associated with increased health risk. People with BMIs greater than 30 are considered obese and have high health risk (see Figure 8.2 and Table 8.1).

# RISK FACTORS FOR OBESITY

It would seem that the cause of obesity is quite simple: when you take in more calories than you burn, you will gain weight—most often in the form of fat. If you do this frequently throughout your life, you will become obese. If we know what the cause is, we should be able to offer a simple prescription for preventing the problem. Right?

Wrong. Although the calorie balance equation (or, if calories in equals calories out then there is no weight gain) explanation of obesity is valid, it offers only one possible reason for a person's weight problem. It does not explain the many other factors that may be involved and reduce the likelihood of permanent weight loss. It also fails to answer many other critical questions. If we know that eating too much will cause us to gain weight, why do we continue to eat too much? Is pushing yourself away from the table the best exercise for maintaining your weight? Is there a metabolic explanation for obesity? Why do people who use weight-loss programs have difficulty achieving permanent success (i.e., permanent weight loss).

# Heredity

## Body Type and Genes

In some animal species, the shape and size of the individual's body is largely determined by the shape and size of its parents' bodies. Many scientists have explored the role of heredity in determining human body shapes or physiques. As early as 1940, Harvard psychologist William Sheldon analyzed weight problems in terms of *somatotypes*.[11] The somatotype provides a classification of an individual's physique or body as a whole and comprises three components: endomorphy, mesomorphy, and ectomorphy.[12] Endomorphy describes the relative fatness of the body, specifically referring to the roundness and soft appearance. In Sheldon's work, individuals with a high endomorphic rating often had a large abdomen and typically reported a history of weight problems beginning in childhood. Mesomorphy refers to the relative muscularity of the body; individuals with a high mesomophic rating have a strong tendency to gain weight later in life. Ectomorphy describes the relative linearity of the body, with individuals rating high in this component characterized as tall with slender frames and generally experiencing few difficulties with weight control.

Although somatotype may play a role in the development of obesity, most researchers contend that heredity plays a more subtle role. These researchers argue that obesity has a strong genetic determinant (it tends to run in families) and cite statistics suggesting that 40 percent of children with one obese parent and 80 percent of children with two obese parents are also likely to be obese.[13] But why is this the case? Can you really blame your genetics for your problems with weight? What is the role of your environment?

**Skinfold measurements:** A method of determining body fat where double folds of skin and the underlying tissue (subcutaneous fat) are grasped between the thumb and forefinger and are measured with skinfold calipers.

**Waist circumference:** A method of assessing abdominal body fat where a measuring tape is used to measure the girth at the narrowest point of the waist.

**Bioelectrical impedance analysis (BIA):** A technique of body fat assessment in which the resistance to a weak electrical current is measured when it passes through the body.

**Body mass index (BMI):** A technique of weight assessment based on the relationship of weight to height.

## Body Mass Index

**Height (feet / inches)**

| Weight (pounds) | Weight (kilograms) | 5'0" | 5'1" | 5'2" | 5'3" | 5'4" | 5'5" | 5'6" | 5'7" | 5'8" | 5'9" | 5'10" | 5'11" | 6'0" | 6'1" | 6'2" | 6'3" | 6'4" |
|---|---|---|---|---|---|---|---|---|---|---|---|---|---|---|---|---|---|---|
| 100 | 45 | 20 | 19 | 18 | 18 | 17 | 17 | 16 | 16 | 15 | 15 | 14 | 14 | 14 | 13 | 13 | 12 | 12 |
| 105 | 47 | 21 | 20 | 19 | 19 | 18 | 17 | 17 | 16 | 16 | 16 | 15 | 15 | 14 | 14 | 13 | 13 | 13 |
| 110 | 50 | 21 | 21 | 20 | 19 | 19 | 18 | 18 | 17 | 17 | 16 | 16 | 15 | 15 | 15 | 14 | 14 | 13 |
| 115 | 52 | 22 | 22 | 21 | 20 | 20 | 19 | 19 | 18 | 17 | 17 | 17 | 16 | 16 | 15 | 15 | 14 | 14 |
| 120 | 54 | 23 | 23 | 22 | 21 | 21 | 20 | 19 | 19 | 18 | 18 | 17 | 17 | 16 | 16 | 15 | 15 | 15 |
| 125 | 57 | 24 | 24 | 23 | 22 | 21 | 21 | 20 | 20 | 19 | 18 | 18 | 17 | 17 | 16 | 16 | 16 | 15 |
| 130 | 59 | 25 | 25 | 24 | 23 | 22 | 22 | 21 | 20 | 20 | 19 | 19 | 18 | 18 | 17 | 17 | 16 | 16 |
| 135 | 61 | 26 | 26 | 25 | 24 | 23 | 23 | 22 | 21 | 21 | 20 | 19 | 19 | 18 | 18 | 17 | 17 | 16 |
| 140 | 63 | 27 | 26 | 26 | 25 | 24 | 23 | 23 | 22 | 21 | 21 | 20 | 20 | 19 | 18 | 18 | 17 | 17 |
| 145 | 66 | 28 | 27 | 26 | 26 | 25 | 24 | 23 | 23 | 22 | 21 | 21 | 20 | 20 | 19 | 19 | 18 | 18 |
| 150 | 68 | 29 | 28 | 27 | 27 | 26 | 25 | 24 | 24 | 23 | 22 | 22 | 21 | 20 | 20 | 19 | 19 | 18 |
| 155 | 70 | 30 | 29 | 28 | 27 | 27 | 26 | 25 | 24 | 24 | 23 | 22 | 22 | 21 | 20 | 20 | 19 | 19 |
| 160 | 72 | 31 | 30 | 29 | 28 | 27 | 27 | 26 | 25 | 24 | 24 | 23 | 22 | 22 | 21 | 21 | 20 | 19 |
| 165 | 75 | 32 | 31 | 30 | 29 | 28 | 27 | 27 | 26 | 25 | 24 | 24 | 23 | 22 | 22 | 21 | 21 | 20 |
| 170 | 77 | 33 | 32 | 31 | 30 | 29 | 28 | 27 | 27 | 26 | 25 | 24 | 24 | 23 | 22 | 22 | 21 | 21 |
| 175 | 79 | 34 | 33 | 32 | 31 | 30 | 29 | 28 | 27 | 27 | 26 | 25 | 24 | 24 | 23 | 22 | 22 | 21 |
| 180 | 82 | 35 | 34 | 33 | 32 | 31 | 30 | 29 | 28 | 27 | 27 | 26 | 25 | 24 | 24 | 23 | 22 | 22 |
| 185 | 84 | 36 | 35 | 34 | 33 | 32 | 31 | 30 | 29 | 28 | 27 | 27 | 26 | 25 | 24 | 24 | 23 | 23 |
| 190 | 86 | 37 | 36 | 35 | 34 | 33 | 32 | 31 | 30 | 29 | 28 | 27 | 26 | 26 | 25 | 24 | 24 | 23 |
| 195 | 88 | 38 | 37 | 36 | 35 | 33 | 32 | 31 | 31 | 30 | 29 | 28 | 27 | 26 | 26 | 25 | 24 | 24 |
| 200 | 91 | 39 | 38 | 37 | 36 | 34 | 33 | 32 | 31 | 30 | 30 | 29 | 28 | 27 | 26 | 26 | 25 | 24 |
| 205 | 93 | 40 | 39 | 37 | 37 | 35 | 34 | 33 | 32 | 31 | 30 | 29 | 28 | 28 | 27 | 26 | 26 | 25 |
| 210 | 95 | 41 | 40 | 38 | 37 | 36 | 35 | 34 | 33 | 32 | 31 | 30 | 29 | 28 | 28 | 27 | 26 | 26 |
| 215 | 98 | 42 | 41 | 39 | 38 | 37 | 36 | 35 | 34 | 33 | 32 | 31 | 30 | 29 | 28 | 28 | 27 | 26 |
| 220 | 100 | 43 | 42 | 40 | 39 | 38 | 37 | 36 | 34 | 33 | 32 | 32 | 31 | 30 | 29 | 28 | 27 | 27 |
| 225 | 102 | 44 | 43 | 41 | 40 | 39 | 37 | 36 | 35 | 34 | 33 | 32 | 31 | 31 | 30 | 29 | 28 | 27 |
| 230 | 104 | 45 | 43 | 42 | 41 | 40 | 38 | 37 | 36 | 35 | 34 | 33 | 32 | 31 | 30 | 30 | 29 | 28 |
| 235 | 107 | 46 | 44 | 43 | 42 | 40 | 39 | 38 | 37 | 36 | 35 | 34 | 33 | 32 | 31 | 30 | 29 | 29 |
| 240 | 109 | 47 | 45 | 44 | 43 | 41 | 40 | 39 | 38 | 36 | 36 | 34 | 33 | 33 | 32 | 31 | 30 | 29 |
| 245 | 111 | 48 | 46 | 45 | 43 | 42 | 41 | 40 | 38 | 37 | 36 | 35 | 34 | 33 | 32 | 31 | 31 | 30 |
| 250 | 114 | 49 | 47 | 46 | 44 | 43 | 42 | 40 | 39 | 38 | 37 | 36 | 35 | 34 | 33 | 32 | 31 | 30 |
| | | **150.0** | **152.5** | **155.0** | **157.5** | **160.0** | **162.5** | **165.0** | **167.5** | **170.0** | **172.5** | **175.0** | **177.5** | **180.0** | **182.5** | **185.0** | **187.5** | **190.0** |

**Height (centimetres)**

Legend:
- Underweight
- Weight appropriate
- Overweight
- Obese

FIGURE 8.2

Are you overweight? To find out, find your height (either at the top [in feet and inches] or bottom [in centimetres]) and your weight (at the right [in kilograms] or left [in pounds]) and see where these two intersect.

## Twin Studies

Studies of identical twins separated at birth and raised in different environments have provided some of the most compelling evidence to date that obesity may be genetically determined. Whether raised in environments with fat or thin family members, twins with obese birth parents tended to be obese in later life.[14] According to another study, identical twins separated and raised in different families who ate widely different diets still grew up to weigh about the same.[15] These studies contain the strongest evidence yet that the genes a person inherits are the major factor determining overweight, leanness, or average weight. Although the exact mechanics remain unknown, it is believed that genes set metabolic rates, influencing how the body handles calories.

## Genetic Predisposition and Environmental Factors

Health professionals are concerned that these studies will convince many overweight people that they are doomed to be fat. However, Albert Stunkard, a psychiatrist at the University of Pennsylvania and author of one of these studies, believes that, on the contrary, their conclusions simply indicate that you are more vulnerable than others. As a result your lifestyle choices in regard to dietary intake and physical activity may be even more important than those of your thin friends with a genetic advantage.[16]

It should be pointed out that the link between genetics and obesity is still not completely understood. Researchers continue to search for an obesity gene. One such investigation, the Heritage Family Study, indicates that the genetic predisposition to obesity is a result of deficiencies in many different genes and that the predisposition varies from low to high. Further, these researchers suggest that the predisposition can be challenged by reducing caloric intake and increasing caloric expenditure.[17]

## Thrifty Genes and a Genetic Appetite

Researchers reported that they had discovered a defective gene that disrupts the body's "I've had enough to eat" signalling system and may be responsible for a least some types of obesity.[18] Other research on Pima Indians, a group with a very high incidence of obesity (estimated at 75 percent; 90 percent are overweight), seems to point to an obesity gene that is a "thrifty gene." It is theorized that as certain groups had to struggle during hard times and famines over the centuries, those people who had slower metabolic activity, which allowed them to store precious fat, survived. They passed their genes on to their descendants, which may predispose these descendants to be slow burners.[19] In times of plenty, it seems inevitable that these people will gain weight, unless they eat much less or do much more physical activity than the norm.

## Sex and Obesity

Throughout a woman's life, issues of appearance and beauty dominate her surroundings. Researchers continue to investigate the cultural issues surrounding a woman's quest for beauty and the ideal body shape and size.

Compared with men, women have a lower ratio of lean body mass to fatty mass, in part due to the genetic differences in bone size and mass, muscle size, and other variables. Women also experience greater weight fluctuation due to hormonal changes, pregnancy, and menopause. Following puberty, men have higher metabolic rates and thus require a greater number of calories to maintain bodily functions. Also, as a group, men are socialized more into physically active lifestyles from birth. Strenuous physical activity in work and play are encouraged for men, while women are typically socialized into roles that require a lower level of caloric expenditure.

Not only are women more vulnerable to weight gain, but pressures to maintain or lose weight also make them more likely to take dramatic measures. The predominance of eating disorders among women and the greater numbers of women than men taking diet pills are indicators of the female obsession with thinness and the belief that thin is beautiful. However, males are also increasingly becoming victims of body image issues. As the male image becomes more associated with the bodybuilder shape and size and as men become more preoccupied with their own physical form, eating disorders, exercise addictions, and other maladaptive responses among men will continue to rise.

## Hunger, Appetite, and Satiety

Theories abound concerning the mechanisms that regulate food intake. Some sources indicate that the hypothalamus (the part of the brain that regulates appetite) closely monitors levels of certain nutrients in the blood. When these levels begin to fall, the brain signals us to eat. In the obese person, it is possible that the monitoring system does not work properly and that the cues to eat are more frequent and intense than in people of normal weight.

Other sources indicate that thin people may send more effective messages to the hypothalamus. This concept, known as **adaptive thermogenesis,** states that thin people can often consume large amounts of food without gaining weight because the appetite centre of their brains speeds up metabolic activity to compensate for the increased consumption. More recent studies indicated the possibility that specialized types of fat cells, called **brown fat cells,** may send signals to the brain, which controls the thermogenesis response.

The hypothesis that food tastes better to obese people, thus causing them to eat more, has largely been refuted. Scientists do distinguish, however, between **hunger,** an inborn physiological response to nutritional needs, and **appetite,** a learned response to food tied to an emotional or psychological craving for food often unrelated to nutritional need. Obese people may be more likely than thin people to satisfy their appetite and eat for reasons other than nutrition.

In some instances, the problem with overconsumption may be more related to **satiety** than to appetite or hunger. People generally feel satiated, or full, when they have satisfied their nutritional needs and their stomach signals "no more." For undetermined reasons, obese people may not feel full until much later than thin people.

## Developmental Factors

Some obese people may have an excessive number of fat cells. **Hyperplasia,** which refers to an increase in the number of cells, normally occurs only during specific periods of the growth process.[20] The only time fat cells normally increase in numbers is during infancy and the rapid growth period of puberty. However, fat cells can also increase in number when an individual is under chronic positive energy balance (that is, they continuously consume more calories than they burn) and their current fat cells are "full." Fat cells also have the ability to increase in size. This process is called **hypertrophy,** and can occur at any time in childhood, adolescence, and adulthood—if calorie intake exceeds calorie output. Thus, fat gain is tied to the number of fat cells in the body (during infancy and puberty) and the capacity of the fat cells to increase in size (childhood, adolescence, and adulthood).

An average-weight adult has approximately 30 to 50 billion fat cells,[21] a moderately obese adult about 60 billion to 100 billion, and an extremely obese adult as many as 200 billion.[22] The size of fat cells in a young, normal-weight adult is about 80 to 100 μm.

People with a large number of fat cells may have difficulty with long-term fat loss because there may be a trigger released once they have substantially decreased the size of each fat cell, resulting in a calorie binge and thus sabotaging their fat-loss efforts (see Figure 8.3). Additional research must be conducted to better understand hyperplasia and hypertrophy in fat cells.

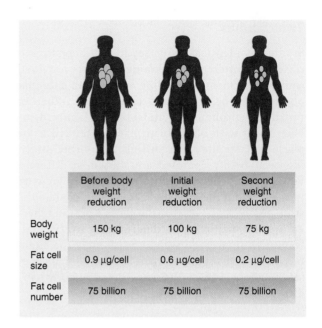

| | Before body weight reduction | Initial weight reduction | Second weight reduction |
|---|---|---|---|
| Body weight | 150 kg | 100 kg | 75 kg |
| Fat cell size | 0.9 μg/cell | 0.6 μg/cell | 0.2 μg/cell |
| Fat cell number | 75 billion | 75 billion | 75 billion |

### FIGURE 8.3

The figure depicts one person at various stages of fat loss. Note that the number of fat cells remains constant but their size decreases.

## Setpoint Theory

In 1982, nutritional researchers William Bennett and Joel Gurin presented a highly controversial theory known as the **setpoint theory.** It states that a person's body has a setpoint of weight at which it is programmed to be comfortable. If your setpoint is around 70 kilograms, you will gain and lose weight fairly easily within a given range around that point. For example, if you gain 2 to 5 kilograms on vacation, it will be fairly easy to lose that weight and remain around the 70-kilogram mark for a long period of time. Related to this concept is the **plateau** often reached after a person on a diet loses a certain amount of weight. The setpoint theory proposes that after losing a predetermined amount of weight, the body will actually sabotage additional weight loss by slowing down metabolism. In extreme cases, the metabolic rate will decrease to a point at which the body will maintain its weight on as little as 1,000 calories per day. Can a person change this predetermined setpoint? Proponents of this theory argue that it is possible to raise one's setpoint over time by continually gaining weight and failing to engage in regular physical activity. Conversely, reducing caloric intake and being physically active over a long period of time may slowly decrease one's setpoint.

This theory, too, remains controversial. Perhaps its greatest impact was the sense of relief it provided for people who lost weight, plateaued, and regained weight time and time again. It told them that their failure was not due to a lack of willpower alone. The setpoint theory also prompted nutritional experts to look more carefully at popular methods of weight loss. If the setpoint theory is correct, a low-calorie or starvation diet, besides being dangerous, may cause the body to protect itself from "starvation" by slowing down metabolism and preventing further weight loss.

## Endocrine Influence

Over the years, many people have attributed their obesity to problems with their thyroid glands. They claimed that an underactive thyroid impeded their ability to burn calories. How many obesity problems may justifiably be blamed on a poorly functioning thyroid? Most agree that fewer than 5 percent of the obese population have a thyroid problem.

## Psychosocial Factors

The relationship of weight problems to deeply rooted emotional insecurities, needs, and wants remains uncertain. Food is often used as a reward for good behaviour in childhood. As adults face unemployment, broken relationships, financial uncertainty, and fears about health and other problems, the bright spot in the day is often "what's on the table for dinner," or, "we're going to that restaurant tonight." In other words, food is often used as a comforting mechanism. Again, the research underlying this theory is controversial. What is certain is that in mainstream Canada eating tends to be a focal point of people's lives—a major part of our socialization, a social ritual associated with companionship, celebration, and enjoyment.

## Eating Cues

At least one major factor in our preoccupation with food is the pressure placed on us by the highly sophisticated, heavily advertised "eating" campaigns launched by the food industry. Although salads and other lower-fat, lower-calorie options are now available at fast-food restaurants, we still have the gauntlet of starchy, beefy delights and tasty high-fat fries to choose from. Food-related messages permeate the media, particularly for children and youth.[23,24] Compared to Canada's Food Guide to Healthy Eating, most advertised foods are lower in nutrient density, fibre, and complex carbohydrates and higher in fat, sodium, simple carbohydrates, caffeine, and alcohol.

A large percentage of the foods we eat are from fast-food restaurants. We eat at fast-food restaurants for a number of reasons, including the relatively low cost and the perceived time that is saved. This is unfortunate because: (1) fast food is high in calories, fat, sodium, and carbohydrates; (2) it tends to all be eaten, even though portions are often much bigger than needed; and (3) it tends to be eaten quickly, so there isn't enough time for the "I'm full" signal to get to your mouth before the last bite of food is consumed.[25] This is a particular problem for post-secondary students, who often encounter fast-food restaurants right on campus.

## Dietary Myth and Misperception

You've all heard the story: "I eat like a bird, but I can't lose weight." Should you believe the person who says this? Probably not, according to a study that analyzed the self-reported and actual caloric intakes and physical activity expenditures of a group of obese adults.[26] The researchers carefully followed obese people who had been unsuccessful after as many as 20 diets, though they claimed to consume fewer than 1,200 calories per day. They blamed their failure on "metabolism." It turned out that their metabolism levels were normal, but that they were actually eating nearly twice as much as they thought and engaging in only three-quarters as much physical activity as they reported. Does this mean that obesity is simply the result of gluttony and sloth? No. In fact, many studies have shown that obese individuals do not eat much, if any, more than their normal-weight counterparts. However, the majority of obese individuals are less physically active than people of normal weight. Of course, it could be argued that their obesity led to their sedentary lifestyle. Much more research is necessary to clearly understand dietary intake and physical activity in obese and nonobese individuals.

---

**Adaptive thermogenesis:** Theoretical mechanism by which the brain regulates metabolic activity according to caloric intake.

**Brown fat cells:** Specialized type of fat cell that affects the ability to regulate fat metabolism.

**Hunger:** An inborn physiological response to nutritional needs.

**Appetite:** A learned response tied to an emotional or psychological craving for food often unrelated to nutritional need.

**Satiety:** The feeling of fullness or satisfaction after eating.

**Hyperplasia:** An increase in the number of cells.

**Hypertrophy:** An increase in the size of cells.

**Setpoint theory:** A theory that suggests fat storage is determined by a thermostatic mechanism in the body that acts to maintain a specific amount of body fat.

**Plateau:** That point in a weight-loss program at which weight loss ceases.

## Metabolic Changes

Even when completely at rest, the body needs a certain amount of energy. The amount of energy your body requires at complete rest is called **basal metabolic rate (BMR).** In physically active individuals, about 60 to 70 percent of all the calories consumed support *basal metabolism*, which provides the energy (that is, calories) needed for bodily functions such as heartbeat, breathing, maintaining body temperature, and so on. So if you consume 2,000 calories per day, between 1,200 and 1,400 of those calories are used for regular body maintenance. The remaining 600 to 800 calories supply the energy required for your physical activities. The key factor here is the amount of physical activity you do. In sedentary individuals BMR may account for as much as 90 percent of their caloric needs. Conversely, in very active individuals BMR may account for only 50 to 60 percent of their caloric needs.

BMR can fluctuate considerably. In general, the younger you are, the higher your BMR, partly because in young people cells undergo rapid subdivision, which requires a good deal of energy. BMR is highest during infancy, puberty, and pregnancy, when bodily changes are most rapid. BMR is also influenced by body composition.

The amount of lean body mass you have also influences your BMR. Muscle tissue is highly active—even at rest—compared to fat tissue. In essence, the more lean tissue you have, the greater your BMR; the more fat tissue you have, the lower your BMR. Thus, men usually have a higher BMR than women, because they have more lean body mass.

Age is another factor that may greatly affect BMR. After the age of 30, your BMR slows down by about one to two percent a year. Therefore, people over 30 commonly find that they either have to eat less or do more physical activity to maintain their body weight. "Middle-age spread," a reference to the tendency to put on weight or fat after the age of 30, is partly related to this change. A slower BMR, coupled with an inclination to be less physically active, puts many middle-aged people's weight in jeopardy.

In addition, the body has a number of self-protective mechanisms that signal BMR to speed up or slow down. For example, when you have a fever, the energy needs of your cells increase, and this increased activity generates heat and increases your BMR. In starvation situations, the body tries to protect itself by slowing down BMR to conserve precious energy. Thus, when people repeatedly resort to low-calorie diets, their bodies "reset" their BMRs to lower rates. **Yo-yo diets,** in which people repeatedly gain and lose weight, lower their BMR in the process, and as a result are doomed to failure. When they begin to eat again after the weight loss, their BMR is set lower, making it almost certain that they will regain the weight they just lost and more. After repeated cycles of such dieting/regaining, these people find it increasingly hard to lose weight and increasingly easy to regain it, and so they become heavier and fatter. Besides an increase in fat, weight cycling may also have a negative effect on risk for heart disease. Specifically, other health risks research indicates that middle-aged men who maintained a steady weight (even if they were overweight) had a lower risk of heart attack than men whose weight cycled up and down in a yo-yo pattern.[27] Furthermore, it was noted that smaller, well-maintained weight losses were more beneficial for reducing cardiovascular risk than larger, poorly maintained weight losses.

Finally, certain hormones, particularly the stress hormones, may cause BMR to rise in response to increased nervous activity and energy requirements by the cells.

## Lifestyle

Of all the factors affecting obesity, perhaps the most critical is the relationship between level of physical activity and caloric intake. Obesity rates are rising. How can this be happening? Aren't more people physically active than ever before? While it may look like it, the facts are not so positive. According to the most recent Canadian Community Health Survey (2003), only 50 percent of the population aged 12 and over were classified as active or moderately active in their leisure time.[28] Similarly, the Canadian Fitness and Lifestyle Research Institute reported in 2004 that 49 percent of Canadians aged 20 and older were at least moderately active during their leisure time.[29] Meanwhile, physical education is optional in most high schools and seldom offered daily in elementary and junior schools. Furthermore, many children and youth are transported to and from school on a daily basis.

You probably know someone who seems to be able to eat a lot and does not appear to do any more physical activity than you, yet never seems to gain weight. You don't understand how this person maintains his or her weight. With few exceptions, if you were to follow this person around for a typical day and monitor their level and intensity of activity, you would discover the answer to your question. Although the person's schedule may not include running or strenuous exercise, it probably includes a high level of physical activity. Walking up a flight of stairs rather than taking the elevator, speeding up the pace while mowing the lawn, getting up to change the TV channel rather than using the remote, and doing housework vigorously all burn extra calories. A major cause of low physical activity levels is the abundance of labour-saving devices in the modern household. Using a blender instead of chopping vegetables or pushing remote-control buttons on television and stereo equipment cause us to expend fewer calories than did previous generations. The automobile is a great convenience, but using it has significantly reduced our daily physical activity.

Clearly, any form of physical activity that helps your body burn additional calories helps you maintain your weight. In fact, in one study a group of men who lost weight through exercise were far more successful at maintaining the weight loss than a similar group who lost weight through dieting.

## WHAT WOULD YOU DO?

Based on the risk factors for obesity discussed thus far, which ones do you think pose the greatest risk for you? Which ones can you do something about? What actions can you take to reduce your risk? What actions will you take to reduce your risk?

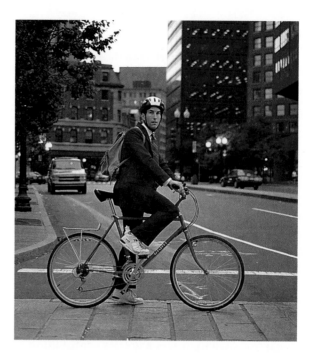

*A physically active lifestyle is key to balancing caloric intake and body weight.*

# MANAGING YOUR WEIGHT

At some point in our lives, almost all of us will decide to go on a diet. Whether dieting for vanity or for your health, it's important to begin by finding the combination of physical activity and healthy eating behaviours that will work for you now and in the long term. You are undoubtedly familiar with the saga of Oprah Winfrey's weight loss: Starting at 86 kilograms, she quickly lost 30 kilograms on a liquid diet. But failure to continue the maintenance program led to a weight gain of 38 kilograms. This example clearly illustrates the need to approach weight loss with behavioural modifications that can be maintained for a lifetime.

## What Is a Calorie?

A *calorie* is a unit of measure that indicates the amount of energy obtained from a particular food. A kilogram of body fat contains approximately 7,500 calories. So each time you consume 7,500 calories more than your body needs, you gain a kilogram (or, roughly, two pounds). Conversely, each time your body expends an extra 7,500 calories, you lose a kilogram. If you add a can of Coca-Cola (140 calories) to your diet and make no other changes in your dietary intake or physical activity, you would gain a kilogram in approximately 54 days (7,500 calories ÷ 140 calories/day = 53.6 days). Conversely, if you walked for half an hour each day at a pace of 9 minutes per kilometre (172 calories burned), you would lose a kilogram in 44 days (7,500 calories ÷ 172 calories/day = 43.6 days).

To lose weight, then, you need to lower caloric intake (through reduced or improved dietary habits) or expend more calories (through increased physical activity). First, determine your daily caloric intake. Then you can identify your daily intake and expenditure of calories until you reach a balance (to maintain weight), a decrease (for weight loss), or an increase (for weight gain). Table 8.3 lists the caloric output of various physical activities. Don't forget, it took time to gain weight; it will take time to lose it. Don't plan on losing more than 500 grams a week if you want to be able to maintain your weight loss.

## Physical Activity

Approximately 90 percent of the daily calorie expenditures of most people occurs as a result of the **resting metabolic rate (RMR).** The RMR is slightly higher than the BMR; it includes the BMR plus any additional energy expended through daily sedentary activities, such as food digestion, sitting, studying,

**Basal metabolic rate (BMR):** The energy expenditure of the body under resting conditions at normal room temperature.

**Yo-yo diets:** Cycles in which people repeatedly gain weight and lose weight. This lowers their BMR, which favours the weight gain process.

**Resting metabolic rate (RMR):** The energy expenditure of the body under BMR conditions plus all other daily sedentary activities.

or standing. The **exercise metabolic rate (EMR)** accounts for the remaining 10 percent of all daily calorie expenditures; it refers to the energy expenditure that occurs during physical activity. For most of us, these calories come from light daily activities, such as walking, climbing stairs, and mowing the lawn. If we increase the level and intensity of our physical activity to moderate or heavy, however, our EMR may be 10 to 20 times greater than typical resting metabolic rates and contribute substantially to our energy needs.

Increasing BMR, RMR, or EMR levels will use more calories. An increase in the intensity, frequency, and time (that is, duration) of your daily physical activity will have a significant impact on your total calorie expenditure and ability to manage or control your weight. Current estimates are that engaging in 60 minutes of moderate-intensity physical activity each day will help with weight management.

Physical activity makes a greater contribution to BMR when large muscle groups are used. The energy spent on physical activity is the energy used to move the body's muscles—the muscles of the arms, back, abdomen, legs, and so on—and the extra energy required to increase heartbeat and respiration rate. The number of calories expended depends on three factors:

1. the amount of muscle mass being moved
2. the amount of weight being moved
3. the amount of time the activity takes

An activity involving the arms and the legs burns more calories than one involving only the legs, an activity performed by a heavy person burns more calories than one performed by a lighter person, and an activity performed for 40 minutes requires twice as much energy as the same activity performed for 20 minutes. Thus, obese persons walking one kilometre burn more calories than slim people walking the same distance. It may also take obese people longer to walk one kilometre, which means they are burning energy for a longer time and therefore expending more overall calories than thin walkers.[30]

## WHAT WOULD YOU DO?

Which of the methods for weight maintenance or weight loss discussed above do you think offers you the lowest risk and the greatest chance for success?

# Determining the Caloric Output of Your Physical Activity

The amount of calories required to do a physical activity depends on a number of factors. First, the amount of calories required depends on how much you weigh. The more you weigh, the greater the caloric cost of the physical activity. In other words, you use more calories when you weigh more. Second, the number of calories required to do a physical activity is based on how intensely or how hard you participate in that physical activity. More intense physical activities require more energy to be performed. The third factor that influences the number of calories required to do a particular physical activity is time. Obviously, the longer you do the physical activity, the more energy is required. The latter two factors, intensity of activity and time, interact. Most often, more intense physical activities (e.g., running) can only be done for shorter periods of time and less intense physical activities (e.g., walking) can be done for longer periods of time.

The following physical activities each require about 150 calories of energy to be performed (with an average body weight of ~68 kilograms)[31]:

- gardening for 30 to 45 minutes
- raking leaves for 30 minutes
- shovelling snow for 15 minutes
- walking 3 kilometres in approximately 30 minutes
- pushing a stroller when walking for 30 minutes
- running 2.25 kilometres in 15 minutes
- climbing the stairs for 15 minutes
- playing touch football for 30 to 45 minutes
- playing basketball (i.e., shooting baskets) for 30 minutes
- playing basketball (i.e., a game) for 15 to 20 minutes
- playing wheelchair basketball for 20 minutes
- bicycling 7.5 kilometres in 30 minutes
- dancing (social) for 30 minutes
- swimming laps for 20 minutes
- water fitness classes for 30 minutes
- jumping rope for 30 minutes

Another way to determine the amount of calories required by a particular physical activity is to use established energy costs for that physical

## TABLE 8.3

**Energy Costs of Selected Physical Activities (min/kg)**

| Physical Activity | Time | Cal/min/kg |
|---|---|---|
| Walking (on a grassy surface) | 10.5 min/km | 0.0794 |
| Cycling | 4 min/km | 0.0985 |
| Cycling | 3.1 min/km | 0.1559 |
| Swimming | 55 min/km | 0.1333 |
| Running | 3.7 min/km | 0.2350 |
| Running | 5 min/km | 0.1856 |

Source: Adapted from B. Getchell, *Physical Fitness: A Way of Life* (Benjamin Cummings, 1992).

activity, along with your body weight (in kilograms) and the time you engaged in that physical activity, to calculate your energy costs. This method takes into account the three factors that are involved in determining the energy costs of physical activity: body weight, intensity, and time. Table 8.3 provides a sample of the energy costs of selected physical activities per minute per kilogram.

Thus, if you weigh 65 kilograms and go for a 30-minute run at a pace of 5 minutes per kilometre, you will use 362 calories (65 kg × 0.1856 cal/min/kg × 30 minutes = 362 calories). You would only need to run for 24 minutes at a pace of 3.7 minutes per kilometre to use the same approximate number of calories (i.e., 65 kg × 0.2350 cal/min/kg × 24 minutes = 367 calories).

## Is Dieting Healthy?

Dieting can lead to improved health. It can also lead to serious physical problems and battered self-esteem. What seems to make the difference is whether a diet is part of an overall reappraisal of a person's attitudes about food and weight and part of an action plan that integrates improved nutrition and physical activity rather than just a quick fix.

Most experts agree that the ultimate goal of a weight-loss program should be improved quality of life and lifetime weight maintenance.[32] Weight goals should be set to reduce health risks and address medical problems and to help people improve their ability to perform daily tasks without undue stress and strain rather than to achieve an "ideal" weight or shape. In addition, experts agree that weight-loss programs that promote qualitative rather than quantitative changes in food intake improve health and long-term weight maintenance and are more easily sustained than those that force people to severely restrict intake of calories or specific foods.[33] While the experts seem to agree on these points, many weight-loss programs fail to follow these basic premises. What happens to people who get caught up in "lose weight fast and furiously" campaigns? Researchers are increasingly concerned that:

- dieting to lose weight may be more harmful than helpful in promoting health and psychological well-being[34]

- because dieting only rarely produces successful weight loss, the physical and psychological stress, damage to self-esteem, and other emotional disturbances associated with it are without purpose[35]

**Exercise metabolic rate (EMR):** The energy expenditure that occurs during physical activity.

- dieting causes repeated cycles of weight loss and regain, changes in metabolic rates, increased risk for cardiovascular problems, and other conditions hazardous to health[36]
- dieting contributes to the development of eating disorders such as anorexia and bulimia nervosa[37]

Most health authorities recommend that, rather than going on a diet, a person should adopt dietary changes and a program of increased physical activity aimed at changing metabolic rates and increasing muscle mass.

## Changing Your Eating Habits

Before you can change a given behaviour, you must first determine what causes that behaviour. Why do you suddenly find yourself at the refrigerator door eating? Why do you take that second and third helping of potatoes or dessert when you know that as a result you will gain weight? Our eating is influenced by a number of things including individual and environmental determinants.[38] Specifically, individual determinants include our physiological state (that is, whether or not we are hungry), food preferences, nutritional knowledge, perceptions of healthy eating, and psychological factors. Environmental factors that influence our eating include the interpersonal environment created by our family and peers, the physical environment, which determines food accessibility and availability, the economic and social environment, and the cultural milieu surrounding food choices. Further, food policy has an overarching influence on our personal and the environmental factors influencing our eating behaviours.

Many people have discovered that one of the best ways of assessing their eating behaviours is to chart exactly when they feel like eating, where they are when they decide to eat, the amount of time they spend eating, other activities they engage in while eating (watching television, reading, or something else), whether they eat alone or with others, what and how much they eat, and how they felt before they took their first bite. If you keep a detailed log each day for at least a week, you will discover useful clues about what in your environment or in your emotional makeup causes you to eat. Typically, these dietary "triggers" centre on problems in everyday living rather than on real hunger pangs. As you record this information, your reasons for eating will often become apparent. Many people find that they eat compulsively when stressed or when they have problems in their relationships. For others, it is the smell of a particular food (for example, popcorn) or routine (for example, eating while studying) that causes them to eat rather than hunger itself.

Once you recognize the factors that cause you to eat, removing the triggers or substituting other activities for them will help you develop more sensible eating behaviours. Here are some examples of substitute behaviours:

1. When eating dinner, turn off all distractions, including the television and radio.
2. Replace snack breaks or coffee breaks with physically active breaks.
3. Instead of gulping your food, chew slowly, putting your fork down between bites.
4. Vary the time of day when you eat. Instead of eating by the clock, eat when you are truly hungry.
5. If you find that you generally eat all that is on a plate, use smaller plates.
6. If you find that you are continually seeking your favourite foods in the cupboard, stop buying them or buy them in smaller quantities and store them in an inconvenient spot.

### WHAT WOULD YOU DO?

Based on what you have read so far, what triggers your eating? Is it certain people? Places? Situations? What can you do to manage these triggers?

## Selecting a Nutritional Plan

Once you have discovered what factors tend to sabotage your weight-loss efforts, you will be well on your way to successful weight maintenance. To be successful, however, you must plan for success. By setting goals that are too far in the future or unrealistic for your current lifestyle, you will doom yourself to failure. Don't try to lose 20 kilograms in four months. Remember, you didn't gain 20 kilograms in four months, so it is unrealistic to expect to lose that amount of weight in such a short time. Try instead to lose a healthy 500 grams to 1 kilogram during the first week, and keep with this slow and easy regimen. Reward yourself when you lose weight—but not with food. If you binge and go off your dietary plan, get right back on it as soon as possible (later that day or the next day).

Seek help from reputable sources in choosing a dietary plan that is easy to follow and includes adequate amounts of the basic nutrients. Registered dietitians, holistic physicians (only holistic physicians have strong backgrounds in nutrition, which includes some M.D.s), health educators, exercise physiologists with nutritional backgrounds, and other health professionals can provide reliable information. Avoid quick weight-loss programs that promise miracle results. The majority are expensive, and most people regain the weight soon after

# General Tips for Managing Your Weight

## WHEN EATING AT HOME

- Eat only in the kitchen or dining room. Keep food out of the living room, bedroom, and study spaces.
- Eat smaller meals four to five times a day rather than gorging yourself at dinner.
- Use a smaller plate and fill it with low-calorie, nutrient-dense foods such as salad without dressing and pasta with a low-fat sauce.
- Take more time to eat; at least 20 minutes per meal is recommended. Chew each bit of food carefully, setting your fork down between bites and enjoying the taste of the food.
- Drink a glass or two of water before your meal.
- Brush your teeth after eating to limit the temptation to take a second helping or have something sweet.
- Limit your purchases of high-calorie and high-fat foods, even for guests.
- When having desserts, limit yourself to a small taste or make yourself go out for them.
- Get in tune with your true feelings of hunger. Eat when you are really hungry, not by the clock.
- Develop stress-management skills that do not involve eating.
- Obtain adequate sleep, there is some research suggesting that individuals with a "sleep debt" are at a greater risk for obesity.
- Try not to skip meals or allow yourself to get too hungry before eating.
- Limit the amount of food you eat before going to bed.
- Put serving dishes on the counter or stove while you are eating. Leaving them on the table will tempt you to take seconds even when you are no longer hungry.

## WHEN EATING OUT

- Don't be afraid to ask for it "your way." Request that the cheese be left off, the sauce cut in half, and so on.
- Ask for salad dressings, gravies, and sauces on the side. Then use only a little to flavour the food.
- Ask that entrées be broiled, steamed, baked, grilled, poached, or roasted, with only a small amount of fat used for the cooking process.
- When ordering omelettes, ask for a one- or two-egg-yolk version containing only the whites of the other eggs. Limit meat and cheese fillings. Choose low-fat vegetable fillings whenever possible.
- Reduce portion size. Order à la carte if possible, with a salad or fresh vegetable on the side.
- Limit the times you eat at an all-you-can-eat restaurant. Overeating also occurs at all-you-can-eat salad bars because of the many toppings loaded with fat and calories.
- Drink at least one glass of water before starting your meal. Try to relax while eating and make your mealtime last. Talk more, put your fork down more frequently, chew more, and generally slow down.
- Order fresh fruits in place of heavy desserts. Limit dessert to smaller portions and to having it one or two times per week.
- Frequent restaurants that offer low-fat, high-complex-carbohydrate meals. All of us make better choices when there are more good options to choose from.

completing the program. Ask questions about the credentials of the adviser in any weight-loss program, assess the nutrient value of the prescribed diet, verify that dietary guidelines are consistent with information from reliable dietary research, and analyze how suitable the dietary plan is for your tastes, budget, and lifestyle to avoid putting yourself in a risky, expensive, or unhealthy dietary situation. Any diet that requires radical behaviour changes is doomed to fail. Dietary plans that do not ask you to sacrifice everything you enjoy and that allow you to make choices are usually the most successful.

Ultimately, it is your decision to practise responsible weight management. Choose a combination of physi-cal activity and eating that fits your needs and lifestyle, find a workable plan, stick to it, and you will succeed.

## "Miracle" Diets

Fasting, starvation diets, and other forms of **very low-calorie diets (VLCDs)** have been shown to cause significant health risks. Typically, when you deprive your body of food for prolonged periods, your body makes adjustments to save you from

**Very-low-calorie diets (VLCDs):** Diets with caloric value of 400 to 700 calories.

inevitable organ shutdown. It begins to deplete its energy reserves to obtain necessary fuels. One of the first reserves to which the body turns to maintain its supply of glucose is lean, protein tissue. When this occurs you lose weight rapidly, because protein contains only half as many calories per kilogram as fat. At the same time, significant water stores are lost. Over time, the body begins to run out of liver tissue, heart muscle, blood, and so on, as these readily available substances are used to supply energy. Only after the readily available proteins from these sources are depleted will your body begin to use fat reserves. In this process, known as **ketosis,** the body adapts to prolonged fasting or carbohydrate deprivation by converting body fat to ketones, which can be used as fuel for some brain cells. Within about ten days after the typical adult begins a complete fast, the body has used many of its energy stores and death may occur.

In very-low-calorie diets, powdered formulas are usually given to patients under medical supervision. These formulas have daily values ranging from 400 to 700 calories plus vitamin and mineral supplements. Although these diets may be beneficial for people who have failed at all conventional weight-loss methods and who face severe threats to their health that are complicated by their obesity, they should never be undertaken without close medical supervision. Problems associated with fasting, VLCDs, and other forms of severe calorie deprivation include blood sugar imbalances, cold intolerance, constipation, decreased BMR, dehydration, diarrhea, emotional problems, fatigue, headaches, heart irregularity, ketosis, kidney infections and failure, loss of lean body tissue, weakness, and weight gain due to the yo-yo effect and other variables.

## Trying to Gain Weight

Although trying to lose weight poses a major challenge for many, there is a smaller group of people who, for a variety of metabolic, hereditary, psychological, and other reasons, can't seem to gain weight no matter how hard they try. If you are one of these individuals, you must determine why you have difficulty in gaining weight. Once you know that, there are several things you can do to help yourself:

- *Control your physical activity.* Cut back if you are doing too much, slow down, and keep a careful record of calories burned.
- *Eat more.* Obviously, you are not taking in enough calories to support whatever is happening in your body. Eat more frequently, spend more time eating, eat high-calorie, nutrient-dense foods first if you tend to fill up fast, and start with the main course. Take time to shop and to cook, and eat slowly. Make your sandwiches with extra-thick slices of bread and add more filling such as peanut

butter, cream cheese, or cheese. Take seconds whenever possible and eat high-calorie, nutrient-dense snacks during the day.

- *Try to relax.* Many people who are underweight also suffer from anxiety and the "hurry syndrome." Slow down and try to manage your reactions to stress.

# EATING DISORDERS

Obesity itself is neither a psychiatric disorder nor an **eating disorder.** An eating disorder consists of severe disturbances in eating behaviours, unhealthy efforts to control body weight, and abnormal attitudes about one's body and shape. The three main eating disorders are anorexia nervosa, bulimia nervosa, and binge eating disorder. These eating disorders are mostly associated with females.

Those with eating disorders often suffer from low self-esteem. However, contrary to popular stereotypes, eating disorders are not restricted to middle-class white females with overprotective or over-perfectionist parents. Eating disorders span social classes and ethnic groups.

Eating disorders have been reported to occur with roughly similar frequencies in most industrialized countries, including Canada, the United States, Europe, Australia, Japan, New Zealand, and South Africa. Emigrants from cultures in which the disorders are rare to cultures where the disorders are more prevalent may develop anorexia nervosa as they assimilate thin-body ideals. The disorders usually begin during early adolescence, although rare cases occur even after the age of 40. More than 90 percent of cases occur in women.

## Anorexia Nervosa

**Anorexia nervosa** is characterized by self-starvation motivated by an intense fear of gaining weight and a severe disturbance in the perception of one's body. When anorexia nervosa develops in childhood or early adolescence, an indication is the failure to gain weight associated with normal growth rather than the loss of weight. About one-half to one percent of females in late adolescence or early adulthood meet the diagnostic criteria of anorexia nervosa.

Those diagnosed with anorexia nervosa weigh less than 85 percent of normal weight. Their unusual weight is accomplished primarily through reducing their total food intake. Usually, they begin by restricting high-calorie foods, and eventually exclude almost all foods from their diet. In addition, they lose weight through *purging*—self-induced vomiting or the misuse of laxatives or diuretics—and through exercise.

Individuals with this disorder have an intense fear of gaining weight or becoming fat. This intense fear is usually

## Anorexia Athletica (Compulsive Exercising)

Anorexia athletica is not a recognized diagnosis in the same way that anorexia, bulimia, and binge eating disorder are. However, many people preoccupied with food and weight exercise compulsively to try to control their weight in a misguided attempt to gain a sense of power, control, and self-respect.

Symptoms of anorexia athletica include:

■ exercising beyond the requirements for good health

■ being fanatical about weight and dietary intake

■ stealing time from work, school, and relationships to exercise

■ focusing on challenge and forgetting that physical activity can be fun

■ defining self-worth in terms of performance

■ rarely or never being satisfied with athletic achievements

■ always pushing on to the next challenge

■ justifying excessive behaviours by defining self as an athlete or insisting that their behaviour is healthy

Source: National Eating Disorder Information Centre, www.nedic.ca/qa.html#16 416-340-4156.

not alleviated by weight loss. In fact, concern about weight gain often increases as actual weight decreases.

People with this illness have a distorted view of the experience and significance of body weight and shape. Some feel globally overweight; others feel that parts (particularly the abdomen, buttocks, and thighs) are "too fat." They may constantly weigh themselves, measure themselves, and look at themselves in the mirror to check for fat. This is because their self-esteem is highly dependent on their body shape and weight. Weight loss is viewed as an impressive achievement and a sign of extraordinary self-discipline; weight gain is perceived as unacceptable failure of self-control.[39]

The medical problems associated with anorexia nervosa are appalling. Starvation can damage the bones, the muscles, and the organs as well as the immune, nervous, and digestive systems. The acid in vomit may cause tooth enamel to dissolve. People with anorexia nervosa often lose hair or develop excessive, fine facial and body hair. Worse, between 10 and 15 percent of individuals with anorexia nervosa die as a result of the disorder.[40]

## Bulimia Nervosa

The essential features of **bulimia nervosa** are binge eating followed by inappropriate compensating

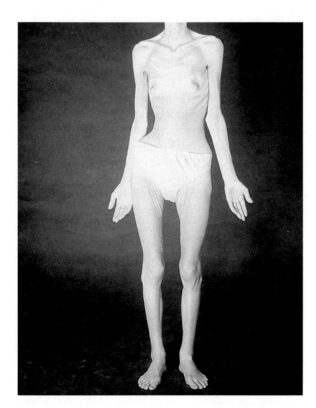

*The self-starvation associated with eating disorders like anorexia nervosa can damage bones, muscles, and organs and create a host of other serious and, in some cases, life-threatening medical problems.*

**Ketosis:** A condition in which the body adapts to prolonged fasting or carbohydrate deprivation by converting body fat to ketones, which can be used as fuel for some brain activity.

**Eating disorder:** Disorder consisting of severe disturbances in eating behaviours, unhealthy efforts to control body weight, and abnormal attitudes toward one's body and shape.

**Anorexia nervosa:** Eating disorder characterized by excessive preoccupation with food, self-starvation, and/or extreme exercising to achieve weight loss.

**Bulimia nervosa:** Eating disorder characterized by binge eating followed by inappropriate compensating measures taken to prevent weight gain.

# Helping Someone with an Eating Disorder

When a family member or a friend has an eating disorder, that person needs serious medical help. You can take a proactive role in getting help. Here are some suggestions:

- Speak up. Don't encourage denial of the problem by ignoring it.
- Base what you say on your own observations and keep the tone affectionate, not accusing: "I've noticed you're skipping a lot of meals, and I'm worried about you." Or, "I can smell that you have been vomiting, and I'm concerned about your health." Make yourself available to the individual to discuss emotional concerns and anxieties.
- Inform yourself about the disorder, and share your information with the person who you suspect has the disorder. For many women, recovery starts with a book or a pamphlet provided by a friend or relative. Consult an eating disorders clinic in your area. Clinics in teaching hospitals are the most likely to offer counselling and programs free or at a low cost.
- Attend a support group for help with your own pain resulting from the situation and for advice on how to interact with your family member or friend.
- If the person with the disorder agrees to seek help, be supportive in constructive ways. Offer to accompany him or her to appointments; express interest and concern without trying to take over.

- If a relative has an eating disorder, consider family therapy to explore some of the emotional roots of the disorder. Jean Rubel, Ph.D., founder of an organization dealing with anorexia nervosa and related eating disorders, says, "Ignore tears, tantrums, and promises." If the relative is younger than 18, get him or her to a doctor and tell the doctor what you suspect; this is no time for guessing games. Get educational counselling and therapy. Rubel also believes that the whole family should be involved in the therapy to deal with the root issues: "You can't send her or him off to be fixed like a car to a garage."
- Do not nag or bully. You can't recover for someone else, and you may create more problems by monitoring someone else's eating habits.
- Do not tell a person recovering from anorexia or bulimia nervosa that he or she is looking better. No matter how carefully you phrase it, he or she will hear, "You got fat."

Source: Adapted with permission from Suanne Kelman, "The Way Back," *Shape,* March 1995, 113.

---

measures taken to prevent weight gain, such as induced vomiting. Binge eating normally occurs in secrecy and is accompanied by a lack of control. It is difficult for a person with bulimia nervosa to stop the binge once it has started. About 1 to 3 percent of adolescent and young adult females have bulimia nervosa; the rate among men is about 10 percent of that among females.

Similar to individuals with anorexia nervosa, those with bulimia nervosa place an excessive emphasis on body shape and weight in their self-evaluation, and these factors are critical in determining their self-esteem. Unlike individuals with anorexia nervosa, the body weight of individuals with bulimia nervosa is typically within the normal weight range (some may be underweight or overweight). In addition, treatment of bulimia nervosa is effective in the majority of cases, with good prospects for a full and lasting recovery.[41]

## Binge Eating Disorder

People afflicted with **binge eating disorder (BED)** engage in recurrent binge eating but, unlike those with bulimia, do not take excessive measures to lose the weight gained during binges. Neither do BED patients report abnormal attitudes about dieting or body weight and shape. Binge eating disorder occurs predominantly in obese patients. This disorder is often referred to in the popular literature as "compulsive overeating." Studies show that obese patients with BED consume significantly more food than obese people who don't binge.

## Who's at Risk?

Disordered eating patterns are the result of many factors besides low self-esteem or an addiction to food. Often they are partially the result of poor self-concept, but other factors, such as a perceived lack of control in a person's life, may trigger these problems. To win social approval by maintaining a thin body and to gain

**Binge eating disorder (BED):** Eating disorder characterized by recurrent binge eating. Individuals with BED do not take excessive measures to lose weight gained from binges.

# Managing Your Weight

Managing your weight is not an easy task. To ensure success, you must make a real change in the way you eat and consider it a lifelong commitment rather than a diet—that is, something you follow for a few weeks and then return to previous dietary behaviours. Analyzing where you are right now and then taking the steps outlined below will help you lose excess weight.

## MAKING DECISIONS FOR YOU

The first step in managing your weight is an honest self-assessment of where you are. You don't need sophisticated fat-measurement techniques. What you need is a scale. Next, you need to set a realistic goal. Ask yourself, why do I want to meet this goal? What will I do when I reach this goal? Then set out a plan to reach your goal. Keep in mind what you enjoy doing. If you like taking walks, you might make walking part of your program. If you absolutely love chocolate chip cookies, you might consider limiting yourself to two cookies per day.

## CHECKLIST FOR CHANGE: MAKING PERSONAL CHOICES

■ *Design your plan to meet your needs.* Your plan must fit your personality, your priorities, and your work and recreation schedules. It should also allow for sufficient rest and relaxation.

■ *Plan for nutrient-dense foods.* Attempt to get the most from the foods you eat by selecting foods with high nutritional value.

■ *Spread caloric intake throughout the day.* Although the evidence is controversial, research indicates that the body may burn calories more efficiently in small amounts than in large quantities.

■ *Plan for plateaus.* If you prepare yourself psychologically for plateaus you will be less likely to become discouraged. Physical activity is likely the critical factor in getting past a plateau.

■ *Chart your progress.* For many people, the daily "weigh-in" is a critical factor in maintaining their program. However, for others, the daily monitoring of weight negatively influences self-esteem. It should also be kept in mind that body weight normally fluctuates throughout the week and a once per week "weigh-in" may be more appropriate, particularly for those who have reached a weight plateau, to avoid frustration or disappointment.

■ *Chart your setbacks.* Rather than thinking in terms of failure and punishment, think in terms of temporary setbacks and how to accommodate them. By carefully recording your emotional states when eating, eating habits, environmental cues, and feelings, you may determine why you needed that ice cream cone or that extra slice of pizza. Successful weight-loss plans accommodate for hormonal fluctuations and their potential influence on dietary habits.

■ *Become aware of your feelings of hunger and fullness.* For many of us, eating is time-dependent, and we stop eating only when the food is gone (the "clean your plate" syndrome). Long years of "eating when it is time" instead of eating when it is necessary cost us the ability to tell when we really are hungry and when we really are full. By training yourself to become more aware of the eating process, by learning to recognize true hunger pangs and the first signals that you have eaten enough, you will be able to change your eating patterns.

■ *Accept yourself.* For many people, this is the most important aspect of successful weight management. Although our culture may oppress fat people, many obese people are their own worst enemies. It is important to keep your weight in perspective. Unless you feel good about who you are inside, exterior changes will not help you very much.

■ *Exercise, exercise, exercise.* Different people benefit from different types of physical activities. Just because your friends are into jogging or jazzercise does not mean that that type of physical activity is best for you. Select physical activities that you consider fun, not a daily form of punishment for overeating. Variety may be the key here. Planning physical activities that include friends and family may also improve your chances of success. It is important to remember that every little effort contributes toward long-term results.

## CHECKLIST FOR CHANGE: MAKING COMMUNITY CHOICES

■ Identify volunteer organizations that provide physically active opportunities for teens.

■ What opportunities for volunteering at nutrition- or weight-related programs does your campus provide?

## CRITICAL THINKING

Until post-secondary school, your girlfriend Tami had taken ballet very seriously, practising several hours a day. Now that the time pressures of school, a part-time job, and your relationship are starting to get to her, Tami rarely has time to work out on the dance floor. You notice that she has consequently been more and more concerned about her weight. She rarely eats on your dates because she wants the two of you to save money for a trip during spring break. When you find a laxative hidden under her pillow, she says, "Doesn't everyone get constipated now and then?" Then a mutual female friend tells you that she's heard Tami in the bathroom throwing up on several occasions after meals. Tami denies it.

Using the DECIDE model in Chapter 1, decide how you can approach Tami with your concern that she has an eating disorder. What help is available in your local area? Should you involve Tami's family? If Tami denies she has an eating disorder, what can you do?

# From Atkins to the Glycemic Index: Getting the "Skinny" on Carbohydrates

Low-carbohydrate diets have attracted millions of North Americans with reports of massive, quick weight loss. Bookstores struggle to keep the latest editions of *The Atkins Diet, The South Beach Diet,* and other bestsellers on their shelves. Restaurants have added "low-carb" items to their menus, and a multimillion dollar industry of low-carb food products has emerged. The promise? Eliminate nearly all of the bread, pasta, sweets, and high-carbohydrate foods from your diet, eat red meat and other high-protein and high-fat foods until you are satisfied, and lose weight.

Many health professionals have spent the past 20 years criticizing low-carb diets as dangerous, ineffective, and unhealthy. The American Heart Association and the American Dietetic Association were just two of many professional health groups that issued warnings about the craze. Yet several well-designed clinical trials indicated that low-carbohydrate diets were as good as—and in many cases, better than—low-fat diets in helping very overweight people shed pounds.

In these studies, more people stayed with the low-carb diet than the low-fat one, and, although they ate more fat, they did not experience the harmful changes in blood cholesterol that many expected. In fact, their LDL ("bad") cholesterol and triglycerides were reduced and their HDL ("good") cholesterol increased.

However, these benefits were only short term, and reports of problems with low-carb diets began to surface. A study by the Stanford University Medical Center in conjunction with researchers at Yale University found that although low-carbohydrate diets cause weight loss, it's the total caloric reduction and the duration of the reduction that causes the loss, not the reduction in carbohydrate intake per se. The take-home message was that any low-calorie diet that a person can stay on long enough will have similar results. Furthermore, people had difficulty in sticking to the rigid dietary requirements. When they lost weight, they gained it back nearly as quickly as they had lost it. People with diabetes had problems because whole grains, beans, and other fibre-rich foods were not allowed. And rather than remembering to cut back on saturated fats, people were gulping down bacon and eggs, eating huge steaks, and feeling good about the guilt-free diet.

A major problem with the Atkins and similar diets is that they assume that virtually any carbohydrate is bad for you. However, they do not account for the vast difference in nutrient value among carbohydrates and their *glycemic index*, a ranking of foods according to how quickly their sugars are released into the bloodstream. The body converts a food's sugars into glucose, which is released slowly or rapidly into the bloodstream.

Insulin is secreted to counter glucose levels and return the body to healthy levels. The amount of insulin a food triggers is referred to as *glycemic load*, which considers both a food's glycemic index and how much carbohydrate the food delivers in one hit in a single serving.

Most fruits, vegetables, beans, and whole grains have low glycemic loads; their sugars enter the bloodstream gradually and trigger only a moderate rise in insulin. High-calorie sugars cause insulin levels to rise, triggering a chain of reactions that ultimately make you sluggish, bloated, and feeling hungry, driving you to eat more and continuing the cycle. Ultimately, these high insulin levels can lead to diabetes.

Given this new understanding of carbohydrates, should you do what Atkins suggests and follow a diet that avoids most carbs? No. The bulk of scientific evidence suggests that you should choose foods with low glycemic loads and continue to reduce your total caloric intake and saturated fat intake.

A few examples of the glycemic load of common foods demonstrates the range you may find in your daily diet: a serving of high-quality orange juice has nearly three times the glycemic load (13) as an orange; a serving of cornflakes has five times the load (21) as a serving of All Bran (4). Listings for many foods can be found online, particularly in connection with diabetes resources.

However, instead of memorizing glycemic load values for all your favourite foods, try following these general guidelines:

- *Choose plants*. Pick the fruit rather than its sugar-laden juice counterpart. Eating the skin of apples adds fibre and slows the entry of glucose into the bloodstream. If you must eat potatoes, eat them with the skin on and cut back on other starches. Instead of potatoes and corn, try sweet potatoes and yams.

- *Forgo meat in favour of beans*. It isn't necessary to cut all meat-based protein from your diet. However, when you eat meat, opt for the lean cuts and choose poultry over pork or beef. Learn to cook and flavour beans. They are high in protein and other nutrients and have very little effect on blood sugar and insulin.

- *Go nuts several times a week*. Almonds, hazelnuts, peanuts, pecans, and others are healthy low-carbohydrate alternatives to snacking on chips and desserts made from white flour. They are not calorie free, though, so manage your intake based on exercise patterns and calorie needs.

- *Mix your carbs with other foods*. Eating carbohydrates with other foods such as monounsaturated oils (olive or canola) can slow the rate of carbohydrate absorption. Milk or yogurt with cereal is one example; bananas and cottage cheese in cereal is another.

- *Make whole-grain breads a staple*. Avoid white bread and look for brown breads with 100-percent whole wheat or other grains. Consider options such as brown rice and whole-wheat pizza dough and pasta. These are good choices for slowing your blood sugar.

- *Exercise regularly*. Most people would be shocked if they ate a normal meal, measured their blood sugar, then noted how dramatically their blood sugars go down after a 30-minute walk. It may seem simple, but one of the best ways to keep yourself healthy and still consume the carbs you want is through exercise.

These recommendations hold true no matter what low-fat, low-carb, low-calorie diet or other plan you choose to follow.

*Sources:* W. Willet and P. Skerrett, "Going Beyond Atkins," *Newsweek*, January 19, 2004, 46; S. Conner et al., "Should a Low Fat, High-Carb Diet be Recommended for Everyone?" *New England Journal of Medicine* 350 (2004): 1691–1692. F. F. Samaha et al., "A Low-Carbohydrate as Compared with a Low-Fat Diet in Severe Obesity," *New England* Journal of Medicine 348, no. 21 (2003): 2074–2081; G.D. Foster et al., "A Randomized Trial of Low Carbohydrate Diet for Obesity," *New England Journal of Medicine* 348, no. 21 (2003): 2082–2090; D.M. Bravata et al., "Efficacy and Safety of Low-Carbohydrate Diets," *Journal of the American Medical Association* 289, no. 14 (2003): 1837–1850.

control of some aspects of their lives, those with anorexia or bulimia nervosa take rigid control over eating. Increasing numbers of males also suffer from various forms of eating disorders.

Some studies using identical twins have shown a possible association between heredity and eating disorders, as have others that point to the proportionally large number of eating-disordered persons who have a mother or sister with a like disease. Many persons with disordered eating patterns also suffer from other problems such as clinical depression, alcohol abuse, compulsive stealing, gambling, or other addictions.[42]

## Treating Eating Disorders

The most effective treatments for eating disorders combine different approaches into a package that involves the patient and his or her family and friends. Eating disorder patients usually come to the attention of medical personnel because someone else shows concern. To learn about how you could help someone you suspect has a disorder see the Building Communication Skills box.

Treatment options for eating disorders vary. Due to the medical complications brought on by excessive weight loss, anorexia nervosa often requires hospitalization with the first goal of treatment being to restore patients to near-normal body weight. For all eating disorders, individual psychotherapy provides an opportunity for the patient to enhance self-confidence, self-esteem, and feelings of power and control. In therapy, the person learns new, more effective ways to handle stress so that it is no longer necessary to turn to or away from food to deal with problems. In addition, individuals with an eating disorder often exhibit depression and other clinical illnesses, and these problems can also be treated.

Support groups are useful for providing a social network, emotional support, and self-help techniques. Family therapy can also be useful.

### WHAT WOULD YOU DO?

Why do post-secondary students in particular seem to have so many problems with eating disorders? What factors place young women at risk? Why do you think there are fewer eating disorders among men? What programs or services on your campus would you recommend for a friend with an eating disorder?

# SUMMARY

- Overweight, obesity, and weight-related problems appear to be on the rise in Canada. Obesity is defined in terms of fat content rather than in terms of weight alone. There are many different methods of assessing body fat.

- Many factors contribute to your risk for obesity. Included among these factors are heredity, sex, developmental factors, setpoint, endocrine influences, psychosocial factors, eating cues, lack of awareness, metabolic changes, and lifestyle.

- Physical activity, dieting, diet pills, and other strategies are used to maintain or lose weight. However, sensible eating behaviours and adequate physical activity probably offer the best options.
- Eating disorders consist of severe disturbances in eating behaviours, unhealthy efforts to control body weight, and abnormal attitudes about body and shape. Anorexia nervosa, bulimia nervosa, and binge eating disorder are the three main eating disorders. Eating disorders occur mainly in adolescent and young adult women in industrialized countries.

# DISCUSSION QUESTIONS

1. Discuss the pressures, if any, you feel to improve your body image. Where do these pressures come from? How have the media influenced your thoughts about your body?

2. List the risk factors for obesity. Identify the factors that seem to be most important in determining whether you will be obese in middle age.

3. How is it possible that a person can be classified as obese (BMI greater than 30) and yet not be overfat (that is, percent body fat within the normal range)? Similarly how can a person be overfat (that is, percent fat above the normal range) and not be classified as obese (that is, BMI<30)?

4. Create a plan to help someone lose the weight he has put on over the year during his summer vacation. Assume that this person is male, weighs 82 kilograms, and wants to lose 7 kilograms over 15 weeks.

5. Differentiate among the three eating disorders. Then give reasons why females might be more prone than males to anorexia and bulimia nervosa.

6. Why are popular diets not always the best way to lose body fat over the long term? Which popular diets might have better long-term success? Why?

# APPLICATION EXERCISE

Reread the What Do You Think? scenario at the beginning of the chapter and answer the following questions.

1. What motivates someone like Ray to spiff up and look good at certain times of the year? How could someone like Ray change his behaviours so he can be healthier nutritionally and avoid the diet syndrome so many of us find ourselves in?

2. How can the Food Guide help Ray to manage his weight?

3. Why is dieting to lose weight probably not such a good idea in the long run?

# HEALTH ON THE NET

American Council on Science and Health
**www.acsh.org**

Centre for Science in the Public Interest (Canada)
**www.cspinet.org/canada/**

Health Canada: Food & Nutrition
**www.hc-sc.gc.ca/food-aliment/**

Nutritional Supplements Review
**www.mckinley.uiuc.edu/Handouts/ergogenic_aids.html**

# CHAPTER 9

# PERSONAL FITNESS

*Improving Your Health through Physical Activity*

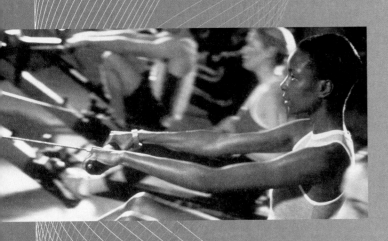

## CHAPTER OBJECTIVES

- Describe the benefits of physical activity, including improved cardiorespiratory efficiency, bone health, weight management, mental health and stress management, and physical fitness.

- Identify the health-related components of physical fitness and the importance of each component.

- Describe the components of an aerobic exercise program and how to determine the exercise frequency, intensity, time (duration), and type of activity.

- Compare the various types of resistance training programs, including the methods of providing external resistance and intended physiological benefits.

- Describe the different stretching exercises designed to improve flexibility.

- Describe common physical activity-related injuries, suggest ways to prevent these injuries, and outline the treatment process.

- Summarize the key components of a personal physical fitness training program.

Regular physical activity results in a wide range of physical, social, and mental health benefits.[1] These health benefits are a result of increased energy expenditure that relates to an overall improvement in quality of life as well as more efficient body functioning, weight management, and reduced risk of chronic diseases including cardiovascular diseases, type 2 diabetes, osteoporosis, and depression.[2] The vast majority of Canadians are aware of the health benefits of physical activity and that they need to be more active, yet almost half the population is considered physically inactive—that is, expends less than 3 cal/kg/day in physical activity.[3] Even more disturbing is that only 21 percent of Canadian teenagers are sufficiently active to meet the international standards for optimal growth and development, with boys twice as likely to make the standard than girls (27 vs. 14 percent).[4] At all ages, men are more active than women. Further, people become less active the older they get: children are more active than adolescents,[5] and adolescents are more active than adults. Research also indicates that your physical activity level as a child and adolescent influences your attitudes and behaviours toward physical activity as an adult.[6] But

if your physical activity experiences as a child or adolescent were negative, don't despair. University or college is an excellent place to make a break with the past and develop positive physical activity attitudes and behaviours that can increase the quality and quantity of your life. Regular physical activity, especially when combined with a healthy dietary intake, may prevent obesity and reduce the likelihood of coronary artery disease, high blood pressure, type 2 diabetes, and other chronic diseases.[7] Further, regular physical activity helps to control stress, increases self-esteem, and contributes to that "feel-good" feeling. Thus, it is no wonder that physical activity is often viewed as the key to health.

# BENEFITS OF REGULAR PHYSICAL ACTIVITY

**Physical activity** refers to all body movements produced by skeletal muscles resulting in energy expenditure.[8] As previously mentioned, higher levels of physical activity have been associated with a lower incidence of cardiovascular disease, the leading cause of death in Canada for men and women.[9] Regular physical activity has also been linked to a lower incidence of high blood pressure (hypertension), cancers of the colon and reproductive organs, bone fractures produced by osteoporosis, and depression.[10] Furthermore, research suggests that regular physical activity (four or more hours accumulated over a week) beginning in adolescence and continuing into adulthood significantly reduced the risk of breast cancer in women 40 years of age and younger.[11]

Many of the risk factors for coronary artery disease, hypertension, and osteoporosis first appear during childhood and adolescence[12] and are often magnified by a child's overweight status. One study reported that almost 60 percent of overweight 5- to 10-year-old children had at least one risk factor for cardiovascular disease (that is, high blood pressure, elevated LDLs, inactivity).[13] Fortunately, if identified during childhood, adolescence, or young adulthood, many of the risks for chronic diseases can be reduced by engaging regularly in moderate-intensity physical activity and eating a low-fat, high-fibre dietary intake.

# Improved Cardiorespiratory Endurance

A regular program of moderately intense aerobic physical activity improves the efficiency of your cardiovascular and respiratory systems: it enables the heart to pump more blood with each stroke, thus lowering resting heart rate; it improves the body's capacity to distribute oxygen to working muscles; and it strengthens the muscles responsible for respiration.

### Reduced Risk of Heart Disease

Your heart is a muscle made up of highly specialized tissue. Because muscles become stronger and more efficient with use, regular physical activity of sufficient intensity strengthens the heart, enabling it to pump more blood with each beat. This increased efficiency means that your heart requires fewer beats per minute to circulate blood throughout your body to maintain function. Thus, a stronger, more efficient heart is better able to meet the ordinary and extraordinary demands of life.

### Prevention of Hypertension

**Hypertension** is the medical term for chronic high blood pressure. It is a cardiovascular disease itself and it increases risk of coronary heart disease and stroke. High blood pressure occurs when the force exerted by the heart (**systolic blood pressure**) or the pressure of the blood on the arterial walls (**diastolic blood pressure**) is greater than normal. A blood pressure reading of 120 over 80 millimetres of mercury (mm Hg) is generally considered normal. Systolic values between 120 and 139 mm Hg or diastolic values of 80 to 89 mm Hg are considered pre-hypertensive, and a blood pressure reading greater than 140 over 90 mm Hg is classified as hypertensive.[14]

Moderate-intensity physical activity lowers systolic and diastolic blood pressure by about 10 mm Hg in people with mild to moderate hypertension.[15] Regular physical activity can also reduce systolic and diastolic blood pressure in people with normal blood pressure.[16]

### Improved Blood Lipid and Lipoprotein Profile

Lipids are fats that circulate in the bloodstream and are stored in various places in your body. A high level of

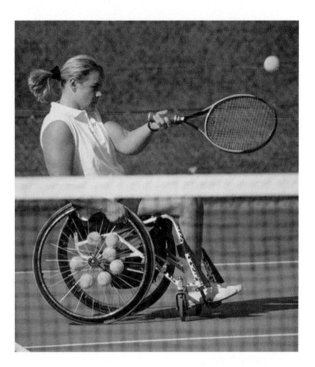

*Reduced risk of chronic disease and improved quality of life are among the benefits of regular physical activity available to people of all ages and all capabilities.*

blood lipids (cholesterol and triglycerides) increases risk of coronary heart disease.[17] Regular physical activity reduces the levels of low-density lipoproteins (LDLs—"bad cholesterol"), while increasing the number of high-density lipoproteins (HDLs—"good cholesterol") in the blood. Higher HDL levels are associated with lower risk for coronary artery disease because they remove some of the "bad cholesterol," thus reducing fatty plaque accumulation from coronary artery walls.

## WHAT WOULD YOU DO?

Do you know your resting heart rate? Body composition? Blood pressure? Cholesterol level? Who could provide you with this information?

**Physical activity:** Body movements produced by skeletal muscles resulting in energy expenditure.

**Hypertension:** Chronic high blood pressure; generally, blood pressure readings consistently greater than 140 over 90 mm Hg.

**Systolic blood pressure:** The pressure of the blood on the arterial walls during a heartbeat.

**Diastolic blood pressure:** The pressure of the blood on the arterial walls between heartbeats.

# Test Your Physical Activity Awareness

To check your understanding of physical activity and its health-related benefits, see how many of the following questions you can answer correctly.

1. People of all ages need to be active to be healthy. How many Canadians are not active enough to achieve health benefits?
   a. All
   b. One-third
   c. One-half
   d. Two-thirds

2. Benefits of regular physical activity include improved health, fitness, and weight management; better posture, balance, and self-esteem; stronger muscles and bones; more energy, greater relaxation, and reduced stress; and continued independent living.
   a. True
   b. False

3. Physical inactivity is as dangerous to your health as smoking.
   a. True
   b. False

4. People who are inactive face a greater risk of premature death, cardiovascular diseases, obesity, type 2 diabetes, osteoporosis, depression, and colon and reproductive organ cancers.
   a. True
   b. False

5. How much physical activity do experts say people should do to stay healthy?
   a. Accumulate 20–30 minutes of vigorous intensity physical activity, 3 days per week
   b. Accumulate 30 minutes of moderate physical activity at least 4 and preferably all days of the week
   c. Accumulate 60 minutes of light physical activity every day
   d. Any of the above

6. You have to join a gym in order to become physically active.
   a. True
   b. False

7. If you're not physically active for at least 30 minutes at a time, you will not gain health benefits.
   a. True
   b. False

8. To stay healthy, people should choose a variety and range of physical activities to maintain cardiorespiratory endurance, muscular strength and endurance, flexibility, and body composition.
   a. True
   b. False

9. Brisk walking is one of the best physical activities to improve health for a majority of people.
   a. True
   b. False

10. Becoming more physically active is safe for most people.
    a. True
    b. False

11. More than half of Canada's children and youth are not physically active enough for optimal growth and development.
    a. True
    b. False

12. To protect your health, physical activity should be as routine as wearing a seat belt or brushing your teeth.
    a. True
    b. False

13. It costs a lot of money to build physical activity into your daily life.
    a. True
    b. False

14. Physical inactivity results in unnecessary costs to Canada's health system.
    a. True
    b. False

15. Many people are inactive because they think regular physical activity takes too much time.
    a. True
    b. False

16. People with physical or mental disabilities can be physically active and participate in a wide range of activities.
    a. True
    b. False

17. Physical activity is an investment in your health and quality of life, and pays real dividends as you get older.
    a. True
    b. False

The correct answers for the above questions are: 1-c, 2–4-a, 5-d, 6–7-b, 8–12-a, 13-b, 14–16-a, 17-a.

Source: Adapted from Health Canada "Canada's Physical Activity Guide—Quiz," 1998.

# Improved Bone Health

**Osteoarthritis** is a nonfatal but incurable disease characterized by degeneration of joint cartilage and irritation of surrounding bone and soft tissues. Affecting one in ten Canadians, osteoarthritis is the most prevalent chronic joint condition in Canada. Women are afflicted more frequently than men.[18] Supervised walking and weight-loss programs can improve physical capacity while reducing knee-joint osteoarthritis symptoms.[19]

A common affliction for the older population is **osteoporosis,** a disease characterized by low bone mass and deterioration of bone tissue, which increases fracture risk. Although men and women are both negatively affected by osteoporosis, the prevalence is greater in women. Weight-bearing and strength-building physical activities are recommended to maintain bone health and to prevent osteoporotic fractures. Bone, like other human tissues, responds to the demands placed upon it (the overload principle), and unless the mechanical stresses placed on bone by a particular physical activity exceed the level of stress the bone has adapted to, bone mass and structure will not adapt.[20] Women (and men) have much to gain by remaining physically active as they age—bone mass levels have been found to be significantly higher among physically active women than among those who are sedentary.[21] However, it appears that the full bone-related benefits of physical activity can be achieved only with sufficient hormone levels (estrogen in women, testosterone in men) and adequate calcium, vitamin D, and total caloric intakes.

# Improved Weight Management

For many people, the desire to lose weight is the main reason for their physical activity. Physical activity has a direct positive effect on metabolic rate and keeps it elevated for a few hours following vigorous physical activities. As previously noted, research suggests that 60 minutes of moderate-intensity physical activity each day should help in maintaining body weight. An effective method for losing weight should combine regular endurance-type physical activities with a moderate decrease (about 500 calories per day) in dietary intake. Decreasing daily caloric intake beyond this may decrease metabolic rate by as much as 20 percent, making short- and long-term weight loss more difficult.

# Improved Health and Life Span

## Prevention of Type 2 Diabetes

Diabetes is a complex metabolic disorder that affects many Canadians. Most Canadians diagnosed with this disorder (90 percent) have type 2 diabetes (also called non–insulin dependent diabetes, although people with this disorder may indeed need insulin). The strongest predisposing factors for this type of diabetes are inactivity, obesity, increasing age, and a family history. Lesser risk factors include high blood pressure and high cholesterol.[22] It is believed that a healthy dietary intake combined with sufficient physical activity could have prevented many of the current cases of type 2 diabetes.[23] A recent large epidemiological study found that for every 2,000 calories of energy expended during leisure-time physical activities, the incidence of diabetes was reduced by 24 percent. Perhaps the most encouraging finding was that the protective effect of physical activity was greatest among individuals at the highest risk for type 2 diabetes.[24]

## Increased Longevity

Experts have long debated the relationship between physical activity and longevity. For decades, most research failed to show that we could increase our life expectancy through physical activity alone. Then a classic prospective study of the Harvard alumni of more than 30 years reported that inactive men were at a greater risk of premature death from all causes than men who engaged in regular physical activity.[25] How much physical activity was required to produce this effect? Men who changed from a sedentary lifestyle to one that included a brisk 30- to 60-minute walk each day experienced the most significant increases in their life expectancies.[26]

## Improved Immunity to Disease

Will regular physical activity make you more immune to disease? Research suggests that regular moderate-intensity physical activity makes people less susceptible to disease, but that this potential benefit may depend upon whether they perceive their physical activity as pleasurable or stressful.[27] Often the relationship of physical activity to immunity, or more specifically to disease susceptibility, is described as a J-shaped curve. In other words, susceptibility to disease decreases as you move from sedentary to moderately active, then increases again as you move to more extreme levels of physical

**Osteoarthritis:** A disease characterized by degeneration of joint cartilage and irritation of surrounding bone and soft tissue.

**Osteoporosis:** A disease characterized by low bone mass and deterioration of bone tissue, which increases fracture risk.

activity or exercise. Research supports the increased susceptibility to disease. Specifically, athletes engaging in marathon-type events or very intense physical training programs have been shown to be at a greater risk of upper respiratory tract infections (colds and flu).[28] In a study of 2,300 marathon runners, those who ran more than 100 kilometres per week suffered twice as many upper respiratory tract infections as those who ran fewer than 35 kilometres per week.[29]

Just how physical activity alters immunity is not well understood. We do know that moderate-intensity physical activity temporarily increases the number of white blood cells (WBCs), the blood cells responsible for fighting infection. An increased number of WBCs suggests increased immunity to disease and infection. How long does one have increased immunity? It is suggested that after 30 minutes or more of physical activity, WBCs may be elevated for 24 hours or more before returning to normal levels.[30]

## WHAT WOULD YOU DO?

Does your participation in physical activity benefit your immune system? How do you know?

## Improved Mental Health and Stress Management

People who engage in regular physical activity may be unaware of the beneficial physiological changes, but most notice the psychological benefits. While these psychological benefits are difficult to quantify, they are frequently mentioned as reasons for continuing to be physically active. Regular vigorous physical activity has been shown to "burn off" the chemical byproducts released by our nervous system during its normal response to stress. Elimination of these biochemicals reduces our stress response by accelerating the neurological system's return to a balanced state. For this reason, regular physical activity should be an integral component of your stress prevention and management plan.

Regular physical activity can improve physical appearance by toning and developing muscles and, combined with a healthy dietary intake, reducing body fat. Feeling good about personal appearance can provide a tremendous boost to self-esteem. Other improvements to self esteem are a result of learning new skills, developing increased ability in recreational activities, and "sticking" with a physical activity plan.

## WHAT WOULD YOU DO?

What makes you feel good about your participation in physical activity? Do you find it difficult to put into words or explain to others why it is that you regularly participate in physical activity?

## Improved Physical Fitness

**Physical fitness** is often defined as a set of health- or performance-related attributes related to the ability to engage in physical activity.[31] These health- and performance-related components are listed and described in Table 9.1. **Exercise** is a form of leisure physical activity that is planned, structured, and repetitive. Generally, exercise is done at a specified frequency and intensity, for a certain length of time, to achieve a desired level of physical fitness.[32] Although physical fitness has many facets, it is most commonly measured by the five interdependent health-related components: (1) cardiorespiratory endurance, (2) muscular strength, (3) muscular endurance, (4) flexibility, and (5) body composition.

## WHAT WOULD YOU DO?

Have you had your physical fitness assessed recently? Do you know where you can go to have it measured? Which components of your physical fitness would you like to improve or develop? What physical activities or exercises will you do to improve your physical fitness?

# IMPROVING CARDIORESPIRATORY ENDURANCE

The number of walkers, joggers, inline skaters, bicyclists, fitness class participants, and swimmers is tangible evidence of the awareness of an important aspect of physical fitness: **cardiorespiratory endurance.** Cardiorespiratory endurance or *cardiovascular fitness* refers to the ability of the heart, lungs, and blood vessels to function efficiently. Our very lives depend on our cardiorespiratory system's ability to deliver oxygenated blood and nutrients to our body tissues and to remove carbon dioxide and other metabolic waste

**TABLE 9.1**

**Health- and Performance-Related Components of Physical Fitness**

**Health**

| | |
|---|---|
| Cardiorespiratory endurance | Ability to sustain moderate-intensity whole-body activity for extended time periods |
| Muscular strength | Ability to apply maximum force with a single muscle contraction |
| Muscular endurance | Ability to perform muscle contractions repeatedly |
| Flexibility | Range of motion in a joint or series of joints |
| Body composition | Ratio of fat to total body weight |

**Performance**

| | |
|---|---|
| Agility | Speed in changing direction or in changing body positions |
| Power | Combination of strength and speed |
| Balance | Maintenance of a stable body position |
| Coordination | Ability to have things work together |
| Reaction time | Ability to adjust or "react" to stimuli |
| Speed | Ability to move quickly |

Source: Adapted from T. Baranowski, et al., "Assessment, Prevalence, and Cardiovascular Benefits of Physical Activity and Fitness in Youth," *Medicine and Science in Sports and Exercise* 24 (June 1992): supplement, S238.

products. The primary category of physical activity known to improve cardiorespiratory fitness is aerobic exercise. The term aerobic means "with oxygen" and describes any type of exercise, typically performed at moderate levels of intensity for extended periods of time, that increases your heart rate. Aerobic activities such as walking, jogging, bicycling, and swimming are among the best exercises for improving cardiorespiratory fitness.

**Aerobic power** is a term used to describe the current functional status of the cardiovascular system (that is, the heart, lungs, blood vessels) and refers specifically to the volume of oxygen consumed by the muscles during exercise. Maximal aerobic power (often referred to as $VO_2max$) refers to the maximal capacity of the cardiorespiratory system. The most common measure of maximal aerobic capacity is determined from a walk or run on a treadmill. In this test, an exercise physiologist or physician will initially ask you to walk or run at an easy pace, and then, at set time intervals gradually increase the workload (that is, a **graded exercise test** in which a combination of running speed and the angle of incline is used) to the point of maximal exertion. The higher your

cardiorespiratory endurance, the more oxygen you can transport to exercising muscles (higher $VO_2max$) and the longer you can maintain a high intensity of exercise before exhaustion. Other less valid, but reliable and safer, methods of measuring aerobic capacity are frequently employed and then used to estimate $VO_2max$. These submaximal tests may use stationary bicycles, walk/run tests, shuttle runs, or walk tests to quantify the aerobic fitness levels in people of all ages and of all abilities. You may have performed one of these aerobic capacity tests.

**Physical fitness:** A set of health- or performance-related attributes related to the ability to engage in physical activity.

**Exercise:** A form of leisure physical activity that is planned, structured, and repetitive.

**Cardiorespiratory endurance:** The ability of the heart, lungs, and blood vessels to function efficiently.

**Aerobic power:** The current functional status of a person's cardiorespiratory system; measured as $VO_2$ max and refers specifically to the volume of oxygen consumed by the muscles during exercise.

**Graded exercise test:** A test of aerobic capacity administered by a physician, exercise physiologist, or other trained person.

Progress slowly through a walking/jogging program at low intensities before you attempt to measure your aerobic capacity with one of these tests.

It is important for you to complete the Physical Activity Readiness Questionnaire (PAR-Q; available at www.csep.ca) prior to engaging in physical activity or any tests to measure your physical fitness.[33] If you answer yes to any of the questions on the PAR-Q or if you have certain medical conditions, such as asthma, diabetes, heart disease, or obesity, you should consult a physician to ensure that physical activity is safe for you.

# AEROBIC FITNESS PROGRAMS

Researchers tell us that a physically active lifestyle is the key to improved cardiorespiratory health, but what level of physical activity is required? There are many variables to consider: generally a comfortable aerobic physical activity that works your heart at a vigorous intensity (approximately 70 to 90 percent of your maximum heart rate, or about 140 to 180 beats per minute if you are a 20-year-old male) for prolonged periods of time (20 to 30 minutes of continuous activity) at least three days per week will improve your cardiorespiratory endurance. A heart rate between 70 and 90 percent of your heart rate maximum corresponds to a workload between 55 and 85 percent of your $VO_2max$.[34]

The most effective aerobic exercises for building cardiorespiratory endurance are total body activities involving the large muscle groups of your body. If you have been sedentary for quite a while, initiating a physical activity program may be a difficult challenge. The key is to begin slowly at a low intensity, progress . . . and stay with it! To start slowly, for example, if jogging is the physical activity you choose, you should alternate jogging and walking until you develop a fitness level that enables you to jog continuously for 15 to 30 minutes.

## Determining Exercise Frequency

If you are a newcomer to regular physical activity, the frequency of your aerobic exercise bouts should begin at three times per week. If you exercise less frequently, you will achieve fewer health benefits. Exercising three to five days per week is the general recommendation for improving cardiorespiratory endurance. Your ultimate goal should be to exercise five days a week. To avoid overuse injuries and monotony, vary your activities and take a day off when needed.

## Determining Exercise Intensity

An aerobic exercise program must employ prolonged, moderate-intensity physical activity to improve cardiorespiratory endurance. A common measure of exercise intensity is your heart rate. The exercise intensity required to improve cardiorespiratory endurance is a heart rate between 70 and 90 percent of your maximum heart rate. To calculate your **target heart rate,** subtract your age from 220 (for males) or 226 (for females). The result is your maximum heart rate ($HR_{max}$). You then determine your target heart rate by calculating the desired percentage of maximum heart rate; that is, 70 to 90 percent. If you are a 20-year-old male, your estimated maximum heart rate is 200 ($220 - 20 = 200$). Your target heart rate would be somewhere between 140 ($200 \times 0.70 = 140$) and 180 ($200 \times 0.90 = 180$). It is recommended that people who have been sedentary for a long time should set a lower target heart rate somewhere between 50 and 60 percent of their maximum. As their cardiorespiratory fitness improves, they can gradually increase their

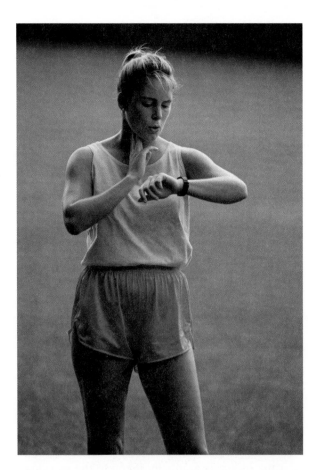

*Measure your heart rate during aerobic exercise to ensure that the intensity is sufficient to attain cardiorespiratory endurance benefits.*

target heart rate using small increments—for example, from 50 to 55 percent, then from 55 to 60 percent. It is not recommended for most people to exceed 90 percent of maximum heart rate.

Once you know your target heart rate, you can determine how close you are to this value during your workout. You'll need to stop exercising briefly to measure your heart rate. To take your pulse, lightly place your index and middle fingers (not your thumb) over one of the major (carotid) arteries in your neck, along either side of your Adam's apple, or on the artery on the inside of your wrist. Be sure to start counting your pulse immediately—the first count is "0"—after you stop exercising, as your heart rate decreases quickly. Using a watch or clock, take your pulse for 6 seconds and multiply this number by 10 (just add a zero to your count) to get the number of beats per minute. If necessary, increase or decrease the pace or intensity of your workout to achieve your target heart rate.

Another way to monitor your heart rate while exercising is to use a heart rate monitor. Various pieces of exercise equipment (treadmill, stepper, etc.) show your heart rate while you are using them. Keep in mind that there is a substantial percentage of error with this type of heart rate monitoring. It still may be useful to stop briefly and check your heart rate to ensure you are exercising in the target heart rate zone.

A target heart rate of 70 percent of maximum is sometimes called the "conversational level of exercise" because you are able to talk with a partner while exercising.[35] If you are breathing so hard that talking is difficult, the intensity of your exercise is too high. Conversely, if you are able to sing or laugh heartily while exercising, the intensity of your exercise is not sufficient for improving or maintaining cardiorespiratory endurance.

## Determining Exercise Time

*Time* refers to the number of minutes of exercise performed at the specified intensity during any one session. Every adult should accumulate 30 minutes or more of moderate-intensity physical activity over the course of most days of the week.[36] Activities that contribute to this 30-minute total include dancing, walking up stairs (instead of taking the elevator), gardening, and raking leaves as well as planned physical activities such as jogging, swimming, and cycling. One way to meet this recommendation is to walk three kilometres briskly every day.

You will need to adjust the frequency, intensity, and time of your aerobic activity program to accommodate your improving cardiorespiratory endurance. As you progress and are able to exercise for 20 minutes at 70 percent of your heart rate maximum for three days

per week, increase the frequency, time, or intensity of your exercise—but not all three at the same time. Generally, it is recommended to first increase the frequency of your workouts from 3 to 4 days per week, then from 4 to 5 days per week. Once you have adjusted to that change, it is recommended to increase the length of your exercise period from 20 to 25 minutes; then from 25 to 30 minutes. Again, once you have adjusted to that change, it is recommended that you increase the intensity of your workout from 70 to 90 percent of $HR_{max}$.

Your goal should be to expend 300 to 500 calories per day through leisure-time physical activity, with an eventual weekly goal of 1,500 to 2,100 calories. The lower the intensity of the activity, the longer the time you'll need to get the same caloric expenditure. If your preference is for lower-intensity physical activity, the recommendation changes to 60 minutes every day of the week.[37] It should be pointed out that whether the recommendation is for 30 minutes of moderate-intensity physical activity most days of the week or 60 minutes of light-intensity physical activity every day of the week, it is possible to accumulate these activities in 10-minute spurts. See the Focus on Canada box.

A physical activity program over several months or years—exercise training—improves the way your cardiorespiratory system meets your body's oxygen requirements at rest and during exercise and helps you to feel good about yourself. Keep in mind that the physiological health benefits associated with cardiorespiratory endurance activities (reduced blood pressure, decreased resting heart rate, etc.) take about one year of regular exercise to achieve.[38] However, any physical activity, even if it does not meet all the exercise characteristics mentioned in this chapter, will benefit your overall health and help you to feel better about yourself almost immediately.

### WHAT WOULD YOU DO?

Calculate your target heart rate for 50, 70, and 90 percent of your maximum heart rate. Engaging in a familiar physical activity and monitoring your pulse, experiment by exercising at the three different calculated intensities of exercise. Did you notice any difference in the way you felt while exercising? Afterward?

**Target heart rate:** Calculated as a percentage of maximum heart rate (220 [for males] 226 [for females] minus age); heart rate (pulse) is taken during aerobic exercise to check if exercise intensity is at the desired level (e.g., 70 percent of maximum heart rate).

# Physical Activity for Healthy Living: How Much Is Enough?

Similar to Canada's Food Guide to Healthy Eating, Canada's Physical Activity Guide to Healthy Active Living uses a rainbow approach to describe the amount and type of physical activities Canadians need for optimal health benefits.

The outside of the rainbow includes physical activities we need the most of—endurance activities. These activities should be engaged in 4 to 7 days per week, dependent upon the intensity of the activity, and are continuous in nature thus providing benefits to the heart, lungs, and circulatory system. Examples include cross-country skiing, taking the stairs instead of the elevator, cycling, walking, and mowing the lawn.

The intensity of the physical activities engaged in for cardiorespiratory endurance significantly influences the frequency and time needed for health benefits. If your preferred physical activities involve light effort such as slow-paced walking, stretching, or easy gardening, you need 60 minutes 7 days a week. If the physical activities you engage in are of a moderate effort, such as brisk walking, biking, raking leaves, swimming, or dancing, you need 30 to 60 minutes at least 4 days per week. If your preference is for "workout" kinds of physical activities, then you need 20 to 30 minutes 3 days per week. Examples of workout activities include fitness classes, jogging, fast swimming, or fast dancing. Combinations of physical activities of various intensities can also lead to optimal health benefits.

The next arc of the rainbow describes the type of physical activity that we need the next most of—flexibility activities. It is also recommended that we obtain these types of activities 4 to 7 times per week. These types of physical activities are described as "gentle reaching, bending and stretching activities to keep your muscles relaxed and joints mobile." Examples include various stretches that are often done after other types of physical activities.

The third arc of the rainbow is for strength activities, which should be done 2 to 4 days per week. These activities will strengthen muscles and bones as well as improve posture. Examples include weight training with hand-held weights, body-weight resistance exercise (curl-ups and push-ups), as well as walking with backpacks.

The last arc of the rainbow describes activities we should try to reduce. Examples included in this arc of the rainbow are sedentary activities such as watching television or movies, and working or playing on a computer.

## STUDY QUESTIONS

1. Identify the practical, economic, and environmental roadblocks that make it difficult to maintain a physically active lifestyle in Canada. Suggest potential solutions.

2. Describe ways that Canadians of all ages—children, adolescents, young adults, and older adults—could begin to incorporate more physical activity into their lives. When answering this question, consider each demographic group in a rural, urban, and suburban environment.

3. What could the various levels of government (federal, provincial, municipal) do to enhance the physical activity of Canadians? Should the private sector also get involved? How?

Source: Adapted from Public Health Agency of Canada, *Canada's Physical Activity Guide to Healthy Living*, Cat. No. H39-429/1998-2E. Canada's Physical Activity Guide to Healthy Living can be downloaded from www.phac-aspc.gc.ca/pau-uap/paguide/index.html.

# IMPROVING MUSCULAR STRENGTH AND ENDURANCE

**Muscular strength** refers to the maximal amount of force a muscle is capable of exerting in one contraction. The most common way to assess strength is to measure the maximum amount of weight you can lift one time. This value is known as the **one repetition maximum (1RM).** Your 1RM can also be predicted from a 10RM test.[39] **Muscular endurance** is defined as a muscle's ability to exert force repeatedly without fatiguing or the ability to sustain a muscular contraction. The more repetitions of a certain resistance exercise you can perform successfully (for example, push-ups) or the longer you can hold a certain position (for example, flexed arm hang), the greater your muscular endurance. Muscular endurance is often measured from the number of curl-ups or push-ups an individual can do.

# Principles of Strength Development

There are three key principles to follow if you intend to train or exercise to increase your muscular strength and endurance.[40]

## The Tension Principle

The key to developing strength is to create sufficient tension within a muscle. The more tension you can create in a muscle, the greater your strength gain will be. The most common recreational way to create tension in a muscle is by lifting weights. While weight lifting is one method of producing tension in a muscle, any activity that creates muscle tension—for example, using your body weight (push-ups or pull-ups) or riding a bicycle up a steep hill—will result in greater strength. It really does not matter what type of resistance you choose to develop tension in your muscles; what matters is that you use the resistance in such a way as to produce the desired improvements in muscular strength and endurance.

## The Overload Principle

The overload principle is the most important of the three key principles for improving muscular strength. Everyone begins a resistance training program with an initial level of strength. To increase that level of strength, you must regularly create a degree of tension in your muscles greater than what they are accustomed to. This overloading of your muscles will cause them to adapt to the level of overload by getting larger (**hypertrophy**) and stronger, thus capable of generating more tension. Figure 9.1 illustrates how a continual process of overload and adaptation to the overload improves strength. If you fail to provide an overload—if you "underload" your muscles—you will not increase your strength. Alternatively, if you create too great an overload, you may experience muscle injury, muscle fatigue, and even a loss of strength. Once you reach your strength goal, no further overloading is necessary. Your next challenge is to maintain that level of strength by continuing to engage in a regular (once or twice per week) total-body resistance exercise program.

## The Specificity of Training Principle

This principle refers to the manner in which a specific body system responds to the physiological demands placed upon it. According to the specificity principle, you'll get a very specific response to the physical

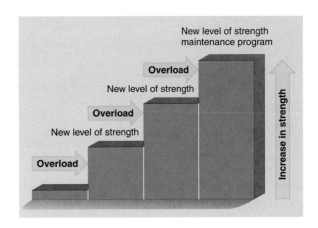

## FIGURE 9.1

The overload principle must be followed to increase strength or endurance. Notice that once the muscle has adapted to the original overload, a new overload must be placed on the muscle for subsequent gains in strength or endurance to occur.

Source: From Philip A. Sienna, *One Rep Max: A Guide to Beginning Weight Training*, Fig. 2.1, 8. © 1989. Wm. C. Brown Communications, Inc., Dubuque, Iowa. Reprinted by permission of Times Mirror Higher Education Group, Inc., Dubuque, Iowa. All rights reserved.

activities or exercises you do. If the specific overload you impose is designed to improve strength in the muscles of your chest and back, the response to that demand (overload) will be improved strength in the chest and back, not in the overall body. Therefore, to improve overall or total body strength, you must include exercises for all the major muscle groups. You must also ensure your overload is sufficient to increase strength rather than endurance.

# Types of Muscle Contractions

When your skeletal muscles receive a stimulus from your nervous system to contract, they respond by developing tension and producing a measurable force.

**Muscular strength:** The maximal amount of force that a muscle is capable of exerting.

**One repetition maximum (1RM):** The amount of weight/resistance that can be lifted/moved only once; a common measure of strength.

**Muscular endurance:** A muscle's ability to exert force repeatedly or to sustain a contraction without fatiguing.

**Hypertrophy:** Increased size (girth) of a muscle.

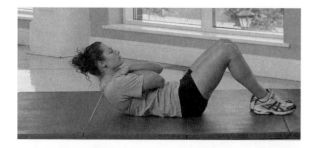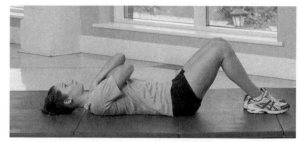

*These photographs illustrate concentric and eccentric muscle actions. In the first photo, the abdominal muscles lengthen while producing tension as the body returns to its starting position. This is known as an eccentric muscle action. In the second photo, the abdominal muscles shorten while producing tension in the lifting phase of a curl-up. This is called a concentric muscle action.*

Your skeletal muscles contract in three different modes—isometric, concentric, and eccentric—to produce this force.[41] An **isometric muscle contraction** is one in which force is produced by the muscle without any muscle movement. Isometric muscle actions do not create joint motion. Muscles act isometrically to stabilize a particular body part while another body part is moving, or when a maximal resistance is met and the force produced by your muscles cannot overcome the resistance. One example of an isometric muscle action is the unsuccessful attempt to push a car out of snow or mud. Although you push with all your might, the car (as well as your joints) does not move. The muscles involved are producing force in an isometric way. Another example related to resistance training is trying to lift a barbell that's too heavy for you. The more you try, the more tired your muscles become, but the barbell never leaves the floor. Isometric muscle contractions are important because they are involved in maintaining body stability. Maintaining your balance and body alignments while holding the top part of a push-up is another example of isometric muscle contractions.

A **concentric muscle contraction** is one in which force is produced while the muscle shortens. Joint movement is always produced during concentric muscle actions. Raising the body in a curl-up is an example of a concentric action of the abdominal muscles. Usually, but not always, concentric muscle contractions produce movement in a direction opposite to the downward pull of gravity.

**Eccentric muscle contraction** describes a muscle's ability to produce force while lengthening. Typically, eccentric muscle contractions occur when movement is in the same direction as the pull of gravity. If you want to be sure that a given resistance exercise has an eccentric phase, you must use the type of resistance that requires you to achieve the starting position

before your next repetition. For example, in a curl-up, you lower your upper body slowly to the starting point of the exercise in an eccentric contraction of the abdominal muscles.

All factors being equal, the greatest amount of force is produced during eccentric muscle contractions, followed by isometric and then concentric muscle contractions. Changes in muscle size and strength are affected by the type of resistance exercise and by the type of muscle contraction(s) you use during your workout. When using free weights (barbells, dumbbells), the typical sequential pattern of concentric–eccentric muscle contractions during resistance training contributes to improved muscle strength and muscle fibre size. If your resistance exercise program uses only concentric muscle contractions, you'll need to perform at least twice as many concentric-only repetitions to achieve the same results as you would attain by using concentric–eccentric combinations.[42]

## Methods of Providing Resistance

There are four commonly used methods of applying resistance to develop muscular strength and endurance.

### Body Weight Resistance

Many different techniques can be used to develop skeletal muscle fitness without relying on exercise equipment. Most of these methods use part or all of your body weight as resistance during exercise. For many individuals these techniques can be as effective as external resistance in developing and maintaining muscular strength and endurance. Most of these exercises (curl-ups, push-ups, and pull-ups) require your muscles to lift your body weight off the floor and involve concentric and eccentric muscle contractions.

## Fixed Resistance

Fixed resistance exercises provide a constant resistance throughout the full range of movement. Barbells and dumbbells provide fixed resistance because their weight (amount of resistance) does not change as you exercise. However, due to the biomechanics of human motion, the muscle forces that must be exerted to move the weight are lower at some joint angles and higher at others. Any given muscle generates its least amount of force at the beginning and ending positions of a resistance exercise and can create the most force when the joint involved in the exercise approximates a right angle (90 degrees). As a result, the disadvantage of fixed resistance exercises is that the extent to which a muscle is overloaded varies throughout the exercise, and the exercise may not fully develop the muscle.

## Variable Resistance

Whether found at a health club or in your home workout area, variable resistance equipment alters the resistance encountered by a muscle at all joint angles so that the effort by the muscle is consistent throughout the full range of motion. Variable resistance machines are typically single-station devices (for example, Nautilus), but some have multiple stations at which muscles of the upper and lower extremities can be exercised (for example, Soloflex).

## Accommodating Resistance

With accommodating resistance devices, the resistance changes according to the amount of force generated by the individual. There is no external weight to move or overcome. Resistance is provided by having the exerciser perform at maximal level of effort, while the exercise machine controls the speed of the exercise and does not allow any faster motion. The body segment being exercised must move at a rate faster than or equal to the set speed to encounter resistance. One way to distinguish between accommodating and variable resistance is to recall that with variable resistance, the resistance increases from the beginning to the end of the repetition. In contrast, accommodating resistance can become more or less difficult depending on the input (muscular force exerted by the exerciser) into the machine.[43]

# Getting Started

You will find some general principles useful whatever your strength training goals. If sufficient tension is generated within a muscle, it will respond by becoming stronger regardless of the type of muscle action or resistance used. To design your program, you need to determine your 1RM for each muscle or muscle group you plan to exercise. Then, using your results, you need to develop specific training goals as well as the strategies to achieve those goals.

## Strength Training

There are almost as many ways to develop muscular strength as there are participants in strength training programs. Given the specificity principle, it is important to select at least one resistance exercise for each major muscle group in the body to develop total body strength. Generally, strength training exercises are done in a set, or a series of multiple repetitions using the same resistance. For increases in muscular strength, you should perform a relatively low number of repetitions of each exercise using relatively high resistance. Therefore, to improve strength, the amount of resistance should be at least 60 percent or greater of the 1RM for a given exercise, with 3 to 6 repetitions of the exercise performed per set.[44] Generally, a resistance that you can move or lift only 8 to 10 times is a good place to start.

Since resistance training exercises cause microscopic damage (tears) to muscle fibres and the rebuilding process that increases the size and capacity of the muscle takes about 24 to 48 hours, resistance training programs should incorporate at least one day of rest (and recovery) between workouts to allow the muscle groups to adapt. Thus, the recommended frequency of programs to build muscular strength is 2 to 4 days per week.[45]

## Muscular Endurance Training

In contrast to improving strength, increases in muscular endurance are achieved by performing a relatively high number of repetitions with a relatively low resistance. Thus, muscular endurance is improved from 10 to 15 repetitions of exercises with an intensity of less than 60 percent of 1RM.[46] Instead of using traditional resistance exercise equipment to develop muscular endurance, consider adding variety to your training program with devices equipped with an ergometer,

---

**Isometric muscle contraction:** Force produced without muscle movement.

**Concentric muscle contraction:** Force produced while shortening the muscle.

**Eccentric muscle contraction:** Force produced while lengthening the muscle.

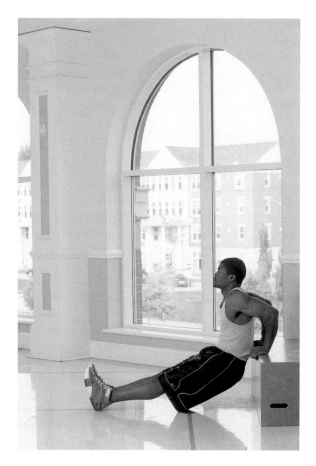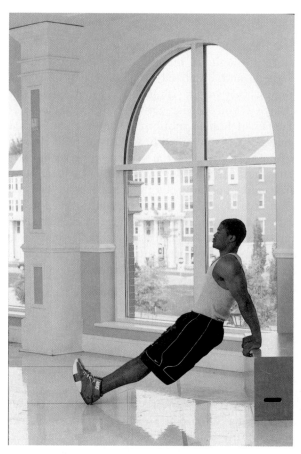

*Using your body weight can be an effective way to build or maintain muscular strength and endurance.*

such as a stationary bicycle, rowing machine, or stair-climbing machine. With these and other devices, you can control the cadence of the activity and/or adjust the amount of resistance you encounter. Performing numerous repetitions during a 20-minute (or longer) workout using a relatively low resistance will quickly develop muscular endurance in the muscles exercised. Other activities that build muscular endurance include hiking, wall climbing, jogging, and cycling. This type of workout will also have cardiorespiratory benefits if you select an intensity that allows you to reach your target heart rate.

No one resistance-exercise program is perfect for everyone. Experiment with different types of resistance exercises and programs to find what works best for you. Once you gain strength and endurance, they are fairly easy to maintain. Maintenance resistance training consists of one to two total body workouts per week. You can consult a fitness professional or hire a credentialed personal trainer to set up a program to meet your personal needs.

## WHAT WOULD YOU DO?

Why is it important to focus on your muscular strength and endurance? What daily activities require strength and endurance? What type of resistance training program would work best for you? Do you require access to equipment and facilities to engage in this type of program? If so, do you know where to go?

# IMPROVING YOUR FLEXIBILITY

**Flexibility** refers to the range of motion, or the amount of movement possible, at a particular joint or series of joints. Although this component of fitness is

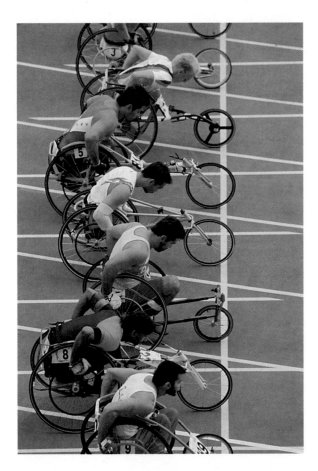

It is important for people with physical disabilities to develop optimal levels of cardiorespiratory endurance, muscular strength and endurance, and flexibility to enable participation in physical activities they enjoy—including competitive sports.

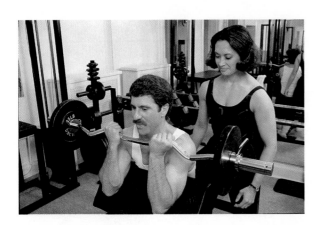

Lifting free weights to build muscular strength and endurance has many advantages

often overshadowed by muscular strength and aerobic capacity, it should not be overlooked given that muscles that lack elasticity and resiliency are more susceptible to injury. Improving your range of motion through stretching exercises will enhance your efficiency of movement and your posture. A regular program of stretching exercises can also enhance psychological well-being.

## Types of Stretching Exercises

Flexibility is enhanced by the controlled stretching of muscles that act on a particular joint. The primary strategy is to decrease the resistance to stretch (tension) within a tight muscle that you have targeted for increased range of motion.[47] To do this, you repeatedly stretch the muscle and its two tendons of attachment to elongate them.

The safest exercises for improving flexibility use **static stretching.** Static stretching techniques involve the slow, gradual lengthening of a muscle or group of muscles. Various positions and postures are used to lengthen the tight muscle or muscle group to a point where tension (mild discomfort) is felt within the muscle. This end position is held for 10 to 30 seconds, and is repeated two or three times in close succession for each muscle or muscle group. With each repetition of a static stretch, range of motion improves temporarily and when this static stretching is done regularly range of motion increases for longer periods of time. Stretching regularly (on at least four, and preferably seven, days a week) will effectively result in this permanent elongation of the targeted muscle or muscle group and permit a greater range of motion at a given joint. See the diagrams in Figure 9.2 for suggested exercises to stretch all the major muscle groups of your body.

### WHAT WOULD YOU DO?

Why is it important to have good flexibility throughout life? What are some situations in which a better range of motion would help you perform daily activities with less effort? What specific actions will you take to improve your flexibility?

**Flexibility:** The range of motion, or the amount of movement possible, at a particular joint or series of joints.

**Static stretching:** Assuming a position for 10 to 30 seconds in which there is a gradual lengthening of a muscle (to the point of tension).

# FITNESS INJURIES

Overtraining is the most frequent cause of injuries associated with developing physical fitness. While participating in your personal fitness program, listen to your body's warning signs. Muscle stiffness and soreness, bone and joint pains, and whole-body fatigue are a few of the common warning signs of an impending overuse injury. One strategy to prevent overuse injury is to vary your physical activities throughout the week to give muscles and joints a rest. Setting appropriate and realistic short- and long-term training goals is another good strategy that may help prevent overtraining.

## Causes of Fitness-Related Injuries

There are two basic types of injuries stemming from participation in fitness training–related activities: overuse and traumatic. **Overuse injuries** occur because of cumulative, day-after-day stresses placed on body parts (tendons, bones, and ligaments). The forces that occur normally during physical activity are not enough to cause a ligament sprain or muscle strain, but when these forces are applied on a daily basis for weeks or months they can result in an injury. That is why people who sustain this type of injury typically cannot pinpoint a particular time or day when they were injured. Common sites of overuse injuries are the leg, knee, shoulder, and elbow joints.

**Traumatic injuries,** which occur suddenly and violently, typically by accident, are the second major type of fitness training–related injuries. Typical traumatic injuries are broken bones, torn ligaments and muscles, contusions, and lacerations. Most traumatic injuries are unavoidable—for example, spraining your ankle by landing on another person's foot after jumping up for a rebound in basketball. If your traumatic injury causes a noticeable loss of function and immediate pain or pain that does not go away after 30 minutes, you should have a physician examine it.

## Prevention

To prevent overuse or traumatic injuries, it is important to examine the equipment that you use—both the actual exercise equipment, and the footwear that you exercise in.

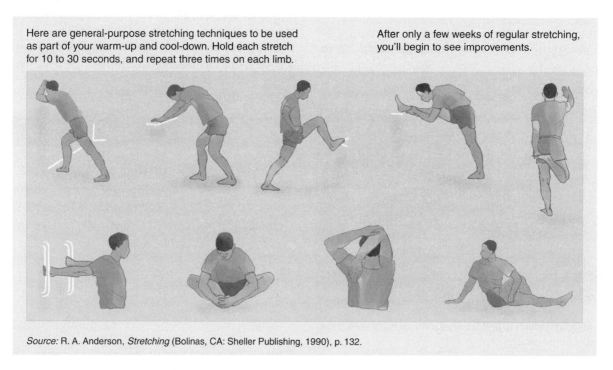

Here are general-purpose stretching techniques to be used as part of your warm-up and cool-down. Hold each stretch for 10 to 30 seconds, and repeat three times on each limb.

After only a few weeks of regular stretching, you'll begin to see improvements.

*Source:* R. A. Anderson, *Stretching* (Bolinas, CA: Sheller Publishing, 1990), p. 132.

## FIGURE 9.2

### Stretching Exercises That Will Help You Improve Your Flexibility

Source: Excerpted from *Stretching,* © 1980 by Bob and Jean Anderson. $12.00 Shelter Publications, Inc., P.O. Box 279, Bolinas, CA 94924. Distributed in bookstores by Random House. Reprinted by permission.

## Appropriate Footwear

When you purchase running shoes, look for several key components. Biomechanics research has revealed that running is a "collision" sport—that is, the runner's foot collides with the ground with a force three to five times the runner's body weight with each stride.[48] The 68-kilogram runner who takes 620 strides per kilometre might apply a cumulative force to his or her body of 127,000 kilograms per kilometre. The force not absorbed by the running shoe is transmitted upward into the foot, leg, thigh, and back. Our bodies are able to absorb forces such as these, but may be injured by the cumulative effects of repetitive impacts (for example, running 65 kilometres per week). Therefore, the ability of running shoes to absorb shock is a critical factor to consider when you purchase footwear for your physical activities. It is also important to replace footwear regularly (after running 1,000 or so kilometres) to ensure the shock absorbency is still effective. Other physical activities or sports (basketball, soccer, cycling, mountain climbing) require different footwear performance, and the requirements of the physical activity or sport should be considered when you prepare yourself to engage in that activity or sport.

## Appropriate Exercise Equipment

It is essential to use correctly fitted, appropriate athletic equipment for your physical activities. For some activities, there is specialized protective equipment that will reduce your chances of injury. In tennis, for example, the use of proper equipment helps prevent the general inflammatory condition known as tennis elbow. Excessive racquet string tension, repetitive use of the forearm muscles during hours of daily practice, and poor flexibility cause this problem in experienced tennis players. To avoid tennis elbow, consult an instructor or skilled salesperson to assist you in selecting the correct tennis racquet and string tension for you.

Eye injuries can occur in virtually all physical activities, though the risk of injury is much greater in some activities than others. As many as 90 percent of the eye injuries resulting from racquetball and squash are preventable with appropriate eye protection—for example, goggles with polycarbonate lenses.[49]

According to the Canadian Cycling Association, cycling is one of the most popular recreational activities in Canada and continues to grow every year. The selection of the right-size bicycle frame and seat height, coupled with the use of a bicycle helmet, padded grips/handlebars, and padded biking gloves, can significantly reduce injuries. In the past, head injuries accounted for 85 percent of all deaths attributable to bicycle accidents; however, the wearing of bicycle helmets has significantly reduced the number of skull fractures and facial injuries among recreational cyclists.[50] All cyclists should wear bicycle helmets that meet the criteria established by the Canadian Standards Association.

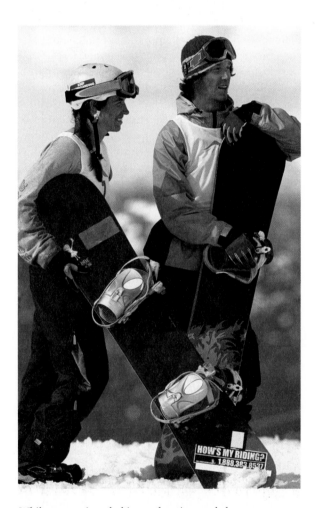

*While appropriate clothing and equipment help prevent injuries in any physical activity, a workout partner is also an important safeguard.*

**Overuse injuries:** Injuries that result from the cumulative effects of day-after-day stresses placed on tendons, muscles, and joints.

**Traumatic injuries:** Injuries that are usually accidental in nature and occur suddenly and violently (e.g., fractured bones, ruptured tendons, and sprained ligaments).

# Common Overuse Injuries

Body movements in physical activities such as running, swimming, and bicycling are highly repetitive, so participants who engage regularly in these activities are susceptible to overuse injuries. In most physical activities, the joints of the lower extremities (foot, ankle, knee, and hip) tend to be injured more frequently than the upper-extremity joints (shoulder, elbow, wrist, and hand). Three most common injuries from repetitive strain during physical activity are plantar fasciitis, "shin splints," and "runner's knee."

## Plantar Fasciitis

Plantar fasciitis is an inflammation of the plantar fascia, a broad band of dense, inelastic tissue (fascia) that runs from the heel to the toe on the bottom of your foot. The main function of the plantar fascia is to protect the nerves, blood vessels, and muscles of the foot from injury. In repetitive, weight-bearing activities such as walking and running, the plantar fascia may become inflamed. Common symptoms of this condition are pain and tenderness under the ball of the foot, at the heel, or at both locations. The pain of plantar fasciitis is particularly noticeable during your first steps out of bed in the morning. If not treated properly, this injury may progress in severity to the point that weight-bearing exercise is too painful to endure. Uphill running is not advised for anyone suffering from this condition, since each uphill stride severely stretches (and thus irritates) the already inflamed plantar fascia. This injury can often be prevented by regularly stretching the plantar fascia prior to exercise and by wearing athletic shoes with good arch support and shock absorbency. The plantar fascia are stretched by slowly pulling all five toes upward toward your head, holding for 10 to 15 seconds, and repeating this three to five times on each foot before exercising.

## Shin Splints

Shin splints is a general term for any pain that occurs on the front part of the lower legs. More than 20 different medical conditions have been identified within the broad description of shin splints. Problems range from stress fractures of the tibia (shinbone) to severe inflammation in the muscular compartments of the lower leg, which can interrupt the flow of blood and nerve supply to the foot. The most common type of shin splints occurs along the inner side of the tibia and is usually a combination of a muscle irritation and irritation of the tissues that attach the muscles to the bone in this region. Typically, there is pain and swelling along the middle one-third of the postero-medial tibia in the soft tissues, not the bone.

Sedentary people who start a new weight-bearing physical activity program are at the greatest risk for shin splints, though well-conditioned aerobic exercisers who rapidly increase their distance or pace may also develop them.[51] Running and exercise classes are the most frequent cause of shin splints, but those who do a great deal of walking (for example, restaurant wait staff) may also develop this injury.

To help prevent shin splints, wear shoes with good arch support and shock absorbency. If the severity of this lower-leg condition increases to the point that you cannot comfortably complete your desired physical activity, see your physician. Specific pain on the tibia or on the fibula (the adjacent, smaller bone) should be examined by a doctor for possible stress fracture. Reducing the frequency, intensity, and time of weight-bearing exercises may be required. You may also be advised to substitute a non–weight bearing activity such as swimming, cycling, or rowing during your recovery period.

## Runner's Knee

An overuse condition known as runner's knee describes a series of problems involving the muscles, tendons, and ligaments of the knee. The most common problem identified as runner's knee is abnormal movement of the patella (kneecap).[52] Women are more commonly affected by this condition than men because of their anatomical structure. Specifically, their wider pelvis results in a lateral pull on the patella by the muscles that act at the knee. In women (and some men), this causes irritation to the cartilage on the back of the patella as well as to the nearby tendons and ligaments.

The main symptom of this kind of runner's knee is the pain experienced when downward pressure is applied to the patella after the knee is straightened fully. Additional symptoms may include swelling, redness, and tenderness around the patella, and a dull, aching pain felt in the centre of the knee.[53] If you have these symptoms, your physician will probably recommend that you stop running for a few weeks and reduce daily physical activities that put compressive forces on the patella (for example, exercise on a stair-climbing machine or doing squats with heavy resistance) until you no longer feel any pain around your kneecap.

## Treatment

First-aid treatment for virtually all physical activity-related injuries involves **RICE:** rest, ice, compression, and elevation. *Rest* is required to eliminate the risk of further irritating the injured body part. *Ice* is applied to relieve the pain of the injury and to

# Evaluating Sources of Health Information

A quick glance at national newspaper headlines, magazine cover stories, nightly television news programs, and the Internet shows how popular it has become to engage in exercises not only to improve health but also to shape one's body. Led by the desire of our aging population to remain physically fit and healthy, there is seemingly no end to the information available. However, the quality of information runs the gamut from physical activity trends, exercise fads, and weight-loss gadgets, to increasingly simplified ways to get fit in the shortest amount of time possible. Take time to carefully consider the original source of the information and the context in which it is presented.

Popular health and fitness magazines can be good sources of information about exercise techniques, program design variables, and training regimens for individuals at all skill levels. However, you must closely examine a magazine's masthead to identify whether or not the editors, staff, and writers have relevant qualifications. A high-quality, reputable health and fitness magazine will complement its staff of professional journalists with a variety of experts in the field—exercise editors, science editors, medical editors, and/or health editors—who hold advanced degrees in their fields and maintain their credentials through membership in highly regarded professional associations. The same goes for television, newspapers, and the Internet. The quality of the experts associated with each story or media outlet will be a fairly accurate indicator of the quality of the information. Are the "experts" celebrities and/or consumers who have experienced tremendous results from a particular product? Or are they top researchers and scientists with recognized credentials from universities, colleges, and professional associations?

Look for these credentials when assessing the expertise of a source on physical activity and exercise:

B.Sc. or B.A.—Bachelor of Science or Bachelor of Arts degree in human kinetics, kinesiology, human movement, or related exercise science fields.

M.Sc. (M.S. if U.S. source)—Master of Science in an exercise science–related field

Ph.D.—Doctor of Philosophy in an exercise science–related field

M.D.—Medical doctor

C.S.C.S.—Certified Strength and Conditioning Specialist (National Strength and Conditioning Association www.nsca-cc.org)

ACSM (American College of Sports Medicine)—Exercise Specialist (www.acsm.org)

CSEP (Canadian Society of Exercise Physiology)—Exercise Specialist (www.csep.ca).

constrict the blood vessels to reduce internal or external bleeding associated with the injury. To prevent frost bite or other irritation to the skin, do not apply ice cubes, reusable gel ice packs, chemical cold packs, or other forms of cold directly to your skin. Instead, place a layer of wet towelling between the ice and your skin. Ice should be applied to a new injury for approximately 20 minutes every hour for the first 24 to 72 hours. *Compression* of the injured body part can be accomplished with a 10- or 15-centimetre-wide elastic bandage; this applies indirect pressure to damaged blood vessels to help stop bleeding. Be careful, though, that the compression wrap does not interfere with normal blood flow. A throbbing, painful hand or foot indicates that the compression wrap was applied too tightly and should be loosened. *Elevation* of the injured extremity above the level of the heart also helps to control internal or external bleeding by making the blood flow uphill to reach the injured area.

## WHAT WOULD YOU DO?

Given what you've read about the symptoms of common physical activity–related injuries, are you currently at risk of developing any overuse injuries? If so, what specific actions can you take to prevent these problems from getting more serious?

**RICE:** Acronym for the standard first-aid treatment for injuries: rest, ice, compression, and elevation.

## Exercising in the Heat

For physical activities outside, the function of your exercise clothing should be far more important than the fashion statement it makes. For some types of physical activity, you will need clothing that allows maximal body heat dissipation—for example, light-coloured nylon shorts and mesh tank top while running in hot weather. For other types, you will need clothing that permits significant heat retention without getting you sweat-soaked—for example, layers of polypropylene and/or wool clothing while cross-country skiing.

Exercising in hot or humid temperatures increases your risk of a heat-related injury. However, if you are in good physical condition, wear appropriate clothing, and drink plenty of fluids, you can safely withstand a wide range of temperatures and humidity levels when engaging in physical activity. Heat stress, which includes several potentially fatal illnesses resulting from elevated core body temperatures, should be a concern when exercising in warm, humid weather. In these conditions, your body's rate of heat production often exceeds its ability to cool itself. You can prevent heat stress by following certain precautions. First, acclimatize yourself properly to hot and/or humid climate. The process of heat acclimatization, which increases your body's cooling efficiency, requires about 10 to 14 days of gradually increased exercise in a hot environment. Second, avoid dehydration by replacing fluids before, during, and after exercise. Third, wear clothing appropriate for the activity and the environment. Finally, use common sense when exercising in hot and humid conditions—for example, when the temperature is 30°C and the humidity 90 percent, postpone your usual lunchtime run until the cool of evening or re-schedule for the early morning.

The three different heat stress illnesses progressive in their level of severity are: heat cramps, heat exhaustion, and heat stroke. The least serious problem, heat-related muscle cramps (**heat cramps**), is easily prevented by adequate fluid replacement and a dietary intake that includes the electrolytes lost during sweating (sodium and potassium). **Heat exhaustion** is most often caused by excessive water loss because of intense or prolonged exercise or work in a warm and/or humid environment. Symptoms of heat exhaustion include nausea, headache, fatigue, dizziness and faintness, and, paradoxically, "goosebumps" and chills. If you are suffering from heat exhaustion, your skin will be cool and moist. Heat exhaustion is actually a mild form of shock, in which the blood pools in the arms and legs away from the brain and major organs of the body, causing nausea and fainting. **Heat stroke,** often called sunstroke, is a

life-threatening emergency condition with a 20- to 70-percent death rate.[54] Heat stroke occurs during vigorous exercise when the body's heat production significantly exceeds its cooling capacity. Body core temperature can rise from normal (37°C) to 40.5°C to 43°C within minutes after the body's cooling mechanism shuts down. With no cooling taking place, rapidly increasing core temperatures can cause brain damage, permanent disability, and death. Common signs of heat stroke are dry, hot, and usually red skin, very high body temperature, and a very rapid heart rate.

Heat stress illnesses may occur in situations in which the danger is not obvious. Serious or fatal heat stroke may result from prolonged sauna or steam baths, prolonged total immersion in a hot tub or spa, or by exercising in a plastic or rubber head-to-toe "sauna suit." If you experience any of the symptoms mentioned here while exercising, stop immediately, move to the shade or a cool spot to rest, and drink plenty of cool fluids.

## Exercising in the Cold

When you are physically active in cool or cold weather, especially in windy conditions, your body's heat loss is frequently greater than its heat production. Under these conditions, **hypothermia**—a potentially fatal condition resulting from abnormally low body core temperature, which occurs when body heat is lost faster than it is produced—may result. Hypothermia can occur as a result of prolonged, vigorous exercise (for example, snowboarding or rugby) in 4°C to 10°C temperatures, particularly if there is rain, snow, or a strong wind.

As your body core temperature drops from the normal 37°C to 34°C, you will begin to shiver. Shivering—the involuntary contraction of nearly every muscle in your body—is designed to increase your body temperature by generating heat through muscle activity. During this first stage of hypothermia, you may also experience cold hands and feet, poor judgment, apathy, and amnesia.[55] Shivering ceases in most hypothermia victims as their body core temperatures drop to between 32°C and 30°C, a sign that the body has lost its ability to generate heat. Death from hypothermia usually occurs at core body temperatures between 26.5°C and 24°C.

To prevent hypothermia, follow these common-sense guidelines: analyze weather conditions and your risk of hypothermia before you undertake your planned outdoor physical activity, remembering that wind and humidity are as significant as temperature; use the "buddy system"—that is, have a friend join you for your cold-weather outdoor activities; wear layers of appropriate clothing to prevent excessive heat loss (for example, polypropylene or woolen undergarments, Gore-Tex® windbreaker, and wool hat and gloves); and, finally, don't allow yourself to become dehydrated.

# PLANNING YOUR PHYSICAL FITNESS TRAINING PROGRAM

## Identifying Your Physical Fitness Goals

Before you start a physical fitness training program, take the time to analyze your individual health and fitness needs, limitations, physical activity likes and dislikes, daily schedule, and goals. Whatever your primary reason is, your most important goal should be to become committed to physical activity and physical fitness for the long haul, by establishing a realistic schedule of diverse physical activities that you can maintain and enjoy throughout your life.

Once you commit yourself to being physically active, you must decide what type of program is best suited to your needs. The amounts and types of exercises required to yield beneficial results vary with the age and physical condition of the exerciser. (Regardless of age, it is wise before engaging in physical activity to complete the PAR-Q and consult your physician if you respond yes to any of the questions.) Fitness can be viewed as a continuum running from low levels to peak performance (in athletic, health-related, work-related, or functional day-to-day activities). You can further categorize your training level as basic, intermediate, or advanced. Thus, you should achieve an intermediate to advanced level of general fitness before moving on to peak performance-related goals.

It is useful to map your journey by identifying your current physical fitness and indicating your end goal. Your program should reflect your initial positioning while addressing your individual strengths and weaknesses so that you can move along the chart stage by stage as you pursue your goals.

## Designing Your Physical Fitness Program

To optimize your physical fitness training, you need to develop a workout schedule that is challenging yet realistic. An important step in adopting a new behaviour is developing a routine, and care must be taken to ensure that you do not set yourself up for failure before you begin by choosing an overly ambitious schedule. If you decide to walk six times per week, but are able to complete only four sessions, you might feel you failed to achieve what you set out to accomplish. However, if you walk four times per week for several months, you would have achieved a significant change in behaviours and success. It is very important to set yourself up for success by making your goals realistic and achievable—success in meeting and exceeding your short-term goals will give you the positive energy and confidence to move forward with your program and reach your long-term goals.

It is also important to keep a record of your workouts. Even something as simple as putting checkmarks on your calendar on the days you exercise will help to keep you motivated. You will quickly see whether or not you are sticking to your schedule. More detailed records will provide positive feedback and motivation by allowing you to look back to see where you started and how much you have progressed over time. Also, it is important to regularly reassess your progress—about every six to eight weeks—and adjust your program accordingly. The human body is incredibly good at adapting to stress, and unless you keep overloading your body on a continuous basis your initial progress will quickly plateau. You must consciously increase the intensity or volume (quantity) of your workouts over time to continue to make gains. Detailed records allow you to make good decisions about the direction of your training program.

Your training program can be as simple as outlining which days you will exercise each week, and for how long—leaving the decision as to what type of activity you will do, or where, for that day. Alternately, you can develop a long-term program where nothing is left to chance, and each set of variables is carefully calculated and managed. Whatever your approach, all good fitness programs should address the major components of physical fitness—cardiorespiratory endurance, muscle strength and endurance, and flexibility. For additional information on putting together a physical activity program, download or view Canada's Physical Activity Guide at www.phac-aspc.gc.ca/pau-uap/paguide/index.html.

**Heat cramps:** Muscle cramps that occur during or following exercise in warm/hot conditions.

**Heat exhaustion:** A heat stress illness caused by significant dehydration resulting from exercise in warm/hot conditions; frequent precursor to heat stroke.

**Heat stroke:** A deadly heat stress illness resulting from dehydration and overexertion in warm/hot conditions; can cause body core temperature to rise from normal to 40.5°C to 43°C in just a few minutes.

**Hypothermia:** A potentially fatal condition resulting from abnormally low body core temperature.

## Warm-up and Cool-down

Every exercise session should begin with a warm-up and end with a cool-down. Your warm-up should include 5 to 15 minutes of moderate-intensity large body movements, followed by some light stretching for the muscle groups you are about to work. The length of your warm-up is often dependent upon how psychologically prepared you are to move; if you are geared up and ready to go the warm-up may not take as long (say, only 5 minutes), whereas if you are not quite in the mood to exercise the warm-up may take longer (say, 15 minutes). A warm-up should gradually increase heart rate and core body temperature, improve joint lubrication, make muscles and tendons more elastic and flexible, and enhance your performance during the workout that follows, making it easier to maintain a higher intensity of exercise for a longer time.

The cool-down should be similar to the warm-up, with 5 to 10 minutes of moderate- to low-intensity cardiorespiratory activity, followed by 5 to 10 minutes of stretching exercises. The purpose of the cool-down is to gradually reduce your heart rate, blood pressure, and body temperature to pre-exercising levels. In addition, a cool-down reduces the risk of blood pooling in the extremities, and facilitates quicker recovery between exercise sessions. Because of the body's increased temperature, the cool-down is an excellent time to stretch and increase flexibility.

## Cardiorespiratory Endurance

An effective cardiorespiratory workout is characterized by repetitive, vigorous, continuous physical activity performed at least three times per week on alternating days, at an intensity of 70 to 90 percent of your $HR_{max}$, for 20–30 minutes per session. As your cardiorespiratory endurance improves, gradually increase the number of workouts per week, the time spent exercising, and then the intensity level or speed of your activity. However, don't change more than one of these parameters at a time and don't increase any of these variables (frequency, time, or intensity) by more than 10 percent per week. Thus, if you started with 20 minutes of jogging in your first week, you would increase to 22 minutes the next week, and so on until you reach your goal time.

## Resistance Training

Progressively overloading your muscles will improve your strength, endurance, and power. Resistance training also builds lean body mass, which will improve your body composition and increase your metabolic rate at rest and during activity. Construct your program using exercises, sets, repetitions, intensity (amount of resistance), and rest interval length. You can also increase the number of reps done at a given resistance, the number of sets in a workout, and the number of exercises; decrease recovery time between sets; or increase the length of time the muscle is under tension during a set. Three days of resistance training per week should provide ample stimulus for strength gains, while allowing for the needed 24 to 48 hours of recovery between workouts. Since improvements in muscle strength and size occur during the recovery period between workouts, not while you are training, the recovery time between training sessions is as important as your workouts (see Table 9.2). Different exercises using free weights, body weight, or machines can be combined in many ways to create an effective resistance-training workout.

## Flexibility

For optimal flexibility, static stretching exercises should be performed every day following a general warm-up to raise the core body temperature and increase the elasticity of muscles and tendons. Stretch all of the major muscle groups, holding each position for 10 to 30 seconds. Perform three repetitions of each stretch for best results. Many people find that stretching between sets during their resistance training sessions is quite effective. The target muscles are already warm, and since the stretches are performed during the rest time between sets no additional time for stretching is required at the beginning or end of the workout. Refer to Figure 9.2 to see some sample stretches.

TABLE 9.2

### Guide to Manipulating Training Variables to Achieve Different Strength Training Goals

|  | Endurance | Strength |
| --- | --- | --- |
| Sets | 2–3 | 3–5 |
| Repetitions | 10–15 | 3–6 |
| Resistance (% of maximum) | < 60% | > 60% |
| Rest between sets (seconds) | 30–60 | 120 |
| Frequency per week (days) | 2–4 | 2–4 |
| Rest between workouts (days) | 1–2 | 1–2 |

Source: Adapted from *Basic Weight Training Guide,* National Strength and Conditioning Association, 1997.

# Managing Your Physical Activity Behaviours

The decision to become physically active is easy to make but not always easy to put into action. Physical activity should be enjoyable, so in addition to considering the health benefits you should choose activities that you enjoy.

## MAKING DECISIONS FOR YOU

Begin by making a list of your favourite physical activities. Which of these increases cardiorespiratory efficiency, strength, endurance, and flexibility? Your list may include walking, gardening, or mowing the lawn, as well as exercises such as weight lifting and swimming. Which would you like to make part of your program? Next, you need to find time to exercise and be physically active. Do you have extra time you could set aside? If not, how could physical activity become part of your daily activities? Could you, for example, leave for class a few minutes earlier and walk a few blocks instead of taking the bus all the way; or rather than watch TV or have a coffee for a study break, do some stretching activities?

## CHECKLIST FOR CHANGE: MAKING PERSONAL CHOICES

- *Start slowly.* For the sedentary, first-time exerciser, any type and amount of physical activity is a step in the right direction. If you have been inactive for a long time or are extremely overweight you may be able to walk for only five minutes at a time. Don't be discouraged: start there and progress as your fitness improves.

- *Make only one lifestyle change at a time.* Attempting too many major changes at once invites failure. Success at one major behaviour change will encourage you to make other positive changes.

- *Have reasonable expectations of yourself and your training program.* Many people become exercise dropouts because their expectations were too high. Have patience with yourself and your body. Allow sufficient time to reach your physical fitness goals.

- *Choose a specific time to be physically active and stick with it.* Learning to establish priorities and keeping to a schedule are vital steps toward improved physical fitness. Experiment by exercising at different times of the day to learn what time works and feels best for you.

- *Be physically active with a friend.* Reneging on an exercise commitment is more difficult if your plans include a friend. Enjoy the social aspects of exercising with a friend. Partners can motivate and encourage one another, provided they remember that progress will not be the same for each of them.

- *Make physical activity a positive habit.* Usually, if you are able to practise a desired activity for three weeks, you will be able to incorporate it into your lifestyle. But also be aware that for some individuals exercise can become a negative habit (addiction).

- *Keep a record of your progress.* A personal journal can be a good motivator. Your journal could include various facts about your physical activities (frequency, intensity, time, type) and chronicle your emotions and personal achievements as you progress in your training.

- *Take lapses in stride.* Physical deconditioning—a decline in fitness level—occurs at about the same rate as does physical conditioning. If you have not exercised for three or more weeks after regular training, you will notice lower levels of cardiorespiratory and muscular fitness. First, renew your commitment, and then restart your exercise program.

## CHECKLIST FOR CHANGE: MAKING COMMUNITY CHOICES

- Does your campus have facilities for physical activity and physical fitness training? Where are these facilities? Are they conveniently located? Is the use of facilities included in your student fees? What hours are those facilities available?

- What community facilities does your home town have available for physical activity? Where are these facilities? Are they conveniently located? Have you ever considered using these facilities?

- What opportunities are available for you to volunteer at a local fitness or wellness facility? Have you considered volunteering to help out low-income individuals or individuals with a physical or mental disability? Why or why not?

## CRITICAL THINKING

Your friend Joan catches everyone's eye: five years of intense bodybuilding have created a sleek, "jacked," hard body. She plans to enter bodybuilding contests within the next year. Joan started working out in high school after her father had a heart attack at age 38. Her family doctor pointed out that her family had a history of cardiovascular disease and that she should take steps to lower her own risk.

Although aerobic exercise was his suggestion, Joan works out two to three hours a day in the weight room, usually powerlifting to build bigger muscles for competition. When she had a higher-than-normal blood pressure reading last week, she became convinced that she had to train harder. From what you have learned in your health class, you want to suggest that she add aerobic exercise and flexibility training to her workout. However, because you do little more than jog 20 minutes a day, you are afraid she won't take your suggestion seriously.

Using the DECIDE model described in Chapter 1, decide how you could approach Joan to urge her to take a more balanced and perhaps realistic approach to her workout regime.

# SUMMARY

- The physiological benefits of regular physical activity include reduced risk of heart disease, prevention of hypertension, improved blood profile, improved skeletal mass, improved weight management, prevention of type 2 diabetes, increased life span, improved immunity to disease, improved mental health and stress management, and the maintenance of physical fitness.

- An aerobic exercise program improves cardiorespiratory endurance. Exercise frequency begins with three days per week and eventually moves up to five. Exercise intensity involves working out at your target heart rate. Exercise time (at the target heart rate) should be between 20 and 30 minutes. Exercise activities should be vigorous, rhythmic, and continuous.

- The key principles for developing muscular strength and endurance are the tension principle, the overload principle, and the specificity of training principle. The different types of muscle contractions include isometric, concentric, and eccentric. Resistance training programs include fixed, variable, and accommodating resistance.

- Flexibility exercises should involve static stretching performed in sets of three repetitions held for 10 to 30 seconds daily for optimal development.

- Physical activity–related injuries are generally caused by overuse or trauma; the most common overuse injuries are plantar fasciitis, shin splints, and runner's knee. Some prevention can be achieved with proper footwear and equipment. Exercise in the heat or cold requires special precautions including attire and sufficient hydration.

- Planning your physical fitness training program involves setting goals and designing a program to achieve these goals.

# DISCUSSION QUESTIONS

1. What is the difference between physical activity and physical fitness? How do each relate to health? What are the physiological and psychological benefits?

2. What are the key components of a physical fitness program? What should you consider when you begin a program?

3. When exercising to improve your cardiorespiratory endurance, how can you monitor the intensity of your exercise? How frequently do you need to exercise? For how long? What kind of physical activities would you do?

4. Compare and contrast strength training using your body resistance versus weight training machines or free weights.

5. When is the most effective time to improve flexibility? Why?

6. How can you prevent physical activity–related injuries?

# APPLICATION EXERCISE

Reread the What Do You Think? scenario at the beginning of the chapter and answer the following questions:

1. Assuming that Georgia's workouts were about 30 to 45 minutes long and alternated each day between cardiorespiratory and muscular strength training, was there really anything wrong with what she was doing? What amount of workout is too much? Too little? Just right?

2. Given that Georgia is still tired and stressed even though she regularly works out, what advice would you give her? Is stress simply a part of university or college life, or can it be managed?

# HEALTH ON THE NET

Canadian Heritage Sport Canada
**www.pch.gc.ca/sportcanada**

Canadian Fitness and Lifestyle Research Institute
**www.cflri.ca/**

Statistics Canada
**www.statcan.ca/**

Canada's Physical Activity Guide
**www.paguide.com**

Canadian Institute for Health Information
**www.cihi.ca**

Canadian Society for Exercise Physiology
**www.csep.ca**

Ontario Association of Sport and Exercise Sciences
**www.oases.on.ca**

Active Living Canada
**www.activeliving.ca**

Health Canada
**www.hc-sc.gc.ca**

# CHAPTER 10

# Licit and Illicit Drug Use

*Understanding Addictions*

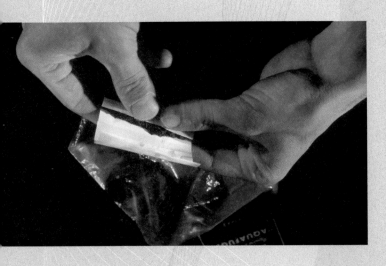

## CHAPTER OBJECTIVES

- Define drug use, misuse, and abuse.

- Define and identify the signs of addiction.

- Explain how drugs can be taken.

- Identify drug interactions. Include general precautions when taking over-the-counter drugs.

- Identify the patterns of illicit drug use, including who uses them and why they do.

- Describe the use and abuse of controlled substances, including cocaine, amphetamines, marijuana, opiates, psychedelics, deliriants, designer drugs, inhalants, and steroids.

- Describe illegal drug use in Canada, including frequency, financial impact, arrests for drug offences, and the impact on the workplace.

The company for which Richard works as a machine operator recently introduced random drug testing for all employees. At a party last weekend, Richard smoked marijuana, unaware that the drug would remain in his body for a few days. At work on Monday, he tested positive for drug use and was suspended without pay for a week. He was informed that he would receive a dismissal warning if he tested positive again. Richard argues that his personal life is his own business as long as he can perform his job.

■ Is Richard justified in maintaining that his use of drugs off the job is his own business? Is his attitude toward drug use a potential danger to co-workers? Is random drug testing in the workplace a viable deterrent? Are an individual's human rights violated by random drug tests at work? Why or why not?

If you pick up the newspaper, watch TV, or listen to the radio, you're certain to hear about the devastating personal and social consequences of substance abuse. Few people would challenge the idea that chemical dependency is a major health threat in Canada. But while the war on drugs rages on, it is increasingly clear that chemical dependency represents only one part of Canada's problem with addiction. Indeed, it seems that millions of Canadians struggle with compulsive and harmful behaviours that not only are conventional but also enhance the lives of people who can engage in them moderately. For example, some people become addicted to shopping or exercise, while others can engage in these behaviours without causing personal, social, or financial harm.

# DRUG USE, MISUSE, AND ABUSE

Many people fail to take the time needed to make intelligent decisions when considering using a drug. Although drug abuse is usually referred to in connection with illicit psychoactive drugs, many people abuse and misuse prescription and over-the-counter medications as well as recreational drugs. While **drug use** is considered taking a drug for the reason it was intended, **drug misuse** is generally considered the use of a drug for a purpose for which it was not intended. For example, taking an over-the-counter pain reliever when you have a headache is an example of drug use, while taking a friend's high-powered prescription painkiller for your headache is considered misuse. **Drug abuse** is usually

defined as the excessive use of any drug. *Excessive use*, however, is difficulty to quantify. Further, what is excessive use for one person may not be for another.

There are risks and benefits to the use of any type of chemical substance. Intelligent decision making requires a clear-headed evaluation of these risks and benefits and the realization that unforeseeable reactions or problems could arise. In order to compare drug risks to benefits, you may want to create a profile for each drug you use or are considering using. A drug profile consists of a set of answers to specific questions about a drug. You should identify the active ingredients in the drug, receptor sites that will be affected, main effects, side effects, and any potential adverse reactions.

## Individual Response to Psychoactive Drugs: Set and Setting

Individuals differ in how they respond to psychoactive drugs. Set and setting are two factors that influence the main side effects of psychoactive drugs. **Set** is the total internal environment, or mindset, of a person at the time a drug is taken. Physical, emotional, and social factors interact to influence the drug's effect on that particular person. Expectations of what the drug will or will not do are also part of the set. For example, a young woman who reads two pages of reported side effects for a particular drug may experience more side effects after taking that drug than someone who chose not to read this information. In other cases, set may be related to the user's mood. Someone who is "pumped" for the party and plans to get drunk is likely to feel the effects of alcohol faster than when they are not as much in the mood to party. The elderly are particularly susceptible to their set.

Whereas set refers to the drug user's internal environment, **setting** refers to the drug user's total external environment. It encompasses the physical and social aspects of that environment at the time the person takes the psychoactive drug. If the user is surrounded by wild colours, heavy-metal rock music, and a noisy crowd of people, the drug will generally produce a very different effect than when it is taken in a quiet place with soft music, soothing colours, and relaxed company.

---

**Drug use:** The use of a drug in a way that it was intended.

**Drug misuse:** The use of a drug for a purpose for which it was not intended.

**Drug abuse:** The excessive use of a drug.

**Set:** The total internal environment, or mindset, of a person at the time a drug is taken.

**Setting:** The total external environment of a person at the time a drug is taken.

---

# DEFINING ADDICTION

The Addiction Foundation of Manitoba[1] defines a "dependency syndrome," commonly called **addiction,** as patterned use that carries with it a dependence on mind- or mood-altering substances that has attained such a degree as to disrupt academic or work performance, interfere with family and interpersonal relationships, disrupt social and economic functioning, and impair the user's state of physical and/or mental health. A person with a dependency syndrome will generally exhibit at least three of the following behaviour patterns:

- over-use a substance; that is, use a larger quantity or over a longer period than intended

- express a persistent desire or make unsuccessful efforts to cut down or control use

- spend a great deal of time to get or use the substance, or to recover from its aftereffects

- frequently be too intoxicated or incapacitated by the aftereffects to fulfill major obligations

- give up activities for substance use

- continue to use the substance despite problems with it

- develop a physical tolerance for the substance

- display signs of withdrawal when not using the substance

- use the substance to relieve or avoid withdrawal symptoms

Physiological dependence is only one indicator of addiction. Psychological dynamics play an important role, which explains why behaviours not related to the use of chemicals—gambling, for example—can also be addictive. In fact, psychological and physiological dependence are so intertwined that it is not possible to separate the two. For every psychological state, there is a corresponding physiological state. In other words, everything you feel is tied to a chemical process occurring in your body.[2]

Chemicals are responsible for the most profound addictions, not only because they produce dramatic mood changes, but also because they cause cellular changes to which the body adapts so well that it eventually requires the chemical in order to function normally. For a behaviour to be addictive, it must have the potential to produce a positive mood state. Since behaviours such as gambling, spending, working, and sex also create changes at the cellular level along with positive mood changes, a person can become addicted to them. Although the mechanism is not well understood, all forms of addiction probably reflect dysfunction of certain biochemical systems in the brain.[3]

## The Physiology of Addiction

Virtually all mental, emotional, and behavioural functions occur as a result of biochemical interactions between nerve cells in the body. Biochemical messengers, called neurotransmitters, exert their influence at specific receptor sites on nerve cells. Drug use and chronic stress can alter these receptor sites and cause the production and breakdown of neurotransmitters.

Mood-altering chemicals, for example, fill up the receptor sites for the body's natural "feel-good" neurotransmitters (endorphins) so that nerve cells are fooled into believing they have enough neurotransmitters and shut down production of these substances temporarily. When the drug use is stopped, those receptor sites become emptied, resulting in uncomfortable feelings that remain until the body resumes neurotransmitter production or the person consumes more of the drug. Some people's bodies always produce insufficient quantities of these neurotransmitters, so they naturally seek out chemicals like alcohol as substitutes, or they pursue behaviours like moderate or vigorous physical activities or thrill-seeking activities such as sky diving or riding a rollercoaster that increase natural production. Thus we may be "wired" to seek substances or experiences that increase pleasure or reduce discomfort.

Engaging in mood-altering substances and experiences results in **tolerance,** a phenomenon in which progressively larger doses of a drug or more intense involvement in an experience are needed to obtain the desired effects. All of us develop some degree of tolerance to mood-altering substances and experiences. Individuals who are addicted generally require amounts of mood-altering substances or experiences large enough to cause negative side effects.

**Withdrawal** is another phenomenon associated with mood-altering substances and experiences. The drug or activity replaces or causes an effect that the

# Early Spirituality Deters Alcohol Abuse

Teens who have an active spiritual life are 50 percent less likely to become addicted to drugs or alcohol or even try illegal drugs than those with no religious beliefs or training, a new study reports.

"Alcoholism, in addition to being a biological disorder, is a spiritual disorder," lead author Dr. Lisa Miller told Reuters Health. "Adolescents who claim to have a personal relationship with the divine are only half as likely to become alcoholics or drug addicts, or for that matter even to try contraband drugs (marijuana and cocaine). This is particularly important because onset of alcoholism and drug addiction usually occurs in adolescents."

To determine the relationship between their religiosity and substance use of 676 adolescents aged 15 to 19, Miller and colleagues conducted a study using survey data. This was the first study to show that personal spirituality strongly protected against developing alcoholism or drug abuse.

## SPIRITUAL, NOT RELIGIOUS

"The findings show that a personal sense of spirituality helps adolescents avoid alcohol and drug use and abuse," Miller told Reuters. "Unlike adults in [Alcoholics Anonymous], adolescents in this study were shown not to be helped by a rigid or forced adherence to religion."

In other words, "religion" forced upon adolescents by their parents or others had little effect, but if teens have made a personal choice to pursue a spiritual life, they were much less likely to drink and take drugs.

"Spirituality . . . is the most central bearing in an adolescent's life," Miller emphasized. "It cannot be ignored by parents, or the adolescent will go 'shopping' for meaning, communion and transcendence," she said.

The study authors concluded that adolescents at high risk might be protected from substance dependence or abuse if they engaged with a higher power or became involved in a religious community.

The survey questioned teens about their personal devotion, personal conservatism, and institutional conservatism, defined as "representing an active personal relationship with the divine, representing a personal choice to teach and adhere closely to creed, in some cases initiated through a 'born-again' experience, and as the degree of fundamentalism in a religious denomination."

The study was published in the September 2000 issue of the *Journal of the American Academy of Child and Adolescent Psychiatry*.

body normally provides on its own. If the experience is repeated often enough or the substance ingested frequently enough, the body makes an adjustment: it comes to require the drug or experience to obtain the effect it previously produced itself, but no longer can. Stopping the behaviour will therefore result in withdrawal. Withdrawal symptoms of chemical dependencies are generally the opposite of the effects of the drug taken. For example, withdrawal from cocaine includes a characteristic "crash" (depression and lethargy), while withdrawal from barbiturates involves trembling, irritability, and convulsions. Withdrawal symptoms for addictive behaviours are usually less dramatic. They usually involve psychic discomforts such as anxiety, depression, irritability, guilt, anger, and frustration, with an underlying preoccupation with or craving for another exposure to the behaviour. Withdrawal syndromes range from mild to severe. The severest form of withdrawal syndrome is delirium tremens (DTs), which occurs in approximately 5 percent of individuals withdrawing from alcohol.

## WHAT WOULD YOU DO?

Since the path to addiction is most often gradual and is not defined by the amount or frequency of consumption, how can you monitor your behaviours in order to avoid addiction? How much is too much? How frequent is too frequent?

**Addiction:** Patterned use resulting in dependence on mind- or mood-altering substances that has a negative influence on academic/work performance, family and interpersonal relationships, social and economic functioning, and/or physical and mental health.

**Tolerance:** Phenomenon in which progressively larger dose of a drug or more intense involvement in a behaviour is needed to produce the desired effects.

**Withdrawal:** A phenomenon experienced by individuals addicted to a substance or behaviour when they no longer use the drug or engage in that activity. Generally the symptoms of withdrawal are opposite to the mood- or mind-altering effects experienced when engaging in the substance or behaviour.

## The Addictive Process

Addiction is a process that evolves over time. It begins when a person repeatedly seeks the illusion of relief to avoid unpleasant feelings or situations. This pattern is known as **nurturing through avoidance** and is a maladaptive way of taking care of emotional needs.[4] As a person becomes increasingly dependent on the addictive behaviours, there is a corresponding deterioration in relationships with family, friends, and co-workers, in performance at work or school, and in personal life. Eventually, these individuals do not find the addictive behaviours pleasurable but consider them preferable to the unhappy realities they are seeking to escape.

## Signs of Addiction

Although different opinions exist as to the cause, most experts agree that there are universal signs of addiction. Addictions are characterized by four common symptoms: (1) **compulsion,** which is described by obsession, or excessive preoccupation, with the behaviours or substance and an overwhelming need to engage in it; (2) **loss of control,** or the inability to predict reliably whether any isolated occurrence of the behaviours or use of the substance will be healthy or damaging; (3) **negative consequences,** such as physical damage, legal trouble, financial problems, academic failure, relationship difficulties, and family dissolution, which do not occur with healthy involvement in any behaviours or substance use; and (4) **denial,** or the inability to perceive that the behaviours or substance use are self-destructive. These four components are present in all addictions, whether chemical or behavioural.

Traditionally, diagnosis of an addiction was limited to drug addiction and was based on three criteria: (1) the presence of an abstinence syndrome, or withdrawal; (2) an associated pattern of pathological behaviours (deterioration in work or academic performance, relationships, and social interaction); and (3) **relapse,** the tendency to return to the addictive behaviours or substance use after a period of abstinence. Furthermore, until recently, health professionals were unwilling to diagnose an addiction until medical symptoms appeared in the patient. Now we know that although withdrawal, pathological behaviours, relapse, and medical symptoms are valid indicators of addiction, they do not characterize all addictive behaviours.

# DRUG DYNAMICS

Have you ever walked into a drugstore looking for some cough syrup or a pain reliever and become overwhelmed by the number of choices available?

Although there are literally tens of thousands of drugs at our disposal, these choices should not be made lightly. All drugs are chemical substances that have the potential to alter the structure and function of our bodies. Quite simply, all drug use involves risks. You can minimize these risks by asking appropriate questions of health providers and by being a critical consumer of all drugs.

Drugs work because they physically resemble the chemicals produced naturally within the body (see Figure 10.1). For example, many painkillers resemble the endorphins (literally "morphine within") that are manufactured in the body. Most bodily processes result from chemical reactions or changes in electrical charge. Because drugs possess an electrical charge and a chemical structure similar to chemicals that occur naturally in the body, they can affect physiological and psychological functions in many different ways.

A current explanation of drug actions is the receptor site theory, which states that drugs attach themselves to specific **receptor sites** in the body. These sites are specialized cells to which a drug is able to attach because of its size, shape, electrical charge, and chemical properties. Most drugs can attach at multiple receptor sites located throughout the body in such places as the heart and blood system, the lungs, liver, kidneys, brain, and gonads (testicles or ovaries). The physiology of drug activity and its effect on human behaviours is very complex.

# TYPES OF DRUGS

Drugs are divided into six categories: prescription drugs, recreational drugs, over-the-counter (OTC) drugs, herbal preparations, illicit drugs, and commercial drugs. Each category includes drugs that either stimulate the body, depress body functions, produce hallucinations, or have the potential to alter a person's mood or behaviours (that is, **psychoactive drugs**).

- **Prescription drugs** can be obtained only with a written prescription from a licensed physician. In 2002, the cost of prescription medicine was $14.8 billion. It was forecast that prescribed drug expenditure would increase to $18.0 billion and account for 82.5 percent (versus 80.5 percent) of total drug expenditure in Canada.[5]

- **Recreational drugs** belong to a vague category with boundaries dependent upon how the term recreation is defined. Generally, these drugs contain

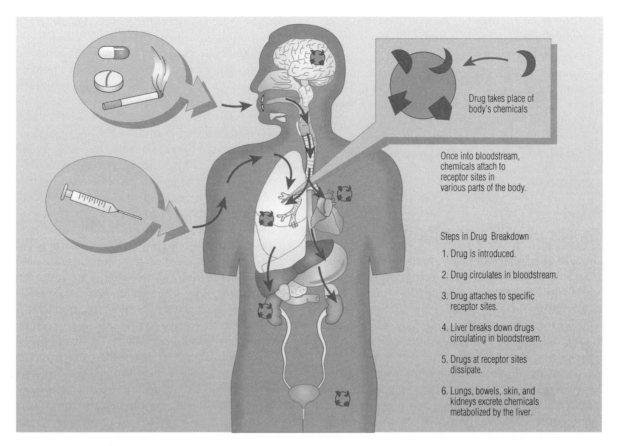

FIGURE 10.1

How the Body Metabolizes Drugs

chemicals that people use to help them relax or socialize. These drugs are legal even though they are psychoactive. Alcohol, tobacco, and caffeine (in coffee, tea, and chocolate) are included in this category.

- **Over-the-counter (OTC) drugs** can be purchased in pharmacies, supermarkets, and discount stores without a physician's prescription. Expenditures specifically on OTC products (which are not usually covered by health care) were more than $1.9 billion in 2002, and when combined with personal health supplies totalled $3.6 billion.[6] Combined, expenditures on non-prescribed drugs (that is, OTC drugs and personal health supplies) were forecast to reach $3.8 billion in 2004.[7]

- **Herbal preparations** form another vague category that includes approximately 750 substances such as herbal teas and other products of botanical origin believed to have medicinal properties.

- **Illicit (illegal) drugs** are the most notorious substances. Although laws governing their use, possession, cultivation, manufacture, and sale

**Nurturing through avoidance:** Repeatedly seeking the illusion of relief to avoid unpleasant feelings or situations.

**Compulsion:** Obsessive preoccupation with a behaviour or substance and an overwhelming need to engage in it.

**Loss of control:** Inability to predict reliably whether any isolated involvement with the addictive substance or behaviour will be healthy or damaging.

**Negative consequences:** Difficulties such as physical damage, legal trouble, financial ruin, academic failure, relationship difficulties, family dissolution, and others as a result of continued engagement in a substance or behaviour.

**Denial:** Inability to perceive or accurately interpret the negative effects of substance use or a behaviour.

**Relapse:** The tendency to return to the addictive behaviours after a period of abstinence.

**Receptor sites:** Specialized cells to which drugs can attach themselves.

**Psychoactive drugs:** Drugs that have the potential to alter mood or behaviours.

**Prescription drugs:** Drugs that can be obtained only with a written prescription from a licensed physician.

**Recreational drugs:** Legal drugs that people use to relax or socialize.

differ from country to country, illicit drugs are generally recognized as harmful. These drugs are psychoactive.

- **Commercial preparations** are the most universally used yet least commonly recognized as chemical substances with a drug action. More than 1,000 of these substances exist, including seemingly benign items as perfumes, cosmetics, household cleansers, paints, glues, inks, dyes, gardening chemicals, pesticides, and industrial byproducts.

## Routes of Administration of Drugs

**Route of administration** refers to the way in which a drug is taken into the body. Common routes include oral ingestion, injection, inhalation, inunction, and suppository.

**Oral ingestion** is the most common method used to take drugs. Drugs that you swallow include tablets, capsules, and liquids. Oral ingestion of a drug generally results in relatively slow absorption compared to other methods, because the drug must pass through the stomach, where it is acted on by digestive juices, and then move on to the small intestine before it enters the bloodstream. Alcohol is the one exception to this rule since the majority of it is absorbed into the bloodstream without digestion.

Many oral preparations are coated to keep them from being dissolved by corrosive stomach acids before they reach the intestine as well as to protect the stomach lining from irritation. If your stomach contains food, absorption will be slower than if your stomach is empty. Some drugs should not be taken with certain foods because the food will inhibit the drug's action. Others must be taken with food to prevent stomach irritation.

**Injection,** another common method of taking a drug, involves the use of a hypodermic syringe. This method usually results in rapid absorption, depending on the type of injection. **Intravenous injection,** or injection directly into a vein, puts the chemical in its most concentrated form directly into the bloodstream. Effects will be felt within three minutes, making this route extremely effective, particularly in medical emergencies. But injection of many substances into the bloodstream may cause serious or even fatal reactions. In addition, some serious diseases, such as hepatitis and HIV infection, can be transferred in this way. For this reason, intravenous injection can also be one of the most dangerous routes of administration. **Intramuscular injection** results in much slower absorption of the drug than intravenous injection. This type of injection places the hypodermic needle into muscular tissue, usually in the buttocks or in the triceps on the back of the upper arm. Normally used to administer antibiotics and vaccinations, this route of administration ensures a slow and consistent dispersion of the drug into the body tissues. **Subcutaneous injection** puts the drug into the layer of fat directly beneath the

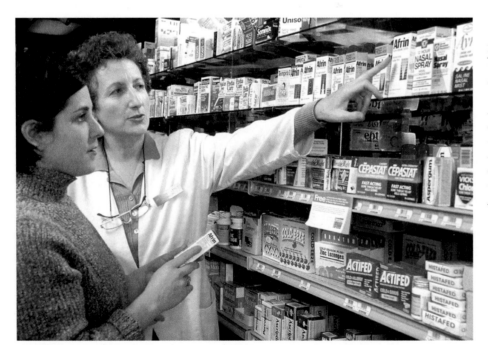

*Whenever you take more than one drug at a time, you should consider how they will interact. For example, women who take oral contraceptives should strictly follow the dosage instructions and be aware that medicines such as penicillin may alter the contraceptive's effectiveness. Asking a pharmacist is a good way to learn about drug interactions.*

skin. Its common medical uses are for administration of local anesthetics and for insulin replacement therapy. A drug injected subcutaneously will circulate even more slowly than an intramuscularly injected drug because it takes longer to be absorbed into the bloodstream.

**Inhalation** refers to the ingestion of drugs through the nostrils. This method transfers the drug rapidly into the bloodstream through the alveoli (air sacs) in the lungs. Some examples of inhalation include nasal sprays, cocaine snorting, and the inhalation of aerosol sprays, gases, or fumes from solvents. The drug effects are usually noticed immediately after inhalation, but they do not last as long because only small amounts of the drug can be absorbed and metabolized in the lungs.

**Inunction** introduces chemicals into the body through the skin. Common examples of this method of taking drugs include the small adhesive patches used to alleviate motion sickness or nicotine patches used to assist individuals when they stop smoking. These patches slowly release their chemicals for a consistent dispersal.

**Suppositories** are drugs mixed with a waxy medium that are designed to melt at body temperature. The most common type of suppository is inserted into the anus past the rectal sphincter muscles. As the wax melts, the drug is released and absorbed through the rectal walls into the bloodstream. Since this area of the anatomy contains many blood vessels, the effects of the drug are usually felt within 15 minutes. Other types of suppositories are inserted in the vagina. Vaginal suppositories usually release drugs, such as antifungal agents, that treat problems in the vagina itself as opposed to drugs meant to travel in the bloodstream.

---

### WHAT WOULD YOU DO?

What types of drugs have you used or experimented with? How do you usually take these drugs? Are you aware of how quickly these work?

---

# DRUG INTERACTIONS

Most people are aware that sharing medications, using outdated prescriptions, taking higher doses than recommended, or using drugs as a substitute for dealing with personal problems may result in serious health consequences. However, many are not aware of the risks of taking several drugs simultaneously.

The most dangerous interactions are synergism, antagonism, inhibition, and intolerance. Hazardous interactions may also occur between drugs and nutrients.

**Synergism,** also known as potentiation, is an interaction of two or more drugs in which the effects of the individual drugs are multiplied beyond what would normally be expected. Synergism can be expressed mathematically as $2 + 2 = 10$. A synergistic interaction is most likely to occur when central nervous system depressants are combined. Included in this category are alcohol, opiates (morphine, heroin), antihistamines (cold remedies), sedative hypnotics (Quaaludes), minor tranquillizers (Valium, Librium, and Xanax), and barbiturates. The worst possible combination is alcohol and barbiturates (sleeping preparations such as Seconal and phenobarbital) because the combination of these depressants leads to a slowdown of the brain centres that normally control vital functions. Respiration, heart rate, and blood pressure can drop to the point of inducing coma or death.

Prescription drugs carry special labels warning the user of any potential drug interactions. Many OTC preparations carry similar warning labels. Because

**Over-the-counter (OTC) drugs:** Drugs that can be purchased without a physician's prescription.

**Herbal preparations:** Substances of plant origin believed to have medicinal properties.

**Illicit (illegal) drugs:** Drugs whose use, possession, cultivation, manufacture, and/or sale are illegal.

**Commercial preparations:** Commonly used chemical substances with a drug action. Examples include cosmetics, household cleaning products, and industrial byproducts.

**Route of administration:** The manner in which a drug is taken into the body.

**Oral ingestion:** Intake of drugs through the mouth.

**Injection:** The introduction of drugs into the body via a hypodermic needle.

**Intravenous injection:** The introduction of drugs directly into a vein.

**Intramuscular injection:** The introduction of drugs into muscles.

**Subcutaneous injection:** The introduction of drugs into the layer of fat directly beneath the skin.

**Inhalation:** The introduction of drugs through the nostrils.

**Inunction:** The introduction of drugs through the skin.

**Suppositories:** Mixtures of drugs and a waxy medium designed to melt at body temperature; usually inserted into the anus or vagina.

**Synergism:** An interaction of two or more drugs in which the effects of the individual drugs are magnified beyond what is expected of their combination.

the dangers associated with synergism are so great, you should always check for possible drug interactions before using a prescribed or OTC drug. Pharmacists, physicians, drug information centres, or community drug education centres can answer your questions. Even if one of the drugs in question is an illegal substance, you should still try to determine the dangers involved in combining it with other drugs. Healthcare professionals are legally bound to maintain confidentiality even when they know that a client is using illegal substances. The Building Communication Skills box suggests questions you should ask before taking any drug.

**Antagonism,** although not usually as serious as synergism, can produce unwanted and unpleasant effects. In an antagonistic reaction, drugs work at the same receptor site where one drug blocks the action of the other. The "blocking" drug occupies the receptor site, preventing the second drug from attaching, and this alters its absorption and action.

**Inhibition** is a type of interaction in which the effects of one drug are eliminated or reduced by the presence of another drug at the receptor site. A common inhibitory reaction occurs between antacid tablets and Aspirin. The antacid inhibits the absorption of Aspirin, making it less effective as a pain reliever. Other inhibitory reactions occur between alcohol and contraceptive pills and between antibiotics and contraceptive pills. Specifically, alcohol and antibiotics may diminish the effectiveness of birth control pills in some women.

**Intolerance** occurs when drugs combine in the body to produce extremely uncomfortable reactions. The drug Antabuse, used to help alcoholics give up alcohol, works by producing this type of interaction. It binds liver enzymes (the chemicals the liver produces to break down alcohol), making it impossible for the body to metabolize alcohol. As a result, the user of Antabuse who drinks alcohol experiences nausea, vomiting, and, occasionally, fever.

**Cross-tolerance** occurs when a person develops a physiological tolerance to one drug and shows a similar tolerance to other drugs with similar effects as a result. For example, cross-tolerance can develop between alcohol and barbiturates, two depressant drugs.

---

## WHAT WOULD YOU DO?

What is the difference between drug use, misuse, and abuse? Give examples of each. Are people who abuse or misuse drugs addicted to them? Is it possible to use illicit drugs without becoming addicted to them?

---

# PRESCRIPTION DRUGS

Even though prescription drugs are administered under medical supervision, the critical consumer still takes precautions. Complications and serious negative health consequences arising from the use of prescription drugs are common. Responsible decision making about prescription drug use requires the consumer to acquire basic drug knowledge.

## Types of Prescription Drugs

**Antibiotics** are drugs used to fight bacterial infection. Bacterial infections continue to be among the most common serious diseases in the world, with the vast majority cured by antibiotics. There are almost 100 different antibiotics available that are dispensed by intramuscular injection or in tablet or capsule form. Some, called broad-spectrum antibiotics, are designed to control disease caused by a number of bacterial species. These medications may also kill off helpful bacteria in the body, thus triggering secondary infections. For example, some vaginal infections are related to long-term use of antibiotics. Further, it is believed that the misuse of antibiotics has led to an increase in drug-resistant bacteria.

**Sedatives** are central nervous system depressants that induce sleep and relieve anxiety. Used heavily in the 1950s and 1960s in the form of phenobarbital or Seconal, they gradually fell out of favour because of the risks involved. Further, the potential for addiction is high. Detoxification can be life-threatening and must be medically supervised. Because doctors do not prescribe sedatives as frequently as they did in the past, users often purchase them illegally.

**Tranquillizers** are another form of central nervous system depressant. They are classified either as major or minor tranquillizers. The most powerful tranquillizers are used in the treatment of major psychiatric illnesses. When used appropriately, these strong sedatives are capable of reducing violent aggressiveness and self-destructive impulses. About 5 percent of Canadians aged 15 and older report using sleeping pills, and 5 percent report using tranquillizers.[8] Women and older Canadians were more likely to report using these medications.[9]

**Antidepressants** are powerful substances used to treat clinically diagnosed cases of depression. These drugs inhibit the release of certain neurotransmitters in the brain, thereby moderating the user's mood.

**Amphetamines** are stimulants prescribed less commonly now than in the past. Like other psychoactive drugs, they are purchased legally and illegally. Amphetamines suppress appetite and elevate respiration, blood pressure, and pulse rate. Tolerance to these

# Asking the Right Questions

At one time or another you will probably use prescription or OTC drugs to restore or maintain your health. How can you be certain that you need a medication in the first place, that you are taking the right medication for you, and that your medication is not robbing you of vital nutrients or being rendered ineffective by other drugs you are taking or foods you are ingesting? Only by asking the right questions of the right people can you be sure. Listed below are questions to pose to your physician, your pharmacist, or yourself before you take any drug.

1. Do you know the diagnosis of your condition?

2. Is your physician or pharmacist aware of all the other drugs you are taking, including prescription drugs (don't forget, birth control pills are drugs), OTCs, recreational drugs, and any others?

3. Do you know the name of the medication you are taking? Is it the chemical name, a generic name, or a brand name?

4. Are you certain of how often you should take the medication, for how long you should take it, and in what dosage?

5. Do you know when your medication should be taken in relation to food intake?

6. Do you know if you can drink alcohol while on your medication?

7. What are the known side effects of the medication? What should you do if you experience any of the side effects?

8. Can you stop taking your medication when you start feeling better, or is it important that you continue taking the drug until the prescription is finished?

9. Do you know what you should do if you forget to take your medication at the scheduled time?

10. Do you know what signs and symptoms signal that you are allergic to the medication?

11. Do you know how and where to store your medication properly?

12. Are there any drug–nutrient interactions that you should be aware of?

13. Are there any potential drug interactions that you should be aware of?

14. Are there any adverse consequences of long-term use of the medication?

---

powerful stimulants develops rapidly, and the user trying to cut down or quit may experience unpleasant **rebound effects.** These severe withdrawal symptoms, peculiar to stimulants, include depression, irritability, violent behaviours, headaches, nausea, and deep fatigue.

## Use of Generic Drugs

**Generic drugs,** medications sold under a chemical name rather than a brand name, have gained popularity in recent years. These alternatives to more expensive brand-name drugs contain the same active ingredients as their brand-name counterparts. There is, however, some controversy about the effectiveness of some generic drugs because substitutions made in minor ingredients can affect the way the drug is absorbed, which may cause discomfort or even an allergic reaction in some users. If you experience any allergic reactions to a prescribed generic drug tell your pharmacist or doctor, who can recommend an alternative drug. A list of medicines that can be interchanged has been approved in Canada. If your doctor or pharmacist fails to offer you the option of using a generic drug, you should ask if such a substitute exists and if it would be safe for you to use it.

**Antagonism:** A type of interaction in which two or more drugs work at the same receptor site with one drug blocking the action of the other.

**Inhibition:** A type of interaction in which the effects of one drug are eliminated or reduced by the presence of another drug at the receptor site.

**Intolerance:** A type of interaction in which two or more drugs taken together produce extremely uncomfortable symptoms.

**Cross-tolerance:** The development of a tolerance to one drug that carries over to another similar drug.

**Antibiotics:** Prescription drugs designed to fight bacterial infection.

**Sedatives:** Central nervous system depressants that induce sleep and relieve anxiety.

**Tranquillizers:** Central nervous system depressants that relax the body and relieve anxiety.

**Antidepressants:** Prescription drugs used to treat clinically diagnosed depression.

**Amphetamines:** Prescription stimulants that suppress appetite and increase breathing rate, blood pressure, and heart rate.

**Rebound effects:** Severe withdrawal effects experienced by users of stimulants, including depression, nausea, and violent behaviours.

**Generic drugs:** Drugs marketed by their chemical name rather than a brand name.

# OxyContin

OxyContin™ is the trade name for the long-lasting form of the prescription opioid (pain reliever) oxycodone. Oxycodone is also an ingredient in Percocet™ and Percodan™. OxyContin™ contains much higher doses, at 10 to 80 mg. OxyContin™ is specially formulated for slow release and as such is intended to provide relief from moderate to severe pain for up to 12 hours. Individuals prescribed OxyContin™ swallow one tablet twice daily. Although most users take this medication appropriately, they need to be monitored closely because of their high risk of dependency.

How is OxyContin™ abused? OxyContin™ is formulated to be swallowed whole to provide the slow release into the blood stream; however, when it is chewed or crushed, the slow release properties are destroyed. Thus, when users chew or crush tablets the oxycodone effects occur very rapidly causing a high or euphoria which users describe as similar to the high from heroin.

Oxycodone is a potent opioid. When large amounts of oxycodone are released into the body all at once (whether the tablets are chewed, crushed tablets are snorted, or dissolved tablets are injected), there is a high risk of overdose and death similar to a heroin overdose. Symptoms of overdose include laboured or slow breathing, extreme somnolence progressing to coma, cardiac arrest, and death. OxyContin™ users who inject the drug have the additional risks associated with sharing needles.

Addiction is also a very real problem with the user requiring larger and larger doses because of tolerance. Tolerance occurs quickly and eventually the drug is needed to simply prevent feeling sick. Withdrawal symptoms include muscle aches, nausea, diarrhea, loss of appetite, restlessness, insomnia, runny nose, teary eyes, and sweating.

Source: Centre for Addiction and Mental Health, "What Is OxyContin," 2004. Retrieved March 2, 2006, from www.camh.net/About_Addiction_Mental_Health/Drug_and_Addiction_Information/oxycontin.

# OVER-THE-COUNTER (OTC) DRUGS

Over-the-counter (OTC) drugs are nonprescription drugs used in the course of self-diagnosis and self-medication. In an effort to cure themselves, Canadians spend many millions yearly on OTC preparations for relief of everything from runny noses to ingrown toenails. Most OTC drugs are manufactured from a basic group of 1,000 chemicals. Combinations of as few as two and as many as ten of these chemicals result in the many different OTC drugs available today. Perhaps because of the common belief that OTC products are safe and effective, indiscriminate use, misuse, and abuse often occurs with these drugs. OTC drugs, like any other drugs, have the potential to produce dependency, tolerance, and addiction as well as adverse toxic reactions.

## Types of OTC Drugs

**Analgesics** are pain relievers. The earliest pain relievers were made of derivatives manufactured from the opium poppy. Today, pain relievers ranging from Aspirin to morphine are among the most commonly used drugs. In fact, in 1998–1999 approximately 65 percent of Canadians said they had taken pain relievers in the past month.[10] Although these pain relievers come in several forms, Aspirin, acetaminophen (Tylenol, Pamprin, Pandol), ibuprofen (Advil, Motrin, Nuprin), and ibuprofen-like drugs such as naproxen sodium (Aleve, Anaprox) and ketoprofen (Orudis) are the most common.

Most pain relievers work at the receptor sites by interrupting pain signals. Some are categorized as non-steroidal anti-inflammatory drugs (NSAIDS), also called **prostaglandin inhibitors.** Prostaglandins are chemicals that resemble hormones and are released by the body in response to pain. Scientists believe that the additional pain caused by the release of prostaglandins signals the body to begin the healing process. Prostaglandin inhibitors restrain the release of prostaglandins, thereby reducing the pain. Common NSAIDS include ibuprofen, naproxen sodium, and Aspirin.

Acetylsalicylic acid or Aspirin (ASA) relieves pain by inhibiting the body's production of prostaglandins. It brings down fever by increasing the flow of blood to the skin's surface, which causes sweating and therefore cooling of the body. ASA is also commonly used to reduce the inflammation and swelling of arthritis. Furthermore, ASA's anticoagulant (interference with blood clotting) effects make it a useful medication for reducing the risk of heart attacks.

Most analgesics have side effects, the most common of which is drowsiness due to the depression of the central nervous system. Label warnings are, as usual, important. Some labels caution specifically against driving or operating heavy machinery when using analgesics, and most state they should not be taken with alcohol. Specific to ASA, possible side effects include allergic reactions, ringing in the ears, stomach bleeding, and ulcers. In addition, research has linked ASA to a potentially fatal condition called Reye's syndrome. Therefore, children, teenagers, and young adults (up to age 25) who are at risk for developing this syndrome are recommended to use an alternative analgesic.

Acetaminophen is the active ingredient found in Tylenol and related medications. Like ASA, acetaminophen is an effective analgesic and antipyretic (fever-reducing) drug. It does not, however, provide relief from inflamed or swollen joints. The side effects associated with acetaminophen are generally minimal, though overdose can cause liver damage.

## Cold, Cough, Allergy, and Asthma Relievers

These substances are popular OTC drugs for the symptoms that affect millions of sufferers. The operative word in their titles is reliever. Most of these medications are designed to alleviate or reduce some or all of the discomforting symptoms associated with upper-respiratory-tract maladies. Unfortunately, no drugs exist to actually cure these conditions. The drugs available provide only temporary relief until the sufferer's immune system prevails. Aspirin or acetaminophen are used in some cold preparations, as are several other ingredients. The basic types of OTC cold, cough, and allergy relievers are:

- *Expectorants.* These drugs are formulated to loosen phlegm, allowing the user to cough it up and clear congested respiratory passages.

- *Antitussives.* These OTC drugs are used to calm or curtail the cough reflex. They are most effective when the cough is "dry," or does not produce phlegm.

- *Antihistamines.* These are central nervous system depressants that dry runny noses, clear postnasal drip, clear sinus congestion, and reduce tears.

- *Decongestants.* These remedies are designed to reduce nasal stuffiness due to colds.

- *Anticholinergics.* These substances are often added to cold preparations to reduce nasal secretions and tears.

It is important to read the labels of cough, cold, allergy, and asthma relievers for a number of reasons. First, some cold compounds contain alcohol in concentrations that may exceed 40 percent, while others contain a lot of sugar. Equally important to consider is the various drug ingredients included. In fact, many cough and cold medications contain expectorants and antitussives, which means there could be conflicting actions occurring in the body (that is, phlegm loosened to be coughed up and cleared combined with a curtailed cough reflex).

## Stimulants

Nonprescription stimulants are sometimes used by post-secondary students in the last minute panic to complete assignments or in "all-nighter" study sessions. The active ingredient in most OTC stimulants is caffeine. Although caffeine heightens wakefulness, increases alertness, and relieves fatigue, it also can result in increased nervousness, irritability, anxiety, and involuntary muscle twitches (see Chapter 11).

## Sleeping Aids and Relaxants

These drugs are often used to induce the drowsy feelings that precede sleep. The principal ingredient is an antihistamine called pyrilamine maleate. Chronic reliance on sleeping aids may lead to addiction; people accustomed to using these products may find it difficult to sleep without them.

## Dieting Aids

Some people rely on **laxatives** and **diuretics** ("water pills") to aid in weight loss. Frequent use of laxatives disrupts the body's natural elimination patterns and may cause constipation or even obstipation (inability to have a bowel movement). The use of laxatives to produce weight loss has generally unspectacular results and can rob the body of needed fluids, salts, and minerals. Use of diuretics as part of a weight-loss plan is also dangerous. Not only will the user gain the weight back upon drinking fluids, but diuretic use may also contribute to dangerous chemical imbalances. The potassium and sodium eliminated by diuretics have important roles in maintaining electrolyte balance. Depletion of these vital minerals may cause weakness, dizziness, fatigue, and sometimes death.

**Analgesics:** Pain relievers.

**Prostaglandin inhibitors:** Drugs that inhibit the production and release of prostaglandins.

**Laxatives:** Medications used to soften stool and relieve constipation.

**Diuretics:** Drugs that increase the excretion of urine from the body.

# ILLICIT DRUGS

Illicit drug use is a problem in our society. We need to understand how these drugs work and why people use them. The drug problem touches us all. In this section, we focus our attention on **illicit drugs**—drugs that are illegal to possess, produce, or sell.

On June 19, 1996, the Senate passed Bill C-8, the Controlled Drugs and Substances Act. The Act came into force on May 14, 1997. It replaced Canada's main laws on illicit drugs—the Narcotic Control Act and parts of the Food and Drugs Act. The Controlled Drugs and Substances Act significantly expanded the reach of Canada's drug laws and continued Canada's heavy reliance on a failed policy of criminal prohibition.[11]

Illicit drug users come from all walks of life. Most illicit drug use occurs elsewhere than dilapidated crack houses, and few users fit the stereotype of the crazed junkie. The reasons for using drugs vary from one situation to another and from one person to another. Age, sex, genetic background, physiology, personality, experiences, and expectations are factors that play a role in a person's choice to use or not use illicit drugs.

Health Canada and the Canadian Executive Council on Addictions sponsored the Canadian Addiction Survey (CAS), which included a random sample of almost 14,000 Canadians aged 15 or older interviewed by telephone between December 16, 2003, and April 19, 2004.[12] In this survey, 44.5 percent of Canadians reported use of marijuana in their lifetime, with 14.1 percent indicating use in the past year. The reported lifetime use of cocaine/crack was 10.6 percent, with 1.9 percent of Canadians indicating use in the past year. Only lifetime use of speed, ecstasy, hallucinogens, and inhalants was reported, with 6.4 percent of Canadians indicating use of speed; 4.1 percent reported ecstasy use, 11.4 percent hallucinogen use, and 1.3 percent inhalant use.

In 1995, there were 804 deaths (695 men and 108 women) in Canada attributed to illicit drugs. Suicides (329 deaths) and opiate poisoning (160 deaths) accounted for almost two-thirds of all drug-related deaths. The 804 deaths resulted in 33,669 potential years of life lost. In 1995–96 there were 6,947 hospitalizations attributable to illicit drugs.[13]

It is estimated that 185 million people worldwide—or 4.3 percent of the population aged 15 and older—used illicit drugs in the late 1990s.[14] Globally, 0.4 percent of deaths and 0.8 percent of "disability adjusted life years" were attributed to illicit drug use.[15] Further, the World Health Organization suggested that, "illicit drugs account for the highest proportion of disease burden among low mortality, industrialized countries in the Americas, Eastern Mediterranean, and European regions [and that the] economic reliance on the drug trade, and drug dependence leaves many individuals open to exploitation by criminals and criminal organizations; threatening the health of men, women and children, the rule of law, and ultimately, the vitality and strength of all our communities."[16]

Why do so many Canadians choose to use illicit drugs? There is no clear answer. Economic despair, collapse of the family and community, and a general sense of hopelessness or boredom may be powerful engines of use. These factors combined with increased availability and diversity as well as potentially liberal parental attitudes may explain the use of illicit drugs.

Social policy also affects drug use, although its effects are extremely hard to measure and evaluate. However, it was noted that drug use declined significantly during the first five years of Canada's Drug Strategy, when the focus was on the general public. It started rising again during Phase II, when the focus shifted to street youth and high-risk groups. The resurgence of drug use we are now witnessing is led largely by mainstream youth, indicating that we may be paying a heavy price for changing our focus and neglecting this group in Phase II. Ultimately, we must aim our prevention messages at all youth. According to the Canadian Centre on Substance Abuse, all young people—dropouts and A students alike—are vulnerable to drug use and should be viewed as an at-risk population.[17]

Antidrug programs have been developed to deal with the problems of illegal drug use. The major drawback of most of these programs is their failure to take a multi-dimensional approach. The tendency has been to focus on only one aspect of drug use rather than to examine the many interrelated factors that contribute to the problem. For example, many programs consider the drugs themselves the culprits. Others oversimplify the problem by exhorting potential users to "just say no," ignoring the fact that drugs are an integral part of many people's social or cultural lives. The pressures to take drugs are often tremendous, and the reasons for using them complex.

People who develop drug problems generally begin with the belief that they can control their use. Initially, they view drug taking as a fun and controllable pastime. Peer influence is a strong motivator, especially among adolescents, who fear not being accepted as part of the group. Other people use drugs to cope with feelings of worthlessness and despair or to battle depression and anxiety. Drugs are seen as the quick answer to life's difficulties. Since the majority of illegal drugs produce physiological and psychological dependence, the idea that a person can use these substances regularly without becoming addicted is foolish. To find out if you are controlled by drugs, see the Rate Yourself box.

# Recognizing a Drug Problem

## ARE YOU CONTROLLED BY DRUGS?

How do you know if you are chemically dependent? A person dependent on drugs can't stop using them; this use hurts the user and those around him or her. Take the following assessment. The more times you respond "yes," the more likely you have a problem.

Do you use drugs to handle stress or escape from life's problems?

Have you unsuccessfully tried to cut down or quit using your drug?

Have you ever been in trouble with the law or been arrested because of your drug use?

Do you think a party or social gathering isn't fun unless drugs are available?

Do you avoid people or places that do not support your drug usage?

Do you neglect your responsibilities because you'd rather use your drug?

Have your friends, family, or employer expressed concern about your drug use?

Do you do things under the influence of drugs that you would not normally do?

Have you seriously thought that you might have a chemical dependency problem?

## ARE YOU CONTROLLED BY A DRUG USER?

Is your life controlled by a drug user? Your love and care (codependency) may actually be enabling the drug user to continue his or her use, hurting you and others. Take this assessment; the more "yes" checks you make, the more likely there's a problem.

Do you often have to lie or cover up for the drug user?

Do you spend time counselling the person about the problem?

Have you taken on additional financial or family responsibilities?

Do you feel that you have to control the drug user's behaviour?

At the office, have you done work or attended meetings for the user?

Do you often put your own needs and desires after the user's?

Do you spend time each day worrying about your situation?

Do you analyze your behaviour to find clues to how it might affect the drug user?

Do you feel powerless and at your wits' end about the user's problem?

Source: Reprinted by permission of Krames Communications, 1100 Grundy Lane, San Bruno, CA 94066–3030.

## WHAT WOULD YOU DO?

Would you change the current laws governing drugs? Why or why not? What do you think is needed to reduce the level of illicit substance use and abuse in Canada?

# CONTROLLED SUBSTANCES

Hundreds of illegal drugs exist. For general purposes, they can be divided into five representative categories: stimulants, marijuana and its derivatives, depressants, psychedelics and deliriants, and so-called designer drugs.

## Cocaine

**Cocaine** is a crystalline white alkaloid powder derived from the leaves of the South American coca shrub (not related to cocoa plants).[18] The leaves had been chewed for thousands of years by people in Peru and Bolivia to lessen hunger and fatigue. Pure cocaine was isolated in 1860, by a German pharmacology graduate student. In the 1880s, Freud praised the powerful stimulant effects of cocaine as the treatment for a variety of illnesses including depression and alcohol and opioid addiction. Cocaine use then increased and it was widely and

**Illicit drugs:** Drugs illegal to possess, produce, or sell.

**Cocaine:** A powerful stimulant drug made from the leaves of the South American coca shrub.

legally available in Canada in medicine and soft drinks. With increased use the risks of cocaine became clear, and in 1911 Canada passed laws restricting its importation, manufacture, sale, and possession.

Cocaine is generally sold on the street as a hydrochloride salt—a fine, white crystalline powder known as blow, C, coke, crack, flake, freebase, rock, and snow.[19] Street dealers dilute it with inert (non-psychoactive) but similar-looking substances such as cornstarch, talcum powder, and sugar, or with active drugs such as procaine and benzocaine (used as local anesthetics), or other central nervous system (CNS) stimulants such as amphetamines.

According to the 2003–2004 Canadian Addiction Survey, 10.6 percent of the population used cocaine or crack at some point in their lives and 1.9 percent reported use in the past 12 months.[20]

Cocaine can affect mood, judgment, and motor skills. The most dramatic effects of cocaine are on vision. Cocaine may cause a higher sensitivity to light, halos around bright objects, and difficulty focusing. Users have also reported blurred vision, glare problems, and hallucinations, particularly "snow lights"—weak flashes or movements of light in the peripheral field of vision, which tend to make drivers swerve toward or away from the lights. Some users have also reported auditory hallucinations (for example, ringing bells) and olfactory hallucinations (for example, the smell of smoke or gasoline).

Cocaine can also heighten irritability, excitability, and startle response. Users have reported that sudden sounds, such as horns or sirens, have caused them severe anxiety coupled with rapid steering or braking reactions, even when the source of the sound was not in the immediate vicinity of their vehicles. Suspiciousness, distrust, and paranoia—other reactions to cocaine—have prompted users to flee in their cars or drive evasively. Everyone surveyed reported attention lapses while driving, and ignoring relevant stimuli such as changes in traffic signals.[21]

## Methods of Cocaine Use

Cocaine can be taken in several ways. The powdered form of the drug is "snorted" through the nose. Smoking (freebasing) and intravenous injections are more dangerous means of ingesting cocaine. When cocaine is snorted, it can cause damage to the mucous membranes in the nose and sinusitis. It can damage the user's sense of smell, and occasionally it creates a hole in the septum. Smoking cocaine can result in lung and liver damage. Freebasing has become more popular than injecting in recent years because people fear contracting diseases such as AIDS and hepatitis by sharing contaminated needles. However, since the volatile mixes freebasing requires

are very explosive, some people have been killed or seriously burned as a result.

Many cocaine users still occasionally "shoot up." Injecting allows the user to introduce large amounts of cocaine rapidly into the body. Within seconds, there is an incredible sense of euphoria. This intense high lasts only 15 to 20 minutes, and then the user heads into a "crash." To prevent the unpleasant effects of the crash, users often shoot up frequently, which can severely damage their veins. Besides AIDS and hepatitis, injecting users place themselves at risk for skin infections, inflammation of the arteries, and infection of the lining of the heart.

## Physical Effects of Cocaine

The effects of cocaine are felt rapidly. Snorted cocaine enters the bloodstream through the lungs in less than one minute and reaches the brain in less than three minutes. When cocaine binds at its receptor sites in the central nervous system, it produces intense pleasure. The euphoria quickly abates, however, and the desire to regain the pleasurable feelings makes the user want more.

Cocaine is an anesthetic and a central nervous system stimulant. In tiny doses, it can slow heart rate. In larger doses, the physical effects are dramatic: increased heart rate and blood pressure, loss of appetite that can lead to dramatic weight loss, convulsions, muscle twitching, irregular heartbeat, even death due to overdose. Other effects of cocaine include temporary relief of depression, decreased fatigue, talkativeness, increased alertness, and heightened self-confidence. Again, however, as the dose increases users become irritable and apprehensive and their behaviours may turn paranoid or violent.

## Cocaine-Affected Babies

Because cocaine rapidly crosses the placenta (as virtually all drugs do), the fetus is vulnerable when a pregnant women uses. The most threatening problem during pregnancy is the increased risk of a miscarriage. Should the pregnant users reach full term, their babies are usually born with brain damage, heart defects, kidney problems, and malformed heads, arms, and fingers. These babies tend to show signs of withdrawal at birth, including irritability, jitteriness, and the inability to eat or sleep properly. They seem to be unable to respond or to relate to people the way normal babies do, and are difficult to console and comfort. Because it is so difficult for adults to interact with them, their social and emotional development is negatively affected. Cocaine is also transmitted from a using mother to her breast-fed baby. The baby is then exposed to all the physical and mental effects of cocaine use.[22]

## Freebase Cocaine

**Freebase** is a form of cocaine that is more powerful and costly than the powder or chip (crack) form. Street cocaine (cocaine hydrochloride) is converted to pure base by removing the hydrochloride salt and many of the "cutting agents." The end product, freebase, is smoked through a water pipe. Because freebase cocaine reaches the brain within seconds, it is more dangerous than cocaine that is snorted. It produces a quick, intense high that disappears quickly, leaving an intense craving for more. Freebasers typically increase the amount and frequency of the dose. They often become severely addicted and experience serious health problems and financial ruin.[23] Side effects of freebasing cocaine include weight loss, increased heart rate and blood pressure, depression, paranoia, and hallucinations. Freebase is an extremely dangerous drug and is responsible for a large number of cocaine-related hospital emergency-room visits and deaths.

## Crack

**Crack** is the street name given to freebase cocaine that has been processed from cocaine hydrochloride using ammonia or sodium bicarbonate (baking soda) and water and heating the substance to remove the hydrochloride. Crack can also be processed with ether, but this is much riskier because ether is a flammable solvent. The mixture (90-percent-pure cocaine) is then dried. The soapy-looking substance that results can be broken up into "rocks" and smoked. These rocks are approximately five times as strong as cocaine. Crack gets its name from the popping noises it makes when burned. A crack user may quickly become addicted to the drug. Addiction is accelerated by the speed at which crack is absorbed through the lungs (it hits the brain within seconds after use) and by the intensity of the high.

> ### WHAT WOULD YOU DO?
>
> Why do you think young people choose to use cocaine? In what circumstances would you consider using cocaine?

## Amphetamines

The **amphetamines** include a large and varied group of synthetic agents that stimulate the central nervous system. Small doses of amphetamines act like adrenaline (a hormone that naturally stimulates the body) and improve alertness, lessen fatigue, and generally elevate mood.[24] With repeated use, however, physiological and psychological dependence develops. Sleep patterns

are affected (insomnia); heart rate, breathing rate, and blood pressure increase; restlessness, anxiety, appetite suppression, and vision problems are common. High doses over long time periods can produce hallucinations, delusions, and disorganized behaviours. Abusers become paranoid, fearing everything and everyone. Some become very aggressive or antisocial.

Amphetamines are sold under a variety of names. "Bennies" (amphetamine/Benzedrine), "dex" (dextroamphetamine/Dexedrine), and "meth" or "speed" (methamphetamine/Methedrine) are some of the most common. Other street terms for amphetamines are "cross tops," "crank," "uppers," "wake-ups," "lid poppers," "cartwheels," and "blackies." Amphetamines do have therapeutic uses in the treatment of attention deficit hyperactivity disorder in children (Ritalin®, Cylert) and of obesity (Pondimin).

## Methamphetamine

An increasingly common form of amphetamine, **methamphetamine** (meth) is a potent, long-acting, addictive drug that strongly activates the brain's reward centre by producing a sense of euphoria.[25] "Crystal meth" can cause brain damage resulting in impaired motor skills and cognitive functions, psychosis, and increased risk for heart attack and stroke. Methamphetamine can be snorted, smoked, injected, or orally ingested. Depending on the method of use, the drug will affect the user in different ways. Users often experience tolerance immediately, making meth a highly addictive drug from the very first time it is used. When snorted, the effects can be felt in 3 to 5 minutes; if orally ingested, the user will experience effects within 15 to 20 minutes. The pleasurable effects of meth are typically an intense rush lasting only a few minutes when snorted or a high lasting over 8 hours when smoked.

## Physical Effects of Methamphetamine

Smaller doses of methamphetamine produce increased physical activity, alertness, and a decreased appetite. However, the drug's effects quickly wear off, and the user seeks more. Long-term use of meth can cause severe dependence, psychosis, paranoia, aggression, weight loss, and stroke. Abusers often do not sleep or

---

**Freebase:** The most powerful distillate of cocaine.

**Crack:** A distillate of powdered cocaine that comes in small, hard "chips" or "rocks."

**Amphetamines** A large and varied group of synthetic agents that stimulate the central nervous system.

**Methamphetamine (meth):** A powerfully addictive drug that strongly activates certain areas of the brain and affects the central nervous system.

eat for days, as they continually inject up to 1 gram of the drug every 2 to 3 hours. A high state of irritability and agitation has been associated with violent behaviours among some users. Use of meth is an increasingly serious problem. A possible contributing factor to the increasing rate of meth use is that it is relatively easy to make. Meth is produced by "cookers" using recipes that often include common OTC ingredients such as ephedrine and pseudoephedrine, found in cold and allergy medication as well as lethal ingredients such as drain cleaner, battery acid, and others.

**Ice** is a potent form of methamphetamine created in Canada and imported primarily from Asia, particularly from South Korea and Taiwan. Ice when smoked is odourless, and its effects can last for more than 12 hours. Like other methamphetamines, the "down" side of this drug is devastating. Prolonged use can cause fatal lung and kidney damage, as well as long-lasting psychological damage. In some instances, major psychological dysfunction can persist as long as two and a half years after last use.

# Marijuana

Although archaeological evidence documents **marijuana** (also known as grass, weed, pot, dope, ganja, and others[26]) use as far back as 6,000 years ago, the drug did not become popular in North America until the 1960s. Marijuana remains by far the most extensively used illicit drug, with 44.5 percent of Canadians over the age of 15 years reporting use in their lifetime and 14.1 percent indicating use in the past 12 months.[27]

### Physical Effects of Marijuana

Marijuana is derived from either the *cannabis sativa* or *cannabis indica* (hemp) plants. Today's top-grade cannabis packs a punch similar to hashish. **Tetrahydrocannabinol (THC)** is the psychoactive substance in marijuana, and the key to determining how powerful a high the marijuana will produce. Two decades ago, marijuana ranged in potency from 1 to 5 percent THC, while today's crop averages 8 to 15 percent.

**Hashish,** a potent cannabis preparation derived mainly from the thick, sticky resin of the plant, contains high concentrations of THC. Hash oil, a substance produced by percolating a solvent such as ether through dried marijuana to extract the THC, is a tarry liquid that may contain up to 70 percent THC.

Marijuana can be brewed and drunk in tea or baked into quick breads or brownies. THC concentrations in such products are impossible to estimate. Most of the time, however, marijuana is rolled into cigarettes (joints) or packed firmly into a pipe. Some people smoke marijuana through water pipes called bongs.

Effects are generally felt within 10 to 30 minutes and wear off within three hours.

The most noticeable effect of THC is the dilation of the eyes' blood vessels, which produces the characteristic bloodshot eyes. Smokers of the drug also exhibit coughing, dry mouth and throat ("cotton mouth"), increased thirst and appetite, lowered blood pressure, and mild muscular weakness, primarily exhibited in drooping eyelids. Users who take a high dose in an unfamiliar or uncomfortable setting are more likely to experience anxiety and the paranoid belief that their companions are ridiculing or threatening them.

### Effects of Chronic Marijuana Use

Potential long-term effects of heavy or regular marijuana use include (1) an increased risk of cancer because of the tar and other known cancer-causing agents in cannabis, (2) irritation to the respiratory system (in fact, smoking 3 to 4 joints per day has a similar effect as 20 cigarettes), (3) reduced motivation for work and study, (4) schizophrenia, and (5) impaired attention, memory, and ability to process complex information.[28] Other risks associated with marijuana include suppression of the immune system and blood pressure changes. Research suggests that pregnant women who smoke marijuana are at a higher risk for stillbirth or miscarriage and for delivering low-birthweight babies and babies with abnormalities of the nervous system. Babies born to women who use marijuana during pregnancy are five times more likely to have features similar to those exhibited by children with fetal alcohol spectrum disorders.

Debates concerning the effects of marijuana on the reproductive system have yet to be resolved. Studies conducted in the mid-1970s suggested that marijuana inhibited testosterone (and thus sperm) production in males and caused chromosomal breakage in ova and sperm. Subsequent research in these areas was inconclusive. The question of whether the high-level THC plants currently available will increase the risks associated with this drug is, as yet, unanswered.

### Marijuana and Medicine

Although recognized as a dangerous drug by the Canadian government, marijuana has several medical purposes. It helps control side effects such as the severe nausea and vomiting produced by chemotherapy, the chemical treatment for cancer. It also improves appetite and forestalls the loss of lean muscle mass associated with AIDS-wasting syndrome. Marijuana reduces the muscle pain and spasticity caused by diseases such as multiple sclerosis. It also temporarily relieves the eye pressure of glaucoma (a progressive disease characterized by increased fluid pressure in the eyeball).

## Marijuana and Driving

Marijuana use presents clear hazards for drivers of motor vehicles as well as for others on the road. The drug substantially reduces a driver's ability to react and to make quick decisions. Studies reveal that 60 to 80 percent of marijuana users sometimes drive while high.[29] Studies of automobile accident victims show that 6 to 12 percent of nonfatally injured drivers and 4 to 16 percent of fatally injured drivers had THC in their bloodstreams. Perceptual and other performance deficits resulting from marijuana use may persist for some time after the high subsides. Users who attempt to drive, fly, or operate heavy machinery often fail to recognize their impairment.

# Opiates

The opiates are among the oldest analgesics known. These drugs cause drowsiness, relieve pain, and induce euphoria. Also called **narcotics,** they are derived from the parent drug **opium,** a dark, resinous substance made from the milky juice of the opium poppy. Other opiates include morphine, codeine, heroin, and black tar heroin.

The word *narcotic* comes from the Greek word for "stupor" and is generally used to describe sleep-inducing substances. For many years, opiates were widely used by the medical community to relieve pain, induce sleep, curb nausea and vomiting, stop diarrhea, and sedate psychiatric patients. During the late nineteenth and early twentieth centuries, many patent medicines contained opiates. Suppliers advertised these concoctions as cures for everything from menstrual cramps to teething pains.

Among the opiates once widely used by medical practitioners was **morphine.** First manufactured in the early nineteenth century, morphine was named after Morpheus, the Greek god of sleep, and is more powerful than opium. **Codeine,** a less powerful analgesic derived from morphine, also became popular.

All opiates are highly addictive. Growing concern about addiction led to government controls of narcotic use. Subsequent legislation required physicians prescribing opiates to keep careful records. Physicians are still subject to audits of their prescriptions of these agents. Some opiates are still used today for medical purposes. Morphine is sometimes prescribed by doctors in hospital settings for relief of severe pain. Codeine is found in prescription cough syrups and in other painkillers. Several prescription drugs, including Percodan, Demerol, and Dilaudid, contain synthetic opiates. All opiate use is strictly regulated.

## Physical Effects of Opiates

Opiates are powerful central nervous system depressants. In addition to relieving pain, these drugs lower heart rate, respiration, and blood pressure. Side effects include weakness, dizziness, nausea, vomiting, euphoria, decreased sex drive, visual disturbances, and lack of coordination. Of all the opiates, heroin is the most notorious. Because all opiate addiction follows a similar progression, we will use heroin as a model for narcotic abuse.

## Heroin Addiction

**Heroin** and black tar heroin are powerful opiates. Heroin is a white powder derived from morphine. Black tar heroin is a sticky, dark brown, foul-smelling substance, also made from morphine. Heroin is a depressant. It produces a dreamy, mentally slow feeling and drowsiness in the user. It also can cause drastic mood swings, with euphoric highs followed by depressive lows. Heroin also slows respiration and urinary output and constricts the pupils of the eyes (hence the image of the stereotypical drug user hiding his eyes behind a pair of dark sunglasses). Symptoms of tolerance and withdrawal can appear within three weeks of first use.

The most common route of administration for heroin addicts is "mainlining"—intravenous injection of powdered heroin mixed in a solution—though fear of HIV and hepatitis infection has resulted in some avoiding needles. Many users describe the "rush" they feel when injecting themselves as intensely pleasurable, whereas others report unpredictable and unpleasant effects. The temporary nature of the rush contributes to the drug's high potential for addiction—many addicts shoot up four or five times a day. Mainlining can cause veins to

**Ice:** A potent, inexpensive stimulant that has long-lasting effects.

**Marijuana:** Chopped leaves and flowers of the *cannabis indica* (hemp) or *cannabis sativa* plant; a psychoactive stimulant that intensifies reactions to environmental stimuli.

**Tetrahydrocannabinol (THC):** The chemical name for the active ingredient in marijuana.

**Hashish:** The sticky resin of the cannabis plant, which is high in THC.

**Narcotics:** Drugs that induce sleep and relieve pain; primarily the opiates.

**Opium:** The parent drug of the opiates; made from the milky juice of the opium poppy.

**Morphine:** A derivative of opium; sometimes used by medical practitioners to relieve pain.

**Codeine:** A drug derived from morphine; used in cough syrups and certain painkillers.

**Heroin:** An illegally manufactured derivative of morphine, usually injected into the bloodstream.

# Battling Addictions

Recognizing that a problem exists is one of the most difficult steps in the process of battling addictions due to individual levels of denial. Intervention is a planned process of confrontation by significant others to break down the denial compassionately so that the individual can see the destructive nature of the addiction. The individual must come to perceive that the addiction is destructive and requires treatment. Once this has been accomplished, treatment and recovery can begin.

Treatment and recovery for any addiction begin with abstinence—refraining from the addictive behaviours. But abstinence does little to change the personality and psychological dynamics or the biological and environmental influences behind the addictive behaviours. Recovery involves learning new ways of looking at oneself, others, and the world. It may require exploration of a traumatic past so that psychological wounds can be healed. It requires new ways of taking care of oneself, physically and emotionally. It involves developing communication skills and new ways of having fun. Recovery programs are the fuel that gives addicts the energy to resist relapsing. For a large number of addicts, recovery begins with a period of formal treatment. A good treatment program should have the following characteristics:

- professional staff familiar with the specific addictive disorder for which help is being sought
- a flexible schedule of inpatient and outpatient services
- access to medical personnel who can assess the addict's medical status and provide treatment for all medical concerns as needed
- medical supervision of addicts at high risk for a complicated detoxification
- a team approach to treatment of the addictive disorders (for example, medical personnel, counsellors, psychotherapists, social workers, clergy, educators, dietitians, fitness counsellors, and family members)
- group and individual therapy options
- integration of peer-led support groups and encouragement to continue involvement after treatment ends
- structured after-care and relapse-prevention programs
- a clean and attractive environment
- a cordial and helping staff

Highly structured treatment programs help their clients get started on a lifetime program of personal recovery. They include wellness programs to teach critical self-care skills, educational programs to formulate a deep understanding of the addiction, self-help groups to provide a foundation of support after treatment, and several forms of therapy, including those listed below.

- *Individual therapy.* Addicts can identify and experience feelings they have been chronically medicating with their addictive behaviours. During sessions, addicts begin to deal with issues related to their addiction.
- *Group therapy.* The group provides an opportunity for developing communication skills and offers an environment where addicts learn how to be honest with themselves and others. The standard care in a treatment program is to combine group therapy with individual therapy.
- *Family therapy.* Family therapy helps all members of the family to recover from their codependant role.
- *12-step programs.* One of the most common types of peer support groups is a 12-step program, patterned after Alcoholics Anonymous. They are designed to keep individuals free of their addictions through honest acknowledgment of their shortcomings and through the mutual support of others who have had similar experiences. There are 12-step programs for every addiction, including Narcotics Anonymous, as well as for families and others who have a relationship with an addict.
- *Alternatives to 12-step programs.* Because many 12-step programs adhere to a spiritual basis in the recovery process, some recovering addicts have sought out or started alternative groups.

become scarred, and if this practice is frequent enough the veins collapse. Once a vein has collapsed, it can no longer be used to introduce heroin into the bloodstream. Addicts become expert at locating new veins to use: in the feet, the legs, and the temples. When they do not want their needle tracks (scars) to show, they inject themselves under the tongue or in the groin.

## Treatment for Heroin Addiction

Programs to help individuals addicted to heroin have not been very successful. The rate of recidivism (tendency to return to previous behaviours) is high. Some individuals resume their drug use even after years of drug-free living because the craving for the injection rush is so strong. It takes a great deal of discipline to seek alternative, non-drug highs. Individuals addicted to heroin experience a distinct pattern of withdrawal. They begin to crave another dose four to six hours after their last dose. Symptoms of withdrawal include intense desire for the drug, yawning, a runny nose, sweating, and crying. About 12 hours after the last dose, addicts experience sleep disturbance, dilated pupils, loss of appetite, irritability, goosebumps, and muscle tremors. The most difficult time in the withdrawal process occurs 24 to 72 hours following last use. All the preceding symptoms continue, along with nausea, abdominal cramps, restlessness, insomnia, vomiting, diarrhea, extreme anxiety, hot and cold flashes, elevated blood pressure, and rapid heartbeat and respiration. Once the peak of withdrawal has passed, these symptoms begin to subside. Still, the recovering addict has many hurdles to jump.

**Methadone maintenance** is one type of treatment available for people addicted to heroin or other opiates. Methadone is a synthetic narcotic that blocks the effects of opiate withdrawal. It is chemically similar enough to the opiates to control the tremors, chills, vomiting, diarrhea, and severe abdominal pains of withdrawal. The methadone dose is decreased over a period of time until the addict is weaned off the drug.

Methadone maintenance is controversial because of its potential for addiction. Critics contend that the program merely substitutes one addiction for another. Proponents argue that people on methadone maintenance are less likely than addicts to engage in criminal activities to support their addictions. For this reason, many methadone maintenance programs are government financed and available to clients free of charge or at reduced costs.

## Psychedelics

**Psychedelics** are a group of drugs whose primary pharmacological effect is to alter feelings, perceptions, and thoughts in the user. The major receptor sites for most of these drugs are in the part of the brain responsible for interpreting outside stimuli before allowing these signals to travel to other parts of the brain. This area is called the **reticular formation** and is located in the brain stem at the upper end of the spinal cord (see Figure 10.2). When a psychedelic drug is present at a reticular formation receptor site, messages become scrambled and the user may see wavy walls instead of straight ones or may smell colours or hear tastes. This mixing of sensory messages is known as *synaesthesia.*

In addition to synaesthetic effects, users may recall events long buried in the subconscious mind or become less inhibited than they are in a non-drug state. Some psychedelic drugs are erroneously labelled

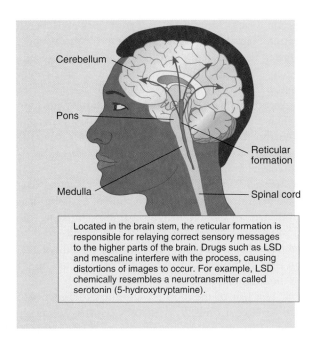

Located in the brain stem, the reticular formation is responsible for relaying correct sensory messages to the higher parts of the brain. Drugs such as LSD and mescaline interfere with the process, causing distortions of images to occur. For example, LSD chemically resembles a neurotransmitter called serotonin (5-hydroxytryptamine).

**FIGURE 10.2**
**The Reticular Formation**

"hallucinogens." Hallucinogens are substances that are capable of creating auditory or visual **hallucinations,** or images that are perceived but are not real. Not all psychedelic drugs are capable of producing hallucinations. The most widely recognized psychedelics are LSD, mescaline, psilocybin, and psilocin. These drugs are illegal and carry severe penalties for manufacture, possession, transportation, or sale.

### LSD

Of all the psychedelics, **lysergic acid diethylamide (LSD)** has achieved the most notoriety. This chemical was first synthesized in the late 1930s by the Swiss chemist Albert Hoffman. It resulted from experiments aimed at deriving medically useful drugs from the ergot fungus found on rye and other cereal grains.

**Methadone maintenance:** A treatment for people addicted to opiates where methadone, a synthetic narcotic, is used to block the withdrawal symptoms.

**Psychedelics:** Drugs that distort the processing of sensory information in the brain.

**Reticular formation:** An area in the brain stem that is responsible for relaying messages to other areas in the brain.

**Hallucination:** An image (auditory or visual) that is perceived but is not real.

**Lysergic acid diethylamide (LSD):** Psychedelic drug causing sensory disruptions; also called acid.

Psychiatrists initially felt it could be beneficial to patients unable to remember and recognize suppressed traumas and the drug was used for such purposes from 1950 through 1968. Known on the street as "acid," LSD continues to be widely available.

An odourless, tasteless, white crystalline powder, LSD is most frequently dissolved in water to make a solution that can then be used to manufacture the street forms of the drug: tablets, blotter acid, and windowpane. What the LSD consumer usually buys is blotter acid—small squares of blotter-like paper that have been impregnated with the liquid. The blotter is swallowed or chewed briefly. LSD also comes in tiny thin squares of gelatin called windowpane and in tablets called microdots, which are less than three millimetres (it would take 10 or more of these to add up to the size of an ASA tablet).

LSD is one of the most powerful drugs known and can produce strong effects in doses as low as 20 micrograms. (To give you an idea of how small a dose this is, the average-sized postage stamp weighs approximately 60,000 micrograms.) The potency of the typical dose of LSD currently ranges from 20 to 80 micrograms, compared to 150 to 300 micrograms commonly used in the 1960s.

Despite its reputation for being primarily a psychedelic, LSD produces a large number of physical effects, including slightly increased heart rate, elevated blood pressure and temperature, goose flesh (roughened skin), increased reflex speeds, muscle tremors and twitches, perspiration, increased salivation, chills, headaches, and mild nausea. Since the drug also stimulates uterine muscle contractions, it can lead to premature labour and miscarriage in pregnant women. Research into the effects of long-term LSD use has been inconclusive. As with any illegally purchased drug, users run the risk of purchasing an impure product.

The psychological effects of LSD vary from person to person. The set and setting in which the drug is used are strong influential factors. Euphoria is the common psychological state produced by the drug, but dysphoria (a sense of evil and foreboding) may also be experienced. The drug also shortens attention span, causing the mind to wander. Thoughts may be interposed and juxtaposed as well. The user may thus be able to experience several different thoughts simultaneously. Synaesthesia occurs occasionally. Users become introspective, and suppressed memories may surface, often taking on bizarre symbolism. Many more effects are possible, including decreased aggressiveness and enhanced sensory experiences.

While there is no evidence of physiological dependence with LSD use, psychological dependence is likely. Many LSD users become depressed for one or two days following a trip and use the drug to relieve this depression. The result is a cycle of LSD use to relieve post-LSD depression, which often leads to psychological addiction.

## Mescaline

**Mescaline** is one of hundreds of chemicals derived from the **peyote** cactus. This small, buttonlike cactus grows in the southwestern United States and parts of Latin America. Natives of these regions have long used the dried peyote buttons during religious ceremonies. In fact, members of the Native American Church (a religion practised by thousands of North American Indians) have been granted special permission to use the drug during ceremonies in some U.S. states.

Users normally swallow 10 to 12 dried peyote buttons. These buttons taste bitter and generally induce immediate nausea or vomiting. Long-time users claim that the nausea becomes less noticeable with frequent use. Those who are able to keep the drug down begin to feel the effects within 30 to 90 minutes, when mescaline reaches maximum concentration in the brain. The effects may persist for up to 9 or 10 hours. Unlike LSD, mescaline is a powerful hallucinogen. It is also a central nervous system stimulant.

Products sold on the street as mescaline are likely synthetic chemical relatives of the true drug. Street names of these products include DOM, STP, TMA, and MMDA. These drugs can be toxic in small quantities.

## Psilocybin

**Psilocybin** and psilocin are the active chemicals in a group of mushrooms sometimes called "magic mushrooms." Psilocybe mushrooms, which grow throughout the world, can be cultivated from spores or can be harvested wild. Because many mushrooms resemble the psilocybe variety, people who use wild mushrooms for any purpose should be certain of what they are doing. Mushroom varieties can easily be misidentified, and mistakes can be fatal. Psilocybin is similar to LSD in its physical effects, which wear off in four to six hours.

# Deliriants

**Delirium** is an agitated mental state characterized by confusion and disorientation. Almost all psychoactive drugs will produce delirium at high doses, with **deliriants** producing this effect at relatively low (subtoxic) levels.

### PCP

**Phencyclidine (PCP)** is one of the best-known deliriants. It is a synthetic substance that became a black-market drug in the early 1970s. PCP was originally developed as a "disassociative anesthetic," which means that patients given this drug could keep their eyes open, apparently remain conscious, and feel no pain during a medical procedure. Patients would afterward experience amnesia for the time the drug was in their system. Such a drug had obvious advantages as an anesthetic during surgery, but its unpredictability and drastic effects (postoperative delirium, confusion, and agitation) made doctors discontinue its use, and it was withdrawn from the legal market.

On the illegal market, PCP is a white, crystalline powder that users often sprinkle onto marijuana cigarettes. It is dangerous and unpredictable regardless of how it is administered. Common street names for PCP are "angel dust" for the crystalline powdered form and "peace pill" and "horse tranquillizer" for the tablet form.

The effects of PCP depend on the dosage. As little as 5 milligrams will produce effects similar to strong central nervous system depressants. These effects include slurred speech, impaired coordination, reduced sensitivity to pain, and reduced heart and respiratory rates. Doses between 5 and 10 milligrams cause fever, salivation, nausea, vomiting, and total loss of sensitivity to pain. Doses greater than 10 milligrams result in a dramatic drop in blood pressure, coma, muscular rigidity, violent outbursts, and possible convulsions and death.

Psychologically, PCP may produce either euphoria or dysphoria. It is also known to produce hallucinations as well as delusions and overall delirium. Some users experience a prolonged state of "nothingness." The long-term effects of PCP use are unknown.

## Designer Drugs

**Designer drugs** are structural analogues (drugs that produce similar effects) of more familiar illicit drugs. These illegal drugs are manufactured by underground chemists to mimic the psychoactive effects of controlled drugs. At present, at least three types of synthetic drugs are available on the illegal drug market: analogues of phencyclidine (PCP), analogues of fentanyl and meperidine (both synthetic narcotic analgesics), and analogues of amphetamine and methamphetamine, which have hallucinogenic and stimulant properties.[30]

Although PCP analogues have been identified in street samples of drugs, they are less frequently used today than other forms of designer drugs. Analogues of fentanyl are much more common. The pharmacological properties of most fentanyl analogues are similar to those of heroin or morphine. These analogues are known as "synthetic heroin" or "new heroin." These designer drugs may be addictive and carry the risk of overdose.

Amphetamine and methamphetamine analogues are the most common forms of designer drugs on campuses today. These analogues often cause hallucinations and euphoria. Ecstasy is one such analogue. It is actually a chemical called methylene dioxymethylamphetamine, or MDMA, and it is similar to the hallucinogen MMDA. In small to moderate doses, ecstasy can produce feelings of energy, confidence, pleasure, well-being, increased sociability, and closeness to others. Larger doses are not likely to enhance these desired effects. In fact, large doses of ecstasy are associated with grinding of teeth, jaw pain, sweating, increased blood pressure and heart rate, anxiety, panic attacks, blurred vision, nausea, vomiting, and convulsions.[31]

## Inhalants

**Inhalants** are chemicals that produce vapours that, when inhaled, can cause hallucinations as well as create intoxicating and euphoric effects. They are not commonly recognized as drugs. They are legal to purchase and universally available but are potentially dangerous when used incorrectly. These drugs appeal to those who can't afford illicit substances.

Included in this category are organic solvents resulting from the distillation of petroleum products (rubber cement, model glue, paint thinner, lighter fluid, varnish, wax, spot removers, and gasoline). Most of these substances are sniffed by users. Because

---

**Mescaline:** A hallucinogenic drug derived from the peyote cactus.

**Peyote:** A cactus with small "buttons" that, when ingested, produce hallucinogenic effects.

**Psilocybin:** The active chemical found in psilocybe mushrooms; it produces hallucinations.

**Delirium:** An agitated mental state characterized by confusion and disorientation produced by psychoactive drugs.

**Deliriant:** Any substance that produces delirium at relatively low doses, including PCP and some herbal substances.

**Phencyclidine (PCP):** A deliriant commonly called "angel dust."

**Designer drug:** A synthetic analogue of an existing illicit drug— that is, a drug that has effects similar to those of an illicit drug.

**Inhalants:** Products sniffed or inhaled in order to produce highs.

they are inhaled, the volatile chemicals in these products reach the bloodstream within seconds. An inhaled substance is not diluted or buffered by stomach acids or other body fluids and thus is more potent and dangerous than the same substance would be if swallowed. This characteristic, along with the fact that dosages are extremely difficult to control because everyone has unique lung and breathing capacities, makes inhalants particularly dangerous. An overdose of fumes from inhalants can cause unconsciousness. If the user's oxygen intake is reduced during the inhaling process, death can result within five minutes.

### Amyl Nitrite

Sometimes called "poppers" or "rush," **amyl nitrite** is often prescribed to alleviate chest pain in heart patients. It is packaged in small, cloth-covered glass capsules that can be crushed to release the active chemical. The drug relieves chest pains because it causes rapid dilation of the small blood vessels and reduces blood pressure. That same dilation of blood vessels in the genital area is thought to enhance sensations or perceptions of orgasm. It also produces fainting, dizziness, warmth, and skin flushing.

### Nitrous Oxide

"Laughing gas" is the popular term for **nitrous oxide.** It is sometimes used as an adjunct to dental anesthesia or minor surgical anesthesia. It is also used as a propellant chemical in aerosol products such as whipped toppings. Users experience a state of euphoria, floating sensations, and illusions. Effects also include pain relief and a "silly" feeling, demonstrated by laughing and giggling (hence the term laughing gas). Regulating dosages of this drug can be difficult. Sustained inhalation can lead to unconsciousness, coma, and death.

## Steroids

Public awareness of **anabolic steroids** has been heightened by media stories about their use by amateur and professional athletes, including Ben Johnson, who lost the gold medal he had won for Canada at the Seoul Olympics when he failed a urine test and then, when he was allowed to return to the sport some years later, promptly failed another test. Anabolic steroids are artificial forms of the male hormone testosterone that promote muscle growth and strength. Although these **ergogenic drugs** are used primarily by young men to increase their strength, power, bulk (weight),

*Steroid acne.*

and speed and thus improve their athletic performance, others not involved in athletics use steroids for the intimidation factor of increased muscle size or simply to improve their physique.

Most steroids are obtained through black-market sources. Steroids are available in two forms: injectable solution and pills.[32] Anabolic steroids produce a state of euphoria, diminished fatigue, and increased bulk and power in both sexes. These qualities give steroids an addictive quality. When users stop, they appear to undergo psychological withdrawal, mainly caused by the disappearance of the physique they have become accustomed to. Steroids cause several adverse effects in men and women. These drugs cause mood swings (aggression and violence), sometimes known as "roid rage," acne, liver tumours, elevated cholesterol levels, hypertension, kidney disease, and immune system disturbances. There is also a danger of HIV transmission through shared needles. In women, large doses of anabolic steroids trigger masculine changes, including lowered voice, increased facial and body hair, male pattern baldness, enlarged clitoris, decreased breast size, and changes in or absence of menstruation. When taken by healthy males, anabolic steroids shut down the body's production of testosterone, causing men's breasts to grow and testicles to atrophy.

A new and alarming trend is the use of other drugs to achieve the "performance-enhancing" effects of steroids. These steroid alternatives are sought in order to avoid the penalties (such as being banned from sports) for illicit use of anabolic steroids. The two most common steroid alternatives are gamma hydroxybutyrate (GHB) and clenbuterol. GHB is a deadly, illegal drug that is a primary ingredient in many of these "performance-enhancing" formulas. GHB does not produce a high. It does, however, cause headaches, nausea, vomiting, diarrhea, seizures and other central nervous system disorders, and possibly death. Another steroid alternative, Nandrolone, has recently been turning up in drug tests, and yet another, Clenbuterol, has become an extremely popular item on the black market. Canada conducts around 2,000 doping control tests per year on premier athletes. Most (70 percent) are random. Excluding body building, power lifting, and junior football (which have a 25-percent positive test result), there is about a 3-percent violation rate. For Olympic sports, the rate is 1 percent.[33]

## WHAT WOULD YOU DO?

How do reports in the media about the use of steroids by athletes affect the popularity of these drugs? Would you consider using such a drug to improve your appearance? Your athletic performance?

# DRUGS IN THE WORKPLACE

The cost of drug and alcohol use in the workplace has been estimated at $18.45 billion—or about 2.7 percent of the total gross domestic product. Illicit drugs cost the Canadian economy $1.4 billion. The balance was due to smoking ($9.6 billion) and alcohol ($7.5 billion). The largest economic costs of substance abuse are for lost productivity due to morbidity and premature mortality, direct health costs, and law enforcement. There is considerable variation in the costs of substance abuse among the provinces.[34] It is becoming more and more common for companies to have employee assistance programs (EAP), which offer drug and personal counselling.

## WHAT WOULD YOU DO?

What is the impact of illicit and licit drug use in society? Why are the costs so high? Have you ever personally known someone addicted to drugs? How was his or her life affected? How did you respond?

# SOLUTIONS TO THE PROBLEM

In 2000, a 9-percent increase in cannabis offences contributed to the 9-percent increase in the overall rate of drug offences, continuing the upward trend that began in 1994. Cannabis offences accounted for three-quarters of all drug-related incidents. More than two-thirds of these were for possession. Increases were also seen in the rate of cocaine offences (+6 percent) and other drug offences (+12 percent). Heroin offences dropped by 8 percent.[35]

In general, researchers in the field of drug education agree that a multimodal approach to drug education is best. Students should be taught the differences in drug use, misuse, and abuse. Factual information that is free from scare tactics must be presented; moralizing about drug use does not work. Critical to these teachings is expanding students' decision making and critical thinking skills. Programs that teach people to control drugs, as opposed to allowing drugs to control them, are needed, as are programs that teach about the influences of set and setting. Reinforcing self-esteem is mandatory. It is not enough to urge people to "just say no." Further, alternatives to drug use should be taught.

All drug abuse prevention approaches probably help up to a point, but neither alone nor in combination do they offer a total solution to the problem. Drug use has been a part of human behaviours for thousands of years, and it is not likely to disappear in the near future. For this reason, we need to educate ourselves and develop the self-discipline necessary to avoid dangerous drug dependencies.

**Amyl nitrite:** A drug that dilates blood vessels and is properly used to relieve chest pain.

**Nitrous oxide:** The chemical name for "laughing gas," a substance used for surgical or dental anesthesia.

**Anabolic steroids:** Artificial forms of the hormone testosterone that promote muscle growth and strength.

**Ergogenic drug:** Substance that enhances athletic performance.

# New Legislation Protects Children Exposed to Drug Manufacturing and Trafficking: First in Canada to Address Emerging Social Issue

*by Jody Korchinski, Alberta Children's Services*

Edmonton—Children exposed to serious drug activity, such as manufacturing and trafficking, will benefit from additional protection under a new law introduced in the Alberta Legislature by Children's Services Minister Heather Forsyth. Bill 2, the *Drug-endangered Children Act* (DECA), was passed on November 1, 2006, and is the first legislation of its kind in Canada.

"Drug manufacturing and trafficking have enormous implications on the well-being and safety of our children," said Forsyth. "We need to keep ahead of this emerging social issue."

The legislation deals with specific drug activity such as manufacturing, particularly crystal methamphetamine labs and indoor marijuana grow operations, and trafficking. It identifies who is a drug-endangered child and makes it clear that a child exposed to a parent or guardian's serious drug activity is a victim of abuse and requires intervention.

This legislation is an excellent tool to help caseworkers and police rescue children endangered by an adult's involvement in serious drug activity. It raises awareness of the plight of drug-endangered children and lets Albertans know the province is committed to taking action. The government expects this will result in an increase in the number of people who report this type of abuse.

"Exposing a child to this type of drug activity is abuse, and it won't be tolerated in Alberta," said Forsyth. "We have a responsibility to take action to protect these children, and that is what this legislation aims to do."

Source: www.ccsa.ca/CCSA/EN/TopNav/Home?Addiction_News/ AddictionNews.htm; Alberta News Release, February 23, 2006; www.gov.ab.ca/acn/200602/1947798C6A2FC-B956-53- AB44F17ADEDDB1CF.html. Alberta Children's Services.

# Managing Drug Use Behaviour

After reading this chapter, you know that addictions can be devastating not only to the user but also to the lives of his or her family and friends. Addictions usually progress gradually, and it is difficult to know for certain when a person crosses the line from habit to addiction. Keep in mind that a behaviour is problematic when it results in negative personal, social, financial, or work-related consequences. If a person continues to use a drug despite negative consequences, chances are that he or she is addicted.

## MAKING DECISIONS FOR YOU

When you have a medical problem (even a minor one such as a headache), you need to decide how best to treat it. What are the symptoms from which you seek relief? What questions should you ask your pharmacist or physician? What drugs (legal or illegal) are you currently using that could cause interactions? What are the pros and cons of each alternative? Which alternative is the best solution for you?

## CHECKLIST FOR CHANGE: MAKING PERSONAL CHOICES

- Do you know what key questions to ask to create a drug profile for any drugs you decide to use?
- Do you read the warning labels on the medications that you use?
- Do you take medication only for the problem for which it is being prescribed?
- Do you ask your doctor or pharmacist if you should avoid alcohol—or any foods, beverages such as coffee or caffeinated soft drinks, or other drugs—while taking an OTC or prescribed medication?
- Do you purchase generic medications instead of brand-name products?
- Do you know what resources exist in the community to help people answer questions about medications?
- What illicit drugs are you familiar with? How did you become familiar with them? What drugs are most popular among your peers? What is it about these drugs that make them popular?
- How do you and your peers feel about illicit drug use? Is it condoned or condemned? Has that changed recently? What has led to these feelings?
- Have you thought of recreational activities that you can do in place of using drugs?
- Are you prepared for the challenge of refusing to use illicit drugs when offered and for dealing with the consequences associated with that decision?

- Do you practise assertiveness? Do you practise speaking up and voicing your opinion regardless of the subject?
- Are you someone who takes pride in your accomplishments? Do you view setbacks as times for growth?
- Do you have strategies for coping with stress? Do you engage in physical activity, meditation, or some other healthy activity as a method of stress reduction?

## CHECKLIST FOR CHANGE: MAKING COMMUNITY CHOICES

- Do you know what comprise the current drug problems on your campus and in your community?
- Would you be willing to assist a friend in combatting his or her substance abuse problem? Would you accompany him or her to support groups?
- Would you be willing to be a role model in community programs such as Big Brothers or Big Sisters?
- Do you volunteer your time for any campus or community organizations that provide opportunities for high-risk youth?
- Would you be willing to volunteer to help at an addiction hotline or community centre?

## CRITICAL THINKING

You have a major term paper due in three days, and you've just completed the reading for it. You are worried about how you'll get it done, and realize you may have to pull an all-nighter. If you don't get at least a B, you'll lose your academic scholarship and will be forced to leave school. A friend tells you that, last semester, she took a few lines of coke; it not only helped her stay awake, but also stimulated her thinking. She got an A– on the paper and experienced no side effects. She suggests you try it, too.

Using the DECIDE model described in Chapter 1, decide how you will keep yourself awake to finish your paper. What stimulant, if any, are you willing to take to stay awake?

# SUMMARY

- Addiction is a process usually evolving over time through a pattern known as nurturing through avoidance. Mood-altering substances and experiences produce biochemical reactions that make the body feel good; when absent, the person feels a withdrawal effect. The addiction process includes biological (genetic) factors as well as social and psychological influences.

- Habits are repetitive behaviours, whereas addiction is behaviour resulting from compulsion; without the behaviours, the addict experiences withdrawal. Addicts have four common symptoms: compulsion, loss of control, negative consequences, and denial.

- The six categories of drugs are prescription drugs, recreational drugs, OTC drugs, herbal preparations, illicit drugs, and commercial preparations. Routes of administration include oral ingestion, injection (intravenous, intramuscular, and subcutaneous), inhalation, inunction, and suppositories.

- Hazardous drug interactions may occur when a person takes several drugs simultaneously. The most hazardous interactions are synergism, antagonism, inhibition, and intolerance.

- Prescription drugs are administered under medical supervision. Categories include antibiotics, sedatives, tranquillizers, antidepressants, and amphetamines. Generic drugs can often be substituted for more expensive brand-name drugs.

- Over-the-counter drug categories include analgesics; cold, cough, allergy, and asthma relievers; stimulants; sleeping aids and relaxants; and dieting aids. Consumers should assume personal responsibility by reading directions for OTC drugs and asking their pharmacist or doctor if any special precautions are advised when taking these substances.

- People from all walks of life use illicit drugs.

- Controlled substances include cocaine and its derivatives, amphetamines and newer-generation stimulants, marijuana, the opiates, the psychedelics, the deliriants, designer drugs, inhalants, and steroids. Users may become addicted quickly to these drugs.

- The drug problem reaches everyone through crime and elevated healthcare costs. Drugs are a major problem in the workplace; workplace drug testing is one proposed solution to this problem.

# DISCUSSION QUESTIONS

1. What factors distinguish a habit from an addiction? Is it possible to gauge your drug use (quantity and frequency) to prevent becoming addicted?

2. Compare and contrast the varied methods of treatment. Which do you think would be most effective for you? For your best friend? For your parents? What accounts for the differences?

3. What environmental factors influence the main effects and side effects of psychoactive drugs?

4. How do analgesics work?

5. What are rebound effects? What are the severe symptoms of withdrawal from stimulants?

6. What general precautions should OTC users consider?

7. Create three antidrug programs aimed at primary, junior, or secondary school children. Think about what antidrug message would have reached you at those particular age levels.

8. List the varied types of drugs. Then discuss their physiological and psychological effects. Why is it that newer, purer forms of drugs (like crack cocaine) are developed?

9. List non-drug alternative behaviours to drug use. Are these realistic? What could make them more enticing?

# APPLICATION EXERCISE

Reread the What Do You Think? scenario at the beginning of the chapter and answer the following questions.

1. Do you think employers have the right to require drug screenings? How about potential employers? Would you want airline pilots or train engineers to be tested regularly? How about cafeteria workers?

2. Do you think that university and college athletes should be tested for drugs? Why or why not? Which drugs would you test for?

# HEALTH ON THE NET

Canadian Centre on Substance Abuse (also has links to various addictions agencies across Canada)
**www.ccsa.ca**

Centre for Addiction and Mental Health
**www.camh.net**

Health Canada — Drugs and Substance Abuse
**www.hc-sc.gc.ca/dhp-mps/substan/index_e.html**

CHAPTER 11

# Alcohol, Tobacco, and Caffeine

*Unacknowledged Drugs with Risk for Addictions*

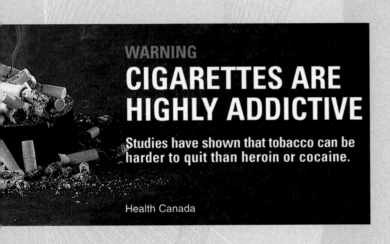

WARNING

## CIGARETTES ARE HIGHLY ADDICTIVE

Studies have shown that tobacco can be harder to quit than heroin or cocaine.

Health Canada

## CHAPTER OBJECTIVES

- Summarize the alcohol-use patterns of post-secondary students and discuss overall trends in consumption.

- Explain the physiological and behavioural effects of alcohol consumption.

- Explain the symptoms and causes of alcoholism, its cost to society, and its effects on the family.

- Explain the treatment of alcoholism, including the family's role and varied treatment methods.

- Discuss the social issues involved in tobacco use.

- Review how regular smoking affects a person.

- Discuss the risks associated with using smokeless tobacco and evaluate the risks to nonsmokers associated with environmental tobacco smoke.

- Describe strategies people adopt to quit using tobacco products, including strategies aimed at breaking the nicotine addiction as well as the habits surrounding the use of tobacco products.

- Compare the benefits and risks associated with caffeine consumption.

When you hear references to the dangers of drugs, what comes to mind? Usually the term "drugs" conjures images of people using cocaine, heroin, marijuana, LSD, PCP, and other illegal substances. Although people use the word *drugs* to refer to one set of dangerous substances, they steadfastly refuse to categorize alcohol as a drug, primarily because its consumption is socially accepted and alcohol sales are booming. In the fiscal year ending March 31, 2004, Canada's beer and liquor sales were $16.1 billion, which is equivalent to almost 2.8 billion litres of alcoholic beverages.[1] Although sales increased by 4.9 percent, this rate of growth was slower than the 6.0 percent reported the previous year.[2] This increase is equivalent to a per capita sale of 107.2 litres for individuals over the age of 15 years.

Most of us think of alcohol the way it is portrayed in ads or in the movies: a way of having fun with company and an important adjunct to a romantic dinner or a cozy evening in front of the fireplace. Moderate use of alcohol can be part of celebrations or special times without health risk. In fact, research shows that low levels of use may actually reduce some health risks. But you should remember that alcohol is a drug that affects your physical and mental behaviours. Further, the tragedies associated with alcohol receive far less attention than cocaine-related deaths, drug busts, and efforts to eradicate marijuana crops. Nevertheless, they are more common and have devastating effects on people of all ages.

# ALCOHOL: AN OVERVIEW

Although 79.3 percent of Canadians reported alcohol consumption in the past year, only 44 percent reported drinking weekly.[3] Males are more likely than females to report drinking in the past year (82.0 vs. 76.8 percent), and the highest past-year drinking rates (~90 percent) are found in the 18- to 24-year-old age group.[4] In the Canadian Addiction Survey, a light infrequent drinker is classified as someone who reported drinking alcohol less than once a week with fewer than five drinks consumed; in contrast, a light frequent drinker consumes fewer than five drinks per occasion more than once a week.[5] A heavy infrequent drinker is someone who consumes five or more drinks at a time less than once a week, while a heavy frequent drinker consumes five or more drinks more than once per week.[6] Using these definitions, 38.7 percent of Canadians aged 15 or older were classified as light infrequent drinkers, 27.7 percent were light frequent drinkers, 5.6 percent were heavy infrequent drinkers, and 7.1 percent were heavy frequent drinkers.[7]

In terms of alcohol sales, beer remains the most popular choice, capturing 50.7 percent of sales.[8] The market share of spirits and wine is almost equivalent, with each accounting for slightly less than 25 percent of sales.[9] When total sales are considered, consumers in Quebec and Newfoundland and Labrador purchased the most (115 litres per capita), while consumers in Saskatchewan purchased the least (94.4 litres).[10] Per capita purchases of beer were also highest in Quebec and Newfoundland and Labrador and lowest in British Columbia.[11] Consumers in Newfoundland and Labrador also bought the most spirits. The greatest wine purchasers came from Quebec, Alberta, and British Columbia.[12]

Alcohol can benefit and harm an individual. Most scientific evidence about the benefit as well as the harm comes from industrialized countries such as Canada, cultures where alcohol consumption is largely accepted and where dietary intake and inactive lifestyles lend themselves to heart diseases. Moderate alcohol consumption has been found to reduce, in certain age groups, the risk of coronary heart disease and ischemic stroke. Despite this individual benefit, the harm associated with the misuse of alcohol still constitutes a major public health problem in developed and developing countries.

Almost 10 percent of current drinkers report some sort of harm to themselves as a result of their drinking in the past year.[13] Of these, 3 percent report negative effects on friendships and social life and 5.4 percent report negative effects to their physical health. More alarming is that 32.7 percent of the respondents to the

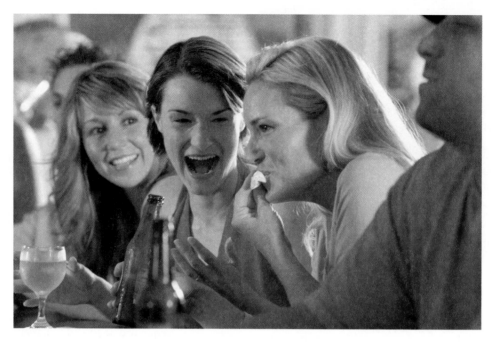

*While alcohol has long been seen as a "social lubricant" by post-secondary students, alcohol abuse and reckless driving continue to be serious problems on many campuses.*

Canadian Addiction Survey reported being harmed the past year because of someone else's drinking.[14] Of these, 10 percent indicated family or marriage difficulties, 22.1 percent reported being insulted or humiliated, 15.5 percent indicated serious arguments or quarrels, 15.8 percent reported verbal abuse, 10.8 percent were pushed or shoved, and 3.2 percent were physically assaulted. Alcohol is a significant factor in hospital admissions, road deaths, industrial accidents, accidental drowning, homicide, and suicide.[15] It is estimated that 6,507 Canadians lost their lives as a result of alcohol consumption in 1995, with the largest number of deaths stemming from impaired driving accidents, and 82,014 Canadians were hospitalized due to alcohol misuse.[16]

## Alcohol and the Post-Secondary Student

Alcohol is the most widely used, misused, and abused recreational drug in our society. It is also the most popular drug on campuses, where approximately 94.5 percent of students consume alcoholic beverages. The Addiction Research Foundation estimates that one-third of Ontario students consume more than 15 drinks per week: this level puts them at health risk. A greater number of alcohol users live in residence (41 percent), are between 17 and 22 years of age (65 percent), and have lower grades (49.5 percent D students, 22.6 percent A students).[17] Interestingly, most students think that other students drink more than they do and use this thought to justify their own drinking habits.

University or college is a critical time to become conscious of and responsible about your drinking. A number of social factors are involved in campus drinking. There is little doubt that alcohol is a part of campus culture and tradition. It is used to help relieve tensions and to celebrate. Its ability to lower inhibitions makes it the "social lubricant" of choice for many students, giving them an easy way to initiate conversations and create friendships.

How do students view the drinking patterns of their peers? Students consistently report that their friends drink much more than they do and that average drinking within their own social living group is higher than actual self-reports. Such misinformation may promote or be used to excuse excessive drinking practices among post-secondary students.

Binge drinking on campuses continues to be a big problem. **Binge drinking** is defined as the consumption of five drinks in a row by men or four in a row by women on a single occasion. The express purpose of binge drinking is to become intoxicated.

### WHAT WOULD YOU DO?

Is binge drinking alcohol abuse? Why or why not? As a post-secondary student, if you drink to get drunk does that indicate a problem? Why or why not?

Although everyone is at some risk for alcoholism and alcohol-related problems, post-secondary students seem to be particularly vulnerable for the following reasons:

- Alcohol exacerbates their already high risk for suicide, automobile crashes, and falls.
- Many university and college customs, norms, traditions, and mores encourage certain dangerous practices and patterns of alcohol use.
- Campuses are heavily targeted by advertising and promotions from the alcohol industry.
- It is more common for post-secondary students than their peers to drink recklessly and to engage in drinking games and other dangerous drinking practices.
- Post-secondary students are particularly vulnerable to peer influences and have a strong need to be accepted by their peers.

In an effort to prevent alcohol abuse, many universities and colleges are instituting strong policies against excessive consumption. At the same time, they are making more help available to students with drinking problems. Today, individual and group counselling are offered on most campuses, and more attention is directed toward the prevention of alcohol abuse. Several student organizations also promote responsible drinking and responsible party hosting.

## Rights versus Responsibilities

Most of us recognize the dangers associated with alcohol consumption in general, yet we tend to deny that such things could happen to us. We are aware of the relationship between alcohol and traffic accidents, spouse battering and child abuse, violent crimes, unprotected sexual activity, and family disruption, but we like to believe that these tragedies happen only to other people. Many people refuse to acknowledge that alcohol is a drug simply because they do not wish to see themselves as drug users. Our society condones, approves, and often encourages the consumption of alcoholic beverages yet neglects to teach how to drink responsibly.

If you make the choice to drink, you should do so judiciously, with complete information about the risks. The physiological and psychological reactions of the human organism to alcohol are strong. For this reason, you should approach the drug carefully. To avoid the devastating effects of alcohol abuse, you must adhere to the same principles of prevention that apply to any potentially harmful substance. The Canadian Centre for Substance Abuse and the Centre for Addiction and Mental Health recommend fewer than 14 standard drinks per week for

men, fewer than 9 standard drinks per week for women, and not more than 2 standard drinks on any one day.[18]

> ### WHAT WOULD YOU DO?
>
> Have you ever thought about how much you drink? Do you compare how much you drink to how much your friends drink? If you are not drinking more than your friends, does that mean your drinking is not a problem? What is a responsible level of alcohol consumption for you? For your friends? What do you do to ensure your safety when drinking? What about the safety of your friends?

# PHYSIOLOGICAL AND BEHAVIOURAL EFFECTS OF ALCOHOL

The intoxicating substance found in beer, wine, liquor, and liqueurs is **ethyl alcohol,** or **ethanol.** It is produced during a process called **fermentation,** whereby plant sugars are broken down by yeast organisms, yielding ethanol and carbon dioxide. Fermentation continues until the solution of plant sugars (called mash) reaches a concentration of 14 percent alcohol. At this point, the alcohol kills the yeast and halts the chemical reactions that produce it.

Manufacturers then add other ingredients that dilute the alcohol content of the beverage, such as in beer and wine. Other alcoholic beverages are produced through further processing called **distillation,** during which alcohol vapours are released from the mash at high temperatures. The vapours are then condensed and mixed with water to make the final product, such as in fortified wines and spirits.

**Binge drinking:** Drinking for the express purpose of becoming intoxicated; five drinks in a single sitting for men and four drinks in a single sitting for women.

**Ethyl alcohol (ethanol):** A drug produced by fermentation and found in many beverages.

**Fermentation:** The process whereby yeast organisms break down plant sugars to yield ethanol.

**Distillation:** The process whereby mash is subjected to high temperatures to release alcohol vapours, which are then condensed and mixed with water to make the final product.

# Contributing Factors to Alcohol Abuse and Related Problems on Campus

Many students are unaware of the reality of alcohol use on their campuses. The following statistics provide a brief glimpse into the issues:

- Alcohol kills more people under the legal drinking age than cocaine, marijuana, and heroin combined.
- Half a million students aged 15 to 24 are unintentionally injured each year while intoxicated.
- One night of heavy drinking can impair the ability to think abstractly for up to 30 days, limiting a student's ability to understand a professor's lecture or think through a football play.
- College and university administrators estimate that alcohol is a factor in 29 percent of dropouts, 38 percent of academic failure, and 64 percent of violent behaviours.
- Over the past decade, there has been a threefold increase in the number of college and university women who report having been drunk on 10 or more occasions in the previous month.
- Areas of a campus offering cheap beer prices have more crime, including trouble between students and police or other campus authorities, arguments, physical fighting, property damage, false fire alarms, and sexual misconduct.
- Alcohol is involved in more than two-thirds of suicides among post-secondary students, 90 percent of campus rapes and sexual assaults, and 95 percent of violent crime on campus.
- The likelihood that a woman will be raped is far greater on campuses with a high rate of binge drinking.
- Each year, more than 100,000 students aged 18 to 24 reported being too intoxicated to know if they consented to having sex.
- College and university binge drinking occurs more often among male students, students who reside on campus, intercollegiate athletes, and members of fraternities and sororities. Approximately 40 percent of fraternity and sorority

members report being frequent binge drinkers, and college or university athletes are 50 percent more likely to binge drink than nonathletes.
- Rates of binge drinking among high-risk students (younger, white males) are lower on more diverse campuses. When high-risk students are together to the exclusion of other groups, there are fewer role models for lighter or nondrinking behaviours.
- Post-secondary students under the legal drinking age are more prone to binge drinking and pay less for their alcohol than their older classmates do. Though underage students drink less often, they consume more per occasion than older students who are allowed to drink legally.
- One risk of binge drinking and excessive alcohol consumption is "passing out." During this time, the drinker who passed out could vomit, choke on their vomit, and die. If someone passes out at a party or later at home, it is important to place them in the recovery position (that is, on his or her side, arm extended with the other arm bent such that the hand is under his or her cheek) and stay with them until they have "slept it off."

Sources: Data were compiled from the numerous studies cited throughout this chapter and from M. Mohler-Kuo et al., "College Rapes Linked to Binge-Drinking Rates," *Journal of Studies on Alcohol* 65.1 (2004); H. Weschler, "Watering Down the Drinks: The Moderating Effect of College Demographics on Alcohol Use in High Risk Groups," *American Journal of Public Health* 93.11 (2003): 1929–1933; T. F. Nelson et al., "Alcohol and Collegiate Sports Fans," *Addictive Behaviors* 28.1 (2003): 1–11; R.W. Hingson et al., "Magnitude of Alcohol-Related Mortality and Morbidity among U.S. College Students Aged 18–24," *Journal of Studies on Alcohol* 63.2 (2002): 136–144.

The **proof** of an alcoholic drink is a measure of the percentage of alcohol in the beverage. "Proof" comes from "gunpowder proof," a reference to the gunpowder test, whereby potential buyers tested the distiller's product by pouring it on gunpowder and attempting to light it. If the alcohol content was at least 50 percent, the gunpowder would burn; otherwise the water in the product would put out the flame. Thus, alcohol percentage is 50 percent of the given proof. For example, 80-proof whiskey or scotch is 40-percent alcohol by volume. The proof of a beverage provides an indication of its strength. Therefore, consuming the same amount

(that is, volume) of lower-proof drinks will produce fewer alcohol effects than higher-proof drinks. Most spirits are 40-percent alcohol, wines are between 12 and 15 percent alcohol, and ales are between 6 and 8 percent. The alcoholic content of most beers is between 2 and 6 percent, varying according to type of beer.

## Behavioural Effects

Behavioural changes caused by alcohol vary with the setting and with the individual. Alcohol may make shy people less inhibited and more willing to talk to others.

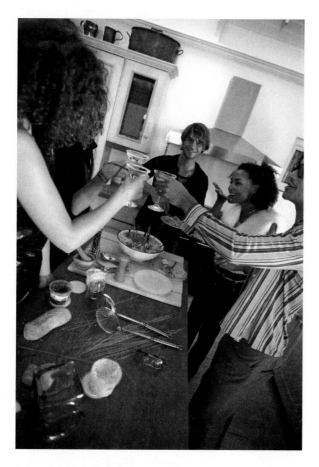

*When drinking alcohol it is important to choose beverages containing a lower percentage of alcohol such as wine or beer, as well as to eat prior to and while drinking to reduce blood alcohol content.*

effects of alcohol become apparent, drowsiness sets in, and motor skills are further impaired, followed by a loss of judgment. Thus a driver may not be able to estimate distances or speed, and some drinkers lose their ability to make value-related decisions and may do things they would not do when sober. As BAC increases, the drinker suffers increased physiological and psychological effects. All these changes are negative; physical and mental functions are impaired.

People can acquire physiological and psychological tolerance to the effects of alcohol through regular use. The nervous system adapts over time, so greater quantities of alcohol are required to produce the same physiological and psychological effects. Furthermore, some people learn to modify their behaviours so that they appear to be sober even when their BAC is quite high. This ability is called **learned behavioural tolerance.**

## Absorption and Metabolism

Alcohol is rapidly absorbed into the bloodstream from the small intestine, and less rapidly from the stomach and colon. In proportion to its concentration in the bloodstream, alcohol decreases activity in parts of the brain and spinal cord. The drinker's blood alcohol concentration depends on:

- the amount consumed in a given time
- the drinker's size, sex, body build, and metabolism
- the type and amount of food in the stomach

Once alcohol has passed into the bloodstream, you cannot slow its absorption by eating or drinking. Mood also influences the rate of absorption, since emotions affect how long it takes for the contents of the stomach to empty into the intestine. Powerful moods, such as stress and tension, are likely to cause the stomach to "dump" its contents into the small intestine. That is why alcohol is absorbed much more rapidly when people are tense than when they are relaxed.

Consuming fruit sugar may shorten the duration of alcohol's effect by increasing the rate of elimination from the blood (that is, metabolism). In the average adult, the rate of metabolism is about 8.5 grams (that is, about two-thirds of a drink) of alcohol per hour. This rate varies dramatically among individuals, however, depending on the user's drinking history, physique, sex, liver size, and genetic factors.[19]

It may make a depressed person even more depressed. In people reluctant to share emotions, it may bring out violence and aggression. In many cases, alcohol will do for the drinker what the drinker expects and wants it to do, making it possible for the user to blame his or her inappropriate behaviours on the alcohol. It is because of this expected effect, combined with reduced inhibitions, that a person who normally does not dance well tears a strip off the dance floor. In other words, a person who normally inhibits dancing behaviours may actually dance better after a drink or two, simply because his or her inhibitions have been reduced.

**Blood alcohol concentration (BAC)** is the ratio of alcohol to total blood volume. It is the factor used to measure the physiological and behavioural effects of alcohol. Despite individual differences, alcohol produces some general behaviour effects based on BAC (see Table 11.1). At a BAC of 0.02, a person feels slightly relaxed and his or her mood will be enhanced. At a BAC of 0.05 relaxation increases, there is some motor impairment, and a willingness to talk becomes apparent. At a BAC of 0.08, the person feels euphoric and there is further motor impairment. At a BAC of 0.10, the depressant

**Proof:** A measure of the percentage of alcohol in a beverage.

**Blood alcohol concentration (BAC):** The ratio of alcohol to total blood volume; the factor used to measure the physiological and behavioural effects of alcohol.

**Learned behavioural tolerance:** The ability of drinkers to modify their behaviours so that they appear sober even when they have high BAC levels.

**TABLE 11.1**

## Psychological and Physiological Effects of Various Blood Alcohol Concentration Levels*

| Number of Drinks† | Blood Alcohol Concentration | Psychological and Physical Effects |
|---|---|---|
| 1 | 0.02%–0.03% | No overt effects, slight mood elevation |
| 2 | 0.05%–0.06% | Feeling of relaxation, warmth; slight decrease in reaction time and in fine-muscle coordination |
| 3 | 0.08%–0.09% | Balance, speech, vision, and hearing slightly impaired; feelings of euphoria, increased confidence; loss of motor coordination |
| 4 | 0.11%–0.12% | Coordination and balance becoming difficult; distinct impairment of mental faculties, judgment |
| 5 | 0.14%–0.15% | Major impairment of mental and physical control; slurred speech, blurred vision, lack of motor skills |
| 7 | 0.20% | Loss of motor control—needs help moving about; mental confusion |
| 10 | 0.30% | Severe intoxication; minimum conscious control of mind and body |
| 14 | 0.40% | Unconsciousness, threshold of coma |
| 17 | 0.50% | Deep coma |
| 20 | 0.60% | Death from respiratory failure |

*For each hour elapsed since the last drink, subtract 0.015% blood alcohol concentration, or approximately one drink.
†One drink = one beer (4–5% alcohol, 375 mL), one highball (31 mL whiskey), or one glass table wine (157 mL).

Source: Modified from data given in Ohio State Police Driver Information Seminars and the National Clearinghouse for Alcohol and Alcoholism Information, Rockville, MD

Alcohol is metabolized in the liver, where it is converted by the enzyme alcohol dehydrogenase to acetaldehyde. It is then rapidly oxidized to acetate, converted to carbon dioxide and water, and eventually excreted from the body. Acetaldehyde is a toxic chemical that can cause immediate symptoms such as nausea and vomiting as well as long-term effects such as liver damage.

Like food, alcohol contains calories. Proteins and carbohydrates (starches and sugars) each contain 4 kilocalories per gram. Fat contains 9 kilocalories per gram. Alcohol, although similar in structure to carbohydrates, contains 7 kilocalories per gram. The body uses the calories in alcohol in the same manner it uses those found in carbohydrates: for immediate energy or for storage as fat.

A drinker's BAC depends on his or her weight and body fat, the water content in the body tissues, the concentration of alcohol in the beverage consumed, the rate of consumption, and the volume of alcohol consumed. Heavier people have larger body surfaces through which to diffuse alcohol; therefore, they have lower concentrations of alcohol in their blood than thin people after drinking the same amount. Because alcohol does not diffuse as rapidly into body fat as into water, alcohol concentration is higher in a person with more body fat. Because a woman is likely to have more body fat and less water in her body tissues than a man of the same weight, she will be more intoxicated than a man after drinking the same amount of alcohol. (See Table 11.2.)

## WHAT WOULD YOU DO?

Did you think that BAC was based only on the amount of alcohol you drink? What other factors contribute to BAC? How are these factors different for men and women? Have you or someone you know ever chosen specifically to alter conditions so as to increase BAC (that is, to get drunk quicker)? Are these wise practices? Why or why not?

# TABLE 11.2

## Calculation of Estimated Blood Alcohol (BAC) for Men and Women

**Number of Drinks: Males**

| Body Weight (kg) | 1 | 2 | 3 | 4 | 5 | 6 | 7 | 8 | 9 | 10 |
|---|---|---|---|---|---|---|---|---|---|---|
| 45.4 | 0.043 | 0.087 | 0.130 | 0.174 | 0.217 | 0.261 | 0.304 | 0.348 | 0.391 | 0.435 |
| 56.8 | 0.034 | 0.069 | 0.103 | 0.139 | 0.173 | 0.209 | 0.242 | 0.278 | 0.312 | 0.346 |
| 68.2 | 0.029 | 0.058 | 0.087 | 0.116 | 0.145 | 0.174 | 0.203 | 0.232 | 0.261 | 0.290 |
| 79.5 | 0.025 | 0.050 | 0.075 | 0.100 | 0.125 | 0.150 | 0.175 | 0.200 | .0225 | 0.250 |
| 90.9 | 0.022 | 0.043 | 0.065 | 0.087 | 0.108 | 0.130 | 0.152 | 0.174 | 0.195 | 0.217 |
| 102.3 | 0.019 | 0.039 | 0.058 | 0.078 | 0.097 | 0.117 | 0.136 | 0.156 | 0.175 | 0.195 |
| 113.6 | 0.017 | 0.035 | 0.052 | 0.070 | 0.087 | 0.105 | 0.122 | 0.139 | 0.156 | 0.173 |

**Number of Drinks: Females**

| Body Weight (kg) | 1 | 2 | 3 | 4 | 5 | 6 | 7 | 8 | 9 | 10 |
|---|---|---|---|---|---|---|---|---|---|---|
| 45.4 | 0.050 | 0.101 | 0.152 | 0.203 | 0.253 | 0.304 | 0.355 | 0.406 | 0.456 | 0.507 |
| 56.8 | 0.040 | 0.080 | 0.120 | 0.162 | 0.202 | 0.244 | 0.282 | 0.324 | 0.364 | 0.404 |
| 68.2 | 0.034 | 0.068 | 0.101 | 0.135 | 0.169 | 0.203 | 0.237 | 0.271 | 0.304 | 0.338 |
| 79.5 | 0.029 | 0.058 | 0.087 | 0.117 | 0.146 | 0.175 | 0.204 | 0.233 | 0.262 | 0.292 |
| 90.9 | 0.026 | 0.050 | 0.076 | 0.101 | 0.126 | 0.152 | 0.177 | 0.203 | 0.227 | 0.253 |
| 102.3 | 0.022 | 0.045 | 0.068 | 0.091 | 0.113 | 0.136 | 0.159 | 0.182 | 0.204 | 0.227 |
| 113.6 | 0.020 | 0.041 | 0.061 | 0.082 | 0.101 | 0.122 | 0.142 | 0.162 | 0.182 | 0.202 |

**Body weight:** Calculations are for people who have a normal body weight for their height, who are free of drugs or other affecting medications, and who are neither unusually thin nor obese.

**Drink equivalents:**

1 drink = 43 mL (1.5 oz) of rum, rye, scotch, brandy, gin, vodka, etc.
1 drink = 341-mL (12-oz) bottle of normal-strength (5%) beer
1 drink = 85 mL (3 oz) of fortified wine
1 drink = 142 mL (5 oz) of table wine

**Using the chart:** Find the appropriate figure using the proper chart (male or female), body weight, and number of drinks consumed. Then subtract the time factor (see Time Factor Table) from the figure on the chart to obtain the approximate BAC. For example, for a 68-kg man who has had 4 drinks in 2 hours, take the figure 0.116 (from the chart for males) and subtract 0.030 (from the Time Factor Table) to obtain a BAC of 0.086 percent.

## Time Factor Table

| Hours since first drink | 1 | 2 | 3 | 4 | 5 | 6 |
|---|---|---|---|---|---|---|
| Subtract from BAC | 0.015 | 0.030 | 0.045 | 0.60 | 0.075 | 0.090 |

Source: From *The Encyclopedia of Alcoholism* by Glen Evans and Robert O'Brien. © 1991 Facts on File and Grennspring Inc. Reprinted with permission of Facts on File, Inc., New York.

## Women and Alcohol

Body fat is not the only contributor to the differences in alcohol's effects on men and women. Compared to men, women appear to have half as much alcohol hydrogenase, the enzyme that breaks down alcohol in the stomach before it has a chance to get to the bloodstream and the brain. Therefore, if a man and a woman drink the same amount of alcohol, the woman's BAC will be approximately 30 percent higher than the man's, leaving her more vulnerable to slurred speech, careless driving, and other drinking-related impairments. Table 11.2 compares blood-alcohol levels by sex, weight, and consumption. Although this table provides an estimate of probable BAC levels, many additional factors may cause considerable variation in these rates. For this reason, you should always err on the side of caution when gauging your blood alcohol level.

### WHAT WOULD YOU DO?

Think about the last time you consumed alcohol. How much did you consume? Over how long? Calculate your blood alcohol content using the information presented in Table 11.2. How long did it take until your BAC was reduced to 0?

## Breathalyzer and Other Tests

The breathalyzer tests used by law enforcement officers are designed to determine BAC based on the amount of alcohol exhaled in the breath. Urinalysis can also yield a BAC based on the concentration of unmetabolized alcohol in the urine. Breath analysis, urinalysis, and blood tests are used to determine whether a driver is over the legal limit, with blood tests providing the most accurate measures.

# Immediate Effects

Alcohol is a central nervous system (CNS) depressant. The primary action of ethanol is to reduce the frequency of nerve transmissions and impulses at synaptic junctions. This reduction of nerve transmissions results in significant depression of CNS functions, with resulting decreases in respiratory rate, pulse rate, and blood pressure. As CNS depression deepens, vital functions become noticeably depressed. In extreme cases, coma and death can result.

Alcohol is a diuretic, increasing urinary output. Although this effect might be expected to lead to automatic **dehydration** (loss of water), the body actually retains water, most of it in the muscles or in the cerebral tissues. This is because water is usually pulled out

of the **cerebrospinal fluid** (fluid within the brain and spinal cord), leading to what is known as mitochondrial dehydration at the cellular level within the nervous system. Mitochondria are miniature organs within cells that are responsible for specific functions. They rely heavily on fluid balance. When mitochondrial dehydration occurs from drinking the mitochondria cannot carry out their normal functions, resulting in symptoms that include the "morning-after" headaches suffered by some drinkers.

Alcohol is also an irritant to the gastrointestinal system and may cause indigestion and heartburn if consumed on an empty stomach. Long-term use of alcohol causes repeated irritation that has been linked to cancers of the esophagus and stomach. In addition, people who engage in brief drinking sprees during which they consume unusually high amounts of alcohol put themselves at risk for irregular heartbeat or even total loss of heart rhythm, which can cause disruption in blood flow and possible damage to the heart muscle.

A **hangover** is sometimes experienced the morning after consuming alcohol. The symptoms of a hangover are familiar to those who drink: headache, upset stomach, anxiety, depression, thirst, and, in severe cases, an almost overwhelming desire to crawl into a hole and die. People who get hangovers often also smoke too much, stay up too late, or engage in other behaviours likely to leave them feeling unwell the next day. The causes of hangovers are not well known, but the effects of congeners are suspected. **Congeners** are more toxic forms of alcohol that are metabolized more slowly than ethanol. Your body metabolizes the congeners after the ethanol is gone from your system, and their toxic byproducts are thought to contribute to the hangover. It usually takes 12 hours to recover from a hangover. Bed rest, plenty of fluids, solid food, and a pain reliever may reduce the discomforts of a hangover, but, unfortunately, nothing cures it but time.

## Drug Interactions

When you use any drug (and alcohol is a drug), you need to be aware of the possible interactions with prescription drugs, over-the-counter drugs, or other drugs you are taking or considering taking. Table 11.3 summarizes some possible interactions. Note that alcohol may cause a negative interaction even with ASA.

# Long-Term Effects
### Effects on the Nervous System

Since alcohol is a CNS depressant, the nervous system is especially sensitive to it. Even people who drink moderately experience shrinkage in brain size and weight and a loss of some degree of intellectual ability.

TABLE 11.3

Drugs and Alcohol: Actions and Interactions

| Drug Class/Name(s) | Effects with Alcohol |
|---|---|
| *Anti-alcohol:* Antabuse | Severe reactions to even small amounts: headache, nausea, blurred vision, convulsions, coma, possible death. |
| *Antibiotics:* Penicillin, Cyantin | Reduces therapeutic effectiveness of antibiotics. |
| *Antidepressants:* Elavil, Sinequan, Tofranil, Nardil | Increased central nervous system (CNS) depression, blood pressure changes. Combined use of alcohol and MAO inhibitors, a specific type of antidepressant, can trigger massive increases in blood pressure, even brain hemorrhage and death. |
| *Antihistamines:* Allerest, Dristan | Drowsiness and CNS depression. Impairs driving ability. |
| *ASA:* Aspirin, Anacin, Excedrin, Bayer | Irritates stomach lining. May cause gastrointestinal pain, bleeding. |
| *Depressants:* Valium, Ativan, Placidyl | Dangerous CNS depression, loss of coordination, coma. High risk of overdose and death. |
| *Narcotics:* Heroin, Codeine, Darvon | Serious CNS depression. Possible respiratory arrest and death. |
| *Stimulants:* Caffeine, Cocaine | Masks depressant action of alcohol. May increase blood pressure, physical tension. |
| Tylenol, Acetaminophen | Risk of liver damage, particularly with heavy alcohol consumption and maximum recommended doses of acetaminophen. |

Source: Adapted by permission from *Drugs and Alcohol: Simple Facts about Alcohol and Drug Combinations* (Phoenix: DIN Publications, 1988), No. 121.

The damage that results from alcohol use is localized primarily in the left side of the brain, which is responsible for written and spoken language, logic, and mathematical skills. The degree of shrinkage appears to be directly related to the amount of alcohol consumed. In terms of memory loss, the evidence suggests that having one drink every day is better than saving up for a binge and consuming seven or eight drinks in a night.

## Cardiovascular Effects

The cardiovascular system is affected by alcohol in a number of ways. Evidence suggests that the effect of alcohol on the heart is not all bad. Some studies suggest that moderate drinkers suffer fewer heart attacks, have less cholesterol buildup, and are less likely to die of heart disease than either nondrinkers or heavy drinkers.[20] However, drinking is not recommended as a preventive measure against heart disease because the benefits do not outweigh the risks. Alcohol contributes to high blood pressure and a slightly increased heart rate and cardiac output. Those who report drinking three to five drinks a day, regardless of race or sex, have higher blood pressure than those who drink less.

People who engage in brief drinking sprees, during which they consume unusually large amounts of alcohol, also suffer some risks, including irregular heartbeat or total loss of heart rhythm. This condition has been called *holiday heart syndrome* because it typically occurs around holidays such as Thanksgiving, Christmas, and New Year's Eve— occasions when drinkers are likely to overindulge. It can cause disruption in blood flow and possible damage to the heart muscle. Prolonged drinking can also lead to deterioration of the heart muscle, a condition called cardiomyopathy.

## Liver Disease

One of the most common diseases related to alcohol abuse is **cirrhosis** of the liver. It is among the top

**Dehydration:** Loss of fluids from body tissues.

**Cerebrospinal fluid:** Fluid within and surrounding the brain and spinal cord tissues.

**Hangover:** The physiological reaction to excessive drinking, including such symptoms as headache, upset stomach, anxiety, depression, diarrhea, and thirst.

**Congeners:** Forms of alcohol that are metabolized more slowly than ethanol and produce toxic byproducts.

**Cirrhosis:** The last stage of liver disease associated with chronic heavy use of alcohol, during which liver cells die and damage is permanent.

ten causes of death in Canada. One result of heavy drinking is that the liver begins to store fat—a condition known as fatty liver. If there is insufficient time between drinking episodes, this fat cannot be transported to storage sites and the fat-filled liver cells stop functioning. Continued drinking can cause a further stage of liver deterioration called fibrosis, in which the damaged area of the liver develops fibrous scar tissue. Cell function can be partially restored at this stage with proper nutrition and abstinence from alcohol. If the person continues to drink, however, cirrhosis results. At this point, the liver cells die and the damage is permanent. **Alcoholic hepatitis** is a serious condition resulting from prolonged use of alcohol. A chronic inflammation of the liver develops, which may be fatal in itself or progress to cirrhosis.

### Cancer

Heavy drinkers are at higher risk for certain types of cancer, particularly cancers of the gastrointestinal tract. The repeated irritation caused by long-term use of alcohol has been linked to cancers of the esophagus, stomach, mouth, tongue, and liver. Research has also shown a link between breast cancer and moderate levels of alcohol consumption in women. A landmark study found that women between the ages of 34 and 59 who consumed between three and nine drinks a week were 30 percent more likely than non-drinkers to develop breast cancer.[21] It is unclear how alcohol exerts its carcinogenic effects, though it is thought that it inhibits the absorption of carcinogenic substances, permitting them to be taken to sensitive organs.

### Other Effects

An irritant to the gastrointestinal system, alcohol may cause indigestion and heartburn if consumed on an empty stomach. It also damages the mucous membranes and can cause inflammation of the esophagus, chronic stomach irritation, problems with intestinal absorption, and chronic diarrhea. Alcohol abuse is a major cause of chronic inflammation of the pancreas, the organ that produces digestive enzymes and insulin. Chronic abuse of alcohol inhibits enzyme production, which further inhibits the absorption of nutrients. Drinking alcohol can block the absorption of calcium, a nutrient that strengthens bones. This should be of particular concern to women, because as women age their risk for osteoporosis (bone thinning and calcium loss) increases. Heavy consumption of alcohol worsens this condition.

Evidence also suggests that alcohol impairs the body's ability to recognize and fight foreign bodies such as bacteria and viruses. The relationship between alcohol and AIDS is unclear, especially since some of the populations at risk for HIV infection are also at risk for alcohol abuse. But any effect on the immune system would probably contribute to the development of the disease.

## Fetal Alcohol Spectrum Disorders

Alcohol can have harmful effects on fetal development. Alcohol consumed during the first trimester poses the greatest threat to organ development, while exposure during the last trimester, when the brain is developing rapidly, is most likely to affect CNS development.

A series of disorders collectively called **fetal alcohol spectrum disorder (FASD)** is caused by prenatal exposure to alcohol and leads to lifelong developmental and cognitive disabilities among Canadian children.[22] FASD occurs when alcohol ingested by the mother passes through the placenta into the infant's bloodstream. Because the fetus is so small, its BAC will be much higher than that of the mother. Thus, consumption of alcohol during pregnancy can affect the infant far more seriously than the mother.

FASD is the leading cause of developmental delay in Canada and North America, with an incidence estimated at 1 to 6 in 1,000 live births.[23] FASD includes the following disorders related to alcohol consumption during pregnancy: **fetal alcohol syndrome (FAS), fetal alcohol effects (FAE),** partial fetal alcohol effects, alcohol-related neurodevelopmental disorders, and neurobehavioural disorder–alcohol exposed. FAS is characterized by retarded growth prenatally and postnatally, facial anomalies, CNS dysfunction as noted by intellectual impairment, structural abnormalities, developmental delay, and complex behavioural problems.[24] One-fifth of FAS children have difficulty sleeping and are hyperactive. Many have severe learning disabilities and are dyslexic. Congenital heart problems are more common than in normal babies, as are genitor-urinary problems. There is an increased incidence of spina bifida, hip dislocation, and delayed skeletal maturation. FAE is used to describe children with prenatal exposure to alcohol but only some FAS characteristics.

As there is no definitive information regarding a safe quantity of alcohol use during pregnancy, women who are or wish to become pregnant should abstain from alcohol. Health professionals should reassure women who have consumed small amounts of alcohol occasionally during pregnancy that the risk is likely minimal. Pregnant women should also know that stopping drinking at any time during a pregnancy will have benefits for the fetus and mother.

# The Public Rates Drinking and Driving as One of Canada's Most Serious Social Issues

According to the 2002 Road Safety Monitor, an annual national opinion poll conducted by the Traffic Injury Research Foundation (TIRF), most Canadians believe that drinking and driving is a priority social issue, and the most important road safety issue that they face.

### Drinking and driving occurrence in Canada:

- 86 percent of Canadians rated drinking and driving as a serious problem
- 16.1 percent of drivers report driving within two hours of consuming alcohol in the 30-day period prior to the survey
- 7.9 percent of drivers admit to driving when they thought they were over the legal limit at some point in 2002
- It is estimated that there were more than 8 million trips during 2002 where the driver was impaired

### A relatively small group of individuals makes our roads particularly dangerous:

- Fewer than 3 percent of drivers account for more than 80 percent of all impaired driving trips
- Young drivers (age 16 to 18) and older drivers (age 65 and over) are least likely to drive after drinking

- Canadians aged 18 to 34 are most likely to report driving after drinking

### Canadian drivers support the following initiatives aimed at decreasing the incidence of drinking and driving:

- Requiring drivers suspected of drinking to perform sobriety tests
- Mandatory breath testing of drivers involved in collisions
- Alcohol ignition interlocks
- Immediate impoundment of vehicles driven by impaired drivers
- A zero blood alcohol content restriction for convicted offenders
- Greater use of police spot checks

Source: Adapted from the Traffic Safety Research Foundation, 2002 Road Safety Monitor.

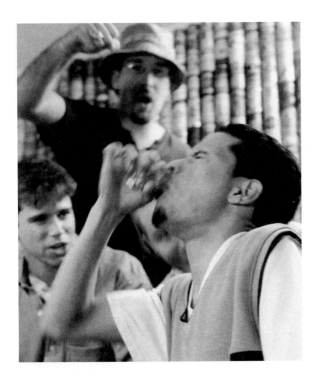

*Deciding when and how much to drink is no simple matter. Irresponsible consumption of alcohol can easily result in disaster.*

In June 1992, the Standing Committee on Health and Welfare, Social Affairs, Seniors, and the Status of Women released its report "Fetal Alcohol Syndrome: A Preventable Tragedy." Since then, Health Canada has worked with healthcare professionals to identify and implement prevention strategies; has produced pamphlets and videos on FAS; and, with the

**Alcoholic hepatitis:** Condition resulting from prolonged use of alcohol in which the liver is inflamed. It can result in death.

**Fetal alcohol spectrum disorder (FASD):** A broad category of disorders relating to consumption of alcohol during pregnancy; includes fetal alcohol syndrome, fetal alcohol effects, partial fetal alcohol effects, alcohol-related neurodevelopmental disorders, and neurobehavioural disorder–alcohol exposed.

**Fetal alcohol syndrome (FAS):** A disorder that may affect the fetus when the mother consumes alcohol during pregnancy. Among its effects are mental retardation, small head, tremors, and abnormalities of the face, limbs, heart, and brain.

**Fetal alcohol effects (FAE):** A syndrome describing children with a history of prenatal alcohol exposure but without all the physical or behavioural symptoms of FAS. Among its symptoms are low birthweight, irritability, and possible permanent mental impairment.

## The Emotional Trauma of Losing a Loved One to Impaired Driving

The loss of someone you love is always devastating. When the death is sudden and violent, it can be even more traumatic. Hurt, anger, sadness, and frustration are just some of the emotions a senseless and violent death causes. The loss of a loved one because of an impaired driving crash brings an abrupt end to all future dreams and aspirations. There is no chance to say good-bye, no time to say thank you or I'm sorry. There are loose ends that will never be tied. In particular, someone who has lost a child or a partner often feels guilty that he or she couldn't protect them.

The violence of auto accidents often leaves the victims unrecognizable. The hospital or funeral home may not permit viewing of the body, which can lead families into painful fantasies about how their loved one looked; or they may doubt that the person has actually died. For many families, seeing the body gives them closure that the person they loved is really gone.

Central to the trauma that families and friends experience after a crash is the senselessness of the death. The fact that the death could have been prevented and is clearly someone's fault is one of the most painful parts of grieving. Knowing that someone chose to be negligent is hard to understand. Many people report feelings of intense anger, even rage, at the offender.

Anger is a theme that can sometimes be central to the grieving process. There is anger not only at the offender and sometimes "the system" but also at other family members. Because people experience the sudden loss differently, some may feel anger at the way other family members appear to be moving on. Even anger toward the person who has died—due to feelings of abandonment—is not unusual. Anger covers up the underlying sadness that may be more difficult to endure.

Anxiety and fear are also common. Suddenly families realize their vulnerability, a concept they may not have fully understood before. Often people hold on to the belief that bad things don't happen to good people. When that idea is destroyed, it may be replaced with fear and a sense of powerlessness that is overwhelming.

The emotional aftermath of losing a loved one to impaired driving is filled with feelings and experiences not even touched upon in this short discussion. The road to feeling better is often blocked; many people feel they will never be happy again. While it is true that life will never again be the same, families do survive the ordeal. Many manage to gain strength and find happiness again. Ultimately, what people are left with is sorrow. Sorrow encompasses the knowledge that you will always feel sadness over the tragic loss of your loved one; however, it is also a step away from being overwhelmed by grief.

Source: Mothers Against Drunk Driving (MADD) Canada (retrieved from the Transport Canada Web site: www.tc.gc.ca/roadsafety/tp1535/smashed/senseless.htm).

---

Association of Canadian Distillers and the Brewers' Association of Canada, sponsors a national information service resource centre providing links to support groups, prevention projects, and experts on FASD (1-800-559-4514).

### WHAT WOULD YOU DO?

Why do we hear so little about FASD when it is the leading cause of developmental delay in North America? Is this a reflection of our society's denial of alcohol as a dangerous drug?

## Drinking and Driving

The leading cause of death for all age groups from 5 to 34 years old (including university and college students) is traffic accidents. Young people between 15 and 29 years old account for 38 percent of motor vehicle fatalities. The rate is highest for 20- to 24-year-olds, at 14.7 percent.[25] Impaired driving is a major cause of death, killing about 1,350 Canadians each year and injuring many more.[26]

## ALCOHOLISM

Alcohol use becomes **alcohol abuse** or **alcoholism** when there is excessive consumption or other use that interferes with work, school, or social and family relationships. Alcoholism is one of many addictions or dependencies on substances or behaviours that have mood-altering consequences.

According to the 2003–04 Canadian Addiction Survey of almost 14,000 Canadians between the ages of 15 and 65, 8.8 percent reported harm to self in the past year as a result of their drinking. Of the past-year drinkers, 6.2 percent indicated heavy drinking (five or more drinks for males and four or more drinks for females on a single occasion) at least once per week, with males between the ages of 18 and 24 years to be the most likely to report heavy drinking. Of the past-year drinkers, 22.6 percent exceeded the low-risk drinking guidelines (that is, consuming no more than 14 standard drinks for males or 9 standard drinks for females per week). Again, males between the ages of 18 and 24 were most likely to exceed these guidelines.

As previously noted, the most common areas affected by excessive drinking are physical health (5.4 percent), financial position (4.7 percent), and social health (3.0 percent). Almost one-third (32.7 percent) of Canadians say they have had problems from other people's drinking, such as being disturbed by loud parties (23.8 percent), being insulted or humiliated (22.1 percent), having a serious argument (15.5 percent), being physically abused (14.0 percent), and experiencing marital difficulties (10.0 percent). There were 6,507 deaths and 82,014 hospitalizations attributed to alcohol in 1995.[27] Motor vehicle accidents accounted for the largest number of alcohol-related deaths, while accidental falls and alcohol dependence syndrome accounted for the largest number of alcohol-related hospitalizations.

## How, Why, Whom?

As with other addictions, tolerance, psychological dependence, and withdrawal symptoms must be present to qualify a drinker as an individual addicted to alcohol. Addiction usually results from chronic use over a period of time that may vary from person to person. Problem drinkers or irresponsible users are not necessarily people addicted to alcohol. The stereotype of the person addicted to alcohol on skid row applies to only 5 percent of those who are affected by alcoholism. The remaining 95 percent of individuals addicted to alcohol live in some type of extended family unit. They can be found at all socioeconomic levels and in all professions, ethnic groups, geographical locations, religions, and races. You have a 1 in 10 risk of becoming addicted to alcohol. Individuals addicted to alcohol tend to have a number of behaviours in common. People who recognize any of these behaviours in themselves should seek professional help to determine whether alcohol has become a controlling factor in their lives.

Women are the fastest-growing component of the population of alcohol abusers. They tend to become addicted to alcohol at a later age and after fewer years of heavy drinking than males. Women at highest risk for alcohol-related problems are those living common-law in their 20s or early 30s, or who have a husband or partner who drinks heavily.

## The Causes of Alcoholism

We know that alcoholism is a disease with biological, psychological, and social/environmental components, but we do not know what role each of these components plays.

### Biological and Family Factors

Research into the hereditary and environmental causes of alcoholism has found higher rates of alcoholism among family members of individuals addicted to alcohol. In fact, according to researchers, alcoholism is four to five times more common among the children of those who are addicted to alcohol than in the general population.

Type 1 alcoholics are drinkers who had at least one parent who was a problem drinker and who grew up in an environment that encouraged heavy drinking. Their drinking is reinforced by family and social events that include heavy drinking. Type 1 alcohol abusers share certain personality characteristics. They avoid novelty and harmful situations and are concerned about the thoughts and feelings of others. Type 2 alcoholism is seen in males only. These alcoholics are typically the biological sons of alcoholic fathers who have a history of violence and drug use. Type 2 alcoholics display the opposite characteristics of type 1 alcoholics. They do not seek social approval, they lack inhibition, and they are prone to novelty-seeking behaviours.[28]

Scientists are on the trail of an "alcohol gene," but so far they have not managed to find one. In 1990, it appeared that a specific gene linked to alcoholism had been discovered. It turned out, however, that not only was the gene not found consistently in every alcoholic studied, but it also existed in some individuals who were not alcoholics.[29]

Because the effects of heredity and environment are so difficult to separate, some researchers have chosen to examine this issue through twin and adoption studies. So far, these studies have produced inconclusive results. However, a slightly higher rate of similar drinking behaviours has been demonstrated among identical twins, and sons living away from their alcoholic parents tend to more nearly resemble them in drinking behaviours than they do their adoptive or foster parents.

### Social and Cultural Factors

There are numerous factors that may mitigate or exacerbate problems with alcohol. Many individuals begin to drink because of peer pressure; because everyone

**Alcohol abuse (alcoholism):** Use of alcohol that interferes with work, school, or personal relationships or that entails violations of the law.

else is doing it. Others may begin drinking as a way to dull the pain of an acute loss or an emotional or social problem. For example, students may drink to escape the stress of university or college life, disappointment over unfulfilled expectations, difficulties in forming relationships, or the loss of the security of home, loved ones, and close friends. Unfortunately, the emotional discomfort that causes many people to turn to alcohol also ultimately causes them to become even more uncomfortable as the depressant effect of the drug begins to take its toll. Thus, the person who is already depressed may become even more depressed, antagonizing friends and other social supports until these supports turn away.

Family attitudes toward alcohol also influence whether or not a person will develop a drinking problem. It has been clearly demonstrated that people raised in cultures in which drinking is a part of religious or ceremonial activities or in which alcohol is a traditional part of the family meal are less prone to alcohol dependency. In contrast, in societies in which alcohol purchase is carefully controlled and drinking is regarded as a rite of passage to adulthood, the tendency for abuse appears to be greater.[30]

Certain social factors have been linked with alcoholism as well. These include urbanization, the weakening of links to the extended family and a general loosening of kinship ties, increased mobility, and changing religious and philosophical values. Apparently, then, some combination of heredity and environment plays a decisive role in the development of alcoholism.

## Effects of Alcoholism on the Family

Recently people have begun to recognize that it is not only the alcoholic but also the alcoholic's entire family that suffers. Although most research focuses on family effects during the late stages of alcoholism, the family unit actually begins to react early on as the person starts to show symptoms of addiction to alcohol.

Many families affected by alcoholism have no idea what normal family life is like. Family members unconsciously adapt to the alcoholic's behaviours by adjusting their own behaviours. To minimize their

feelings about the alcoholic or out of love for him or her, family members take on various abnormal roles. These roles actually help keep the alcoholic drinking. Children in such dysfunctional families generally assume at least one of the following roles:

- *Family hero:* tries to divert attention from the problem by being really good, almost too good to be true
- *Scapegoat:* draws attention away from the family's primary problem through delinquency or misbehaviour
- *Lost child:* becomes passive and quietly withdraws from upsetting situations as well as family life
- *Mascot:* disrupts tense situations by providing comic relief

For children in alcoholic homes, life is a struggle. They have to deal with constant stress, anxiety, and embarrassment. Because the alcoholic is often the centre of attention, the children's wants and needs are usually ignored. It is not uncommon for these children to be victims of violence, abuse, neglect, or incest. As we have seen, when such children grow up they have a greater tendency to become alcoholics themselves than do children from nonalcoholic families.

In the last decade, we have come to recognize the unique problems of adult children of alcoholics whose difficulties in life stem from a lack of parental nurturing during childhood. Among these problems are an inability to develop social attachments, a need to be in control of all emotions and situations, low self-esteem, and depression.

Fortunately, not all individuals who grew up in alcoholic families are doomed to have lifelong problems. Many of these people develop a resiliency in response to their family's problems and enter adulthood armed with positive strengths and valuable career-oriented skills, such as the ability to assume responsibility, strong organizational skills, and realistic expectations of their jobs and those of others.

## Costs to Society

The alcohol industry registered sales of more than $16.1 billion in the fiscal year ending March 31, 2004, providing employment for more than 14,000 persons and generating $4.3 billion in revenue for provincial governments as well as considerable federal revenue. The average Canadian spent $316 on beer, $153 on wine, and $154 on spirits.[31]

The benefits of alcohol sales to the economy should be considered alongside the consequences of alcohol abuse and addiction. Wider society suffers the consequences of individuals' alcohol abuse. The figure of $18.45 billion, or 2.7 percent of GDP, represents the most optimistic estimate of the cost of addiction to society. The actual number could be significantly higher. Of this amount, alcohol accounts for $7.5 billion.[32]

## Women and Alcoholism

In the past, women have consumed less alcohol and had fewer alcohol-related problems than men. Now a greater percentage of women, especially college- and university-aged women, are choosing to drink and many are drinking more heavily.

Studies indicate that there are now almost as many female as male alcoholics. However, there appear to be differences between men and women when it comes to alcohol abuse:[33]

1. Women attribute the onset of problem drinking to a specific life stress or traumatic event more frequently than men.
2. Women's alcoholism starts later and progresses more quickly than men's; this phenomenon is called telescoping.
3. Women tend to be prescribed mood-altering drugs more often than are men; women thus face the risks of drug interaction or cross-tolerance more often.
4. Males who are not addicted to alcohol tend to divorce their spouses who are addicted nine times more often than they do their spouses without an alcohol addiction; women addicted to alcohol are thus not as likely to have a family support system to aid them in their recovery attempts.
5. Females who are addicted to alcohol do not tend to receive as much social support as males in their treatment and recovery.
6. Unmarried, divorced, or single-parent women tend to have significant economic problems that may make entry into a treatment program especially difficult.

---

### WHAT WOULD YOU DO?

Think about your campus and the cultural norms surrounding alcohol use. Do female students drink as frequently as male students? Why? Do women on campus drink heavily? Why or why not? Does the campus culture view men's and women's drinking problems in the same way? What supports are available on campus for men and women with a drinking problem? What supports are available in the local community?

---

# RECOVERY

Most individuals addicted to alcohol and problem drinkers who seek help have experienced a turning point or dramatic occurrence, such as a failed relationship or confrontation at work. Regardless of the reasons for seeking help, the alcoholic has finally recognized that alcohol controls his or her life—this is a critical component of recovery. The first step on the road to recovery is to regain that control and to begin to assume responsibility for personal actions.

## The Family's Role

Family members of an individual addicted to alcohol sometimes take action before that person does. They may go to an organization or a treatment facility to seek help for themselves and their relative. An effective method of helping an individual addicted to alcohol confront the disease is a process called **intervention.** Essentially, an intervention is a planned confrontation with the alcoholic that involves several family members plus professional counsellors. The family members express their love and concern, telling the person with the addiction that they will no longer refrain from acknowledging the problem and affirming their support for appropriate treatment. A family intervention is often the turning point for a growing number of individuals addicted to alcohol.

## Treatment Programs

There are more than 260 residential care facilities in Canada for the treatment of alcohol and drug addiction, funded by a mix of municipal, provincial, and federal sources. There are also outpatient, detox, walk-in, and crisis centres. Treatment programs are based on various models and are offered in many other languages in addition to French and English. Upon admission to a treatment facility, the patient is given a complete physical exam to determine whether there are underlying medical problems that will interfere with treatment. Individuals addicted to alcohol who quit drinking typically experience withdrawal symptoms, such as:

- hyperexcitability
- confusion
- sleep disorders
- convulsions

---

**Intervention:** A planned confrontation with an alcoholic in which family members or friends express their concern about the alcoholic's drinking.

- agitation
- tremors of the hands
- brief hallucinations
- depression
- headache
- seizures

In a small percentage, alcohol withdrawal results in a severe syndrome known as **delirium tremens (DTs).** Delirium tremens is characterized by confusion, delusions, agitated behaviours, and hallucinations.

Withdrawal from alcohol is very difficult and medically risky—more so than for many other addictive substances or behaviours. Thus, for any long-term addiction to alcohol, medical supervision is usually necessary. Detoxification, the process by which individuals addicted to alcohol end their dependence, is commonly carried out in a medical facility where they can be monitored to prevent fatal withdrawal reactions. Withdrawal usually takes 7 to 21 days. Shortly after detoxification, treatment begins for psychological addiction. Most treatment facilities keep their patients from three to six weeks. Treatment at private treatment centres costs several thousand dollars, but some insurance programs or employers will assume most of this expense.

### Family Therapy, Individual Therapy, and Group Therapy

Various individual and group therapies are also available. In family therapy, the person and family members gradually examine the psychological reasons underlying the addiction. In individual and group therapy, alcoholics learn positive coping skills for use in situations that have regularly caused them to turn to alcohol. On some campuses, the problems associated with alcohol abuse are so great that student health centres are opening their own treatment programs.

### Other Types of Treatment

Two other treatments are drug and aversion therapy. Disulfiram (trade name: Antabuse) is the drug of choice for treating alcoholics. If alcohol is consumed, the drug causes unpleasant intolerant effects such as headache, nausea, vomiting, drowsiness, and hangover. These symptoms discourage the alcoholic from drinking. Aversion therapy is based on conditioning therapy. It works on the premise that the sight, smell, and taste of alcohol will acquire aversive properties if repeatedly paired with a noxious stimulus. For a period of 10 days, the alcoholic takes drugs that induce

vomiting when combined with several drinks. These treatments work best in conjunction with counselling.

**Alcoholics Anonymous (AA)** is a private, non-profit, self-help organization founded in 1935. The organization, which relies on group support to help people stop drinking, currently has more than one million members, with branches all over the world. People attending their first AA meeting will find that no last names are ever used. Neither is anyone forced to speak. Members are taught to believe that their alcoholism is a lifetime problem. They share their stories with the group and are asked to place their faith and control of the habit into the hands of a "higher power." The road to recovery is taken one step at a time. AA offers specialized meetings for homosexual, atheist, HIV-positive, and professional individuals with alcohol problems.

Alcoholics Anonymous also has auxiliary groups to help spouses or partners, friends, and children of alcoholics. Al-Anon is the group dedicated to helping adult relatives and friends of alcoholics understand the disease and learn how they can contribute to the recovery process. The support gained from talking with others who have similar problems is one of the greatest benefits derived from participation in Al-Anon. Many members learn how to exert greater control over their own lives. Some are able to rid themselves of the guilt they feel about their participation in their loved one's alcoholism.

Alateen, another AA-related organization, is designed to help adolescents live with an alcoholic parent or parents. Teens are taught that they are not at fault for their parents' problems with alcohol. They learn skills to develop their self-esteem so they can function better socially. Alateen also helps them to overcome their guilt feelings.

## Relapse

Roughly 60 percent of alcoholics relapse (resume drinking) within the first three months of treatment. Why is the relapse rate so high? Treating an addiction requires more than getting the addict to stop using; it also requires getting the person to break a pattern of behaviours that has dominated his or her life—often for some time.

People seeking to regain a healthy lifestyle must not only confront their addiction, but also guard against the tendency to relapse. Drinkers with compulsive personalities need to learn to understand themselves and take control. Others need to view treatment as a long-term process that takes a lot of effort beyond attending a weekly self-help group meeting. In order to work, a recovery program must offer the alcoholic ways to increase self-esteem and resume personal growth.

# SMOKING

Health consequences of the tobacco epidemic in developed and developing countries are devastating. By 2020, tobacco use is expected to kill more people than any single disease. Since the middle of the twentieth century, tobacco products have killed more than 60 million people in developed countries alone.[34]

Canadians have been smoking less since 1966, when 54 percent of men and 28 percent of women were smokers. The Canadian Tobacco Use Monitoring Survey reported (from data collected between February and June 2005) that slightly more than 5 million Canadians were current smokers, representing 20 percent of the population 15 years of age and older.[35] Further, more men than women smoke (22 versus 17 percent). In the 15- to 19-year-old group, 13 percent reported smoking daily (on average 9.6 cigarettes per day) and 7 percent were occasional smokers, with no difference between young men and women. In the 20- to 24-year-old group, 20 percent reported daily smoking with another 7 percent reporting occasionally lighting up. In this age group, males who smoke daily consume more cigarettes per day than do females (14.7 vs. 11.6).[36]

Despite the reduced rate of smoking in the population, it remains the number-one preventable cause of death in Canada. Every year, smoking kills five times more Canadians than car accidents, murder, suicide, and alcohol abuse combined. More than 46,000 Canadians die as a result of illness or disease related to tobacco use each year.

## WHAT WOULD YOU DO?

What would it be like if Canada were smoke-free? Would you support school administration if it made your campus smoke free? What types of repercussions would there be? Who would be affected?

## Tobacco and Its Effects

Tobacco is available in several forms: cigarettes, cigars, and pipes are used for burning and inhaling tobacco. **Snuff** is a finely ground form of tobacco that can be inhaled, chewed, or placed against the gums. **Chewing tobacco,** also known as "smokeless tobacco," is placed between the gums and teeth for sucking or chewing.

The chemical stimulant nicotine is the major psychoactive substance in these products. In its natural form, **nicotine** is a colourless liquid that turns brown upon oxidation (exposure to oxygen). When tobacco leaves are burned in a cigarette, pipe, or cigar, nicotine is released and inhaled into the lungs. Sucking or chewing a quid of tobacco releases nicotine into the saliva, and the nicotine is then absorbed through the mucous membranes in the mouth.

Smoking is the most common form of tobacco use. Smoking delivers a strong dose of nicotine to the user, along with an additional 5,000 chemical substances, 50 of which are known to cause cancer. Among these chemicals are various gases and vapours that carry particulate matter in concentrations that are 500,000 times as great as the most air-polluted cities in the world. Particulate matter condenses in the lungs to form a thick, brownish sludge called tar. **Tar** contains various carcinogenic (cancer-causing) agents such as benzopyrene and chemical irritants such as phenol. Phenol has the potential to combine with other chemicals to contribute to the development of lung cancer.

In healthy lungs, millions of tiny hairlike tissues called cilia sweep away foreign matter. Once the foreign material is swept up and collected by the cilia, it can be expelled from the lungs by coughing. Nicotine impairs the cleansing function of the cilia by paralyzing them for up to one hour following the smoking of a single cigarette. Tars and other solids in tobacco smoke are thus allowed to accumulate and irritate sensitive lung tissue.

Tar and nicotine are not the only harmful chemicals in cigarettes. In fact, tars account for only 8 percent of the components of tobacco smoke. The remaining 92 percent is made up of various gases, the most dangerous of which is **carbon monoxide.** In tobacco smoke, the concentration of carbon monoxide is 800 times higher than the level considered safe. In the human body, carbon monoxide

**Delirium tremens (DTs):** A state of confusion brought on by withdrawal from alcohol. Symptoms include hallucinations, anxiety, and trembling.

**Alcoholics Anonymous:** An organization whose goal is to help alcoholics stop drinking; includes auxiliary branches such as Al-Anon and Alateen.

**Snuff:** A powdered form of tobacco that is sniffed and absorbed through the mucous membranes in the nose or placed inside the cheek and sucked.

**Chewing tobacco:** A stringy type of tobacco that is placed in the mouth and then sucked or chewed.

**Nicotine:** The stimulant chemical in tobacco products.

**Tar:** A thick, brownish substance condensed from particulate matter in smoked tobacco.

**Carbon monoxide:** A gas found in cigarette smoke that binds at oxygen receptor sites in the blood.

reduces the oxygen-carrying capacity of the red blood cells by binding with the receptor sites for oxygen. Smoking thus diminishes the capacity of the circulatory system to carry oxygen, causing oxygen deprivation in many body tissues.

The heat from tobacco smoke, which can reach 880°C, is also harmful to the smoker. Inhaling hot gases and vapours exposes sensitive mucous membranes to irritating chemicals that weaken the tissues and contribute to the development of cancers of the mouth, larynx, and throat.

Filtered cigarettes designed to reduce levels of gases such as hydrogen cyanide and hydrocarbons may actually deliver more hazardous carbon monoxide to the user than do non-filtered brands. Some smokers use low-tar and nicotine products (that is, mild, special, or "lite") thinking these are safer forms of cigarettes. True, they contain 10 percent less carbon monoxide and 8 percent less nicotine, but they contain the same level of the other harmful chemicals. Furthermore, since there is less nicotine, smokers tend to inhale more deeply when smoking this kind of cigarette and actually inhale more of the dangerous chemicals than they would if they smoked regular cigarettes.

Clove cigarettes contain about 40 percent ground cloves (a spice) and about 60 percent tobacco. Many users mistakenly believe that these products are made entirely of ground cloves and that smoking them eliminates the risks associated with tobacco. In fact, clove cigarettes contain higher levels of tar, nicotine, and carbon monoxide than regular cigarettes. In addition, the numbing effect of eugenol, the active ingredient in cloves, allows smokers to inhale the smoke more deeply.

Nicotine is a powerful central nervous system stimulant that produces an aroused, alert mental state. Nicotine also stimulates the adrenal glands, increasing the production of adrenaline. The physical effects of nicotine stimulation include increased heart and respiratory rate, constriction of blood vessels, and subsequent increased blood pressure because the heart must work harder to pump blood through the narrowed vessels. Because smoking increases the "stickiness" of the blood, there is an increased risk of developing blood clots when you smoke. This risk is further elevated when smoking is combined with use of oral contraceptives.

Nicotine decreases the stomach contractions that signal hunger. It also decreases blood sugar levels. These factors, along with decreased sensation in the taste buds, reduce appetite. For this reason, many smokers eat less and weigh, on average, three kilograms less than nonsmokers. Beginning smokers usually feel the effects of nicotine with their first puff. These symptoms, called **nicotine poisoning,** include dizziness, lightheadedness, rapid, erratic pulse, clammy skin, nausea, vomiting, and diarrhea. The effects of nicotine poisoning cease as soon as tolerance

to the chemical develops. Medical research indicates that tolerance develops almost immediately in new users, perhaps after the second or third cigarette. In contrast, tolerance to most other drugs, such as alcohol, develops over a period of months or years.

## Smoking—A Learned Behaviour

Taking up smoking is a gradual process. It begins with forming a predisposition to smoking: that is, a perception that smoking is a normal behaviour acceptable and pervasive in society or one's peer group. Trying smoking can lead to an experimental stage when smoking happens repeatedly but irregularly; regular use and addiction follow. The transition from trying smoking to daily use takes an average of two to three years.

About 85 percent of smokers start before age 16. New smokers do not expect to become addicted, believing instead that they will be able to quit whenever they want to, and tending to discount the prospect of addiction and the potential adverse health effects of that future addiction.

Tobacco product promotions are intended to convey a positive brand image and convey as many "impressions" (exposures to the consumer) as possible in order to create and maintain the perception that tobacco use is desirable, socially acceptable, healthy, sexy, and more pervasive in society than it really is. These promotions are primarily directed to young people, particularly young women, partly because the tobacco companies know that most people make the decision *not* to smoke by the age of 16.

This positive image of tobacco use is precisely the perception that people need in order to feel reassured about smoking. Promotion affects tobacco consumption in three interrelated ways:

- by influencing the smoking decision process among starters through helping to shape and reinforce their belief that it's okay to smoke
- by influencing the amount consumed by smokers
- by hindering the quitting decision process among those who are addicted by acting as a reassuring cue to smoke[37]

### WHAT WOULD YOU DO?

Why do you think the rates of smoking have decreased in recent years? What "antismoking" methods do you think have been successful? Have any of these methods influenced your decision to not smoke (or to smoke)? Why?

## Smokeless Tobacco

Smokeless tobacco is just as addictive as cigarettes due to its nicotine content. There is nicotine in all tobacco products, but smokeless tobacco contains more nicotine than cigarettes. Holding an average-sized dip or chew in your mouth for 30 minutes gives you as much nicotine as smoking four cigarettes. A two-can-a-week snuff dipper gets as much nicotine as a one-and-a-half-pack-a-day smoker.

One of the major risks of chewing tobacco is **leukoplakia,** a condition characterized by leathery white patches inside the mouth produced by contact with irritants in tobacco juice.

Smokeless tobacco also impairs the senses of taste and smell, causing the user to add salt and sugar to food, which may contribute to high blood pressure and obesity. Some smokeless tobacco products contain high levels of sodium (salt), which also contributes to high blood pressure. Another risk of using smokeless tobacco is caused by the addition of fiberglass, which helps cut the lining in the mouth to facilitate the uptake of nicotine by the bloodstream. In addition, dental problems are common among users of smokeless tobacco. Contact with tobacco juice causes receding gums, tooth decay, bad breath, and discoloured teeth. Damage to both the teeth and jawbone can contribute to early loss of teeth. Users of all tobacco products may not be able to use the vitamins and other nutrients in food effectively. In some cases, vitamin supplements may be recommended by a physician.

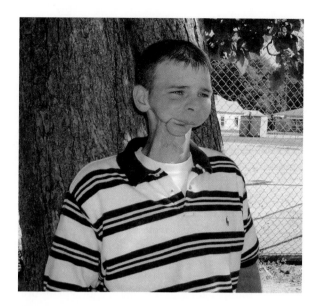

*This 25-year-old cancer survivor has undergone surgery to remove neck muscles, lymph nodes, and his tongue. He began using smokeless tobacco at age 13; by age 17, he was diagnosed with squamous cell carcinoma. He now speaks out about the dangers of smokeless tobacco.*

### WHAT WOULD YOU DO?

Why do people choose to use smokeless tobacco? Do you think the health risks of its use are well understood? Should smokeless tobacco be forbidden in public places just as cigarettes are banned? Why do you think chewing tobacco has attracted athletes? Do you think the use of smokeless tobacco should be banned in high school, college, and university athletics?

## Environmental Tobacco Smoke

As the population of nonsmokers rises, so does the demand for the right to breathe clean air. As a result, smoking is banned in many public places, particularly those that are indoors.

**Environmental tobacco smoke (ETS)** is divided into two categories: mainstream smoke and secondhand smoke (also called sidestream smoke). **Mainstream smoke** refers to smoke drawn through tobacco while inhaling; **secondhand smoke** refers to smoke from the burning end of a cigarette or to smoke exhaled by a smoker. People who breathe smoke from someone else's smoking product are said to be involuntary or passive smokers.

Although involuntary smokers breathe less tobacco than active smokers, they still face risks from exposure to tobacco smoke. Secondhand smoke actually contains more carcinogenic substances than the smoke that a smoker inhales—about twice as much tar and nicotine, five times as much carbon monoxide, and 50 times as much ammonia. There is also evidence that secondhand smoke may pose an even greater risk for death due to heart disease than for death due to lung cancer.[38] Secondhand smoke is estimated to cause more deaths per year than any other environmental pollutant.[39]

**Nicotine poisoning:** Symptoms often experienced by beginning smokers; they include dizziness; diarrhea; lightheadedness; rapid, erratic pulse; clammy skin; nausea; and vomiting.

**Leukoplakia:** A condition characterized by leathery white patches inside the mouth produced by contact with irritants in tobacco juice.

**Environmental tobacco smoke (ETS):** Smoke from tobacco products, including sidestream and mainstream smoke.

**Mainstream smoke:** Smoke that is drawn through tobacco while inhaling.

**Secondhand smoke:** The cigarette, pipe, or cigar smoke breathed by nonsmokers; also called sidestream smoke.

Lung cancer and heart disease are not the only risks involuntary smokers face. Children exposed to secondhand smoke also have a greater chance of developing other respiratory problems, such as cough, wheezing, asthma, and chest colds, along with a decrease in pulmonary performance. The greatest effects of secondhand smoke are seen in children under the age of five.

Cigarette, cigar, and pipe smoke in enclosed areas presents other hazards to nonsmokers. An estimated 10 to 15 percent of nonsmokers are extremely sensitive (hypersensitive) to cigarette smoke.[40] These people experience itchy eyes, difficulty in breathing, painful headaches, nausea, and dizziness in response to minute amounts of smoke. The level of carbon monoxide in cigarette smoke contained in enclosed places is 4,000 times higher than the standard recommended by the U.S. Environmental Protection Agency for a definition of clean air.

Efforts to reduce the hazards associated with passive smoking have been gaining momentum in recent years. Smoking is now illegal in most public places, including government buildings, restaurants, cafés, coffee shops, shopping malls, and universities. Hotels and motels set aside rooms for nonsmokers, and car rental agencies designate certain vehicles for nonsmokers. Smoking has been banned on all domestic airline flights. (See the Building Communication Skills box.)

# QUITTING

From what we know about successful quitters, quitting is often a lengthy process involving several unsuccessful attempts before success is finally achieved. Even successful quitters suffer occasional slips, emphasizing the fact that quitting smoking is a dynamic process that may actually be never-ending.

## Breaking the Nicotine Addiction

Nicotine addiction may be one of the toughest addictions to overcome. Smokers' attempts to quit often lead to **nicotine withdrawal,** which includes irritability, restlessness, nausea, vomiting, and intense cravings for tobacco. The person who wishes to quit has several options.

### Nicotine Replacement Products

Non-tobacco products that replace depleted levels of nicotine in the bloodstream have helped some people stop using tobacco. The two most common nicotine-replacement products are nicotine chewing gum and the nicotine patch, both available by prescription.

Some patients use a prescription chewing gum containing nicotine, called Nicorette, to help them reduce their nicotine consumption over time. Under the guidance of a physician, the user chews between 12 and 24 pieces of gum per day for up to six months. Nicorette delivers about as much nicotine as a cigarette does, but because it is absorbed through the mucous membrane of the mouth, it doesn't produce the same rush as inhaling a cigarette does. Users experience no withdrawal symptoms and fewer cravings for nicotine as the dosage is reduced until completely weaned. There is some controversy surrounding the use of nicotine replacement gum. Opponents believe that it substitutes one addiction for another. Successful users counter that it is a valid way to help break a deadly habit without suffering the unpleasant withdrawal symptoms and cravings that often lead ex-smokers to resume smoking.

The nicotine patch, first marketed in 1991, is a popular method for those attempting to quit smoking. It is generally used in conjunction with a comprehensive smoking-behaviour cessation program. A small, thin 24-hour patch placed on the smoker's upper body delivers a continuous flow of nicotine through the skin, helping to relieve the body's cravings. The patch is worn for 8 to 12 weeks under the guidance of a physician. During this time, the dose of nicotine is gradually reduced until the smoker is fully weaned from nicotine. Occasional side-effects include mild skin irritation, insomnia, dry mouth, and nervousness. The patch is relatively inexpensive compared to the price of a pack of cigarettes, and some insurance plans will pay for it.

## Breaking the Habit

For many smokers, the road to quitting includes some type of antismoking therapy. Among the more common therapy techniques are aversion therapy, operant conditioning, and self-control therapy. Prospective quitters must decide which method or combination of methods will work best for them. Programs that combine several approaches have shown the most promise.

## Benefits of Quitting

Many tissues damaged by smoking can repair themselves. As soon as smokers stop, their bodies begin the repair process. Within eight hours, carbon monoxide and oxygen levels return to normal, and "smoker's breath" disappears. Within a few days of quitting, the mucus clogging airways is broken up and eliminated. Circulation and the senses of taste and smell improve

**Nicotine withdrawal:** Symptoms, including nausea, headaches, and irritability, suffered by smokers who cease using tobacco.

# How to Help Your Family Clear the Air: The Rules and Regulations

Smoking is subject to a patchwork of federal, provincial, and municipal legislation:

- By federal law, it is illegal to sell or supply tobacco products to anyone under 18, with some provinces having raised that age to 19.
- Smoking is banned in most federally regulated workplaces, such as banks and government offices. It is also banned in provincial government workplaces in British Columbia, Saskatchewan, Ontario, New Brunswick, Nova Scotia, and Newfoundland (Newfoundland bans smoking in all workplaces, and has requirements for ventilation for those places with smoking sections, such as restaurants) and in territorial government offices. Federal prisons became smoke-free in 1998.
- About 97 percent of schools have smoking policies, but only 66 percent ban smoking completely, indoors and outdoors, at all times. Sanctions against students are usually stronger than those against staff.
- Almost all licensed day-care centres have policies against smoking, most of them unwritten, but only 62 percent of day-care agencies regulate smoking in private or home day-cares.
- One-quarter of hospitals permit smoking in areas that do not have separate ventilation. In one out of every five health-care institutions that restrict smoking, cigarettes are nevertheless for sale.

## THE PROBLEM WITH VENTILATION

There is only one method to keep an indoor space smoke-free: send smokers outdoors.

The main purposes of indoor ventilation systems are to limit the accumulation of carbon dioxide, which we exhale, and to keep odours down. At an average ventilation rate of one air exchange per hour, it takes three hours to remove 95 percent of the smoke from a single cigarette—and the remaining five percent is still harmful. Electronic air cleaners, air purification systems and "smokeless" ashtrays can double or triple the rate at which the air clears of smoke. But the air-exchange rate would need to increase a thousandfold to be effective. Such a system would have to be so powerful it would create gale-force winds, says Mary Jane Ashley, principal investigator of the Ontario Tobacco Research Unit.

Confining smokers to one room in a house or one section of a workplace doesn't work either, since the laws of physics dictate that the smoke will disperse throughout the area. Garfield Mahood, executive director of the Non-Smokers' Rights Association, compares having nonsmoking sections in restaurants to having nonurinating sections in swimming pools.

Opening a window can help—but depending on which way the wind is blowing, it can also direct the smoke straight to a non-smoker.

## STRATEGIES

- If you live with a smoker be firm about your right to live in a smoke-free home.
- Ask a smoker to smoke outside but agree to sit outside or go for a walk with her or him to show you're not rejecting her or him, just the smoke.
- Let every caregiver (including teenage babysitters) know that you don't allow your children to be in smoke-filled environments. That means no smoking in your home, or any other place that does not restrict smoking.
- Ask about the policy on smoking anywhere that your child spends time: school, community centre, local arena. Be clear that your child requires a smoke-free place to play or learn.
- Ask your kids how they feel about smoking, and, if you're a smoker, try to explain what the addiction is like. Be honest about your own worries and feelings of guilt.
- Accept the fact that kids have a right to a smoke-free home and be open to discussing how, as a family, you will achieve that.
- Encourage your teens to support smoke-free businesses (and do so yourself).
- If your teen is spending time in places where smoking is allowed let the owners know your concerns and ask them to establish a smoke-free policy.
- If your teen is smoking, take her addiction seriously. Offer to help her quit and suggest she contact Quit 4 Life, www.quit4life.com.
- If you are pregnant and you smoke, quit. Every cigarette not smoked helps you and your fetus.
- If pregnant, ask all the smokers you know not to smoke around you, and let people know that your home will continue to be a smoke-free environment after your baby arrives.

Source: *Smoke Gets in Your Eyes, Ears, Nose, and Lungs: How to Help Your Family Clear the Air,* Health Canada, 2002. Adapted and reproduced with the permission of the Minister of Public Works and Government Services Canada, 2006.

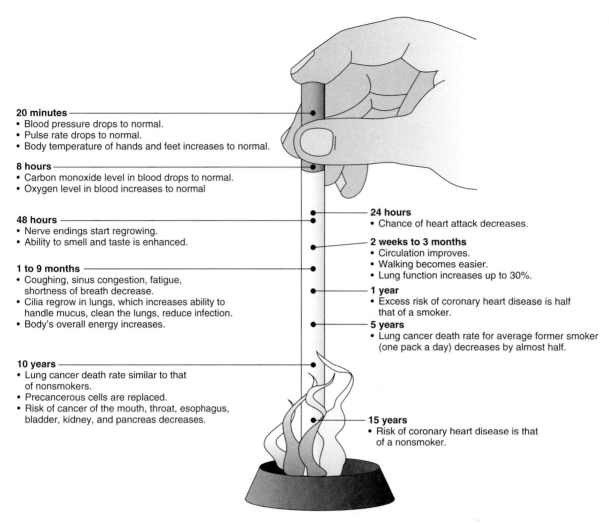

**20 minutes**
- Blood pressure drops to normal.
- Pulse rate drops to normal.
- Body temperature of hands and feet increases to normal.

**8 hours**
- Carbon monoxide level in blood drops to normal.
- Oxygen level in blood increases to normal

**48 hours**
- Nerve endings start regrowing.
- Ability to smell and taste is enhanced.

**1 to 9 months**
- Coughing, sinus congestion, fatigue, shortness of breath decrease.
- Cilia regrow in lungs, which increases ability to handle mucus, clean the lungs, reduce infection.
- Body's overall energy increases.

**10 years**
- Lung cancer death rate similar to that of nonsmokers.
- Precancerous cells are replaced.
- Risk of cancer of the mouth, throat, esophagus, bladder, kidney, and pancreas decreases.

**24 hours**
- Chance of heart attack decreases.

**2 weeks to 3 months**
- Circulation improves.
- Walking becomes easier.
- Lung function increases up to 30%.

**1 year**
- Excess risk of coronary heart disease is half that of a smoker.

**5 years**
- Lung cancer death rate for average former smoker (one pack a day) decreases by almost half.

**15 years**
- Risk of coronary heart disease is that of a nonsmoker.

## FIGURE 11.1

### When Smokers Quit

Within 20 minutes of smoking that last cigarette, the body begins a series of changes that continues for years.

Source: G. Hanson and P. Venturelli, *Drugs and Society,* 5th ed. (Sudbury, MA: Jones and Bartlett, 1998), 320 © Jones and Bartlett, www.jbpub.com. Reprinted with permission.

within weeks. Many ex-smokers who have kicked the cigarette habit say they have more energy, sleep better, and feel more alert. By the end of one year, the risk for lung cancer and stroke decreases. Within two years, the risk for heart attack drops to near-normal. At the end of 10 smoke-free years, the ex-smoker can expect to live out his or her normal life span. Figure 11.1 shows the health benefits of quitting smoking.

### WHAT WOULD YOU DO?

What could you personally do to help someone quit smoking? What are the most common barriers to quitting? When trying to stop smoking, why do people often interpret a relapse as a total failure?

# CAFFEINE

Caffeine is the most popular and widely consumed drug in Canada. Almost half of Canadians drink coffee every day, and many others consume caffeine in some other form (tea, colas, chocolate), mainly for its well-known "wake-up" effect. Drinking coffee is legal, even socially encouraged. Many people believe caffeine is not a drug and not really addictive. Coffee and other caffeine-containing products seem harmless. If you share these attitudes, think again; research has linked caffeine to certain health problems. **Caffeine** is a drug derived from the

**Caffeine:** A stimulant found in coffee, tea, chocolate, and some soft drinks.

chemical family called **xanthines.** Two related chemicals, *theophylline* and *theobromine,* are found in tea and chocolate, respectively. Xanthines are mild CNS stimulants that enhance mental alertness and reduce feelings of fatigue. Other stimulant effects include increases in heart muscle contractions, oxygen consumption, metabolism, and urinary output. These effects are felt within 15 to 45 minutes of ingesting a product that contains caffeine.

Side effects of xanthines include wakefulness, insomnia, irregular heartbeat, dizziness, nausea, indigestion, and sometimes mild delirium. Some people also experience heartburn. As with other drugs, the user's psychological outlook and expectations will influence the effects. Different products contain different concentrations of caffeine. A 156-mL (5-ounce) cup of coffee contains 65 to 115 milligrams. Caffeine concentrations vary with the brand and strength of the brew. Small chocolate bars (28 grams) contain up to 15 milligrams of caffeine and theobromine. Table 11.4 outlines the caffeine content of various products.

## TABLE 11.4
### Caffeine Content of Various Products

| Product | Caffeine Content (average mg per serving) |
| --- | --- |
| *Coffee (156-mL cup)* | |
| Regular brewed | 65–115 |
| Decaffeinated brewed | 3 |
| Decaffeinated instant | 2 |
| *Tea (175-mL cup)* | |
| Hot steeped | 36 |
| Iced | 31 |
| Bottled (375 mL) | 15 |
| *Soft drinks (375-mL serving)* | |
| Jolt Cola | 100 |
| Dr. Pepper | 61 |
| Mountain Dew | 54 |
| Coca-Cola | 46 |
| Pepsi | 36–38 |
| *Chocolate* | |
| 28 grams baking chocolate | 25 |
| 28 grams chocolate candy bar | 15 |
| 1/2 cup chocolate pudding | 4–12 |
| *Over-the-counter drugs* | |
| No Doz (2 tablets) | 200 |
| Excedrin (2 tablets) | 130 |
| Midol (2 tablets) | 65 |
| Anacin (2 tablets) | 64 |

Source: Office of Department of Health and Welfare, October 2001.

## Caffeine Addiction

As the effects of caffeine wear off, users may feel let down—mentally or physically depressed, exhausted, and weak. To counteract this, people commonly choose to drink another cup of coffee. Habitually engaging in this practice leads to tolerance and psychological dependency. Until the mid-1970s, caffeine was not medically recognized as addictive. Chronic caffeine use and its attendant behaviours were called "coffee nerves." This syndrome is now recognized as *caffeine intoxication,* or **caffeinism.** Symptoms of caffeinism include chronic insomnia, jitters, irritability, nervousness, anxiety, and involuntary muscle twitches. Withdrawing the caffeine may compound the effects and produce severe headaches. (Some physicians ask their patients to take a simple test for caffeine addiction: don't consume anything containing caffeine, and if you get a severe headache within four hours, you are addicted.) Because caffeine meets the requirements for addiction—tolerance, psychological dependency, and withdrawal symptoms—it can be classified as addictive. Although you would have to drink 67 to 100 cups of coffee in a day to produce a fatal overdose of caffeine, you may experience sensory disturbances after consuming only ten cups of coffee within a 24-hour period. These symptoms include tinnitus (ringing in the ears), spots before the eyes, numbness in arms and legs, poor circulation, and visual hallucinations. Because ten cups of coffee is not an extraordinary amount to drink in one day, caffeine use clearly poses health threats.

## The Health Consequences of Long-Term Caffeine Use

Long-term caffeine use has been suspected of being linked to a number of serious health problems, ranging from heart disease and cancer to mental dysfunction and birth defects. However, no strong evidence exists to suggest that moderate caffeine use (less than 300 milligrams daily, approximately three cups of coffee) produces harmful effects in healthy, nonpregnant people. It appears that caffeine does not cause long-term high blood pressure and it has not been linked to strokes, nor is there any evidence of a relationship between coffee and heart disease. However, people who suffer from irregular heartbeat are cautioned against using caffeine because the resultant increase in heart rate might be life-threatening. Both decaffeinated and caffeinated coffee products contain ingredients that can irritate the stomach lining and be harmful to people with stomach ulcers. For years, caffeine consumption was linked with fibrocystic breast disease, a condition characterized by painful, noncancerous lumps in the breast. Although these conclusions have been challenged, many clinicians advise patients with mammillary cysts to avoid caffeine use.

---

**Xanthines:** The chemical family of stimulants to which caffeine belongs.

**Caffeinism:** Caffeine intoxication brought on by excessive caffeine use; symptoms include chronic insomnia, irritability, anxiety, muscle twitches, and headaches.

---

# SUMMARY

- Alcohol is a central nervous system depressant. University and college students are under extreme pressure not only to consume alcohol but also to consume large quantities of alcohol.

- Alcohol's effect on the body is measured by the blood alcohol concentration (BAC), the ratio of alcohol to total blood volume. The higher the BAC, the greater the impaired judgment and coordination and drowsiness. Use during pregnancy can cause fetal alcohol spectrum disorder (FASD), including fetal alcohol effects (FAE) and fetal alcohol syndrome (FAS). Alcohol is also a causative factor in many traffic accidents.

- Alcohol use becomes alcoholism when it interferes with school, work, or social and family relationships. Causes of alcoholism include biological and family factors and social and cultural factors. Alcoholism has far-reaching effects on families, especially on children.

- Most individuals addicted to alcohol do not admit to a problem until reaching a major life crisis or having their families intervene. Treatment options include detoxification at private medical facilities, therapy (family, individual, or group), and programs like Alcoholics Anonymous.

- The use of tobacco involves many social issues, including advertising targeted at youth and women, the largest-growing populations of smokers.
- Tobacco is available in smoking and smokeless forms, both containing addictive nicotine (a psychoactive substance). Smoking also delivers 5,000 other chemicals, 50 which are known to cause cancer to the lungs of smokers.
- Smokeless tobacco contains more nicotine than cigarettes and dramatically increases risks for oral cancer and other oral problems.
- Quitting is complicated by the dual nature of smoking: smokers must kick a chemical addiction as well as a habit.
- Although caffeine is the most popular and widely consumed drug in Canada, it is often not recognized as a drug. The active ingredient in caffeine is xanthines. Xanthines are mild CNS stimulants that enhance mental alertness and reduce feelings of fatigue.

# DISCUSSION QUESTIONS

1. When it comes to drinking alcohol, how much is too much? How often is too often? When you see a friend having "too many" drinks at a party, what actions do you normally take? What actions should you take?

2. What factors may cause someone to slip from being a social drinker to being an alcoholic? What effect does alcoholism have on an alcoholic's family?

3. Discuss the varied forms in which you can ingest tobacco. In each form, how do chemicals enter your system? What are the physiological effects of nicotine?

4. Discuss the risks of smokeless tobacco. Do you think that smokeless tobacco should be banned from major league baseball, as it was from the minor leagues?

5. Smokers often claim they have the right to smoke in public places. From what you have learned about secondhand smoke, how would you argue against a smoker's right to smoke in public?

6. Do you drink coffee or other beverages that contain caffeine? Do you limit your consumption of these beverages? Why or why not? Are you addicted to caffeine? How could you find out? What are the risks of caffeine addiction or excessive caffeine consumption?

# APPLICATION EXERCISE

Reread the What Do You Think? scenario at the beginning of the chapter and answer the following questions.

1. What responsibility does the restaurant have in protecting the fetus from a known teratogen?

2. What responsibility does the mother have for protecting the fetus?

3. If you were the waiter/waitress, what would you do?

# HEALTH ON THE NET

Alcoholics Anonymous
**www.alcoholics-anonymous.org**

Canadian Centre on Substance Abuse
**www.ccsa.ca**

The Centre for Addiction and Mental Health
**www.camh.net**

World Health Organization: Tobacco Free Initiative
**www.who.int/tobacco/en/**

# CHAPTER 12

# CARDIOVASCULAR DISEASE AND CANCER

*Reducing Your Risks*

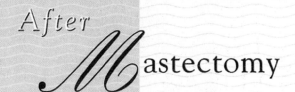

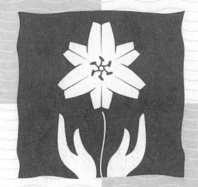

*After* ***Mastectomy***

A Woman's Guide

## CHAPTER OBJECTIVES

- Describe the anatomy and physiology of the heart and the circulatory system.

- Review the various types of heart disease; their diagnoses, treatments, and how to prevent them.

- Identify the controllable risk factors for cardiovascular disease. Examine the risk factors you cannot control.

- Discuss the issues uniquely concerning women in relationship to cardiovascular disease.

- Explain the importance of lifestyle choices in preventing heart disease.

- Define cancer and explain how cancer develops.

- Discuss the probable causes of cancer, including biological, occupational and environmental, social and psychological, chemicals in foods, viral, medical, and combined causes.

- Understand and act in response to self-exams, medical exams, and symptoms related to different types of cancers. Discuss cancer detection and treatment, including radiation therapy, chemotherapy, and immunotherapy.

- Explain the importance of lifestyle choices in preventing cancer.

Kassandra is an avid sunbather. She thinks the glow of a tan makes her look healthy and attractive. In fact, when she cannot get the tan she desires from the sun, she spends time at tanning salons. This year, she has decided to get a jump on her tan and is studying for her final exams outside any minute she can. In her efforts to get tanned as quickly as possible, she has decided to not wear sunscreen.

■ How many others like Kassandra do you know? What is the risk of suntanning—under the sun or in tanning beds? What will it take to change the attitude that a suntan makes a person look healthy and attractive? What can a person do to reduce his or her risk of developing skin cancer? What do you know about sunscreen and how and when to apply it?

Despite many advances in medical technology, heart disease and cancer continue to be two of the leading causes of death in Canada. The actions you take today have a significant impact on reducing your risks for these diseases now and in the future.

# CARDIOVASCULAR DISEASES

During the last century, we consumed more protein-rich, high-fat, high-sugar, high-sodium, and high-calorie foods to the point that, today, more than half of us are overweight (BMI > 25.0) or so out of shape that a simple trip up the stairs leaves us gasping for breath. Escalators and elevators, automobiles, and numerous other labour-saving devices have released us from much physical exertion. In fact, muscular efforts required at work and home accounted for about 30 percent of our daily caloric needs in the late 19th century, whereas today the same tasks account for only about one percent of our energy needs. We sit on plump couches and flip through the TV channels by remote control rather than moving ourselves to change them by hand. We buy blowers to whisk our leaves away rather than use a rake. To compound this lack of physical activity or sedentary lifestyle, millions of us continue to smoke and drink to excess. It is no wonder then that **cardiovascular diseases (CVD)** are the leading cause of death in Canada today, accounting for more than 36 percent of all male deaths and 39 percent of all female deaths.[1] Further, cardiovascular disease is the third leading cause of premature death under

age 75.[2] Death rates from CVD are, however, declining. Since the mid-1950s the death rate for cardiovascular diseases in Canada has decreased by more than 50 percent for males and 60 percent for females.[3]

How do health experts account for this decline? There are no simple answers. Advances in medical techniques, earlier and better diagnostic procedures and treatments, better emergency medical assistance programs, and training of ordinary citizens in cardiopulmonary resuscitation (CPR) have greatly aided individuals with cardiovascular disease. Refinements in surgical techniques and improvements in heart transplants and artificial heart devices have enabled many to live longer lives. Educational programs have promoted public awareness of the role that individual efforts, including a healthy dietary intake and regular physical activity, can play in risk reduction. You can reduce your risk for cardiovascular diseases by taking steps to change certain behaviours. For example, controlling high blood pressure and reducing your intake of saturated fats and cholesterol are two things you can do to lower your chances of heart attack. By maintaining your weight, decreasing your intake of sodium, engaging in regular physical activity, and changing your lifestyle to reduce stress, you can lower your blood pressure. You can also monitor the levels of fat and cholesterol in your blood and adjust your dietary intake to prevent your arteries from becoming clogged. By understanding how your cardiovascular system works, you will have a better chance of understanding your risks and of changing your behaviours to reduce them.

# UNDERSTANDING YOUR CARDIOVASCULAR SYSTEM

The **cardiovascular system** is the network of elastic tubes through which blood flows as it carries oxygen and nutrients to all parts of the body. It includes the heart, lungs, arteries, *arterioles* (small arteries), and *capillaries* (minute blood vessels). It also includes *venules* (small veins) and *veins*, the blood vessels though which blood flows as it returns to the heart and lungs.[4]

Under normal circumstances, the human body contains approximately six litres of blood. This blood transports nutrients, oxygen, waste products, hormones, and enzymes throughout the body. It also regulates body temperature, cellular water levels, and acidity levels of body components, and aids in bodily defence against toxins and harmful microorganisms. An adequate blood supply is essential to health and well-being.

How does the heart ensure that blood is constantly recirculated to body parts? The four chambers of the heart work together to achieve this (see Figure 12.1). The

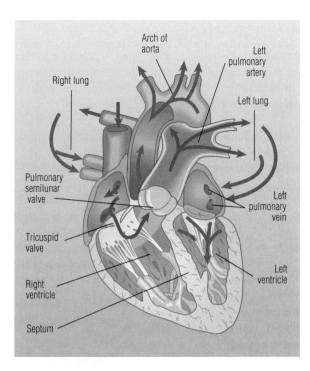

**FIGURE 12.1**
**Anatomy of the Heart**

Image labels:
Arch of aorta
Left pulmonary artery
Right lung
Left lung
Pulmonary semilunar valve
Left pulmonary vein
Tricuspid valve
Right ventricle
Left ventricle
Septum

two upper chambers of the heart, called **atria,** or auricles, are large collecting chambers that receive blood from the rest of the body. The two lower chambers, known as **ventricles,** pump the blood out again. Small valves regulate the steady, rhythmic flow of blood between chambers and prevent inappropriate backwash. The *tricuspid valve,* located between the right atrium and the right ventricle, the *pulmonary (pulmonic) valve,* between the right ventricle and the pulmonary artery, the *mitral valve,* between the left atrium and left ventricle, and the *aortic valve,* between the left ventricle and the aorta, permit blood to flow in only one direction.[5]

Heart activity depends on a complex interaction of biochemical, physiological, and neurological signals. The following is a simplified version of the steps involved in heart function:

1. Deoxygenated blood enters the right atrium after circulating through the body.
2. From the right atrium, blood moves to the right ventricle and is pumped through the pulmonary artery to the lungs, where it receives oxygen.
3. Oxygenated blood from the lungs then returns to the left atrium of the heart.
4. Blood from the left atrium is forced into the left ventricle.
5. The left ventricle pumps blood through the aorta to the body.

Different types of blood vessels are required for different parts of this process. **Arteries** carry blood away from the heart—except for pulmonary arteries, which carry deoxygenated blood to the lungs, where it picks up oxygen and gives off carbon dioxide. As they branch off from the heart, the arteries divide into smaller blood vessels called **arterioles,** and then into even smaller blood vessels called capillaries.

**Capillaries** have thin walls that permit the exchange of oxygen, carbon dioxide, nutrients, and waste products with body cells. The carbon dioxide and waste products are transported to the lungs and kidneys through **veins** and venules (small veins).

For the heart to function properly, the four chambers must beat in an organized manner. This is governed by an electrical impulse that directs the heart muscle to move when the impulse moves across it, which results in a sequential contraction of the four chambers. This signal starts in a small bundle of highly specialized cells, the **sinoatrial node (SA node),** located in the right atrium. The SA node serves as a form of natural pacemaker for the heart.[6] People with damaged or nonfunctional natural pacemaker activity have a mechanical pacemaker inserted to ensure the smooth passage of blood through the sequential phases of the heartbeat.

At rest, the average adult heart beats 70 to 80 times per minute. A well-conditioned heart may beat only 50 to 60 times per minute. The heart beats harder when the body is engaged in physical activity. When stressed, a heart may beat over 200 times per minute, particularly in an individual who is overweight or in poor physical condition. A healthy heart functions more efficiently and is less likely to suffer damage from overwork than an unhealthy one.

**Cardiovascular diseases (CVD):** Diseases of the heart and blood vessels.

**Cardiovascular system:** A complex system comprising the heart and blood vessels that transports nutrients, oxygen, hormones, and enzymes throughout the body and regulates temperature, the water levels of cells, and the acidity levels of body components.

**Atria:** The two upper chambers of the heart, which receive blood.

**Ventricles:** The two lower chambers of the heart, which pump blood through the blood vessels.

**Arteries:** Vessels that carry blood away from the heart to other regions of the body.

**Arterioles:** Branches of the arteries.

**Capillaries:** Minute blood vessels that branch out from the arterioles; their thin walls allow for the exchange of oxygen, carbon dioxide, nutrients, and waste products with body cells.

**Veins:** Vessels that carry blood back to the heart from other regions of the body.

**Sinoatrial node (SA node):** Node serving as a form of natural pacemaker for the heart.

# TYPES OF CARDIOVASCULAR DISEASES

Although most of us associate cardiovascular disease with heart attacks, there are actually a number of different types of cardiovascular diseases. The four most common forms include:

- arteriosclerosis (a group of diseases characterized by a narrowing or hardening of the arteries)
- coronary heart disease (a result of atherosclerotic plaque building up in the arteries such that coronary artery blood flow is reduced; when the blood flow is severely restricted or blocked a heart attack (myocardial infarction) results; when the blood flow is reduced (~ 75 percent), but not blocked, chest pain (angina pectoris) often occurs)
- stroke (cerebrovascular accident that occurs as a result of reduced blood supply to the brain)
- hypertension (chronic high blood pressure)

Other less common forms of cardiovascular disease include irregular heartbeat (arrhythmia), congestive heart failure, and congenital and rheumatic heart disease.

Some individuals are at a greater risk than others for cardiovascular diseases.[7] Generally, risk increases with age; men are at a greater risk than women, and individuals of African, South Asian, and First Nations descent are at greater risk than other ethnicities.

Methods of prevention and treatment of these diseases range from changes in dietary intake and lifestyle (become more physically active, manage stress, and so on) to use of medications and surgery. Timing of treatment is critical as well. Survival rates from a heart attack are highest for those treated within two hours of the first symptom.[8] Similarly, the key to surviving a stroke is to obtain medical treatment within two hours of the first symptom.[9]

# Arteriosclerosis

**Arteriosclerosis** is a general term for the narrowing or "hardening" of the arteries. The end result of arteriosclerosis is reduced blood flow to vital organs. **Atherosclerosis** is a type of arteriosclerosis characterized by deposits of fatty substances, cholesterol, cellular waste products, calcium, and fibrin (a clotting material in the blood) in the inner lining of an artery. The resulting build-up is referred to as atherosclerotic **plaque**.[10]

Plaque may partially or totally block the blood's flow through an artery. When plaque develops, two things that can happen are (1) bleeding (hemorrhage) into the plaque or (2) formation of a blood clot (thrombus) on the plaque's surface. If either of these occurs and an artery is blocked, the chances of a heart attack or stroke are great.[11]

Atherosclerosis does not suddenly occur. In fact, evidence suggests that atherosclerotic plaque actually begins to form while a person is in the womb, and becomes progressively worse as the years pass. As such, atherosclerosis is not an all-or-none disease but occurs in varying degrees. Further, there are lifestyle choices one makes in regards to physical activity and dietary intake that significantly influence the amount of plaque that develops. If the arteries are occluded (blocked with plaque) to about 75 percent, angina pectoris (chest pain) results. When the arteries are 90 to 95 percent occluded and a blood clot attempts to travel through them, a myocardial infarction (heart attack) occurs.

Many scientists believe that the process of plaque buildup begins because the protective inner lining of the artery (endothelium) becomes damaged and that fat, cholesterol, and other substances in the blood are deposited in the damaged area, eventually obstructing blood flow. The three major causes of such damage are (1) dramatic fluctuations in blood pressure, (2) elevated levels of cholesterol and triglycerides in the blood, and (3) cigarette smoking. Cigarette smoke aggravates and speeds up the development of atherosclerosis, particularly in the coronary arteries, the aorta, and the arteries of the legs.[12]

# Coronary Heart Disease

Coronary heart disease (CHD), also called coronary artery disease (CAD), is the major disease of the cardiovascular system. It is the result of atherosclerotic plaque accumulation such that a blockage occurs in one or more of the coronary arteries and blood flow is impeded. Chest pain or angina pectoris results when the blockage is equivalent to 75 percent or more. Complete blockage of a coronary artery results in a heart attack.

Those of you raised on a weekly dose of TV doctor programs will recognize Code Blue as the term for a **myocardial infarction (MI),** or heart attack. However, you may not know exactly what a heart attack is. A **heart attack** involves a blockage of the normal blood supply to an area of the heart. This condition is often brought on by a **coronary thrombosis,** or blood clot in the coronary artery. When blood does not flow readily, there is a corresponding decrease in oxygen flow. If the heart blockage is extremely minor, the otherwise healthy heart will adapt over time by using small unused or underused blood vessels to reroute the needed blood. This system, known as **collateral circulation,** is a form of self-preservation that allows a damaged heart muscle to heal.

When heart blockage is more severe, the body is unable to adapt on its own and outside lifesaving support is critical. The two hours following a heart attack are believed to be the most critical period; more than 40 percent of heart attack victims die within this time.[13] Following this time period, 12 percent of Canadians who experience a heart attack die within 30 days. Long-term survival after 30 days reaches 91 to 93 percent.[14]

It is believed that normal nonatherosclerotic arteries can also go into spasm and cause circulatory impairment. Excessive calcium and potassium are among the suspected causes of these spasms.

As a result of atherosclerosis and other circulatory impairments, the heart's oxygen supply is often reduced, a condition known as ischemia. Individuals with **ischemia** often suffer from varying degrees of **angina pectoris,** or chest pains. Many of these individuals experience short episodes of angina whenever they exert themselves physically. Symptoms may range from a slight feeling of indigestion to a feeling that the heart is being crushed. Generally, the more serious the oxygen deprivation, the more severe the pain.

Currently, there are several methods of treating angina. In mild cases, rest is critical. The most common treatments for more severe cases involve using drugs that affect (1) the supply of blood to the heart muscle or (2) the heart's demand for oxygen. Pain and discomfort are often relieved with *nitroglycerin,* a drug used to relax (dilate) veins, thereby reducing the amount of blood returning to the heart and thus lessening its workload. Patients whose angina is caused by spasms of the coronary arteries are often given drugs called *calcium channel blockers.* These drugs prevent calcium atoms from passing through coronary arteries and causing heart contractions. They also appear to reduce blood pressure and to slow heart rates. **Beta blockers** are another major type of drugs used to treat angina. The chemical action of beta blockers serves to control potential overactivity of the heart muscle.

# Stroke

Like the heart muscle, brain cells must have a continuous and adequate supply of oxygen in order to survive. A **stroke** (also called a *cerebrovascular accident*) occurs when the blood supply to the brain is cut off. Strokes may be caused by a **thrombus** (blood clot), an **embolus** (a wandering clot), or an **aneurysm** (a weakening in a blood vessel that causes it to bulge and, in severe cases, burst). Figure 12.2 illustrates these blood vessel disorders.

When any of these events occurs, the result is the death of brain cells, which do not have the capacity to

---

**Arteriosclerosis:** A general term for narrowing and hardening of the arteries.

**Atherosclerosis:** A type of arteriosclerosis characterized by deposits of fatty substances, cholesterol, cellular waste products, calcium, and fibrin in the inner lining of an artery.

**Plaque:** Accumulation of deposits in the arteries.

**Myocardial infarction (MI):** Heart attack.

**Heart attack:** A blockage of normal blood supply to an area in the heart.

**Coronary thrombosis:** A blood clot occurring in the coronary artery.

**Collateral circulation:** Adaptation of the heart to partial damage accomplished by rerouting the needed blood through unused or underused blood vessels.

**Ischemia:** Reduced oxygen supply to the heart.

**Angina pectoris:** Severe chest pain occurring as a result of reduced oxygen flow to the heart.

**Beta blockers:** A type of drug used to treat angina; they control potential overactivity of the heart muscle.

**Stroke:** A condition occurring when the brain is damaged by disrupted blood supply.

**Thrombus:** Blood clot.

**Embolus:** Blood clot forced through the circulatory system.

**Aneurysm:** A weakened blood vessel that may bulge under pressure and, in severe cases, burst.

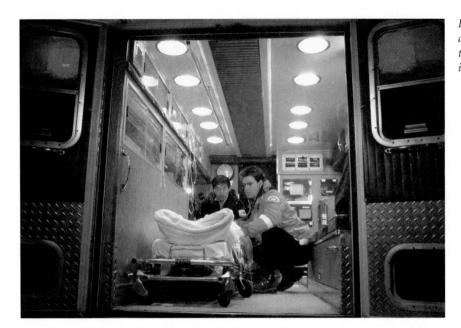

heal or regenerate. Strokes may result in speech impairments, memory loss, and loss of motor control. Although some strokes affect parts of the brain that regulate heart and lung function and kill within minutes, others are mild and cause only temporary dizziness or slight weakness or numbness. Mild forms of strokes are called **transient ischemic attacks (TIAs)** and are often indications of an impending major stroke. Knowing the warning signs or symptoms of stroke may help you or a loved one get medical attention earlier, when treatment may be more effective. As noted previously, survival is greatest when treatment is within the first two hours after a stroke occurs. Among the most common symptoms are:

- sudden weakness or numbness of the face, arm, or leg on one side of the body
- sudden dimness or loss of vision, particularly in only one eye
- loss of speech, or trouble talking or understanding speech
- sudden, severe headaches with no known cause
- unexplained dizziness, unsteadiness, or sudden falls, especially along with any of the previous symptoms

## Hypertension

Hypertension (that is, chronic high blood pressure) is unique because it not only is recognized as a cardiovascular disease itself, but also is a risk factor for coronary heart disease and stroke. When blood pressure is chronically elevated the workload on the heart is greater, which may damage the heart's ability to pump blood effectively throughout the body and may result in heart muscle damage.[15] High blood pressure may also damage the interior walls of the arteries, which facilitates atherosclerotic plaque accumulation.[16]

Sustained high blood pressure, or **hypertension,** that cannot be attributed to any specific cause is known as **essential hypertension.** Approximately 90 percent of all cases of high blood pressure fit this category. **Secondary hypertension** refers to high blood pressure caused by specific factors, such as kidney disease, obesity, or tumours of the adrenal glands.

Blood pressure is measured in two parts and is expressed as two numbers separated by a slash—for

Thrombus

Embolism

Hemorrhage

Aneurysm

FIGURE 12.2
**Common Blood Vessel Disorders**

## TABLE 12.1

### Blood Pressure Classifications

| Classification | Systolic Reading (mm Hg) | Diastolic Reading (mm Hg) |
|---|---|---|
| Normal | < 120 | < 80 |
| Prehypertension | 120–139 | 80–89 |
| Hypertension | | |
| Stage 1 | 140–159 | 90–99 |
| Stage 2 | ≥ 160 | ≥ 100 |

Note: If systolic and diastolic readings fall into different categories, treatment is determined by the highest category. Readings are based on the average of two or more properly measured, seated readings on each of two or more health care provider visits.

Source: National Heart, Lung, and Blood Institute, *The Seventh Report of the Joint National Committee on Prevention, Detection, Evaluation, and Treatment of High Blood Pressure* (NIH Publication No. 03-5233) (Bethesda, MD: National Institutes of Health, May 2003).

example, 120/80, or 120 over 80. Both values are measured in millimetres of mercury (mm Hg). The first number refers to **systolic pressure,** or the pressure on the walls of the arteries when the heart contracts, pumping blood to the rest of the body. The second value refers to **diastolic pressure,** or the pressure on the walls of the arteries during the heart's relaxation phase. During this phase, blood re-enters the chambers of the heart, preparing for the next heartbeat. Normal resting blood pressure is approximately 120 over 80 mmHg (see Table 12.1). A resting blood pressure greater than 140 over 90 mmHg is considered hypertensive.[17] Values between these are considered pre-hypertensive.[18]

### WHAT WOULD YOU DO?

Do you know your blood pressure? Why or why not? How can you tell if you have high blood pressure? What can you do to keep your blood pressure under control?

## Arrhythmia, Congestive Heart Failure, and Congenital and Rheumatic Heart Disease

An **arrhythmia** is an irregularity in heartbeat. It may be suspected, for instance, when a person complains of a racing heart in the absence of physical activity or anxiety; *tachycardia* is the medical term for an abnormally fast heartbeat. On the other end of the continuum is *bradycardia,* or abnormally slow heartbeat. When a heart goes into **fibrillation,** it exhibits a sporadic, quivering pattern of beating resulting in extreme inefficiency in moving blood through the cardiovascular system. If untreated, this condition may be fatal. Not all arrhythmias are life-threatening. Excessive caffeine or nicotine consumption can trigger an arrhythmia episode. For the most part, in the absence of other symptoms, arrhythmias are not serious. However, severe cases may require drug therapy or an external electrical stimulus to prevent serious complications.

**Congestive heart failure** occurs when the heart muscle is damaged or overworked and lacks the strength to keep blood circulating normally through the body. Individuals afflicted with rheumatic fever, pneumonia, or other cardiovascular problems in the past often have weakened heart muscles. In addition, the walls of the heart and the blood vessels may be damaged from previous radiation or chemotherapy treatments for cancer. These weakened muscles respond poorly when stressed; blood flow out of the heart is diminished, and the return flow of blood through the veins begins to back up, causing congestion in the tissues. This pooling of blood causes enlargement of the heart and decreases the amount of blood that can be circulated. Blood begins to accumulate in other body areas, such as in the vessels in the legs and ankles or the lungs, causing swelling or difficulty in breathing. If untreated, congestive heart failure will result in death. Most cases respond well to a treatment

**Transient ischemic attacks (TIAs):** Mild form of stroke; often an indicator of impending major stroke.

**Hypertension:** Chronic high blood pressure; 140/80 mmHg or greater.

**Essential hypertension:** Hypertension that cannot be attributed to any cause.

**Secondary hypertension:** Hypertension caused by specific factors, such as kidney disease, obesity, or tumours of the adrenal glands.

**Systolic pressure:** The upper number in the fraction that measures blood pressure, indicating pressure on the walls of the arteries when the heart contracts.

**Diastolic pressure:** The lower number in the fraction that measures blood pressure, indicating pressure on the walls of the arteries during the relaxation phase of heart activity.

**Arrhythmia:** An irregularity in heartbeat.

**Fibrillation:** A sporadic, quivering pattern of heartbeat resulting in extreme inefficiency in moving blood through the cardiovascular system.

**Congestive heart failure:** Occurs when the heart muscle is damaged or overworked and lacks the strength to keep blood circulating normally through the body.

of *diuretics* (water pills) for relief of fluid accumulation, *digitalis*, a drug that increases the pumping action of the heart, and a vasodilator that expands blood vessels and decreases resistance, allowing blood to flow more easily and reducing the workload on the heart.

Approximately 1 out of every 125 children is born with some form of **congenital heart disease** (heart disease present at birth). These forms may range from slight murmurs caused by valve irregularities, which some children outgrow, to serious complications in heart function that can be corrected only with surgery. Their underlying causes are unknown but are believed to be related to hereditary factors; maternal diseases, such as German measles (rubella), occurring during fetal development; or chemical intake (particularly alcohol) by the mother during pregnancy. Because of advances in pediatric cardiology, the prognosis for children with congenital heart defects is better than ever before.

**Rheumatic heart disease** can cause heart problems in children. It is attributed to rheumatic fever, an inflammatory disease caused by an unresolved *streptococcal infection* of the throat (strep throat) that may affect many connective tissues of the body, especially those of the heart, the joints, the brain, or the skin. In a small number of cases, the streptococcal infection can lead to an immune response in which antibodies attack the heart as well as the bacteria.

# CONTROLLING YOUR RISKS FOR CARDIOVASCULAR DISEASES

Our understanding of the role of not smoking, physical activity, stress management, sodium reduction, low-fat dietary intake, and other preventive actions, coupled with better diagnostic aids, has allowed many people to avoid major circulatory episodes. Figure 12.3 summarizes known ways to reduce your risk for heart attack.

Knowledge of the factors that contribute to cardiovascular disease and how to make lifestyle changes that reduce one's risk can motivate one to make the necessary health-promoting lifestyle changes. Different risks have a compounded effect when combined. For example, if you have high blood pressure, high cholesterol level, a family history of heart disease, and smoke cigarettes, you run a much greater risk of having a heart attack or other cardiovascular disease than someone with only one of these risks. To assess your risks for heart disease, see the Rate Yourself box.

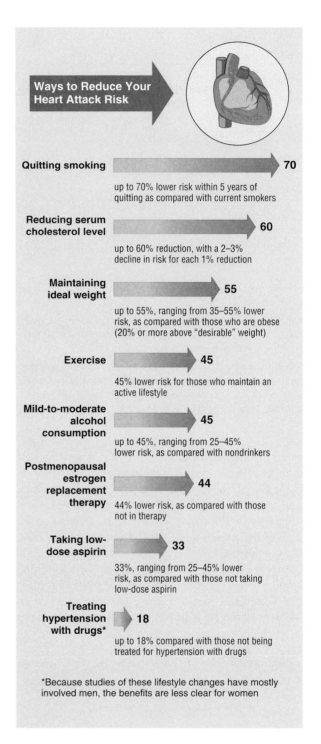

FIGURE 12.3

**Estimated Average Reduction in Risk for Heart Attack\***

\*Estimated risk reductions refer to the independent contribution of each risk factor to heart attack and do not address the wide range of known or hypothesized reactions among them.

Source: Adapted from information appearing in J. E. Mason, "Medical Progress: The Primary Prevention of Myocardial Infarction," *The New England Journal of Medicine* 326 (May 21, 1992): 1406–1416.

# Risks You Can Control

Factors that increase the risk for cardiovascular disease fall into two categories: those that can be controlled and those that cannot. The following risk factors can be controlled. As you read about each factor, ask yourself whether it applies to you and note the steps you can take to reduce its influence.

## Cigarette Smoking

The link between cigarette smoking and heart disease has been firmly established. The risk for cardiovascular disease is 70 percent greater for smokers than for nonsmokers. Further, the more a person smokes, the greater their risk for heart disease. Smokers who have a heart attack are more likely to die suddenly (within one hour) than nonsmokers. Evidence also indicates that chronic exposure to environmental tobacco smoke (*passive smoking or secondhand smoke*) also increases risk of heart disease.[19] If the effects of smoking are combined with other risk factors, the danger is greater than the sum of the added effects.

Cigarette smoking increases your risk of heart disease in several ways. First, the drug nicotine, a CNS stimulant, increases heart rate, heart output, blood pressure, and oxygen use by heart muscles. This causes the heart to work harder. Second, the carbon monoxide in cigarette smoke displaces oxygen in heart tissue, resulting in the heart being forced to work harder. Third, nicotine can lead to irregular heart rates (that is, arrhythmias) that may result in sudden death. Finally, cigarette smoke damages the lining of the coronary arteries, allowing cholesterol and plaque to accumulate more easily. This additional accumulation constricts the vessels, increasing blood pressure and causing the heart to work harder.

## Blood Fat and Cholesterol Levels

A dietary intake high in saturated fats is known to raise cholesterol levels, send the body's blood-clotting system into high gear, and make the blood sludgy in just a few hours, increasing the risk for heart attack or stroke. A fatty diet also increases the amount of cholesterol in the blood, contributing to atherosclerosis. A total cholesterol concentration of less than 5.2 mmol/L (200 mg/dL—milligrams per decilitre) indicates a low risk for heart disease, while values greater than 5.2 mmol/L (or 240 mg/dL) indicate high risk.[20] Values between 200 and 240 mg/dL are considered moderate risk.

Although risk values are established for total cholesterol, it is really the individual components that you need to be concerned about. Cholesterol comes in two varieties: **low-density lipoproteins (LDLs)** and **high-density lipoproteins (HDLs).** Low-density lipoproteins, often referred to as "bad" cholesterol, are believed to build up on artery walls. In contrast, high-density-lipoproteins, or "good" cholesterol, appear to remove cholesterol from artery walls, thus serving as a protector. In theory, if LDL levels get too high ($\geq 3.4$ mmol/L) or HDL levels too low ($< 0.9$ mmol/L)—largely because of too much saturated fat consumed, lack of physical activity, high stress, or genetic predisposition—cholesterol will accumulate inside arteries and lead to cardiovascular disease. The goal is to manage the ratio of HDL to total cholesterol by lowering LDL levels, raising HDL, or both. Regular physical activity and a healthy dietary intake low in saturated fat continue to be the best methods for maintaining healthy ratios.

**Triglycerides,** the type of fat we normally consume, are also manufactured by our bodies. As people get older or fatter or both, their triglyceride and cholesterol levels tend to rise. According to the Heart and Stroke Foundation of Canada,[21] triglycerides greater than or equal to 2.3 mmol/L increase risk for coronary heart disease.

## High Blood Pressure

As mentioned previously, high blood pressure (hypertension) is a unique risk factor for coronary heart disease because it is also a cardiovascular disease itself. In general, the higher your blood pressure, the greater your risk for coronary heart disease. High blood pressure is known as the "silent killer," because it usually has no symptoms. The latest data available from Statistics Canada (2000/01)[22] indicate that 12.6 percent of the population 12 years of age and over have high blood pressure. Very few 12- to 19-year-olds (0.6 percent) or 20- to 34-year-olds (2.3 percent) have high blood pressure. In the 35- to 44-year-old age group, 5.9 percent have high blood pressure. Rates more than double in the 45- to 54-year-old age group with 14.2 percent having high blood pressure. In the older age groups rates increase dramatically,

**Congenital heart disease:** Heart disease present at birth.

**Rheumatic heart disease:** A heart disease caused by untreated streptococcal infection of the throat.

**Low-density lipoproteins (LDLs):** Compounds that facilitate the transport of cholesterol in the blood to the body's cells and accumulate on arterial walls.

**High-density lipoproteins (HDLs):** Compounds that facilitate the transport of cholesterol in the blood to the liver for metabolism and elimination from the body.

**Triglycerides:** The most common form of fat in the body; excess calories are converted into triglycerides and stored as body fat.

# Understanding Your Risk for CVD

Each of us has a unique level of risk for various diseases. Some of these risks are things you can take action to change; others are risks that you need to consider as you plan a lifelong strategy for overall risk reduction. Complete each of the following questions and total your points in each section. If you score between 1 and 5 in any section, consider your risk. The higher the number, the greater your risk. If you answer "don't know" for any question, talk to your parents or other family members as soon as possible to find out if you have any unknown risks.

## PART I: ASSESS YOUR FAMILY RISK FOR CVD

1. Do any of your primary relatives (mother, father, grandparents, siblings) have a history of heart disease or stroke?

   Yes _____ (1 point) No_____ (0 points) Don't Know _____

2. Do any of your primary relatives (mother, father, grandparents, siblings) have diabetes?

   Yes _____ (1 point) No_____ (0 points) Don't Know _____

3. Do any of your primary relatives (mother, father, grandparents, siblings) have high blood pressure?

   Yes _____ (1 point) No_____ (0 points) Don't Know _____

4. Do any of your primary relatives (mother, father, grandparents, siblings) have a history of high cholesterol?

   Yes _____ (1 point) No_____ (0 points) Don't Know _____

5. Would you say that your family consumed a high-fat diet (lots of red meat, dairy, butter/margarine) during your time spent at home?

   Yes _____ (1 point) No_____ (0 points) Don't Know _____

   **Total** _____

## PART II: ASSESS YOUR LIFESTYLE RISK FOR CVD

1. Is your total cholesterol level higher than it should be?

   Yes _____ (1 point) No_____ (0 points) Don't Know _____

2. Do you have high blood pressure?

   Yes _____ (1 point) No_____ (0 points) Don't Know _____

3. Have you been diagnosed as prediabetic or diabetic?

   Yes _____ (1 point) No_____ (0 points) Don't Know _____

4. Do you smoke?

   Yes _____ (1 point) No_____ (0 points) Don't Know _____

5. Would you describe your life as being highly stressful?

   Yes _____ (1 point) No_____ (0 points) Don't Know _____

   **Total** _____

## PART III: ASSESS YOUR ADDITIONAL RISKS FOR CVD

1. How would you best describe your current weight?

   a. Lower than what it should be for my height and weight (0 points)

   b. About what it should be for my height and weight (1 point)

   c. Higher than it should be for my height and weight (1 point)

2. How would you describe the level of exercise that you get each day?

   a. Less than what I should be exercising each day (1 point)

   b. About what I should be exercising each day (0 points)

   c. More than what I should be doing each day (0 points)

3. How would you describe your dietary behaviours?

   a. Eating only the recommended number of calories per day (0 points)

   b. Eating less than the recommended number of calories per day (0 points)

   c. Eating more than the recommended number of calories per day (1 point)

4. Which of the following best describes your typical dietary behaviours?

   a. I eat from the major food groups, trying hard to get the recommended amount of fruits and vegetables (0 points)

   b. I eat too much red meat and consume too much saturated fat from meats and dairy products each day (1 point)

   c. Whenever possible, I try to substitute olive oil or canola oil for other forms of dietary fat (0 points)

5. Which of the following best describes you?

   a. I watch my sodium intake and try to reduce stress in my life (0 points)

   b. I have a history of *Chlamydia* infection (1 point)

   c. I try to eat 5 to 10 milligrams of soluble fibre each day and to substitute a soy product for an animal product in my diet at least once each week (0 points)

   **Total** _____

Source: Lab 9.2, pp. 277–278, from *Total Fitness and Wellness*, 4th ed., by Scott Powers, Stephen L. Dodd, and Virginia J. Noland. Copyright © 2006 by Pearson Education, Inc. Reprinted by permission.

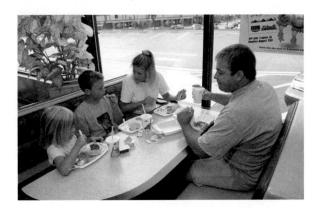

*Controlling the amount and type of fat you eat is one thing you can do to lower your risk for heart disease*

with 26.0 percent of 55- to 64-year-olds and 38.5 percent of all individuals over the age of 65 having high blood pressure. After the age of 45 years more females than males have high blood pressure, with the greatest difference noted in the over-65 group (42.3 vs. 33.8 percent).

Normal blood pressure varies for different individuals depending on weight, physical fitness, sex, and race. For the average person, 120 over 80 is a normal blood pressure level. If your blood pressure exceeds 140 over 90, you should make appropriate lifestyle changes to lower it (engage in regular physical activity, eat healthy, manage your stress, attain a healthy body weight). If these lifestyle changes do not reduce your blood pressure to more normal values, you may need to take medication. Similarly, if your blood pressure is pre-hypertensive (that is, between 120/80 and 140/90), you should adjust your lifestyle first in an attempt to lower your blood pressure.

## Physical Inactivity

Inactivity is a primary risk factor for coronary heart disease. Moreover, physically inactive people also tend to be overweight and are more likely to smoke and to pay less attention to their overall health than active people. The good news is that you don't have to be an exercise fanatic to reduce your risk. Even moderate levels of low-intensity physical activity are beneficial if done regularly and on a long-term basis. Such activities include walking for pleasure, gardening, housework, and dancing.

Engaging in physical activity on a regular basis reduces risk for heart disease in a number of ways. First, physical activity of a sufficient intensity strengthens the heart, improves circulation, and improves your blood profile (that is, increases HDLs). Because of the increases in HDL, there is a reduced level of atherosclerotic plaque development. Third, physical activity plays

an important role in reducing hypertension and maintaining body weight.

## Dietary Intake and Obesity

Dietary intake and obesity also play a role in CVD. Researchers are not certain whether high-fat, high-sugar, high-calorie diets are a direct risk for cardiovascular disease or whether they invite risk by causing obesity, which strains the heart to push blood through the many kilometres of capillaries that supply each kilogram of fat. A heart that continuously has to move blood through an overabundance of vessels may become damaged. In fact, people who are overweight or obese and sedentary are more likely to develop heart disease and stroke even if they have no other risk factors. Moreover, evidence indicates that how fat is distributed on the body may affect a person's risk for CHD. Specifically, if excess fat accumulates around your upper body and waist (apple-shaped), you are at a greater risk than if your excess fat accumulates around your hips and thighs (pear-shaped). A waist girth greater than 102 cm for men and 88 cm for women is significantly related to elevated triglyceride levels, low HDL concentrations, and hypertension.[23]

## Diabetes

Diabetics, particularly those who have taken insulin for a number of years, appear to run an increased risk for the development of CHD. In fact, heart disease is the leading cause of death among individuals with diabetes. Because overweight people have a higher risk for diabetes, distinguishing between the effects of the two conditions is difficult. Individuals with diabetes also tend to have elevated blood fat levels, increased atherosclerosis, and a tendency toward deterioration of small blood vessels, particularly in the eyes and extremities. Through a prescribed regimen of diet, physical activity, and medication, individuals with diabetes can control much of their increased risk for heart disease.

## Individual Response to Stress

Activities of daily living can have substantial and variable effects on blood pressure. These activities result in a variable but high estimate of blood pressure in the "unrested" patient relative to that obtained with a standardized technique.[24] For example, people under stress may start smoking or smoke more than they otherwise would. In one study, one out of five people had an extreme cardiovascular reaction to stressful stimulation (see Chapter 3).[25]

# Obesity Link to Heart Disease Confirmed

Dr. Jean-Pierre Després, Director of Research Cardiology at Laval's University Hospital in Quebec, is a member of the International Day for Evaluation of Abdominal Obesity (IDEA) study, which examined the relationship of abdominal obesity to cardiovascular disease in 170,000 individuals in 63 countries. The results of this study confirmed that abdominal obesity, as measured by waist circumference in men and women, was associated with the presence of cardiovascular disease. More specifically, it was found that a 14- or 14.9-cm increase in waist circumference, in men and women respectively, increased the risk of cardiovascular disease from 21 to 40 percent. Furthermore, this study showed that a 16-year increase in age tripled the likelihood of an adult developing cardiovascular disease.

Dr. Després commented, "this is the first time a study of this magnitude has been conducted worldwide in a primary care population," and "these figures show that patients do not feel that having their waist measured is intrusive. The importance and the clinical significance of these results will stimulate initiation of additional studies that will aid us in identifying patients most at risk and help us to evaluate the impact that new treatments will have on the overall cardiometabolic risk of these patients."

Source: "Obesity Link to Heart Disease Confirmed," report by Jennifer Tyron, Global National, March 14, 2006: www.canada.com/nationalpost/news/story.html?id=5ee25c66-9c9b-4fe7-a05a-be485d60cddc&k=95067.

These people experience alarm and resistance so strongly that, when under stress, their bodies produce large amounts of stress chemicals, which in turn cause tremendous changes in the cardiovascular system, including increases in blood pressure. These people are called *hot reactors*. Although their blood pressure may be normal when they are not under stress—for example, in a doctor's office—it increases dramatically in response to even small amounts of everyday tension. *Cold reactors* are those who are able to experience stress without harmful cardiovascular responses. Cold reactors may internalize stress, but their self-talk and perceptions about the stressful events lead them to a non-response state in which their cardiovascular system remains virtually unaffected.

Research in this area remains inconclusive. However, more recent studies investigating the relationship of personality to heart disease do suggest that personality plays a role in effective coping of the stress response. See Chapter 3 for tips on managing your stress response, whether you are a cold or a hot reactor.

## Risks You Cannot Control

There are some risk factors for CVD that you cannot prevent or control. The most important are:

- *Heredity:* Having a family history of heart disease appears to increase risks significantly. Whether this is because of genetics or environment is an unresolved question.

- *Age:* Eighty percent of all fatal heart attacks occur in people over age 65. The risk for CVD increases with age for both sexes.[26]

- *Sex:* Men are at much greater risk for CVD until old age. Women under 35 have a fairly low risk unless they have high blood pressure, kidney problems, or diabetes. Using oral contraceptives while smoking also increases risk. Hormonal factors appear to reduce risk for women, although after menopause or after estrogen levels are otherwise reduced (for example, hysterectomy), women's LDL levels tend to go up, increasing their risk for CVD. (For a more detailed discussion of the sex factor, see the next section.)

- *Race:* First Nations and Inuit people have three times the rate of heart problems of Canadians in general.[27] Also at greater risk for heart disease are individuals of African and South Asian descent.[28]

## WHAT WOULD YOU DO?

Complete the "Understanding Your Risk" box. What is your biggest risk factor for heart disease right now? What is your second biggest risk factor? What action will you take immediately to reduce your risk? Will it be difficult to take this action? Why or why not? Who can help you in taking this action to improve your health behaviours?

# WOMEN AND CARDIOVASCULAR DISEASE

Cardiovascular disease accounts for the death of more Canadians than any other disease. In Canada, approximately 40 percent of women's deaths are due to heart disease and stroke. Eight times as many women die from heart disease and stroke than from breast cancer. Currently, two in three women have one or more of the major risk factors for heart disease.[29]

While men have more heart attacks and have them earlier in life, women have a much lower chance of survival. Although we understand the mechanisms that cause heart disease in men and women, their experiences in the healthcare system, their reactions to life-threatening diseases, and a host of other technological and environmental factors may play a role in their survival rates.

## Risk Factors for Heart Disease in Women

Premenopausal women are unlikely candidates for heart attacks unless they also have diabetes, high blood pressure, kidney disease, or a genetic predisposition to high cholesterol levels. Family history, oral contraceptive use, and smoking also increase the risk for heart disease in premenopausal women.

### The Estrogen Element

Once her estrogen production drops with menopause, a woman's chance of developing heart disease rises rapidly. A 60-year-old woman has the same heart attack risk as a 50-year-old man. By her late 70s, a woman has the same heart attack risk as a man her age. To date, much of this changing risk has been attributed to the aging process, but the role of estrogen and other hormones remains unclear. Early studies of **hormone replacement therapies (HRT)** indicated that HRT may reduce a woman's risk for CVD by raising HDL cholesterol levels and lowering LDL cholesterol levels. However, other research since has been unable to find a similar reduced risk of heart disease with HRT.[30] Furthermore, the potential benefits for the cardiovascular system must be weighed against the potential risk of breast cancer and endometrial cancer that may be related to prolonged HRT.[31]

Cholesterol is another factor to consider in women's increased risk for heart disease as they age. Although women aged 25 and over tend to have lower cholesterol levels than men of the same age, when they reach 45 things change. Most men's cholesterol levels become more stable, while LDL and total cholesterol levels in women start to rise. And the gap widens further beyond age 55.[32] Before age 45, women's total blood cholesterol levels average below 220 mg/dL. By the time she is 45 to 55, the average woman's blood cholesterol rises to between 223 and 246 mg/dL (~5.2 mmol/L). Studies of men have shown that for every 1-percent drop in cholesterol, there is a 2-percent decrease in CVD risk.[33] If this holds true for women, prevention efforts focusing on dietary interventions and physical activity may significantly help postmenopausal women.

## Symptoms in Postmenopausal Women

Postmenopausal women often do not display the same extreme symptoms of heart disease that men do. The first sign of heart disease in men is generally a myocardial infarction. In women, the first sign is usually uncomplicated angina pectoris. Because chest discomfort rather than pain is the common manifestation of angina in women, and because angina has a much more favourable prognosis in women than in men, many physicians ignore the condition in their female patients or treat it too casually.

A heart attack also results in different symptoms in women than in men. In men, a heart attack usually manifests itself as crushing chest pain radiating to the shoulders, arms, neck, jaw, or back as well as dizziness, paleness, difficulty breathing, sweating, nausea, vomiting, or anxiety.[34] But in women, a heart attack results in much more vague symptoms such as pain in the neck, jaw, or arms; heaviness in the shoulders, back, or the pit of the stomach; and feeling out of breath, tired, sweating, nausea, or vomiting.[35] If these symptoms are experienced for two minutes or longer, it is critical to seek help immediately (call 911) or get to the nearest hospital that offers emergency cardiac care.

## Neglect of Symptoms

In the past decade, three main reasons why signs of heart disease in women may be overlooked have been postulated: (1) physicians may often be sex-biased in their delivery of health care, tending to concentrate on women's reproductive organs rather than on the whole body; (2) physicians tend to view male heart disease as a more severe problem because men traditionally have

**Hormone replacement therapies (HRT):** Therapies that replace estrogen and progestin in postmenopausal women.

a higher incidence of the disease; and (3) women decline major procedures more often than men. Other explanations for diagnostic and therapeutic difficulties encountered by women with heart disease include:[36]

- Delay in diagnosing a possible heart attack due to the complexity of interpreting chest pain and because symptoms of heart attack differ greatly for women compared to men.

- Typically less aggressive treatment of female heart attack victims.

- Their older age, on average, and frequency of other health problems.

- Women's coronary arteries are often smaller than men's, making surgical or diagnostic procedures more difficult technically.

- Their increased incidence of post-infarction angina or heart failure.

---

### WHAT WOULD YOU DO?

How do men and women differ in their experiences with heart disease? How have women played a role in the under-diagnosis of their heart disease? What actions do you think individuals can take to help improve this situation for women? What actions can communities and medical practitioners take?

---

# NEW WEAPONS AGAINST HEART DISEASE

The victim of a heart attack today has a variety of options not available a generation ago. Medications can strengthen heartbeat, control arrhythmias, remove fluids in cases of congestive heart failure, and relieve pain. Further, bypass surgery and angioplasty have become relatively commonplace procedures in hospitals throughout the nation.

## Techniques of Diagnosing Heart Disease

Several techniques can be used to diagnose heart disease, including electrocardiogram, angiography, and positron emission tomography scans. An **electrocardiogram (ECG)** is a record of the electrical activity of the heart measured during a stress test. Patients walk or run on treadmills with their hearts monitored. A more accurate method of testing for heart disease is **angiography** (often referred to as *cardiac catheterization*), in

which a needle-thin tube called a catheter is threaded through blocked heart arteries, a dye is injected, and an X-ray is taken to discover which areas are blocked. A more recent and even more effective method of measuring heart activity is **positron emission tomography,** also called a **PET scan,** which produces three-dimensional images of the heart as blood flows through it. During a PET scan, a patient receives an intravenous injection of a radioactive tracer. As the tracer decays, it emits positrons that are picked up by the scanner and transformed by a computer into colour images of the heart.

Other tests include:

- *Radionuclide imaging* (includes such tests as thallium test, multinucleated gated angiography [MUGA] scan, and acute infarct scintigraphy). In these procedures, substances called *radionuclides* are injected into the bloodstream. Computer-generated pictures can then show them in the heart. These tests can show how well the heart muscle is supplied with blood, how well the heart's chambers are functioning, and which part of the heart has been damaged.

- *Magnetic resonance imaging (MRI).* This test uses powerful magnets to look inside the body. Computer-generated pictures can show the heart muscle, identify damage from a heart attack, diagnose certain congenital heart defects, and evaluate disease of larger blood vessels such as the aorta.

- *Ultrafast computed tomography (CT).* This is an especially fast form of X-ray of the heart designed to evaluate bypass grafts, diagnose ventricular function, and measure calcium deposits.

- *Digital cardiac angiography* (also called DCA or DSA). This modified form of computer-aided imaging records pictures of the heart and its blood vessels.

## Angioplasty versus Bypass Surgery

During the 1980s, **coronary bypass surgery** seemed to be the ultimate technique for treating patients who had coronary blockages or suffered heart attacks. In coronary bypass surgery, a blood vessel taken from another site in the patient's body (usually the saphenous vein in the leg or the internal mammary artery) is implanted to transport blood by bypassing blocked arteries. Recently, experts have begun to question the effectiveness of bypass operations, particularly for elderly people.

A procedure called **angioplasty** (sometimes called balloon angioplasty) has fewer risks and is believed by many to be more effective than bypass surgery in selected cardiovascular cases. This procedure is similar to angiography. A needle-thin catheter is threaded through blocked heart arteries. The catheter has a balloon at the tip, which is inflated to flatten fatty deposits against the artery walls, allowing blood to flow more freely. Angioplasty patients are generally awake but sedated during the procedure and spend only one or two days in the hospital after treatment. Most people can return to work within five days. Only about 1 percent of all angioplasty patients die during or soon after the procedure. However, there are some risks in this procedure. In 3 to 7 percent of cases, the blood vessel that is stretched open by the balloon collapses spontaneously, and a bypass has to be done anyway. In addition, in about 30 percent of all angioplasty patients, the treated arteries become clogged again within six months. Some patients may undergo the procedure as many as three times within a five-year period. Some surgeons argue that given angioplasty's high rate of recurrence, bypass may be a more effective method of treatment.

New research suggests that in many instances, drug treatments may be as effective in prolonging life as invasive surgical techniques, but it is critical that doctors follow an aggressive drug treatment program and that patients comply. Among the most effective are beta blockers and calcium channel blockers to reduce high blood pressure and treat other symptoms. Cholesterol-lowering medications are also effective.

Research indicates that low doses of Aspirin (80 milligrams daily or every other day) are beneficial to heart patients because of their blood-thinning properties. It should be pointed out that higher doses do not provide additional protection. Aspirin is even recommended as a preventive strategy for individuals without current heart disease symptoms. However, given the additional risks from emergency surgery or accidental bleeding, Aspirin should be taken as a preventive measure only if your physician recommends it.

## Thrombolysis

Whenever a heart attack occurs, prompt action is the key factor in the patient's eventual prognosis. When a coronary artery gets blocked, the heart muscle doesn't die immediately, but time determines how much damage occurs. If a victim gets to an emergency room and is diagnosed fast enough, a form of reperfusion therapy called **thrombolysis** can sometimes be performed. Thrombolysis involves injecting an agent such as TPA (tissue plasminogen activator) to dissolve the clot and restore some blood flow, thereby reducing the amount of tissue that dies from ischemia.[37] These drugs must be used within one to three hours of a heart attack for best results.

### WHAT WOULD YOU DO?

With all the new diagnostic procedures, treatments, and differing philosophies about various prevention and intervention techniques, how can the typical health consumer ensure that he or she will get the best treatment when needed? Where can one go for information? Why might women, members of certain minority groups, and the elderly need a "health advocate" who can help them get through the system?

# CANCER INCIDENCE AND MORTALITY

An estimated 153,100 new cases of cancer and 70,400 deaths from cancer will occur in Canada in 2006.[38] It is projected that 38 percent of women and 44 percent of men will develop cancer in their lifetime and that one of every four Canadians will die of cancer (24 percent of women; 29 percent of men). The greater number of new cases of cancer is primarily due to an aging population. Mortality is declining for males of all ages, for women under the age of 70, and most rapidly in children and adolescents.

Lung cancer continues to be the leading cause of premature death due to cancer with mortality estimates for 2006 of 10,700 for males and 8,600 for females. It is also expected that 22,700 new cases (12,100 for males and 10,600 for females) for lung cancer will be diagnosed in 2006.[39] It should be pointed out that although lung cancer is the number one cancer killer of men and women, it is only the second highest for new cases. In men there

---

**Electrocardiogram (ECG):** A record of the electrical activity of the heart measured during a stress test.

**Angiography:** A technique for examining blockages in heart arteries. A catheter is inserted into the arteries, a dye injected, and an X-ray taken to find the blocked areas.

**Positron emission tomography (PET scan):** Method for measuring heart activity by injecting a patient with a radioactive tracer scanned electronically to produce a three-dimensional image of the heart and arteries.

**Coronary bypass surgery:** A surgical technique where a blood vessel is implanted to bypass a clogged coronary artery.

**Angioplasty:** A technique in which a catheter with a balloon at the tip is inserted into a clogged artery; the balloon is inflated to flatten fatty deposits against artery walls, allowing blood to flow more freely.

**Thrombolysis:** Injection of an agent to dissolve clots and restore some blood flow, thereby reducing the amount of tissue that dies from ischemia.

are more new cases of prostate cancer (20,700) expected in 2006, while in women there are more new cases of breast cancer (22,200). The third highest expected cancer incidence for 2006 for men and women is colorectal cancer, with 10,800 and 9,100 new cases, respectively.

Not everyone is equally at risk for all types of cancers. Cancer incidence and mortality vary greatly by age, sex, race, and socioeconomic status. Because cancer risk is strongly associated with lifestyle and behaviours, differences in ethnic and cultural groups can provide clues to factors involved in the development of cancer. Culturally influenced values and belief systems can also affect whether or not a person seeks care, participates in screenings, or follows recommended treatment options. In Canada, cancer incidence and mortality are higher in the Atlantic provinces and Quebec and lowest in British Columbia.[40]

## What Is Cancer?

**Cancer** is the name given to a large group of diseases characterized by the uncontrolled growth and spread of abnormal cells. It may be hard to understand how normal, healthy cells become cancerous, but if you think of a cell as a small computer, programmed to operate in a particular fashion, the process may become clearer. Under normal conditions, healthy cells are protected by the immune system as they perform their daily functions of growing, replicating, and repairing body organs. When something interrupts normal cell programming, uncontrolled growth and abnormal cellular development result in a new growth of tissue. This new tissue serves no physiologic function and is called a **neoplasm.** When this neoplasmic mass forms a clump of cells it is known as a **tumour.**

Not all tumours are **malignant** (cancerous); in fact, most are **benign** (non-cancerous). Benign tumours are generally harmless unless they grow in such a fashion as to obstruct or crowd out normal tissues or organs. A benign tumour of the brain, for instance, is life-threatening when it grows in a manner that causes blood restriction and results in a stroke. The only way to determine whether a given tumour or mass is benign or malignant is through **biopsy,** or microscopic examination of cell development.

Benign and malignant tumours differ in several key ways. Benign tumours are generally composed of ordinary-looking cells enclosed in a fibrous shell or capsule that prevents their spreading to other body areas. Malignant tumours are usually not enclosed in a protective capsule and can therefore spread to other organs. This process, known as **metastasis,** makes some forms of cancer particularly aggressive in their ability to overcome bodily defences. By the time they are diagnosed, malignant tumours have frequently metastasized throughout the body, making treatment

extremely difficult. Unlike benign tumours, which merely expand to take over a given space, malignant cells invade surrounding tissue, emitting clawlike protrusions that disrupt chemical processes within healthy cells. More specifically, malignant cells disturb the ribonucleic acid (RNA) and deoxyribonucleic acid (DNA) within the normal cells. Tampering with these substances, which control cellular metabolism and reproduction, produces mutant cells that differ in form, quality, and function from normal cells.

## What Causes Cancer?

After decades of research, most cancer epidemiologists believe that cancers are preventable, at least in theory, and could be avoided by healthier choices in lifestyle and environment.[41] Many specific causes of cancer are well documented, the most important of which are smoking, obesity, and a few organic viruses. Most research supports the idea that cancer is caused by *external* (chemicals, radiation, viruses, and lifestyle) and *internal* (hormones, immune conditions, and inherited mutations) factors. These causal factors may act together or in sequence to promote cancer development. We do not know why some people have malignant cells in their body and never develop cancer while others may take ten years or more to develop the disease. Many factors are believed to cause cancer, and a combination of these factors can dramatically increase one's risk of the disease.

One theory of cancer development proposes that cancer results from spontaneous errors during cell reproduction. Perhaps cells that are overworked or aged are more likely to break down, causing genetic errors that result in mutant cells. Another theory suggests that cancer is caused by some external agent or agents that enter a normal cell and initiate the cancerous process. Numerous environmental factors, such as radiation, chemicals, hormonal drugs, immunosuppressant drugs (drugs that suppress the normal activity of the immune system), and other toxins are considered possible **carcinogens** (cancer-causing agents) (see Figure 12.4); perhaps the most common carcinogen is the tar found in cigarettes. The greater the dose or exposure to environmental hazards, the greater the degree of risk. Thus, people forced to work, live, and pass through areas that have high levels of environmental toxins may be at greater risk for several types of cancers.

A third theory came out of research on certain viruses believed to cause tumours in animals. This research led to the discovery of **oncogenes,** suspected cancer-causing genes that are present on chromosomes. Although oncogenes are typically dormant, scientists theorize that certain conditions such as age, stress, and exposure to carcinogens, viruses, and radiation may activate these oncogenes. Once activated, they

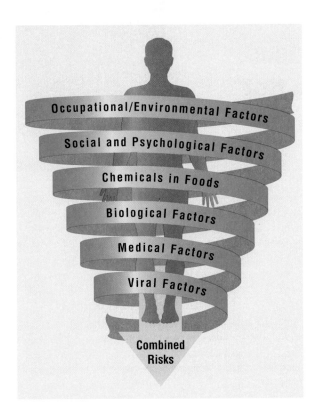

**FIGURE 12.4**
**Suspected Causes of Cancer**

begin to grow and reproduce in an out-of-control manner. Scientists are uncertain whether only people who develop cancer have oncogenes or whether we all have **protooncogenes,** genes that can become oncogenes under certain conditions. Many **oncologists** (physicians who specialize in the treatment of malignancies) believe that the oncogene theory may lead to a greater understanding of how individual cells function and may bring us closer to developing an effective treatment for cancerous cells.

## Risks for Cancer: Lifestyle

Anyone can develop cancer; however, most cases affect adults beginning in middle age. In fact, nearly 80 percent of cancers are diagnosed at ages 55 and over. Cancer researchers refer to one's *cancer risk* when they assess risk factors. *Lifetime risk* refers to the probability that an individual, over the course of a lifetime, will develop cancer or die from it. In 2006, as noted previously, 44 percent of men and 38 percent of women have a lifetime risk of developing cancer.[42]

*Relative risk* is a measure of the strength of the relationship between risk factors and a particular cancer. Basically, relative risk compares your risk if you engage in certain known risk behaviours with that of someone who does not engage in such behaviours.

For example, if you are a male and smoke, you have a 20-fold relative risk of developing lung cancer compared to a nonsmoker. In other words, the chances of getting lung cancer are about 20 times greater in a smoker than a nonsmoker.[43]

Over the years, researchers have found that people who engage in certain behaviours show a higher incidence of cancer. In particular, dietary intake, sedentary lifestyle (and resultant obesity), consumption of alcohol or cigarettes, stress, and other lifestyle factors seem to play a role. Likewise, colon and rectal cancer occur more frequently among persons with a high-fat, low-fibre dietary intake; in those who don't eat enough fruits and vegetables; and in those who are inactive.

Keep in mind that a high relative risk does not guarantee cause and effect. It merely indicates the likelihood of a particular risk factor being related to a particular outcome.

## Smoking and Cancer Risk

Of all the potential risk factors for cancer, smoking is among the greatest; it is the leading cause of preventable death in the world today. In Canada, tobacco is responsible for nearly one in five deaths annually. Recent declines in smoking have likely had a direct effect on the overall decrease in lung cancer rates; however, as previously noted, lung cancer remains the leading cause of cancer death in men and women.

**Cancer:** A large group of diseases characterized by the uncontrolled growth and spread of abnormal cells.

**Neoplasm:** A new growth of tissue that serves no physiological function resulting from uncontrolled, abnormal cellular development.

**Tumour:** A neoplasmic mass that grows more rapidly than surrounding tissues.

**Malignant:** Very dangerous or harmful; refers to a cancerous tumour.

**Benign:** Harmless; refers to a non-cancerous tumour.

**Biopsy:** Microscopic examination of tissue to determine if a cancer is present.

**Metastasis:** Process by which cancer spreads from one area to different areas of the body.

**Carcinogens:** Cancer-causing agents.

**Oncogenes:** Suspected cancer-causing genes present on chromosomes.

**Protooncogenes:** Genes that can become oncogenes under certain conditions.

**Oncologists:** Physicians who specialize in the treatment of malignancies.

# Canadian Cancer Statistics 2006: Cancer Screening in Canada Not Realizing Full Potential

TORONTO—Fewer Canadians would die from cancer if cancer screening in Canada was enhanced and expanded, according to a special report in *Canadian Cancer Statistics 2006* released today by the Canadian Cancer Society.

The report also states that some screening tests can help prevent cancer (e.g., cervical and colorectal cancers) as they detect pre-cancerous conditions, which can then be treated or removed.

"We have solid scientific evidence that screening through an organized program can reduce cancer deaths and, in some cases, even the incidence of certain cancers," says Heather Logan, Director, Cancer Control Policy, Canadian Cancer Society. "Existing cancer screening has helped reduce the cancer toll in Canada. However, we need to do more to make the most of this opportunity, which has the potential to significantly reduce the cancer burden in this country."

The special report—*Progress in Cancer Control: Screening*—says that cancer screening in Canada is not reaching its full potential because:

■ participation in existing cervical and breast cancer screening programs needs to be enhanced. Barriers have to be identified so that effective methods to reach out to women can be developed.

■ an organized colorectal cancer screening program has not been implemented in any province or territory in Canada, despite scientific evidence showing it would be an effective way to reduce both incidence [of] and death [from] this common cancer.

In addition, the special report states more research is needed to identify effective screening tests for prostate, lung and ovarian cancers.

Screening is the early detection of cancer by testing or checking for disease in people who don't show any symptoms of the disease. Detecting cancer early usually improves the likelihood of successful treatment, which leads to fewer Canadians dying from the disease. Screening can also help prevent some cancers by detecting pre-cancerous stages of the disease.

## BREAST CANCER

Current evidence suggests that breast cancer deaths could be reduced by as much as one-quarter if 70 per cent of women in the target age group (50–69 years) participated in organized screening programs. Every province and territory (except Nunavut) had an organized breast-screening program by 2003. However, none of the organized programs have achieved the nationally established target of 70 per cent participation.

"While it's encouraging that the proportion of women in organized breast cancer screening programs has increased over time, in 2003 participation was only 34 per cent nationally," says Logan.

The special report also says that about 61 per cent of Canadian women reported having a screening mammogram within two years. This is likely because mammography is also available through centres not affiliated with organized programs.

"The percentage of women who have been screened is probably somewhere between 34 and 61 per cent, and this is too low," says Logan. "However, breast cancer death rates have been declining and screening is one reason for this downward trend."

The Canadian Cancer Society recommends that women between the ages of 50 and 69 have a screening mammogram and a clinical breast exam every two years.

Women report that barriers to screening include not having a regular doctor or living in rural areas. "It's important to understand the barriers so that effective methods to reach out to women can be developed. For example, for women living in rural areas, a portable mammography unit may encourage women to get screened," says Logan

## COLORECTAL CANCER

In Canada, scientific evidence shows that colorectal cancer deaths could be reduced by 17 per cent if 70 per cent of Canadians between the ages of 50 and 74 had a fecal occult blood test (FOBT) every two years.

"This is a potentially significant drop in deaths from colorectal cancer," says Logan. "Although some informal screening is taking place, there is no organized colorectal screening program in Canada."

In addition, FOBT screening could have an impact on incidence of colorectal cancer as this test can detect blood in the stool from pre-cancerous polyps. Once identified, these polyps can be removed by colonoscopy or sigmoidoscopy before they become cancerous.

## CERVICAL CANCER

Largely as a result of "ad-hoc" (not organized) screening for cervical cancer with the Pap test, incidence rates have declined by 50 per cent and death rates by 60 per cent since 1977. The Pap test can identify pre-cancerous lesions that can then be treated, and can identify cancer at an early stage when treatment is most effective.

"Because of the long history of high-quality cervical cancer screening in Canada, the benefit achieved so far may be close to the maximum," says Logan. "However, it might be possible to see even further reductions in both incidence and death for this cancer if all elements of an organized screening program are incorporated, which would include identifying opportunities to increase participation."

The special report says that screening in Canada could be enhanced and improved if:

- Canada's capacity to review scientific evidence about screening was strengthened so that appropriate health policy recommendations could be developed in a timely fashion;

- adequate funding and support was provided for screening programs that scientific evidence shows are effective at reducing cancer death rates;

- more research was done to identify screening tests for those cancers for which there is not yet sufficient evidence to support an organized cancer screening program (for example, the prostate specific antigen [PSA] test for prostate cancer and CT scans for those at high risk of lung cancer).

"Many Canadians have been touched personally by cancer, and millions more have supported friends and family members in their fight against this devastating disease," says the Honourable Tony Clement, Minister of Health. "This is why the Government of Canada is committed to implementing a five-year Canadian Strategy for Cancer Control.

"We recognize the enormous contribution the Canadian Cancer Society and others in the cancer community have made," he adds. "We are proud to again partner with them in developing this report, and we are pleased to continue our work with the provinces and territories on national quality standards and targets for cancer screening programs."

If funding is allocated from provincial governments, implementing organized cancer screening programs is the responsibility of provincial cancer agencies (not every province has a cancer agency). The federal government is supportive of the development of screening policies and guidelines.

"Achieving maximum benefit from cancer screening across Canada requires continued work by all levels of government, cancer organizations, experts and Canadians," says Logan. "The Canadian Strategy for Cancer Control provides an effective mechanism to bring these groups together so this important issue can be dealt with in a coordinated and collaborative way. By working together we can identify gaps, develop ways to provide more opportunity for people to get screened, and target funding to areas with the most need.

"The Canadian Cancer Society is looking forward to working with the government to implement this important health initiative for Canadians."

For individual Canadians, Logan urges them to take full advantage of current cancer screening programs. "Talk to your doctors about what cancer screening tests are best for you," says Logan. "It could save your life."

Logan adds that the Society will continue its work in developing screening recommendations, getting this information to Canadians, and advocating governments to ensure appropriate screening programs are implemented.

Screening is delivered in two ways in Canada—through organized programs or through what is called "ad-hoc" screening. Screening is most effective and cost-efficient when offered through an organized screening program. There are defined elements for an organized program, which include follow-up guidelines, recruitment strategies, and monitoring and evaluation. Ad-hoc screening may include some of these elements, but not all.

Source: Canadian Cancer Society. Media Release, April 11, 2006, www.cancer.ca/ccs/internet/mediareleaselist/0,,3172_615815452_943322260_langId-en,00.html with permission of the Canadian Cancer Society. National Cancer Institute of Canada: Canadian Cancer Statistics 2005, Toronto, Canada, 2006.

Researchers once believed that cigarettes caused only cancers of the lung, pancreas, bladder, and kidney, and (synergistically with alcohol) the larynx, mouth, pharynx, and esophagus. However, recent evidence indicates that several other types of cancer are also related to tobacco. Most notably, cancers of the stomach, liver, and cervix seem to be directly related to long-term smoking.

## Obesity and Cancer Risk

It is difficult to sort through the accumulated evidence about the role of nutrients, obesity, sedentary lifestyle, and related variables. Nevertheless, research points to a potential cancer link. Cancer is more common among people who are overweight, and risk increases as obesity increases. A recent study of more than 900,000 adults indicates a significant relationship between a high body mass index and death rates for cancers such as esophagus, colon, rectum, liver, kidney, and pancreas. Women with a high BMI have a higher mortality rate from breast, uterine, cervical, and ovarian cancers; men with a high BMI have higher death rates from prostate and stomach cancers. In this study, 34 percent of all cancer deaths were attributable to overweight and obesity.[44] Other findings relevant to the obesity–cancer link are:

- The relative risk of breast cancer in postmenopausal women is 50 percent higher for obese women.

- The relative risk of colon cancer in men is 40 percent higher for obese men.

- The relative risks of gallbladder and endometrial cancer are five times higher in obese individuals compared to individuals of "healthy" weight.

## Biological Factors

Some early cancer theorists believed that we inherit a genetic predisposition toward certain forms of cancer.[45] Cancers of the breast, stomach, colon, prostate, uterus, ovaries, and lungs do appear to run in families. Specifically, a woman runs a much higher risk of having breast cancer if her mother, sisters, or daughters (primary relatives) had the disease, particularly if they had it at a young age. Hodgkin's disease and certain leukemias also show similar familial patterns. Whether these familial patterns are attributable to genetic susceptibility or to the fact that people in the same families experience similar environmental risks remains uncertain.

Sex also affects the likelihood of developing certain forms of cancer. For example, breast cancer occurs primarily among females, although men occasionally get breast cancer. Of the 22,300 new cases expected in 2006, 160 will be in males.[46] Obviously, factors other than heredity and familial relationships affect which sex develops a particular cancer. In the 1950s and 1960s, for example, women rarely contracted lung cancer. But with increases in the number of women who smoked and the length of time they had smoked, lung cancer became a leading cause of cancer deaths for Canadian women in the 1980s. Although sex plays a role in certain cases, other variables, such as lifestyle, are probably more significant.

## Occupational Environmental Factors

Various occupational hazards are known to cause cancer when exposure levels are high or exposure is prolonged. Overall, however, workplace hazards account for only a small percentage of all cancers. One of the most common occupational carcinogens is asbestos, a fibrous substance once widely used in the construction, insulation, and automobile industries. Nickel, chromate, and chemicals such as benzene, arsenic, and vinyl chloride have definitively been shown to be carcinogens for humans. Also, people who routinely work with certain dyes and radioactive substances may have increased risks for cancer. Working with coal tars, as in the mining profession, or working near inhalants, as in the auto-painting business, is also hazardous. Those who work with herbicides and pesticides also appear to be at higher risk, although the evidence is inconclusive to date for low-dose exposures.

Because people are sometimes forced to work near hazardous substances, it is imperative that worksites enact policies and procedures designed to minimize or eliminate toxic exposure to the above substances.

Ionizing radiation—radiation from X-rays, radon, cosmic rays, and ultraviolet radiation (primarily UV-B radiation)—is the only form of radiation proven to cause human cancer. (See the section on skin cancer.)

While reports about cancer-case clusters in communities around nuclear power facilities have raised public concerns, studies show that clusters do not occur more often near nuclear power plants than they do by chance in wider geographical areas.[47]

## Social and Psychological Factors

Although orthodox medical personnel are skeptical of overly simplistic prevention centres that focus on humour and laughter as the way to prevent cancer, we cannot rule out the possibility that negative emotional states contribute to disease development. People who are lonely, depressed, and lack social support have been shown to be more susceptible to cancer than their mentally healthy counterparts. Similarly, people under chronic stress and those with poor nutrition or sleep habits develop cancer at a slightly higher rate than the general population. Experts believe that severe depression or prolonged stress may reduce the activity of the body's immune system, thereby wearing down bodily resistance to cancer. Although psychological factors may play a part in cancer development, exposure to substances such as tobacco and alcohol in our social environment cannot be ignored.

## Chemicals in Foods

Among the food additives suspected of causing cancer is *sodium nitrate*, a chemical used to preserve and give colour to red meat. Research indicates that the actual carcinogen is not sodium nitrate but *nitrosamines*, substances formed when the body digests the sodium nitrates. Sodium nitrate has not been banned, primarily because it kills the bacterium *Clostridium botulin*, which is the cause of the highly virulent food-borne disease known as *botulism*. It should also be noted that the bacteria found in the human intestinal tract may contain more nitrates than a person could ever take in when eating cured meats or other nitrate-containing food products. Nonetheless, concern about the carcinogenic properties of nitrates has led to the introduction of meats that are nitrate-free or that contain reduced nitrate levels.

There is also concern about the possible harm caused by pesticide and herbicide residues. While some of these chemicals cause cancer at high doses in experimental animals, the very low concentrations found in some foods are well within government-established safety levels. Continued research regarding pesticide and herbicide use is essential for maximum food safety and the continuous monitoring of agricultural practices is necessary to ensure a safe food supply. Scientists and consumer groups stress the importance of a balance between chemical use and the production of quality food products.[48]

Policies protecting consumer health and ensuring the continued improvement in food production through development of alternative, low-chemical pest and herbicide control and reduced environmental pollution should be the goal of prevention efforts.

## Infectious Diseases and Cancer

According to recent estimates in 2005, 17 percent of new cancers worldwide will be attributable to infections.[49] Infections are thought to influence cancer development in several ways, most commonly through chronic inflammation, suppression of the immune system, or chronic stimulation.

## HBV, HCV, and Liver Cancer

Viruses such as hepatitis B (HBV) and C (HCV) are believed to stimulate cancer cells in the liver because they are chronic diseases that cause inflammation of liver tissue. This may prime the liver for cancer or make it more hospitable for cancer development. Global increases in HBV and HCV rates and concurrent increases in liver cancer rates provide evidence of such an association.

## HPV and Cervical Cancer

Nearly 100 percent of women with cervical cancer have evidence of human papilloma virus (HPV) infection, believed to be a major cause of cervical cancer. Fortunately, only a small percentage of HPV cases progress to cervical cancer.[50]

### WHAT WOULD YOU DO?

Given what you've read and heard about cancer, how much control do you think you have over your chance of developing it? What lifestyle changes do you need to make to reduce your risk of developing cancer? What will you do to make the necessary lifestyle changes?

## Medical Factors

Some medical treatment increases a person's risk for cancer. One famous example is the widespread use of the prescription drug *diethylstilbestrol (DES)* widely used from 1940 to 1960 to control problems with bleeding during pregnancy and to reduce the risk of miscarriage. It was not until the 1970s that the dangers of this drug became apparent. Although DES caused few side effects in the millions of women who took it, their daughters were found to have an increased risk for cancers of the reproductive organs. Another example is the use of estrogen replacement therapy among postmenopausal women because of the potential risk of increased uterine cancer. Ironically, chemotherapy, which is used to treat cancer, may also increase risk for other forms of cancer.

# TYPES OF CANCER

As noted previously, the term *cancer* refers to hundreds of different diseases. Four broad classifications are made according to the type of tissue from which the cancer arises.

- *Carcinomas*—Epithelial tissues (tissues covering body surfaces and lining most body cavities) are the most common sites for cancers. Carcinoma of the breast, lung, intestines, skin, and mouth are examples. These cancers affect the outer layer of the skin and mouth as well as the mucous membranes. They metastasize through the circulatory or lymphatic system initially and form solid tumours.

- *Sarcomas*—Sarcomas occur in the mesodermal, or middle, layers of tissue—for example, in bones, muscles, and general connective tissue. They metastasize primarily via the blood in the early stages of disease. These cancers are less common but generally more virulent than carcinomas. They also form solid tumours.

- *Lymphomas*—Lymphomas develop in the lymphatic system—the infection-fighting regions of the body—and metastasize through the lymph system. Hodgkin's disease is one type of lymphoma. Lymphomas also form solid tumours.

- *Leukemia*—Cancer of the blood-forming parts of the body, particularly the bone marrow and spleen, is called leukemia. A non-solid tumour, leukemia is characterized by an abnormal increase in the number of white blood cells.

The seriousness and general prognosis of a particular cancer are determined through careful diagnosis by trained oncologists. Once laboratory results and clinical observations have been made, cancers are rated by level and stage of development. Those diagnosed as "carcinoma in situ" are localized and are often curable. Cancers given higher level or stage ratings have spread farther and are less likely to be cured.

## Lung Cancer

Symptoms of lung cancer include a persistent cough, blood-streaked sputum, chest pain, and recurrent attacks of pneumonia or bronchitis. Treatment depends on the type and stage of the cancer. Surgery, radiation therapy, and chemotherapy are treatment options. If the cancer is localized, surgery is usually the treatment of choice. If the cancer has spread, surgery is used in combination with radiation and chemotherapy.

Despite advances in medical technology, survival rates for lung cancer have improved only slightly over the past decade. Just 13 percent of lung cancer patients live five or more years after diagnosis. These rates improve to 47 percent with early detection, but relatively few lung cancers are discovered in their early stages of development.[51]

### Prevention

Smokers, especially those who smoked for more than 20 years, and people exposed to certain industrial substances such as arsenic and asbestos or to radiation from occupational, medical, or environmental sources are at the highest risk for lung cancer. Exposure to secondhand cigarette smoke increases the risk for nonsmokers. Some researchers have theorized that as many as 90 percent of all lung cancers could be prevented if people did not smoke. Quitting smoking—or not starting—are the best measures you can take to prevent lung cancer. Any time is a good time to quit smoking, with health improvements noted almost immediately (see Chapter 11 for more details).

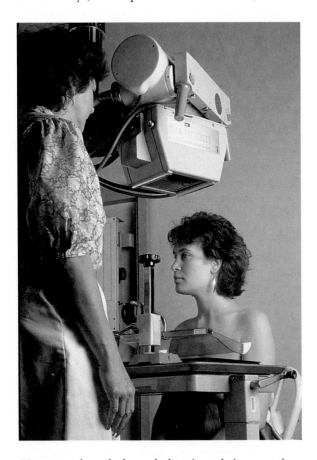

*Mammography and other early detection techniques greatly increase a woman's chance of surviving breast cancer.*

# Breast Cancer

About 1 out of 10 women will develop breast cancer at some time in her life. Although this oft-repeated ratio has frightened many women, it represents a woman's lifetime risk. Thus, not until the age of 80 does a woman's risk of breast cancer rise to 1 in 10.[52] Here are the risks at earlier ages:

- Age 50: 1 in 50
- Age 60: 1 in 24
- Age 70: 1 in 14

Breast cancer incidence among women rose steadily over the past three decades—although the rate of increase is declining somewhat—whereas mortality rates for breast cancer declined slightly since 1986 and particularly since 1990. This pattern of divergent trends is consistent with benefits being achieved through screening programs and improved treatments.[53]

Warning signals of breast cancer include persistent breast changes such as a lump, thickening, swelling, dimpling, skin irritation, distortion, retraction or scaliness of the nipple, nipple discharge, pain, or tenderness. Risk factors for breast cancer may vary considerably.[54] Typically, risk factors include being over the age of 40, having a primary relative (a mother, sister, or daughter) who had breast cancer, never having had children or never having breastfed, having your first child after age 30, early menarche, a late age of menopause, obesity after menopause, consuming two or more drinks of alcohol per day, and a higher education and socioeconomic status. Other potential risk factors include a dietary intake high in saturated fats; exposure to pesticides and other chemicals; weight gain, particularly after menopause; physical inactivity; and a genetic predisposition through BRCA1 and BRCA2 genes.[55]

Although risk factors are useful tools, they do not always adequately predict individual susceptibility. However, because of increased awareness, better diagnostic techniques, and improved treatments, breast cancer victims have a better chance of surviving today than in the past. A key factor in survival rests with individual recognition of early symptoms.[56]

### Prevention

A study of the role of physical activity in reducing the risk for breast cancer has generated excitement in the scientific community. In this study of 1,090 women 40 years or younger (545 with breast cancer, 545 without), exercise patterns were examined. The women who averaged four hours of exercise per week since menstruating had a 58 percent lower risk. Researchers speculated that exercise may protect women by altering

**How to Examine Your Breasts**

Do you know that 95% of breast cancers are discovered first by women themselves? And that the earlier the breast cancer is detected, the better the chance for a complete cure? Of course, most lumps or changes are not cancer. But you can safeguard your health by making a habit of examining your breasts once a month—a day or two after your period or, if you're no longer menstruating, on any given day. And if you notice anything changed or unusual—a lump, thickening, or discharge—contact your doctor right away.

**How to Look for Changes**

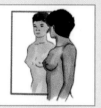

**Step 1**
Sit or stand in front of a mirror with your arms at your sides. Turning slowly from side to side, check your breasts for
• changes in size or shape
• puckering or dimpling of the skin
• changes in size or position of one nipple compared to the other

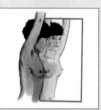

**Step 2**
Raise your arms above your head and repeat the examination in Step 1.

**Step 3**
Gently press each nipple with your fingertips to see if there is any discharge.

**How to Feel for Changes**

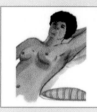

**Step 1**
Lie down and put a pillow or folded bath towel under your left shoulder. Then place your left hand under your head. (From now on you will be feeling for a lump or thickening in your breasts.)

**Step 2**
Imagine that your breast is divided into quarters.

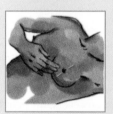

**Step 3**
With the fingers of your right hand held together, press firmly but gently, using small circular motions to feel the inner, upper quarter of your left breast. Start at your breastbone and work toward the nipple. Also examine the area around the nipple. Now do the same for the lower, inner portion of your breast.

**Step 4**
Next, bring your arm to your side and feel under your left armpit for swelling.

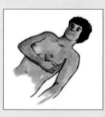

**Step 5**
With your arm still down, feel the upper, outer part of your breast, starting with your nipple and working outwards. Examine the lower, outer quarter in the same way.

**Step 6**
Now place the pillow under your right shoulder and repeat all the steps using your left hand to examine your right breast.

FIGURE 12.5

**The Illustration Demonstrates Breast Self-Examination— the Ten-Minute Habit that Could Save Your Life.**

the production of the ovarian hormones estrogen and progesterone during menstrual cycles.[57]

Regular self-examination (see Figure 12.5) and mammography offer the best hope for early detection of breast cancer. Although breast cancer screening with mammography and clinical breast exam could reduce mortality by nearly one-third in most women aged 50 to 69 if they were regularly screened, only 34 percent participate in organized screening in Canada.[58] All women, regardless of age, should be in the habit of breast self-examination every month. Despite the controversy over the cost-effectiveness and usefulness of a mammogram before the age of 40, many health professionals recommend that if you have any of the risk factors listed above, are prone to fibrous breasts, and are worried about your own condition, a mammogram may be warranted. Consult with your physician if you are in doubt, as it is generally best to be a proactive health consumer.

### Treatment

Today, people with breast cancer (similar to any other type of cancer) have many treatment options. Fortunately, there are services available to help you get the best information, even if you live in a fairly remote area of the country. The important thing to remember is that in most instances, taking the time to thoroughly check your physician's track record and his or her philosophy on the best treatment is always a good idea. Often, cancer support groups can give you invaluable information and advice. Treatments range from the simple lumpectomy to radical mastectomy to various combinations of radiation or chemotherapy. Figure 12.6 reviews these options. Remember that it is always a good idea to seek more than one opinion before making a decision.

### WHAT WOULD YOU DO?

Why do you think so few women get tested for breast cancer? Do you think men are better at seeking recommended screenings for cancers? Why or why not? Do you regularly (that is, monthly) examine your breasts for lumps? Why or why not?

## Colon and Rectum Cancers

Although colorectal cancers (that is, cancer of the colon and rectum) are the second leading cause of cancer deaths in men and women, many people are unaware of their potential risk. Bleeding from the rectum, blood in the stool, and changes in bowel habits are the major warning signals. People over the age of 40, with a family history of colorectal cancer, a personal or family history of polyps (benign growths) in the colon

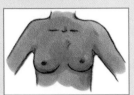

**Lumpectomy**
Performed when tumor is in earliest localized stages. Prognosis for recovery is better than 95 percent. Only tumor itself is removed. Some physicians may also remove normal tissue in surrounding area.

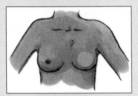

**Simple mastectomy**
Removal of breast and underlying tissue. Prognosis for full recovery better than 80 percent.

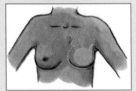

**Modified radical mastectomy**
Breast and lymph nodes in immediate area removed. Prognosis for full recovery dependent on level of spread.

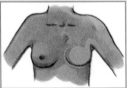

**Radical mastectomy**
Removal of breast, lymph nodes, pectoral muscles, all fat and underlying tissue. Prognosis for recovery may be as low as 60 percent dependent on level of spread.

FIGURE 12.6

The Illustration Depicts Selected Surgical Procedures for Diagnosed Breast Cancer. These Surgeries are Typically Followed By Radiation Treatment and/or Chemotherapy.

colostomy, the creation of an abdominal opening for the elimination of body wastes, is seldom required for people with colon cancer and even less frequently for those with rectum cancer.[60]

## Prostate Cancer

Cancer of the prostate continues to be the most frequently occurring cancer for men. It is the third leading cause of cancer deaths in males. In 2006, it is estimated that 20,700 Canadian men will be diagnosed with prostate cancer and about 4,200 will die of the disease.[61] Beginning in 1994, incidence rates for prostate cancer began to decline after increasing rapidly for several years. It was noted in 2006 that mortality rates due to prostate cancer are declining.[62]

Most signs and symptoms of prostate cancer are nonspecific—that is, they mimic the signs of infection or enlarged prostate. Symptoms include weak or interrupted urine flow or difficulty starting or stopping the urine flow; the need to urinate frequently; pain or difficulty in urinating; blood in the urine; and pain in the lower back, pelvis, or upper thighs. Many males mistake these symptoms for other nonspecific conditions, such as infections, and delay treatment.

Fortunately, even with so many generalized symptoms, most prostate cancers are detected while they are still localized and tend to progress slowly. Prostate patients have an average five-year survival rate of 80 percent. Because the incidence of prostate cancer increases with age, every man over the age of 40 should have an annual prostate examination.[63]

## Skin Cancer

Skin cancer may be one of the most underrated of all cancers, particularly among young people. Although it is true that most people do not die of the common, highly curable *basal* or *squamous cell* skin cancers, many people do not know that another, highly virulent form of skin cancer known as **malignant melanoma** has become a major killer of young women. Rates for men over 50 are

or rectum, or inflammatory bowel problems such as colitis run an increased risk. Further, a dietary intake high in fats or low in fibre may also increase risk.[59]

Because colorectal cancer tends to spread slowly, the prognosis is quite good if it is caught in the early stages. Treatment often consists of radiation or surgery. Chemotherapy, although not used extensively in the past, is a possibility today. A permanent

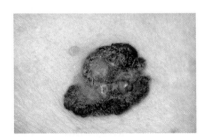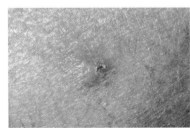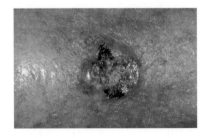

*Prevention of skin cancer includes keeping a careful watch for any new pigmented growths and for changes to any moles. Melanoma symptoms, as shown in the left photo, include scalloped edges, asymmetrical shapes, discolouration, and an increase in size. Basal cell carcinoma and squamous cell carcinoma (middle and right photos) should be brought to your physician's attention but are not as deadly as melanoma.*

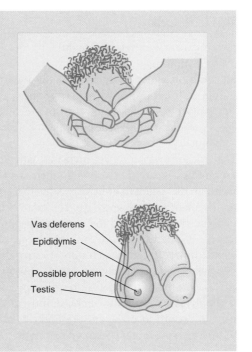

Follow the instructions in the diagram carefully and examine your testes immediately after your next hot bath or shower. Heat causes the testicles to descend and the scrotal skin to relax, making it easier to find unusual lumps.

Examine each testicle by placing the index and middle fingers of both hands on the underside of the testicle and the thumbs on the top. Gently roll the testicle between your thumb and fingers, feeling for small lumps.

Changes or anything abnormal will appear at the front or side of your testicle. Did you find any unusual lumps? Are there any unusual signs of any kind? Are there any markings or lumps at any site?

Keep in mind that not all lumps are a sign of testicular cancer. Unusual lumps at any location, however, should be checked by a physician. Early detection greatly increases your chances of a complete cure. Repeat the examination every month and record your findings.

Vas deferens
Epididymis
Possible problem
Testis

**FIGURE 12.7**
Testicular Self-Exam

also increasing. Yet many people still bask unprotected on beaches, apparently not making the connection between death from melanoma and sunlight overexposure. The perception that health and a well-tanned body go together couldn't be further from the truth.

### Symptoms

Many people do not have any idea what to look for when considering skin cancer. Any unusual skin condition, especially a change in the size or colour of a mole or other darkly pigmented growth or spot, should be considered suspect. Scaliness, oozing, bleeding, the appearance of a bump or nodule, the spread of pigment beyond the border, change in sensation, itchiness, tenderness, and pain are all warning signs of the basal and squamous cell skin cancers. However, melanoma symptoms are slightly different. Often there is a sudden or progressive change in a mole's appearance from a small, mole-like growth to a large, ulcerated, and easily-prone-to-bleeding growth. A simple ABCD rule outlines the warning signals of melanoma:

- **A** is for *asymmetry*. One half of the mole does not match the other half.

- **B** is for *border irregularity*. The edges are ragged, notched, or blurred.

- **C** is for *colour*. The pigmentation is not uniform.

- **D** is for *diameter* greater than 6 millimetres.

Any or all of these symptoms should cause you to visit a physician.[64]

## Testicular Cancer

Testicular cancer is currently one of the most common types of solid tumours found in males entering early adulthood. Those between the ages of 17 and 34 are at greatest risk. There has been a steady increase in tumour frequency over the past several years in this age group. It is estimated that 830 new cases of testicular cancer will be diagnosed in 2006 and 30 men will die as a result of testicular cancer.[65]

Although the exact cause of testicular cancer is unknown, several possible risk factors have been identified. Males with undescended testicles appear to be at greatest risk for the disease. In addition, some studies indicate that there may be a genetic influence. In general, testicular tumours are first noticed as a painless enlargement of the testis or as an apparent thickening in testicular tissue. Because this enlargement is often painless, it is extremely important that all young males practise regular testicular self-examination (see Figure 12.7). If a suspicious lump or thickening is found, medical follow-up should be sought immediately.

**Malignant melanoma:** A virulent cancer of the melanin (pigment-producing portion) of the skin.

## Ovarian Cancer

Ovarian cancer is often silent, showing no obvious signs or symptoms until late in its development. The most common sign is enlargement of the abdomen (or a feeling of bloating) in women over the age of 40. Other symptoms include vague digestive disturbances, such as gas and stomachaches that persist and cannot be explained.[66]

The risk for ovarian cancer increases with age, with the highest rates found in women in their 60s. Women who never had children are twice as likely to develop ovarian cancer as those who have. The main risk factor appears to be exposure to the reproductive hormone estrogen. Women who have multiple pregnancies or use oral contraceptives, which inhibit estrogen, are at lower risk. In addition, having one or more primary relatives (mother, sisters, grandmothers) who have had the disease appears to increase individual risk. With the exception of Japan, the highest incidence rates are reported in industrialized countries.[67]

### Prevention

One study indicated that dietary intake may play a role in ovarian cancer.[68] Researchers found that when comparing 450 Canadian women with newly diagnosed ovarian cancer with 564 demographically similar, healthy women, the women without ovarian cancer had a dietary intake lower in saturated fat. Such results, particularly when combined with cardiovascular risks and other health risks, may provide yet another reason to reduce your overall intake of saturated fats.

The best way to protect yourself is with annual, thorough pelvic examinations. **Pap tests,** although useful in detecting cervical cancer, do not reveal ovarian cancer. Women over the age of 40 should have a cancer-related checkup every year. If you have any of the symptoms of ovarian cancer and they persist, see your doctor. If they continue to persist, get a second opinion.[69]

## Uterine Cancer

Most cervical and endometrial (that is, uterine) cancers develop in the body of the uterus, usually in the endometrium (lining). The rest develop in the cervix, located at the base of the uterus. The overall incidence of early-stage uterine cancer—that is, cervical cancer—has decreased 50 percent since 1977, although it is estimated that 1,350 new cases will still be diagnosed in 2006.[70] Further, invasive, later-stage forms of the disease appear to be decreasing, and mortality rates from cervical cancer have declined by 60 percent since 1977. Much of this apparent trend may be due to more effective regular screenings of younger women using the Pap test, a procedure in which cells taken from the cervical region are examined for abnormal cellular activity. Although these tests are very effective for detecting early-stage cervical cancer, they are less effective for detecting cancers of the uterine lining and are not at all effective for detecting cancers of the fallopian tubes or ovaries.[71]

Risk factors for cervical cancer include early age of first intercourse, multiple sex partners, cigarette smoking, and certain sexually transmitted infections, such as the herpes virus and the human papilloma virus (the cause of genital warts). For endometrial cancer, a history of infertility, failure to ovulate, obesity, and treatment with tamoxifen or unopposed estrogen therapy appear to be major risk factors.[72] Early warning signs of uterine cancer include bleeding outside the normal menstrual period or after menopause or persistent unusual vaginal discharge. These symptoms should be checked by a physician immediately.[73]

## Leukemia

Leukemia is a cancer of the blood-forming tissues that leads to proliferation of millions of immature white blood cells. These abnormal cells crowd out normal white blood cells (which fight infection), platelets (which control hemorrhaging), and red blood cells (which prevent anemia). As a result, symptoms such as fatigue, paleness, weight loss, easy bruising, repeated infections, nosebleeds, and other forms of hemorrhaging occur. In children, these symptoms can appear suddenly.[74]

Leukemia can be acute or chronic in nature and can strike both sexes and all age groups. Chronic leukemia can develop over several months and have few symptoms. Although many people believe that leukemia is a childhood disease, leukemia strikes many more adults than children.[75] Over the last 30 years, there has been a dramatic improvement in survival of patients with acute lymphocytic leukemia.

## Oral Cancer

Cancer may develop in any part of the oral cavity. Most often it is found on the lips, the lining of the cheeks, the gums, and the floor of the mouth. The tongue, the pharynx, and the tonsils are other common sites. Tobacco use—smoking, chewing, or dipping—is the most common risk factor for oral cancer.

### WHAT WOULD YOU DO?

What types of cancers do you think you and your friends are at greatest risk for right now? What part(s) of your lifestyle put you most at risk? What are you willing to change?

# FACING CANCER

As previously mentioned 44 percent of men and 38 percent of women are likely to develop cancer in their lifetime, with approximately one in four Canadians dying as a result. Many factors have contributed to the rise in cancer mortality—one being simply longer life expectancies—but the increase in the incidence of lung cancer is probably the most important reason. However, recent advances in the diagnosis and treatment have reduced much of the fear and mystery that once surrounded cancer.

## Detecting Cancer

The earlier a person is diagnosed as having cancer, the better the prospect for survival. Various high-tech diagnostic techniques exist to detect cancer. New high-technology diagnostic imaging techniques have replaced exploratory surgery for some cancer patients. **Magnetic resonance imaging (MRI)** is one example of such technology. In MRI, a huge electromagnet is used to detect hidden tumours by mapping the vibrations of the various atoms in the body on a computer screen. **Computerized axial tomography scanning (CAT scan)** uses X-rays to examine parts of the body. In both of these painless, noninvasive procedures, cross-section pictures can show a tumour's shape and location more accurately than can conventional X-rays.

*Prostatic ultrasound* (a rectal probe using ultrasonic waves to produce an image of the prostate) is currently being investigated as a potential means to increase the early detection of prostate cancer. Recently, prostatic ultrasound has been combined with a blood test for **prostate-specific antigen (PSA),** an antigen found in prostate cancer patients. Although the reliability of the PSA test for screening has been questioned, it appears to show promise.

These medical techniques, along with regular self-examinations and checkups, play an important role in the early detection and secondary prevention of cancer. Familiarize yourself with the Seven Warning Signals of cancer, as shown in Figure 12.8. If you notice any of these signals, and they don't appear to be related to anything else, you should see a doctor immediately. Make sure that appropriate diagnostic tests are completed whenever any warning signals appear. Also make a realistic assessment of your individual risk factors and try to avoid those you have some control over.

## New Hope in Cancer Treatments

Although cancer treatments have changed dramatically over the last 25 years, surgery, in which the tumour and surrounding tissue are removed, is still

## Cancer's Seven Warning Signals

1 Changes in bowel or bladder habits.
2 A sore that does not heal.
3 Unusual bleeding or discharge.
4 Thickening or lump in breast or elsewhere.
5 Indigestion or difficulty in swallowing.
6 Obvious change in a wart or mole.
7 Nagging cough or hoarseness.

**If you have a warning signal, see your doctor.**

FIGURE 12.8
**Cancer's Seven Warning Signals**

common. Today's surgeons tend to remove less surrounding tissue than previously and to combine surgery with either **radiotherapy** (the use of radiation) or **chemotherapy** (the use of drugs) to kill cancerous cells.

Radiation works by destroying malignant cells or stopping cell growth. It is most effective in treating localized cancer masses. Unfortunately, in the process of destroying malignant cells, radiotherapy also destroys healthy cells. When cancer has spread throughout the body, it is necessary to use some form of chemotherapy. Similar to radiation therapy, chemotherapy attacks and kills healthy and cancerous cells. Ongoing research will result in new, less toxic drugs for normal cells that remain potent against tumour cells.

**Pap test:** A procedure in which cells taken from the cervical region are examined for abnormal cellular activity.

**Magnetic resonance imaging (MRI):** A device that uses magnetic fields, radio waves, and computers to generate an image of internal tissues of the body for diagnostic purposes without the use of radiation.

**Computerized axial tomography (CAT scan):** A machine that uses radiation to view internal organs not normally visible on X-rays.

**Prostate-specific antigen (PSA):** An antigen found in prostate cancer patients.

**Radiotherapy:** The use of radiation to kill cancerous cells.

**Chemotherapy:** The use of drugs to kill cancerous cells.

# Talking with Your Doctor about Cancer

Anytime there is the suspicion of cancer, the person involved is likely to react with great anxiety, fear, and anger. Emotional distress is sometimes so intense that the person involved is unable to serve as his or her own best advocate in making critical healthcare decisions. If you find it difficult to know what to ask your doctor in a routine exam, imagine how hard it would be to discuss life or death options for yourself or a loved one. Having a list of important questions to ask when you appear at the doctor's office may help tremendously. Remember, your healthcare provider should be your partner in making the best decisions for you. Actively challenging, questioning, and letting the physician know your wishes can make difficult decisions easier.

**If the diagnosis is cancer, you may want to ask these questions:**

- What kind of cancer do I have? What stage is it in? Based on my age and stage, what is my prognosis?

- What are my treatment choices? Which do you recommend? Why?

- What are the expected benefits of each kind of treatment?

- What are the long- and short-term risks and possible side effects?

- Would a clinical trial be appropriate for me? (Clinical trials are research studies designed to answer specific questions and to find better ways to prevent or treat cancer. Often new cancer-fighting treatments are used.)

**If surgery is recommended, you may want to ask these questions:**

- What kind of operation will it be and how long will it take? What form of anesthesia will be used? How many similar procedures has this surgeon done in the last month? What is his or her success rate?

- How will I feel after surgery? If I have pain, how will you help me?

- Where will the scars be? What will they look like? Will they cause disability?

- Will I have any activity limitations after surgery? What kind of physical therapy, if any, will I have? When will I get back to normal activities?

**If radiation is recommended, you may want to ask these questions:**

- Why do you think this treatment is better than my other options?

- How long will I need to have treatments and what will the side effects be in the short and long term? What body organs/systems may be damaged?

- What can I do to take care of myself during therapy? Are there services available to help me?

- What is the long-term prognosis for people my age with my type of cancer using this treatment?

**If chemotherapy is recommended, you may want to ask these questions:**

- Why do you think this treatment is better than my other options?

- Which drug combinations pose the least risks and most benefits?

- What are the short- and long-term side effects on my body?

- What are my options?

Before beginning any form of cancer therapy, it is imperative that you be a vigilant and vocal consumer. Read and seek information from cancer support groups. Check the skills of your surgeon, your radiation therapist, and your doctor in terms of clinical work and interpersonal interactions. The time spent asking these questions and seeking information is well worth the effort.

---

Whether used alone or in combination, radiotherapy and chemotherapy have possible side effects, including extreme nausea, nutritional deficiencies, hair loss, and general fatigue. Long-term damage to the cardiovascular system and many other systems of the body can be significant. It is important that you discuss these matters fully with your doctors. The Building Communication Skills box offers advice on how to talk to your doctor about cancer.

**Immunotherapy:** A process that stimulates the body's immune system to combat cancer cells.

## Gilda's Club: A Support Community for Thousands Living with Cancer

Gilda's Club is named in honour of the late comedian Gilda Radner, who, when describing the emotional and social support she received when she had cancer, called for such places of participation, education, hope, and friendship to be made available for people with cancer and their families and friends everywhere.

### WHAT IS GILDA'S CLUB?

A free, non-residential, emotional and social support community for men, women, and children living with cancer. It includes not only people affected with cancer, but their families, caregivers, significant others and friends—because cancer affects everyone, not only the person with the physical disease. Unlike a social service agency, Gilda's Club is a community centre that is driven by its membership. It is open to all, without referral and at no cost. Funding is solicited from private individuals, corporations, and foundations.

### THE UNIQUE VISION OF GILDA'S CLUB

Gilda's Club provides a meeting place where people with cancer can come together to learn how to live with cancer and celebrate the challenges and opportunities of everyday life. Our philosophy is premised on the belief that people gather strength and knowledge from support groups and social interaction in a cancer support community.

The first Gilda's Club, including a worldwide training centre, opened its signature red door in New York City in 1995. Many affiliates are open or under development in different parts of the world. Canada has one in Toronto and one in Montreal. Since 1995, thousands of members now attest to the fact that Gilda's Club has helped change their lives by restoring control and enabling them to plan their own emotional and social support, thus strengthening and enriching the entire family.

Source: www.gildasclubtoronto.org.

Other promising advances in the battle against cancer include the following:[76]

- A large clinical trial that is underway to evaluate the usefulness of an estrogen-blocking drug called tamoxifen to treat women with some forms of breast cancer.
- **Immunotherapy,** a new technique designed to enhance the body's own disease fighting systems to help control cancer.
- A powerful *enzyme inhibitor,* TIMP-2, which is showing promise for slowing the metastasis of tumour cells. A metastasis suppressor gene, NM23, has also been identified.
- *Neoadjuvant chemotherapy* (giving chemotherapy to shrink the cancer and then removing it surgically), which has been tried against various types of cancers, is a promising new treatment approach.

In addition, psychosocial and behavioural research has become increasingly important as health professionals seek the answers to questions concerning complex lifestyle factors that appear to influence risks for cancer as well as the survivability of patients with particular psychological and mental health profiles. Also, healthcare practitioners have become more aware of the psychological needs of patients and families and have begun to tailor treatment programs to meet the diverse needs of different people.

## Life after Cancer

Heightened public awareness and an improved prognosis for cancer victims have made the cancer experience less threatening and isolating than it once was. Assistance for individuals with cancer is more readily available than ever before. Cancer support groups, cancer information workshops, and low-cost medical consultation are just a few of the forms of assistance now offered in many communities. Increasing efforts in cancer research, improvements in diagnostic equipment, and advances in treatment provide hope for the future.

# Managing Your Health

Although it is easy to read through a chapter like this and learn what we should be doing to keep ourselves healthy, few of us ever really think about what it takes to prevent serious illness. Relationships, financial worries, grades, time for fun, and other issues often take precedence over our long-term commitments to wellness.

## MAKING DECISIONS FOR YOU

List the five things that matter to you most right now. Is appearance part of your list? Is being able to get through a day without feeling tired or unusually fatigued important? Are you motivated to change your health behaviours and take action to reduce your circulatory disease and cancer risks by engaging in more physical activity, reducing stress, and eating properly? Was there anything about this chapter that helped you become more concerned about making a change now? Why is this important? What actions do you plan to take?

## CHECKLIST FOR CHANGE: MAKING PERSONAL CHOICES

- Determine your hereditary risks. If they are high, outline the steps that you can take to reduce your overall risk.
- Know about the normal cardiovascular disease risk changes that occur with age. Take the extra steps needed to minimize your risks as you age.
- If you smoke, quit. If you don't smoke, don't start.
- If you chew, dip, or use snuff, quit. If you don't, don't start.
- Find out what your cholesterol level is, including HDL and LDL levels.
- Reduce saturated fat in your diet and take steps to reduce your triglyceride and cholesterol levels.
- Get out and do some physical activity. Even a relaxing walk every day is a good risk reducer. Nobody says you have to run until you drop. Take it easy, but keep it up.
- Control your blood pressure. Monitor it regularly and see your doctor if you have high blood pressure.
- Lose weight if you are overweight. Obesity is a significant risk factor for cardiovascular disease and cancer.
- Manage your stress.
- Avoid excessive sunlight. When in the sun, wear sunscreen that is at least SPF 15.
- Avoid excessive alcohol consumption.
- Properly monitor estrogen use. While estrogen therapy may lower women's risk for heart disease and osteoporosis, it should not be undertaken without careful consideration of a woman's personal risk profile.
- Avoid occupational exposures to carcinogens. Exposure to several different industrial agents (nickel, chromate, asbestos, vinyl chloride, and so on) increases risk for various cancers.
- Eat your fruits and vegetables. Eat at least five servings of fruits and vegetables every day to reduce your risk for lung, colon, pancreatic, stomach, bladder, esophageal, mouth, and throat cancer.
- Be happy; take care of your spiritual self.

## CHECKLIST FOR CHANGE: MAKING COMMUNITY CHOICES

- Take a class in CPR. Your local Red Cross likely offers them; courses may be available on campus. Be prepared to offer bystander CPR.
- Consider becoming an emergency medical technician (EMT). You don't have to make a career of it. But you could be prepared to save people in your dorm, your office building, and your community.
- Does your community have any major sources of carcinogens (toxic waste dumps, chemical factories, and so on)? What precautions are taken to ensure that any environmental risks are reduced?
- Does the Canadian Cancer Society have a local office at which you could volunteer some time?
- Does your community have cancer support groups that you could join if you were found to have cancer? Where would you find out about such support groups?

## CRITICAL THINKING

You've been good friends with one of your 30-something neighbours for some time. Recently, after spending a good deal of time working on a community project together, you start to date. After a few terrific dates, during which you really hit it off socially, you find out that your friend had cancer two years ago, and that there is a 50-percent chance the cancer will return within five years. You truly love this person, but wonder what to do. If you commit yourself to this relationship and the cancer returns, then what? You've always wanted to have children, but are concerned about what would happen if your partner died of cancer while the kids were young. On the other hand, there is a 50-percent chance that the cancer will not return.

Using the DECIDE model described in Chapter 1, decide whether or not you would continue the relationship. Does it make any difference to you whether the cancer survivor described is male or female? Explain why.

# SUMMARY

- The cardiovascular system consists of the heart and circulatory system and is a carefully regulated, integrated network of vessels that supplies the body with the nutrients and oxygen necessary to perform daily functions.

- Cardiovascular diseases combine to be the leading cause of death in Canada today.

- Risk factors for cardiovascular disease include cigarette smoking, high blood fat and cholesterol levels, high blood pressure, inactivity, high-fat and low fibre dietary intake, obesity, diabetes, and emotional stress. Some factors, such as age, sex, and heredity, are risk factors that are not under your control. Many of these factors have a compounded effect when combined.

- Women have a unique challenge in controlling their risk for cardiovascular diseases, particularly after menopause, when estrogen levels are no longer sufficient to be protective.

- Methods developed for treating heart blockages include coronary bypass surgery and angioplasty.

- Cancer is a group of diseases characterized by uncontrolled growth and spread of abnormal cells.

- Early diagnosis of cancer affects your survival rate. Self-exams for breast, testicular, and skin cancer and knowledge of the Seven Warning Signals of cancer aid early diagnosis.

- New types of cancer treatments include various combinations of radiotherapy, chemotherapy, and immunotherapy.

- Various lifestyle behaviours such as eating well, obtaining regular physical activity, managing your stress, getting adequate sleep, and so on may help to prevent heart disease and cancer.

# DISCUSSION QUESTIONS

1. List the different types of cardiovascular diseases. Compare and contrast their symptoms, risk factors, prevention, and treatment.

2. What are the major indicators that cardiovascular disease poses a particularly significant risk to people your age? To the elderly? To people from particular racial or ethnic groups?

3. Discuss the role that physical activity, stress management, dietary changes, checkups, sodium reduction, and other factors can play in reducing your risk for cardiovascular disease.

4. Discuss why age is such an important factor in women's risk for cardiovascular diseases. What can be done to lower women's risks in later life?

5. Describe some of the diagnostic and treatment alternatives for cardiovascular diseases. If you had a heart attack today, which treatment would you prefer? Explain why.

6. What is the difference between a benign and a malignant tumour?

7. List the likely causes of cancer. Do any of these causes put you at greater risk? What can you do to reduce this risk?

8. What are the symptoms of lung, breast, prostate, colorectal, and testicular cancer? What can you do to increase your chances of surviving these cancers?

9. What could signal that you have cancer instead of a minor illness? How soon should you seek treatment for any of the seven warning signs?

# APPLICATION EXERCISE

Reread the What Do You Think? scenario at the beginning of the chapter and answer the following questions.

1. Consider Kassandra's case in the chapter opener. Why do you think so many young Canadians deny their risk for skin cancer?

2. As a friend of Kassandra's, what advice might you give?

3. Think about close friends or people in your family who also are at risk of developing skin cancer or other forms of cancer. What could you do to help them become aware of their risks without preaching to them about their lifestyle choices and turning them off?

4. What kinds of community efforts are needed to change the perceptions that a "healthy glow" results from suntanning?

# HEALTH ON THE NET

Canadian Cancer Society
**www.cancer.ca**

National Cancer Institute of Canada
**www.ncic.cancer.ca**

Heart and Stroke Foundation of Canada
**www.heartandstroke.ca**

World Health Organization
**www.who.org**

# CHAPTER 13

# INFECTIOUS AND NONINFECTIOUS CONDITIONS

*Risks and Responsibilities*

## CHAPTER OBJECTIVES

- Identify the risk factors for infectious diseases, including those you can and cannot control.

- Describe the most common pathogens.

- Summarize the immune system and explain the role of vaccinations in fighting disease.

- Discuss the various sexually transmitted infections, their means of transmission, and actions that prevent the spread of STIs.

- Explain the transmission, symptoms, treatment, and prevention of HIV.

- Identify common respiratory disorders.

- Explain the common neurological disorders, including the varied types of headaches and seizure disorders.

- Identify the common sex disorders, risk factors for these conditions, their symptoms, and methods of their control or prevention.

- Summarize diseases of the digestive system, including their symptoms, prevention, and control.

- Describe the varied musculoskeletal diseases and their effects on the body.

Every moment of every day you are in contact with microscopic organisms that have the ability to make you sick. These disease-causing agents, or **pathogens,** are found in the air you breathe, in the foods you eat, and on nearly every person or object that you come into contact with. Most deaths from infectious diseases—almost 90 percent—are caused by only a handful of diseases. And most of these diseases have plagued humankind throughout history, often ravaging populations more effectively than wars.[1] There is fossil evidence that infections, cancer, heart disease, and a host of other ailments afflicted the earliest human beings. At times, infectious diseases wiped out whole groups of people through **epidemics** such as the Black Death or bubonic plague, which killed up to one-third of the population of Europe in the 1300s. A pandemic, or global epidemic, of influenza killed more than 20 million people in 1918, while strains of tuberculosis and cholera continue to cause premature death throughout the world.

In spite of our best efforts to eradicate them, these diseases continue to be a menace. The news isn't all bad; even though we are bombarded by potential pathogenic threats, our immune systems are remarkably adept at protecting us. *Endogenous microorganisms* are those that live in peaceful coexistence with their human host most of the time. For people in good health, and whose immune systems are functioning well, endogenous organisms are usually harmless; but, in sick people or those with a compromised immune system, these normally harmless pathogenic organisms can cause serious health problems.

*Exogenous microorganisms* are organisms that do not normally inhabit the body. When they do, however, they are apt to produce an infection or illness. The more easily these pathogens can gain a foothold in the body and sustain themselves, the more **virulent** or

aggressive the organism, the higher the probability that it will overcome your body defences and cause disease. However, if your immune system is strong and your internal capacity to ward off disease is substantial, you should be able to fight even the most virulent attacker. Just because you inhale a flu virus does not mean that you will get the flu. Just because your hands are teeming with bacteria does not mean that you will get a bacterial disease. Several factors influence your susceptibility to these diseases.

Infectious diseases in Canada are controlled through ongoing vigilance by public health networks operating at local, regional, provincial, and national levels. Clean food and water, immunizations, and an excellent health-care system have maintained Canadians' health. Good nutrition and engaging in a physically active lifestyle are factors in overall good health. Nutritional status has been found to have an effect on resistance to infectious diseases in certain population groups such as infants, young children, and the elderly. Nutritional status can also affect the course of an infectious disease, as has been shown with individuals who are HIV-positive.[2] Regular physical activity of moderate intensity is also thought to boost the immune system functioning.

# INFECTIOUS DISEASE RISK FACTORS

At one time, it was believed that most diseases were caused by a single factor, but today we recognize that most diseases are **multifactorial,** or caused by the interaction of several factors from inside and outside the person. For a disease to occur, the *host* must be *susceptible,* meaning that the immune system must be in a weakened condition; an *agent* capable of transmitting a disease must be present; and the *environment* must be hospitable to the pathogen in terms of temperature, light, moisture, and other requirements. Other factors also increase or decrease levels of susceptibility.

## Risk Factors You Can't Control

Uncontrollable risk factors are those that increase your susceptibility to a disease and that you may have little or no control over. Some of the most common factors are examined below.

### Heredity

Perhaps the single greatest factor influencing your longevity is your parents' longevity. Being born into a family in which heart disease, cancer, or other illnesses are prevalent increases your risk. Some people with a close relative who has diabetes develop diabetes themselves even though they take precautions, manage their weight, and engage in regular physical activity. Still other diseases are a result of chromosomal inheritance. **Sickle cell anemia,** an inherited blood disease that primarily affects individuals of African descent, is often transmitted to the fetus when both parents carry the sickle cell trait. It remains unclear, though, whether heredity diseases are a result of inherited chromosomal abnormalities or inherited deficiencies in immune system functioning.

### Aging

After the age of 40 we become more vulnerable to many chronic diseases. Moreover, as we age, our immune systems respond less efficiently to invading organisms, increasing our risk for infection and illness. The same flu that produces an afternoon of nausea and diarrhea in a younger person may cause days of illness or even death in an older person. The very young are also at risk for many diseases, particularly if they are not vaccinated against them.

### Environmental Conditions

Unsanitary conditions and the presence of drugs, chemicals, and hazardous pollutants and wastes in our food and water probably have a great effect on our immune systems. That **immunological competence**—the body's ability to defend itself against pathogens—is weakened in such situations has been well documented.[3]

---

#### WHAT WOULD YOU DO?

Examine the risk factors you can and cannot control. How great is your risk of contracting an infection from some form of invading pathogen? Outline a strategy that may help you improve your ability to ward off infectious agents.

---

## Risk Factors You Can Control

On a positive note, we have some degree of personal control over many risk factors for disease. Too much stress, an inadequate dietary intake, inactivity, lack of sleep, misuse or abuse of legal and illegal drugs, poor personal hygiene, high-risk behaviours, and other variables significantly increase the risk for a number of diseases. Factors we can control—at least partly—through lifestyle choices include vigour of immune response; pre-existing level of immunity; pre-existing

disease; use of substances such as cigarettes, chew, dip, alcohol, and drugs; and psychological factors such as stress, depression, and anxiety.[4]

# THE PATHOGENS: ROUTES OF INVASION

Pathogens enter the body in several ways. They may be transmitted by direct contact between infected persons, such as during sexual relations, kissing, or touching, or by indirect contact, such as by touching an object the infected person has had contact with. The hands are probably the greatest source of transmission. You may also **autoinoculate** yourself, or transmit a pathogen from one part of your body to another. For example, you may touch a sore on your lip teeming with viral herpes and then transmit the virus to your eye when you scratch your itchy eyelid.

Pathogens are also transmitted by *airborne contact,* either through inhaling the droplet spray from a sneeze or through breathing in air that carries a particular pathogen. You may become the victim of *food-borne* infection if you eat something contaminated by microorganisms. The *E. coli* bacteria and other virulent pathogens are responsible for a variety of emerging diseases that pose significant threats to humans. Examples of these are found in Table 13.1.

Your "best friend" may be the source of *animal-borne pathogens.* Dogs—as well as cats, livestock, and wild animals—can spread numerous diseases through their bites or feces or by carrying infected insects into your living areas. For example, ticks in some regions carry Lyme disease. *Water-borne* diseases are transmitted directly from drinking water and indirectly from foods washed or sprayed with water containing their pathogens. These pathogens can also invade your body if you wade or swim in contaminated streams, lakes, rivers, and reservoirs.

---

**Pathogen:** A disease-causing agent.

**Epidemic:** Disease outbreak that affects many people in a community or region at the same time.

**Virulent:** Strong enough to overcome host resistance and cause disease.

**Multifactorial disease:** Disease caused by interactions of several factors.

**Sickle cell anemia:** Genetic disease commonly found among individuals of African descent; results in organ damage and premature death.

**Immunological competence:** Ability of the immune system to defend the body from pathogens.

**Autoinoculation:** Transmission of a pathogen from one part of your body to another.

---

TABLE 13.1

## Emerging Diseases: Challenges to Public Health

Over the past few decades more than 30 diseases have been identified in humans for the first time. More than two-thirds of these diseases are known to have originated from animals—wild and domestic species

| Disease/Cause Agent | Description |
|---|---|
| Avian influenza [Type A (H5N1)] | Thought to infect only birds (to whom it can be deadly), avian influenza first jumped to humans in 1997 in Hong Kong. Initial symptoms include fever, cough, and chills; most influenza infections cause only self-limited illness that does not require hospitalization. Symptoms after infection with the H5N1 strain can be severe in all age groups. |
| Ebola virus | A deadly disease concentrated in portions of Africa. Ebola can be transferred only by direct contact with infected blood, organs, secretions, semen, or contaminated needles. Transmission is enhanced by unsanitary, overcrowded conditions and poor preventive practices. No treatment or vaccine is available and 50 to 90 percent of those contracting the disease die. |
| Dengue | More than 200,000 cases in Latin America alone during 1994, of which 5,000 were dengue hemorrhagic fever (DHF), a severe form of the disease that causes high mortality. The type of mosquito that carries the disease is establishing new habitats in the Americas and parts of Africa and Asia. Over the past 40 or so years the number of cases has increased at least 20-fold. |
| *E. coli* bacteria | Illness caused by ingesting undercooked meats tainted by *Escherichia coli* bacteria. |
| Flesh-eating strep | A rare disease caused by a strain of Group A Strep bacterium that produces materials that dissolve tissue. Early diagnosis and treatment with antibiotics stops the disease. |
| Cholera | A bacterial disease affecting the intestinal tract of individuals who eat or drink food or water contaminated by fecal waste of an infected person. In 1992, a new strain of cholera was detected in the Bay of Bengal and spread to 10 other countries. |
| Tuberculosis | A pulmonary disease once thought to be almost eliminated from North America. Depressed social conditions and improper use of antibiotics have revived this airborne disease, which is particularly threatening to people with weakened immune systems. Strict adherence to drug therapy for several months can cure the disease. |
| West Nile virus | A flavivirus commonly found in Africa, West Asia, and the Middle East that can infect mosquitoes, birds, horses, humans, and some other mammals. Increasingly common in North America, most people experience only a mild case, characterized by flu-like symptoms that last for a few days. However, more extreme forms of this disease can cause encephalitis (inflammation of the brain) and meningitis (inflammation of the membrane around the brain and spinal cord), which could prove to be fatal. |

## WHAT WOULD YOU DO?

What are the most common pathogens you are currently exposed to? How can you best protect yourself against them?

Although there are several thousand species of bacteria, only approximately 100 cause diseases in humans. In many cases, it is not the bacteria themselves that cause disease but rather the poisonous substances, called **toxins,** that they produce. Some of these toxins are extremely powerful. Bacterial infections can take many forms. The following are the most common.

## Bacteria

**Bacteria** are single-celled organisms that are plantlike in nature but lack chlorophyll (the pigment that gives plants their green colouring). There are three major types of bacteria: *cocci, bacilli,* and *spirilla.* Bacteria may be viewed under a standard light microscope.

### Staphylococcal Infections

One of the most common forms of bacterial infection is the staph infection. **Staphylococci** are normally present on our skin at all times and seldom cause problems. But when there is a cut or break in the **epidermis,** or outer layer of the skin, staphylococci may enter and cause a localized infection. If you have ever suffered from acne, boils, styes (infections of the eyelids), or infected cuts, you have probably had a staph infection.

At least one staph-caused disorder, **toxic shock syndrome,** is potentially fatal. Media reports in the early 1980s indicated that this disorder was exclusive to menstruating women, particularly those who used high-absorbency tampons for prolonged periods of time. Although tampons are strongly implicated, the actual mechanisms that produce this disease remain uncertain. Even though most cases of toxic shock syndrome occurred in menstruating women, the disease was first reported in 1978 in a group of children and continues to be reported in men, children, and nonmenstruating women. Most cases not related to menstruation occur in individuals recovering from wounds, surgery, and similar incidents.

To reduce the likelihood of contracting toxic shock syndrome, take the following precautions: (1) avoid superabsorbent tampons except during the heaviest menstrual flow; (2) change tampons frequently, at least every four hours; and (3) use pads at night instead of tampons. Call your doctor immediately if you have any of the following symptoms during menstruation: high fever, headache, vomiting, diarrhea and the chills, stomach pains, or shock-like symptoms such as faintness, rapid pulse, pallor (which can be caused by a drop in blood pressure), or a sunburn-like rash, particularly on fingers and toes.

## Streptococcal Infections

Another common form of bacterial infection is caused by microorganisms called **streptococci.** A "strep throat" (severe sore throat characterized by white or yellow pustules at the back of the throat) is the typical streptococcal problem. *Scarlet fever* (characterized by acute fever, sore throat, and rash) and *rheumatic fever* (said to "lick the joints and bite the heart") are serious streptococcal infections.

## Pneumonia

In the late nineteenth century and early twentieth century, **pneumonia** was one of the leading causes of death in North America. This disease is characterized by chronic cough, chest pain, chills, high fever, fluid accumulation, and eventual respiratory failure. One of the most common forms of pneumonia is caused by bacterial infection and responds readily to antibiotic treatment. Other forms are caused by the presence of viruses, chemicals, or other substances in the lungs. In these types of pneumonia, treatment may be more difficult.

## Legionnaire's Disease

This bacterial disorder gained widespread publicity in 1976, when several legionnaires at the American Legion convention in Philadelphia contracted the disease and died before the invading organism was isolated and effective treatment devised. The symptoms are similar to those for pneumonia, which sometimes makes identification difficult. In people whose immunity is compromised, particularly the elderly, delayed identification can have serious consequences. If they are misdiagnosed as suffering from pneumonia, they may be given **penicillin,** which is ineffective as a treatment for Legionnaire's disease, instead of the required erythromycin.

## Tuberculosis

One of the leading fatal diseases in Europe and North America in the early 1900s, **tuberculosis (TB)** was largely controlled by the mid-1900s through improved sanitation, isolation of infected persons, and treatment with drugs such as rifampin or Isoniazid. Although treatable with antibiotics, TB continues to be a worldwide problem, killing almost two million people each year.[5]

**Bacteria:** Single-celled organisms that may cause diseases.

**Toxins:** Poisonous substances produced by certain microorganisms that cause various diseases.

**Staphylococci:** Round, gram-positive bacteria, usually found in clusters.

**Epidermis:** The outermost layer of the skin.

**Toxic shock syndrome:** A potentially life-threatening bacterial infection most common in menstruating women.

**Streptococci:** Round bacteria, usually found in chain formation.

**Pneumonia:** Bacterially caused disease of the lungs.

**Penicillin:** Antibiotic used to fight a variety of bacterially caused ailments.

**Tuberculosis (TB):** A disease caused by bacterial infiltration of the respiratory system.

Switzerland, Italy, and the United States are experiencing a resurgence of new TB cases. Several factors contribute to this resurgence, including the phasing-out of TB surveillance and control programs, the emergence of multiple-drug-resistant TB (MAR-TB), large-scale migration, social and natural disasters, and infection with the human immunodeficiency virus (HIV). The risk of developing clinical TB in tuberculin-positive individuals is very high in HIV-seropositive patients.[6] For most Canadians, the risk of developing TB is low, although there are approximately 1,600 new cases reported each year.[7]

Tuberculosis is caused by bacterial infiltration of the respiratory system. It is transmitted by breathing infected air from an infected person's coughing or sneezing. Many people infected with TB are contagious without actually showing symptoms themselves. Symptoms include persistent coughing, weight loss, fever, and spitting up blood. Fortunately, the average healthy person is not at high risk; however, those who may be fighting other diseases, such as some of the HIV-related diseases, may be at increased risk. A quick test can usually detect TB. If you do have it, you can usually be treated and made noncontagious within two weeks. You can often be cured within six months.

### Periodontal Diseases

Diseases of the tissue around the teeth, called **periodontal diseases,** affect three out of four adults over age 35. Improper home tooth care, including lack of flossing and poor brushing habits, and the failure to obtain regular professional dental care lead to increased bacterial growth, caries (tooth decay), and gum infections. If left untreated, permanent tooth loss may result.

## Viruses

**Viruses** are the smallest of the pathogens, approximately 1/500 the size of bacteria. Because of their tiny size, they are visible only under an electron microscope and therefore were not identified until the twentieth century. At present, more than 150 viruses are known to cause diseases in humans.

A virus consists of a protein structure that contains either *ribonucleic acid (RNA)* or *deoxyribonucleic acid (DNA)*. It is incapable of carrying out the normal cell functions of respiration and metabolism. It cannot reproduce on its own and exists only in a parasitic relationship with the cell it invades.

Treatment of viral diseases is difficult because many viruses can withstand heat, formaldehyde, and large doses of radiation with little effect on their structure. In addition, some viruses may have **incubation periods** (the length of time required to develop fully and cause symptoms in their hosts) measured in years rather than hours or days. Termed **slow-acting viruses,** these viruses infect the host and remain in a semidormant state for years, causing a slowly developing illness. HIV is the most recent example of a slow-acting virus.

Drug treatment for viral infections is limited. Drugs powerful enough to kill viruses also kill the host cells, although some drugs are available that block stages in viral reproduction without damaging the host cells. We have another form of virus protection within our bodies. When exposed to certain viruses, the body begins to produce a protein substance known as **interferon.** Interferon does not destroy the invading microorganisms but sets up a protective mechanism to aid healthy cells in their struggle against the invaders. Although interferon research is promising, it should be noted that not all viruses stimulate interferon production.

### The Common Cold

Caused by any number of viruses (some experts claim there may be more than 100 different viruses responsible for the common cold), colds are **endemic** among peoples throughout the world. Current research indicates that otherwise healthy people carry cold viruses in their noses and throats most of the time. These viruses are held in check until the host's resistance is lowered. In the true sense of the word, it is possible to "catch" a cold—from the airborne droplets of another person's sneeze or from skin-to-skin or mucous membrane contact—though recent studies indicate that the hands may be the greatest source of cold and other viral transmission.

Although numerous ideas exist concerning how to prevent or cure the common cold, including taking megadoses of vitamin C, little hard evidence supports them. The best rule of thumb for preventing the common cold is to keep your resistance level high. Eating well, getting adequate rest, managing your stress, and engaging in regular physical activity appear to be your best bets to fight off infection. Also, limiting contact with people with newly developed colds (colds appear to be most contagious during the first 24 hours of onset) is advisable. Once you contract a cold, bed rest, plenty of fluids, and a pain reliever are the tried-and-true remedies for adults. Keep in mind that children should not be given Aspirin for colds or the flu because of the possibility of Reye's syndrome. Several over-the-counter preparations are available to alleviate various cold symptoms.

### Influenza

In otherwise healthy people, **influenza,** or flu, is usually not serious. Symptoms, including aches and pains,

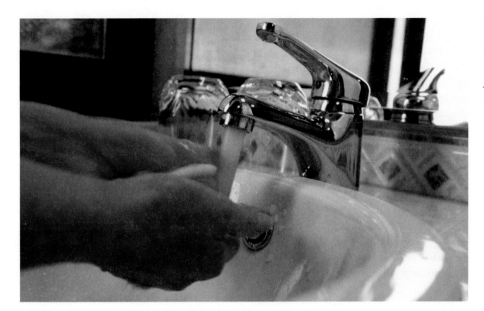

*Hands may be the greatest source of viral transmission, so washing them often and well may help prevent you from catching or transmitting the common cold.*

nausea, diarrhea, fever, and coldlike ailments, generally pass very quickly. However, in combination with other disorders, or among the elderly (people 65+), those with respiratory or heart disease, or the very young (children under the age of 5), the flu can be very serious.

To date, three major varieties of flu virus have been discovered, with many different strains existing within each variety. The "A" form of the virus is generally the most virulent, followed by the "B" and "C" varieties. If you contract one form of influenza you may develop immunity to it, but you may not necessarily be immune to other forms of the disease. There is little that can be done to treat individuals with the flu once the infection has become established. Some vaccines have proven effective for certain strains of flu virus, but are totally ineffective against others. Flu vaccination is recommended for those with a compromised immune system, including adults and children with chronic pulmonary disorders, people of any age who are residents of nursing homes, people 65 years of age or over, and people with diabetes and other metabolic diseases. In many jurisdictions, vaccination for these most vulnerable groups is at no cost to the person. Vaccination for people in essential services is recommended, but usually the person bears the cost. Because flu shots take anywhere from two to three weeks to become effective, you should get these shots in the fall, before the flu season begins.

## Infectious Mononucleosis

This affliction of college- and university-aged people is often jokingly referred to as the "kissing disease." The symptoms of mononucleosis, or "mono," include sore throat, fever, headache, nausea, chills, and a pervasive weakness or tiredness in the initial stages. As the disease progresses, lymph nodes may continue to enlarge, and jaundice, spleen enlargement, aching joints, and body rashes may occur.

Theories on the transmission and treatment of mononucleosis are highly controversial. Caused by the *Epstein-Barr virus,* mononucleosis is readily detected through a *monospot test,* a blood test that measures the percentage of specific forms of white blood cells. Because many viruses are spread by transmission of body fluids, people once believed that young people passed the disease on by kissing. Although this is still considered a possible cause, mononucleosis is not believed to be highly contagious. It does not appear to be easily contracted through normal, everyday personal contact. Multiple cases among family members are rare, as are cases between intimate partners.

Treatment of mononucleosis is often a lengthy process that involves bed rest, balanced nutrition, and medications to control the symptoms of the disease. Gradually, the body develops a form of immunity to the disease and the person returns to normal activity levels.

**Periodontal diseases:** Diseases of the tissue around the teeth.

**Viruses:** Minute parasitic microbes that live inside another cell.

**Incubation period:** The time between exposure to a disease and the appearance of the symptoms.

**Slow-acting viruses:** Viruses having long incubation periods and causing slowly progressive symptoms.

**Interferon:** A protein substance produced by the body that aids the immune system by protecting healthy cells.

**Endemic:** Describing a disease always present to some degree.

**Influenza:** A common viral disease of the respiratory tract.

## Hepatitis

One of the most highly publicized viral diseases is **hepatitis.** Incidence of hepatitis has been rising in Canada, and educational programs have been initiated in the hope of preventing new outbreaks. Hepatitis is generally defined as a virally caused inflammation of the liver, characterized by symptoms that include fever, headache, nausea, loss of appetite, skin rashes, pain in the upper right abdomen, dark yellow (with a brownish tinge) urine, and the possibility of jaundice (it's "the disease your friends diagnose" because of the yellowing of the whites of the eyes and the skin).

Treatment of all the forms of viral hepatitis (see Table 13.2) is somewhat limited. A balanced dietary intake, bed rest, and antibiotics to combat bacterial invaders that may cause additional problems are recommended. Vaccines for hepatitis are available through a series of injections, although costs are high. Many provinces are beginning to require vaccinations against hepatitis B for healthcare workers and others who may be exposed to blood-borne pathogens.

TABLE 13.2

### Forms of Hepatitis: A Comparison

| Disease | Incubation Period | Acute Infectious (% symptomatic) | Outcome |
|---|---|---|---|
| Hepatitis B | 45–180 days | <10% of childhood infections; 50% of adult infections | 1% develop fulminant hepatitis; 1–10% of adults become chronic carriers; >90% perinatal or early childhood infections become carriers |
| Hepatitis A | 15–45 days | <10% of childhood infections; 50% of adult infections | No chronic carriers |
| Hepatitis C | 14–168 days | More often asymptomatic | 50% become chronic carriers |

Source: Canadian Communicable Disease Report, Supplement 21S4, November 1995, Health Canada. © Reproduced with the permission of Minister of Public Works and Government Services Canada, 2007.

## Mumps

Until 1969, mumps was a common viral disorder among children with an average of 30,000 cases per year. That year a vaccine become available and the disease seemed to be largely under control, with reported cases declining to between 1.2 and 3.5 per 100,000 from 1986 to 1995.[8] Approximately one-half of all mumps infections are not apparent because they produce only minor symptoms. Typically, there is an incubation period of 16 to 18 days, followed by symptoms caused by the lodging of the virus in the glands of the neck. The most common symptom is the swelling of the parotid (salivary) glands. One of the greatest dangers associated with mumps is the potential for sterility in men who contract the disease in young adulthood. Also, transient deafness may occur in fewer than one to five cases per 100,000, and may be permanent in some.[9]

## Chicken Pox

Caused by the *herpes zoster varicella* virus, chicken pox produces the characteristic symptoms of fever and tiredness 13 to 17 days after exposure, followed by skin eruptions that itch, blister, and produce a clear fluid. The virus is present in these blisters for approximately one week. Symptoms are generally mild, and immunity to subsequent infection appears to be lifelong. A chicken pox vaccine for use in children aged 12 months and older has been available in Canada since 2000. However, many unvaccinated children still contract the disease, and a small percentage of those vaccinated may still contract chicken pox. Scientists believe that after the initial infection, the virus goes into permanent hibernation and, for most people, there are no further complications. For a small segment of the population, however, the zoster virus may become reactivated. Blisters will develop, usually on only one side of the body and tending to stop abruptly at the midline. Cases in which the disease covers both sides of the body are far more serious. This disease, known as shingles, affects more than 5 percent of the population each year, most often in individuals over 50 years of age.

## Measles

Measles is the most contagious disease known to humans. It is a major childhood killer in developing countries, accounting for about 900,000 deaths a year. The **measles** virus may ultimately be responsible for more child deaths than any other single microbe, due to complications from pneumonia, diarrhea, and malnutrition.[10] Technically referred to as *rubeola*, measles is a viral disorder that often affects young children. Symptoms, appearing about ten days after exposure, include an itchy rash and a high fever.

**Rubella** (or **German measles**), is a milder viral infection believed to be transmitted by inhalation, after which it multiplies in the upper respiratory tract and passes into the bloodstream. It causes a rash, especially on the upper extremities. It is not generally a serious health threat and usually runs its course in three to four days. The major exceptions to this rule are newborns and pregnant women. Rubella can damage a fetus, particularly during the first trimester, creating a condition known as congenital rubella, in which the infant may be born blind, deaf, cognitively impaired, or with heart defects. Immunization has greatly reduced the incidence of measles and German measles. Infections in children not immunized against measles can lead to fever-induced problems such as rheumatic heart disease, kidney damage, and neurological disorders.

## Other Pathogens

### Fungi

Hundreds of species of **fungi,** multi- or unicellular primitive plants, inhabit our environment and serve useful functions. Mouldy breads, cheeses, and mushrooms used for domestic purposes pose no harm to humans. But some species of fungi can produce infections. Candidiasis (a vaginal yeast infection), athlete's foot, ringworm, and jock itch are examples of fungal diseases. Keeping the affected area clean and dry plus treatment with appropriate medications will generally bring prompt relief.

### Protozoa

**Protozoa** are microscopic, single-celled organisms generally associated with tropical diseases such as African sleeping sickness and malaria. Although these pathogens are prevalent in the developing countries of the world, they are largely controlled in Canada. The most common protozoan disease in North America is trichomoniasis, an infection discussed further in the sexually transmitted infections section of this chapter. A common water-borne protozoan disease in many regions of the country is *giardiasis,* sometimes called "beaver fever." Persons who drink or are exposed to the *giardia* pathogen may suffer symptoms of intestinal pain and discomfort weeks after infection. Protection of water supplies is the key to prevention.

### Parasitic Worms

Parasitic worms are the largest of the pathogens. Ranging in size from the relatively small pinworms typically found in children to the relatively large tapeworms found in warm-blooded animals, most parasitic worms are more a nuisance than a threat. Of special note are the new forms of worm infestations commonly associated with eating raw fish (that is, sushi). Cooking fish and other foods to temperatures sufficient to kill the worms or their eggs is an effective means of prevention.

### Rickettsia

Once believed to be closely related to viruses, **rickettsia** are now considered to be bacteria-like organisms. They produce toxins and multiply within small blood vessels, causing vascular blockage and tissue death. Rickettsia require an insect vector (carrier) for transmission to humans. Two common forms of human rickettsia disease are Rocky Mountain spotted fever, carried by ticks, and typhus, carried by lice, fleas, or ticks. Both diseases can be life-threatening. They produce similar symptoms, including high fever, weakness, rash, and coma. You do not actually have to be bitten by a vector to contract either disease. Because the vectors themselves harbour the developing rickettsia in their intestinal tracts, insect excrement deposited on the skin and entering the body through abrasions and scratches may be a common source of infection.

### Prions

A **prion,** or unconventional virus, is a self-replicating, protein-based agent that can infect humans and other animals. Believed to be the underlying cause of spongiform diseases—such as "mad cow disease"— this agent systematically destroys brains cells.

# YOUR BODY'S DEFENCES: KEEPING YOU WELL

Although all the pathogens described in the preceding section pose a threat if they take hold in your body, the chances that they will take hold are actually quite

**Hepatitis:** A virally caused disease in which the liver becomes inflamed, producing symptoms such as fever, headache, and jaundice.

**Measles:** A viral disease that produces symptoms including an itchy rash and a high fever.

**Rubella (German measles):** A milder form of measles that causes a rash and mild fever in children and may cause damage to a fetus or a newborn baby.

**Fungi:** A group of plants that lack chlorophyll and do not produce flowers or seeds; several microscopic varieties are pathogenic.

**Protozoa:** Microscopic, single-celled organisms.

**Rickettsia:** A small form of bacteria that lives inside other living cells.

**Prion:** A self-replicating protein-based agent that systematically destroys brain cells.

small. To do so, they must overcome a number of effective barriers, many of which were established in your body before you were born.

## Physical and Chemical Defences

Perhaps our single most critical early defence system is the skin. Layered to provide an intricate web of barriers, the skin allows few pathogens to enter. **Enzymes,** complex proteins manufactured by the body that appear in body secretions such as sweat, provide additional protection, destroying microorganisms on skin surfaces by producing inhospitable pH levels. Normal body pH is 7.0, but enzymatic or biochemical changes may cause the body chemistry to become more acidic (pH of less than 7.0), or more alkaline (pH of more than 7.0). In either case, microorganisms that flourish at a selected pH will be weakened or destroyed as these changes occur. A third protection is our frequent slight elevations in body temperature, which create an inhospitable environment for many pathogens. Further, only when there are cracks or breaks in the skin can pathogens gain easy access to the body.

The linings of the body provide yet another protection against pathogens. Mucous membranes in the respiratory tract and other linings of the body trap and engulf invading organisms. *Cilia,* hairlike projections in the lungs and respiratory tract, sweep unwanted invaders toward body openings, where they are expelled. Tears, nasal secretions, ear wax, and other secretions found at body entrances contain enzymes designed to destroy or neutralize invading pathogens. Finally, any invading organism that manages to breach these initial lines of defence faces a formidable specialized network of defences from the immune system.

## The Immune System: Your Body Fights Back

*Immunity* is the condition of being able to resist a particular disease by counteracting the substance that produces the disease. Any substance capable of triggering an immune response is called an **antigen.** An antigen can be a virus, a bacterium, a fungus, a parasite, or a tissue or cell from another individual. When invaded by an antigen, the body responds by forming substances called antibodies matched to the specific antigen much as a key is matched to a lock. **Antibodies** belong to a mass of large molecules known as *immunoglobulins,* a group of nine chemically distinct protein substances, each of which plays a role in neutralizing, setting up for destruction, or actually destroying antigens. Once an antigen breaches the body's initial defences, the body begins a careful process of antigen analysis. It considers the size and shape of the invader, verifies that the antigen is not part of the body itself, and then begins to produce a specific antibody to destroy or weaken the antigen. This process, which is much more complex than described here, is part of a system called *humoral immune responses.* Humoral immunity is the body's major defence against many bacteria and bacterial toxins.

*Cell-mediated immunity* is characterized by the formation of a population of lymphocytes that can attack and destroy the foreign invader. These lymphocytes constitute the body's main defence against viruses, fungi, parasites, and some bacteria. Key players in this immune response are specialized groups of white blood cells known as *macrophages* (a type of phagocytic, or cell-eating, cell) and *lymphocytes,* other white blood cells in the blood, lymph nodes, bone marrow, and certain glands.

Two forms of lymphocytes in particular, the *B-lymphocytes* (B-cells) and *T-lymphocytes* (T-cells), are involved in the immune response. There are different types of B-cells, named according to the area of the body in which they develop. Most are manufactured in the soft tissue of the hollow shafts of the long bones. T-cells, in contrast, develop and multiply in the thymus, a multi-lobed organ that lies behind the breastbone. T-cells assist your immune system in several ways. *Regulatory T-cells* help direct the activities of the immune system and assist other cells, particularly B-cells, to produce antibodies. Dubbed "helper Ts," these cells are essential for activating B-cells, other T-cells, and macrophages. Another form of T-cell, known as the "killer Ts" or "cytotoxic Ts," directly attacks infected or malignant cells. Killer Ts enable the body to rid itself of cells infected by viruses or transformed by cancer; they are also responsible for the rejection of tissue and organ grafts. The third type of T-cells, "suppressor Ts," turns off or suppresses the activity of B-cells, killer Ts, and macrophages. Suppressor Ts circulate in the bloodstream and lymphatic system, neutralizing or destroying antigens, enhancing the effects of the immune response, and helping to return the activated immune system to normal levels. After a successful attack on a pathogen, some of the attacker T- and B-cells are preserved as *memory T-* and *B-cells,* enabling the body to quickly recognize and respond to subsequent attacks by the same kind of organism at a later time. Thus macrophages, T- and B-cells, and antibodies are the key factors in mounting an immune response.

Once people have survived certain infectious diseases, they become immune to those diseases, meaning that in all probability they will not develop them again. When the disease-causing microorganism next attacks them, their memory T- and B-cells are quickly activated to come to their defence. Immunization works on the same principle. Vaccines containing an attenuated (weakened) or killed version of the disease-causing microorganism or containing an antigen similar to but not as dangerous as the disease antigen are administered to stimulate the person's immune system to produce antibodies against future attacks—without actually causing the disease.

### Autoimmune Diseases

Although white blood cells and the antigen–antibody response generally work in our favour by neutralizing or destroying harmful antigens, the body sometimes makes a mistake and targets its own tissue as the enemy, builds up antibodies against that tissue, and attempts to destroy it. This is known as autoimmune disease ( *auto* means "self"). Common examples of this type of disease are rheumatoid arthritis, lupus erythematosus, and myasthenia gravis.

In some cases, the antigen–antibody response completely fails to function. The result is a form of *immune deficiency syndrome.* Perhaps the most dramatic case of this syndrome was the "bubble boy," who died in 1984 after living his short life inside a sealed-off environment designed to protect him from all antigens. A much more common immune system disorder is *acquired immune deficiency syndrome (AIDS),* discussed later in this chapter.

## Fever

If an infection is localized, pus formation, redness, swelling, and irritation often occur. These symptoms indicate a systematic response against the invading organisms. Another indication is the development of a fever, or a rise in body temperature above the norm of 37°C. Fever is frequently caused by toxins secreted by pathogens that interfere with the control of body temperature. Although this elevated temperature is often harmful to the body, it is also believed to act as a form of protection. A one- or two-degree elevation in temperature creates an environment that destroys some types of disease-causing organisms. Also, as body temperature rises the body is stimulated to produce more white blood cells, which destroy more invaders.

## Pain

Although pain is not usually thought of as a defence mechanism, it plays a valuable role in the body's response to invasion. Pain is generally a response to injury. Pain may be either direct, caused by the stimulation of nerve endings in an affected area, or referred, meaning it is present in one place while the source is elsewhere. An example of referred pain is the pain in the arm or jaw often experienced by someone having a heart attack. Regardless of the cause of pain, most pain responses are accompanied by inflammation. Pain tends to be the earliest sign that an injury occurred and often causes the person to slow down or stop the activity, thereby protecting against further damage. Because it is often one of the first warnings of disease, persistent pain should not be overlooked or masked with short-term pain relievers.

## Vaccines: Bolstering Your Immunity

Our natural defence mechanisms are our strongest allies in the battle against disease from birth until death. There are periods in our life, however, when either invading organisms are too strong or our own natural immunity is too weak to protect us from catching a given disease. It is at such times that we need outside assistance in developing immunity to an invading organism. Such assistance is generally provided in the form of a **vaccination.** Vaccines are given orally or by injection, and this form of *artificial immunity* is termed acquired immunity, in contrast to *natural immunity,* which a mother passes to her fetus via their shared blood supply.

Today, depending on the virulence of the organism, vaccines containing live, weakened, or dead organisms are given to people for a variety of diseases. In some instances, if a person is already weakened by other diseases, vaccination may provoke an actual case of the disease. This was what happened with the smallpox vaccinations administered routinely in the 1960s. It was believed that the risk of contracting smallpox from the vaccine was actually greater than the chance of contracting the disease in an environment where it had essentially been eradicated. For this reason, routine smallpox inoculations were eliminated in the late 1960s. Currently recommended childhood vaccinations are shown in Table 13.3.

**Enzymes:** Organic substances that cause bodily changes and destruction of microorganisms

**Antigen:** Substance capable of triggering an immune response.

**Antibodies:** Substances produced by the body individually matched to specific antigens.

**Vaccination:** Inoculation with killed or weakened pathogens or similar, less dangerous antigens in order to prevent or lessen the effects of some disease.

**TABLE 13.3**

## Recommended Childhood Immunization Schedule

| Age | Immunization Against |
|---|---|
| 2 months | Diphtheria, pertussis, tetanus, poliomyelitis, haemophilus influenzae b[1], pneumococcal conjugate vaccine, meningococcal C conjugate vaccine |
| 4 months | Diphtheria, pertussis, tetanus, poliomyelitis, haemophilus influenzae b, pneumococcal conjugate vaccine[2], meningococcal C conjugate vaccine |
| 6 months | Diphtheria, pertussis, tetanus, poliomyelitis,[3] haemophilus influenzae b, pneumococcal conjugate vaccine |
| 12 months | Measles, mumps, rubella,[4] varicella,[5] pneumococcal conjugate vaccine |
| 18 months | Diphtheria, pertussis, tetanus, poliomyelitis, haemophilus influenzae b |
| 4–6 years | Diphtheria, pertussis, tetanus, poliomyelitis |
| 9–13 years | Hepatitis B[6] |
| 14–16 years | Diphtheria, tetanus, poliomyelitis, meningococcal C conjugate vaccine[7] |

Notes:

1. Haemophilus influenzae b requires a series of immunizations. The exact number and timing of each may vary with the brand of vaccine used.

2. Recommended schedule, number of doses, and subsequent use of pneumococcal vaccine depends on the age of the child when vaccination is begun.

3. If oral polio virus vaccine is used exclusively in a series of immunizations, this dose may be omitted.

4. A second dose of MMR vaccine is recommended for children and youth. It may be administered any time after a minimum one-month waiting period; provincial schedules differ.

5. Children aged 12 months to 12 years should receive one dose of varicella vaccine. Individuals aged 13 years or older should receive two doses at least 28 days apart.

6. Hepatitis B requires a series of immunizations. In some jurisdictions, they may be administered at a younger age.

7. Recommended schedule and number of doses of meningococcal vaccine depends on the age of the child.

Source: Adapted from *Canadian Immunization Guide,* 6th ed., Health Canada, 2002. Reproduced with the permission of the Minister of Public Works and Government Services Canada, 2007.

# SEXUALLY TRANSMITTED INFECTIONS

There are more than 20 different types of **sexually transmitted infections** (STIs, formerly called *STDs,* or *sexually transmitted diseases*). These infections were once referred to as venereal diseases, but the newer classification is believed to be broader in scope and reflective of the numbers and types of communicable infections, which are sometimes asymptomatic.[11] In Canada, since 1997, the incidence of STIs is rising.[12] Young people today generally become sexually active sooner and marry later and as a result have a greater number of partners, which increases their risk of acquiring an STI. Further, with a higher risk for divorce than in past generations, people are once again more likely to have multiple sex partners during their life and increase their risk of developing an STI.

In many, the early symptoms of an STI are not serious. They may range from mild discomfort to annoying itching or discharge. (See Figure 13.1 for signs that may indicate the presence of an STI.) Left untreated, however, some of these infections can have grave consequences, such as sterility, blindness, central nervous system destruction, disfigurement, and even death. Infants born to mothers carrying the organisms for these infections are at risk for a variety of health problems.

As with many of the communicable diseases, much of the pain, suffering, and anguish associated with STIs could be eliminated or substantially reduced through education, responsible action, and prompt treatment when symptoms first occur. Overcoming the tendency to pass moral judgments on those who contract an STI would certainly lower the barriers to treatment. Being prepared to deal with the pressure to engage in sexual activity can also be helpful.

## Possible Causes: Why Me?

Sexually transmitted infections affect males and females of all socioeconomic levels, ages, ethnicities, and regions of the world. Several reasons have been

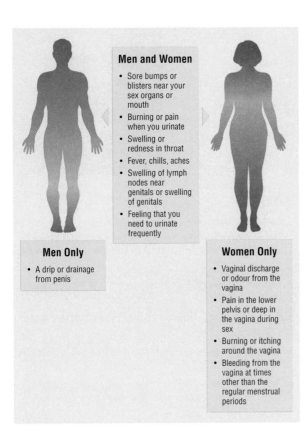

**Men and Women**
- Sore bumps or blisters near your sex organs or mouth
- Burning or pain when you urinate
- Swelling or redness in throat
- Fever, chills, aches
- Swelling of lymph nodes near genitals or swelling of genitals
- Feeling that you need to urinate frequently

**Men Only**
- A drip or drainage from penis

**Women Only**
- Vaginal discharge or odour from the vagina
- Pain in the lower pelvis or deep in the vagina during sex
- Burning or itching around the vagina
- Bleeding from the vagina at times other than the regular menstrual periods

**FIGURE 13.1**

**The illustration lists signs or symptoms of STIs.**

proposed to explain the present high rates of STIs. The first relates to the moral and social stigma associated with these infections. Shame and embarrassment often keep infected people from seeking treatment. Unfortunately, these people usually continue to be sexually active, thereby infecting others. People uncomfortable discussing sexual issues may also be less likely to use or ask their partners to use condoms as a means of protection against STIs and pregnancy.

Another reason proposed for the STI epidemic is our casual attitude about sex. Bombarded by media hype that glamorizes easy sex, many people engage in various sexual activities without considering the consequences. Others are pressured into sexual relationships they don't really want. Generally, the more sexual partners a person has, the greater the risk for contracting an STI. Evaluate your beliefs and attitudes about STIs by taking the Rate Yourself box self-assessment.

Ignorance about the infections themselves and an inability to recognize actual symptoms or to acknowledge that a person may be asymptomatic yet still have an infection are also factors behind the STI epidemic. A person infected but asymptomatic may unknowingly spread an STI to an unsuspecting partner, who may then ignore or misinterpret symptoms that do appear. By the time either partner seeks medical help, he or she may have infected several others.

## Modes of Transmission

Sexually transmitted infections are generally spread through some form of sexual contact. Vaginal and anal intercourse, oral–genital contact, and hand–genital contact are (in decreasing order of likelihood) the most common modes of transmission. More rarely, pathogens for STIs are transmitted mouth to mouth or, even more infrequently, through contact with fluids from body sores. While each STI is a different infection caused by a different pathogen, all STI pathogens prefer dark, moist places, especially the mucous membranes lining the reproductive organs. The majority of these organisms are susceptible to light, excess heat, cold, and dryness, and many die quickly on exposure to air. (The toilet seat is not a likely breeding ground for most bacterial or viral STIs!) Although most STIs are passed on by sexual contact, other kinds of close contact, such as sleeping on the sheets used by someone who has pubic lice, may also result in transmission from one person to another. One method of preventing the spread of STIs is to use a condom during any sexual activity, including vaginal, anal, and oral sex. To fully protect yourself, follow these basic rules:

- Decide ahead of time that you will not have sex without a condom. Make sure you have one with you.
- Never reuse a condom.
- Use only latex condoms.
- Store condoms in a cool, dry place—not in the glove compartment of your car or in your wallet.
- If a condom appears brittle or sticky, don't use it.
- Put the condom on (correctly) before having any sex, including oral sex.
- Apply a water-based lubricant containing spermicide to the condom for additional protection.
- If the condom breaks, tears, or becomes dislodged, wash the genitals thoroughly with soap and water, apply a spermicide to the area, and put on another condom before additional contact. It takes only a fraction of a second to become infected with disease-laden body fluids or to infect someone else if you are a carrier.
- Hold the condom in place during withdrawal to make sure it doesn't come off.

Like other communicable diseases, STIs have both pathogen-specific incubation periods and periods of time during which transmission is most likely, called periods of communicability.

**Sexually transmitted infections (STIs):** Infectious diseases transmitted via vaginal, anal, and oral sexual contact.

# STI Attitude and Belief Scale

The following quiz will help you evaluate whether your beliefs and attitudes about STIs lead you to behaviours that may heighten your risk for contracting an STI.

## DIRECTIONS

Indicate that you believe the following items are true or false by circling the T or the F. Then consult the answer key that follows.

1. You can usually tell whether someone is infected with an STI, especially HIV.

   T                    F

2. Chances are that if you haven't caught an STI by now, you probably have a natural immunity and won't get infected in the future.

   T                    F

3. A person successfully treated for an STI needn't worry about getting it again.

   T                    F

4. So long as you keep yourself fit and healthy, you needn't worry about STIs.

   T                    F

5. The best way for sexually active people to protect themselves from STIs is to practise safer sex.

   T                    F

6. The only way to catch an STI is to have sex with someone who has one.

   T                    F

7. Talking about STIs with a partner is so embarrassing that you're best off not raising the subject and hoping the other person will.

   T                    F

8. STIs are mostly a problem for people who are promiscuous.

   T                    F

9. You don't need to worry about contracting an STI so long as you wash yourself thoroughly with soap and hot water immediately after sex.

   T                    F

10. You don't need to worry about AIDS if no one you know has ever come down with it.

   T                    F

## SCORING KEY

1. **False.** Several STIs, such as chlamydia, gonorrhea (especially in women), internal genital warts, and even HIV infection in its early stages, cause few if any obvious signs or symptoms.

2. **False.** If you practise unprotected sex and have not contracted an STI to this point, count your blessings.

3. **False.** Sorry. Successful treatment does not render immunity against reinfection.

4. **False.** Even people in prime physical condition can be felled by the tiniest of microbes that cause STIs.

5. **True.** If you are sexually active, practising safer sex is the best protection against contracting an STI. Of course, abstinence is the only sure way to not contract an STI through sexual activity.

6. **False.** STIs can also be transmitted through nonsexual means, such as by sharing contaminated needles or, in some cases, through contact with disease-causing organisms on towels and bedsheets or even toilet seats.

7. **False.** Don't let embarrassment prevent you from taking steps to protect your and your partner's welfare.

8. **False.** STIs are a potential problem for anyone who is sexually active.

9. **False.** While washing your genitals immediately after sex may have some limited protective value, it is no substitute for practising safer sex.

10. **False.** Symptoms of HIV infection may not appear for years after initial infection with the virus.

## INTERPRETING YOUR SCORE

First, add up the number of items you got right. A score of 8 or better indicates that your attitudes toward STIs would probably decrease your risk of contracting them. Yet even one wrong response on this test increases your risk of contracting an STI. Knowledge alone isn't sufficient to protect yourself from STIs. You need to ask yourself how you are going to put knowledge into action by changing your behaviours to reduce your chances of contracting an STI.

Source: Adapted from Jeffrey S. Nevid with Fern Gotfried, *Choices: Sex in the Age of STDs*, 10–13. © 1995 by Allyn & Bacon. Reprinted by permission.

Although there are more than 20 different types of sexually transmitted infections, we discuss only those most likely to pose a risk for the average adult.

# Chlamydia

Genital **chlamydia** (*chlamydia trachomatis*) first became nationally reportable in 1990 and emerged as the most prevalent bacterial STI in Canada. Preventable and treatable, genital chlamydia remains high in Canada—in 2004 the chlamydia rate (197.1 per 100,000) was much greater than the national rate for gonorrhea (28.9 per 100,000).[13] Current chlamydia infection rates are slightly higher than in past years. Further, chlamydia rates are expected to rise to 198.5 per 100,000 in 2005, while gonorrhea rates are expected to decline to 26.1 per 100,000.[14] This is likely due to more screening being done with newer, non-invasive technologies (see Table 13.4).

The name of the infection is derived from the Greek verb *chlamys*, meaning "to cloak," because, unlike most bacteria, chlamydia can live and grow only inside other cells. Although many people classify chlamydia as either *nonspecific* or *nongonococcal urethritis (NGU)*, a person may have NGU without having the organism for chlamydia. In more than half of the cases of NGU (infections of the urethra and surrounding tissues not caused by gonococcal bacteria), however, *Chlamydia trachomatis*, the bacterial organism that causes chlamydia, is present. For this reason, the two disease terms tend to be used interchangeably, even though NGU may be caused by other organisms.

In males, early symptoms may include painful and difficult urination, frequent urination, and a watery, puslike discharge from the penis. Symptoms in females may include a yellowish discharge, spotting between periods, and occasional spotting after intercourse. Unfortunately, many individuals with chlamydia display no symptoms and therefore do not seek help until the infection has done secondary damage. Females are especially likely to be asymptomatic; more than 70 percent do not realize they have the infection until secondary damage occurs.

The secondary damage resulting from chlamydia is serious for males and females. Males can suffer damage to the prostate gland, seminal vesicles, and bulbourethral glands, as well as arthritis-like symptoms and damage to the blood vessels and heart. In females, secondary damage from chlamydia may include inflammation that damages the cervix or fallopian tubes, causing sterility, and damage to the inner pelvic structure, leading to pelvic inflammatory disease (PID). If an infected woman becomes pregnant, she has a high risk for miscarriages and stillbirths. Chlamydia may also be responsible for one type of **conjunctivitis,** an eye infection that affects not only

## TABLE 13.4

### Screening for STIs

Screening to detect asymptomatic STI is divided into three categories:

**Case Finding:** A patient-based strategy in individuals with an increased likelihood of one or more STIs, e.g., sexual contacts to gonorrhea

**Focused Screening:** A group-based strategy in subpopulations with high STI prevalence rates, e.g., street youth, core groups, adolescents, and those with a history of STI

**General Screening:** A population-based strategy in certain members of the general public who are not considered to be at increased risk for STI but in whom serious consequences may occur if infected, e.g., syphilis and HIV testing in pregnancy

| | Case Finding | Focused Screening | General Screening |
|---|---|---|---|
| **Procedures** | | | |
| Sexual history | X | X | X |
| **Physical examination** | | | |
| External genital | X | X | X |
| Internal genital | Adults, adolescents | Adults, adolescents | – |
| Targeted extragenital | X | X | X |
| **Laboratory tests** | | | |
| *Neisseria gonorrhoeae* | X | X | – |
| *Chlamydia trachomatis* | X | X | – |
| *Treponema pallidum* | X | X | X |
| Pap smear | Adults, adolescents | Adults, adolescents | – |
| Hepatitis B (HBV) | Optional | Optional | X |
| HIV | X | X | X |

Source: Canada Communicable Disease Report, Supplement 21S4, November 1995, Health Canada. Adapted and reproduced with the permission of the Minister of Public Works and Government Services Canada, 2006.

adults but also infants, who can contract the disease from an infected mother during delivery. Untreated conjunctivitis can cause blindness.

Chlamydia can be controlled through responsible sexual behaviours and familiarity with the early symptoms

**Chlamydia:** Bacterially caused STI of the urogenital tract.

**Conjunctivitis:** Serious inflammation of the eye caused by any number of pathogens or irritants; can be caused by STIs such as chlamydia.

of the disease. If detected early enough, chlamydia is easily treatable with antibiotics such as tetracycline, doxycycline, or erythromycin. In most cases, treatment is successfully completed in two to three weeks. Unfortunately, chlamydia checks are not a routine part of many STI testing procedures. You may have to request a chlamydia check specifically before one is performed on you.

## WHAT WOULD YOU DO?

Why do you think many post-secondary students, even though they have heard of the risks of STIs and HIV disease, fail to use condoms and in general act irresponsibly regarding their sexual health? What actions do you think could be taken to help you and your friends engage in sexually responsible behaviours?

## Pelvic Inflammatory Disease (PID)

**Pelvic inflammatory disease (PID)** is actually not one disease but a term used to describe a number of infections of the uterus, fallopian tubes, and ovaries. Although PID is often the result of an untreated sexually transmitted infection, especially chlamydia or gonorrhea, it is not actually an STI. Nonsexual causes of PID are also common, including excessive vaginal douching, cigarette smoking, and substance abuse. PID is not a notifiable disease in Canada; thus, estimating prevalence is difficult. A study undertaken by Health Canada's Laboratory Centre for Disease Control found that the rate of PID declined appreciably over 10 years. A study done in Manitoba came to a similar conclusion.[15]

Symptoms may include acute inflammation of the pelvic cavity, severe pain in the lower abdomen, menstrual irregularities, fever, nausea, painful intercourse, tubal pregnancies, and severe depression.[16] The major consequences of untreated PID are infertility, ectopic pregnancy, chronic pelvic pain, and recurrent upper genital infections. Risk factors include young age at first sexual intercourse, multiple sex partners, high frequency of sexual intercourse, and change of sexual partners within the last 30 days.[17] Regular gynecological examinations and early treatment for STI symptoms reduce risk.

## Gonorrhea

**Gonorrhea** still exists in Canada, though it has declined more than tenfold since 1980. The most recent data (2004) indicate a national incidence of 28.9 per 100,000, with a lower estimate of 26.1 per 100,000 predicted for 2005.[18] This dramatic decline has been attributed to better control programs involving diagnostic services, contact tracing, and effective treatment.[19]

Currently, the majority of endemic gonococcal infections is thought to reside within core groups: a small subset of the population whose members frequently acquire new sexual partners. Currently, the highest rates of infection are found in the territories, particularly the Northwest Territories (167.5 per 100,000) and the Yukon (103.3 per 100,000), followed by Manitoba (80.5 per 100,000) and Saskatchewan (55.9 per 100,000).[20] More research needs to be conducted to assess and describe core groups within a Canadian context; appropriate prevention and control strategies, aimed at reducing or ideally eliminating indigenous gonococcal infections, can then be implemented.[21]

Caused by the bacterial pathogen *Neisseria gonorrhoea*, this infection primarily infects the linings of the urethra, genital tract, pharynx, and rectum. It may be spread to the eyes or other body regions via the hands or body fluids.

In males, a typical symptom is a white milky discharge from the penis accompanied by painful, burning urination two to nine days after contact. This is usually enough to send most men to their physician for treatment. Only about 20 percent of all males with gonorrhea are asymptomatic.

In females, the situation is just the opposite. Only about 20 percent of all females experience any form of discharge, and few develop a burning sensation upon urinating until much later in the course of the infection (if ever). The organism can remain in the woman's vagina, cervix, uterus, or fallopian tubes for long periods with no apparent symptoms other than an occasional slight fever. Thus, a woman can be unaware that she has been infected and that she may be infecting her sexual partners.

Upon diagnosis, an antibiotic regimen using penicillin, tetracycline, spectiomycin, ceftriaxone, or other drugs is begun. A penicillin-resistant form of gonorrhea may require a particularly strong combination of antibiotics. Treatment is generally completely effective within a short period of time if the disease is detected early.

If the disease goes undetected in a woman, it can spread throughout the genital–urinary tract to the fallopian tubes and ovaries, causing sterility—or, at the very least, severe inflammation and pelvic inflammatory disease symptoms. If an infected woman becomes pregnant, the disease can cause conjunctivitis in her infant. To prevent this, physicians routinely administer silver nitrate or penicillin preparations to the eyes of newborn babies.

Untreated gonorrhea in the male may spread to the prostate, testicles, urinary tract, kidney, and bladder. Blockage of the *vasa deferentia* due to scar tissue formation may cause sterility. In some cases, the penis develops a painful curvature during erection.

# Syphilis

**Syphilis,** the other well-known sexually transmitted infection, is also caused by a bacterial organism, the spirochete known as *Treponema pallidum*. Because it is extremely delicate and dies quickly on exposure to air, dryness, or cold, the organism is generally transferred only through direct sexual contact. Typically this means contact between sexual organs during intercourse, but in rare instances the organism enters the body through a break in the skin, through deep kissing in which body fluids are exchanged, or through some other transmission of body fluids.

With the arrival of HIV in the 1980s, syphilis took on new importance. It increases sexual transmission of HIV by six- to sevenfold, and neurosyphilis in HIV-infected patients is particularly difficult to treat. Scientific evidence has shown that early detection and treatment of STIs can have a major impact on the sexual transmission of HIV2-9. Because of this synergy, syphilis control can have a significant impact on the HIV epidemic in Canada.[22]

Syphilis is called the "great imitator" because its symptoms resemble those of several other diseases. Only an astute physician who has reason to suspect the presence of the disease will order the appropriate tests for a diagnosis. Unlike most of the other STIs, syphilis generally progresses through several distinct stages.

## Primary Syphilis

The first stage of syphilis, particularly for males, is often characterized by the development of a sore known as a **chancre** (pronounced "shank-er"), located most frequently at the site of the initial infection. This chancre is usually about the size of a dime and is painless, but it is oozing with bacteria, ready to spread to an unsuspecting partner. Usually the chancre appears between three and four weeks after contact.

In males, the site of the chancre tends to be the penis or scrotum because this is the site where the organism first makes entry into the body. But, if the infection was contracted through oral sex, the sore can appear in the mouth, throat, or other "first contact" area. In females, the site of infection is often internal, on the vaginal wall or high on the cervix. Because the chancre is not readily apparent, the likelihood of detection is not great. In males and females, the chancre will completely disappear in three to six weeks.

## Secondary Syphilis

From a month to a year after the chancre disappears, secondary symptoms may appear, including a rash or white patches on the skin or on the mucous membranes of the mouth, throat, or genitals. Hair loss may occur, lymph nodes may become enlarged, and the victim may run a slight fever or develop a headache. In rare cases, sores develop around the mouth or genitals. As during the active chancre phase, these sores contain infectious bacteria, and contact with them may spread the disease. In some people, symptoms follow a textbook pattern; in others, there are no symptoms at all. In a few cases, there may be arthritic pain in the joints. Because symptoms vary so much and because the symptoms that do appear are so far removed from previous sexual experience that the individual infected seldom connects the two, the infection often goes undetected even at this second stage. Symptoms may persist for a few weeks or months and then disappear, leaving the infected individual thinking that all is well.

## Latent Syphilis

The syphilis spirochetes begin to invade body organs after the secondary stage. There may be periodic reappearance of previous symptoms, including the presence of infectious lesions, for between two and four years after the secondary period. After this period, the infection is rarely transmitted to others, except during pregnancy, when it can be passed on to the fetus. The child will then be born with *congenital syphilis,* which can cause death or severe birth defects such as blindness, deafness, or disfigurement. Because in most cases the fetus does not become infected until after the first trimester, treatment of the mother during this period will usually prevent infection of the fetus.

In some instances, a child born to an infected mother will show no apparent signs of the disease at birth but within several weeks will develop body rashes, a runny nose, and symptoms of paralysis. Congenital syphilis is usually detected before it progresses much further. But sometimes the child's immune system will ward off the invading organism, and further symptoms may not surface until the teenage years.

In addition to causing congenital syphilis, latent syphilis, if untreated, will continue to progress, infecting more and more organs until the infection reaches its final stage, late syphilis.

---

**Pelvic inflammatory disease (PID):** Term used to describe various infections of the female reproductive tract.

**Gonorrhea:** Second most common STI in Canada; if untreated, may cause sterility.

**Syphilis:** An STI caused by a bacterial infection, cured with antibiotics, spread through direct sexual contact.

**Chancre:** Sore often found at the site of syphilis infection.

### Late Syphilis

Most of the horror stories concerning syphilis involve the late stages of the infection. Years after syphilis has entered the body and progressed through the various organs, its net effects become clearly evident. Late-stage syphilis indications may include heart damage, central nervous system damage, blindness, deafness, paralysis, premature senility, and, ultimately, insanity.

### Treatment for Syphilis

Treatment for syphilis resembles that for gonorrhea. Because the organism is bacterial, it is treated with antibiotics, usually penicillin, benzathine penicillin G, or doxycycline. Blood tests are administered to determine the exact nature of the invading organism, and the doses of antibiotics are much stronger than those taken by the typical gonorrhea patient. The major obstacle to treatment is misdiagnosis of this "imitator" disease.

## Pubic Lice

Often called "crabs," **pubic lice** are more annoying than dangerous. Pubic lice are small parasites usually transmitted during sexual contact. They prefer the dark, moist regions of the body and, during vaginal and anal sex, move easily from partner to partner. Although sexual contact is the most common mode of transmission, you can become infected with pubic lice from lying on sheets an infected person slept on. Sleeping in hotel and dormitory rooms in which blankets and sheets are not washed regularly or sitting on toilet seats where the nits or larvae have been dropped and lie in wait for a new carrier may put you at risk.

## Venereal Warts

**Venereal warts** (also known as *genital warts* or *condylomas*) are caused by a small group of viruses known as *human papilloma viruses (HPVs)*. A person becomes infected when an HPV penetrates the skin and mucous membranes of the genitals or anus through sexual contact. The virus appears to be relatively easy to catch. The typical incubation period is from six to eight weeks. Many people have no apparent symptoms, particularly if the warts are located inside the reproductive tract. Others may develop a series of itchy bumps on the genitals, which may range in size from a small pinhead to large cauliflower-like growths that can obstruct normal urinary or reproductive activity. On dry skin (such as on the shaft of the penis), the warts are commonly small, hard, and yellowish-grey, resembling warts that appear on other parts of the body. Venereal warts are of two different types: (1) *full-blown genital warts* noticeable as tiny bumps or growths, and (2) the much more prevalent *flat warts* not usually visible to the naked eye.

### Risks of Venereal Warts

Many venereal warts will eventually disappear on their own. Others will grow and generate unsightly flaps of irregular flesh on the external genitalia. The greatest threat from venereal warts may lie in the apparent relationship between them and a tendency for *dysplasia,* or changes in cells that may lead to a precancerous condition. Exactly how HPV infection leads to cervical cancer is uncertain. What is known is that within five years after infection, 30 percent of all HPV cases progress to the precancerous stage. Of those cases that become precancerous and are left untreated, 70 percent will eventually result in actual cancer. In addition, venereal warts may pose a threat to a pregnant woman's unborn fetus if the fetus is exposed to the virus during birth. Caesarean deliveries may be considered in serious cases.

### Treatment for Venereal Warts

Treatment for venereal warts may take several forms:

1. Warts are painted with a medication called podophyllin during a visit to the doctor's office. The podophyllin is washed off after about four hours, and a few days later the warts begin to dry up and fall off. Sometimes more than one application is necessary. This procedure is relatively painless.
2. Warts may be removed by *cryosurgery,* a procedure in which an instrument treated with liquid nitrogen is held to the affected area, "freezing" the tissue. Within a few days, the warts fall off.
3. Depending on size and location, some warts are removed by *simple excision.*
4. For larger warts, *laser surgery* is often used. This is a major procedure that generally requires general anesthesia. The frequency of laser use for wart removal is currently questioned by many health experts. (Precautions must also be taken during this procedure to shield medical staff from infection by viral spray.)
5. Creams containing 5-Fluoracil (an anticancer drug) are used to prevent further precancerous cell development.
6. For warts located externally, injections of interferon are sometimes given to keep the virus from spreading to healthy tissue. This treatment shows promise, but it is expensive and, in large doses, may cause flu-like symptoms.

Prevention is clearly a better approach. What is true about protecting yourself from HIV infection is also true about protecting yourself from genital warts and other STIs (see the section on AIDS prevention later in this chapter).

## Candidiasis (Moniliasis)

Unlike many of the other sexually transmitted infections caused by pathogens that come from outside the body, the yeast-like fungus caused by the *Candida albicans* organism normally inhabits the vaginal tract in most women. Only under certain conditions will these organisms multiply to abnormal quantities and begin to cause problems.

The likelihood of **candidiasis** (also known as *moniliasis*) is greatest if a woman has diabetes, if her immune system is overtaxed or malfunctioning, if she is taking birth control pills or other hormones, or if she is taking broad-spectrum antibiotics. All of the above factors decrease the acidity of the vagina, making conditions more favourable for the development of a yeast-like infection.

Symptoms of candidiasis include severe vaginal itching, a white, cheesy discharge, swelling of the vaginal tissue due to irritation, and a burning sensation. These symptoms are often collectively called **vaginitis.** When this microbe infects the mouth, whitish patches form and the condition is referred to as *thrush.* This monilial infection also occurs in males and is easily transmitted between sexual partners.

Antifungal drugs applied on the surface or by suppository usually cure the infection in a few days. For approximately one out of ten women, however, nothing seems to work, and the organism returns again and again. In women with this chronically recurring infection, symptoms are often aggravated by contact of the vagina with soaps, douches, perfumed toilet paper, chlorinated water, and spermicides. Further, tight-fitting jeans and pantyhose can provide the combination of moisture and irritant the organism thrives on.

## Trichomoniasis

Unlike many of the other STIs, **trichomoniasis** is caused by a protozoan. Although many men and women have this organism, most remain free of symptoms until their bodily defences are weakened. Men and women may transmit the disease, but women are the more likely candidates for infection. The "trich" infection may cause a foamy, yellowish discharge with an unpleasant odour that may be accompanied by a burning sensation, itching, and painful urination. These symptoms are most likely to occur during or shortly after menstruation, but they can appear at any time or be absent altogether. Although usually transmitted by sexual contact, the "trich" organism may be easily spread by toilet seats, wet towels, or other items that have discharged fluids on them. You can also contract trichomoniasis by sitting naked on the bench of the dressing room of your local health spa or locker room. Treatment includes oral metronidazole, usually given to both sexual partners to avoid the possible "ping-pong" effect of repeated cross-infection typical of STIs.

## General Urinary Tract Infections

Although *general urinary tract infections (UTIs)* can be caused by various factors, some forms are sexually transmitted. Any time invading organisms enter the genital area, there is a risk that they may travel up the urethra and enter the bladder. Similarly, organisms normally living in the rectum, urethra, or bladder may travel to the sexual organs and eventually be transmitted to another person.

You can also get a UTI through autoinoculation (transmission to yourself by yourself). This frequently occurs during the simple task of wiping yourself after defecating. Wiping from the anus forward may transmit organisms found in feces to the vaginal opening or to the urethra. Contact between the hands and the urethra and between the urethra and other objects are also common means of autoinoculation of bacterial and viral pathogens. Women, with their shorter urethras, are more likely to contract UTIs. Treatment depends on the nature and type of pathogen.

## Herpes

Herpes is a general term for a family of diseases characterized by sores or eruptions on the skin. Herpes infections range from mildly uncomfortable to extremely serious. One subcategory, *herpes simplex,* is caused by a virus. Herpes simplex virus type 1 (HSV-1) causes the cold sores and fever blisters that most of us have experienced at one time or another. The *herpes simplex virus (HSV)* is one of the most common infectious agents in Canada; in 1994, more than 14,000 cases were identified in laboratory tests, and many more undoubtedly went unreported.[23] HSV infection has overtaken bacterial STI infection as the most common cause of genital ulceration worldwide.[24] HSV-2

**Pubic lice:** Parasites that inhabit various body areas, especially the genitals; also called "crabs."

**Venereal warts:** Warts that appear in the genital area or the anus; caused by the human papilloma viruses (HPVs).

**Candidiasis:** Yeast-like fungal disease often transmitted sexually.

**Vaginitis:** Set of symptoms characterized by vaginal itching, swelling, and burning.

**Trichomoniasis:** Protozoan infection characterized by foamy, yellowish discharge and unpleasant odour.

(genital herpes) is not a reportable STI in Canada; therefore, we have little baseline data available. The data we do have suggest that genital herpes is as great a concern in Canada as in the rest of the world.[25]

**Genital herpes,** caused by *herpes simplex virus type 2 (HSV-2),* is one of the most widespread STIs in the world. Typically, genital herpes is characterized by distinct phases. First, the herpes virus must gain entrance to the body, which it usually does through the mucous membranes of the genital area. Once these organisms invade, the infected individual will experience the *prodromal* (precursor) phase of the disease, characterized by a burning sensation and redness at the site of the infection. This phase is typically followed by the formation of a small blister filled with a clear fluid containing the virus. If you pick at this blister or otherwise spread this clear fluid by your hands, you can autoinoculate other body parts. Particularly dangerous is the possibility of spreading the infection to your eyes this way, because a herpes lesion on the eye may cause blindness.

Over a period of days, this unsightly blister will crust, dry, disappear, and the virus will travel to the base of an affected nerve supplying the area and become dormant. Only when the individual infected becomes overly stressed, when dietary intake is inadequate, when the immune system is overworked, or when there is excessive exposure to sunlight or other stressors will the virus reactivate (at the same site every time) and begin the blistering cycle all over again. This cyclical recurrence can be painful, unsightly, and, most important, highly contagious. Fluids from these blisters may readily be transmitted to sexual partners. Through oral sex, herpes simplex type 2 may be transmitted to the mouth. Symptoms are similar to those of herpes simplex type 1. Figure 13.2 summarizes the herpes cycle.

Genital herpes is especially serious in pregnant women because of the danger of infecting the baby as it passes through the vagina during birth. For that reason, many physicians recommend caesarean deliveries for infected women. Additionally, women with a history of genital herpes also appear to have a greater risk of developing cervical cancer.

Although there is no cure for herpes at present, certain drugs have shown some success in reducing symptoms. Unfortunately, they seem to work only if the infection is confirmed during the first few hours after contact. As you may guess, this is rather rare. The effectiveness of other treatments, such as L-lysine, is largely unsubstantiated to date. Although lip balms and cold-sore medications may provide temporary anesthetic relief, it is useful to remember that rubbing anything on a herpes blister may spread herpes-laden fluids to other tissues or, via the hands, to other body parts.

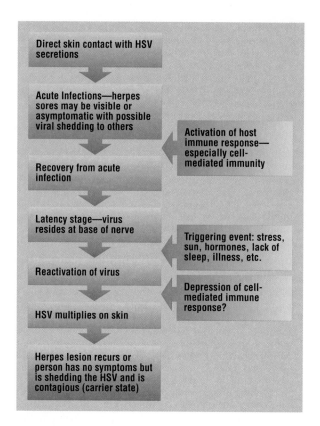

## FIGURE 13.2

### The Herpes Cycle

Source: Adapted by permission of J. B. Lippincott from "Sexually Transmitted Diseases in the 1990's," *STD Bulletin* 11 (1992): 4.

## Preventing Herpes

If you are worried about contracting herpes, there are several precautions that you should take:

- Avoid any form of kissing if you notice a sore or blister on your partner's mouth. Kiss no one, not even a peck on the cheek, if you know that you have a herpes lesion. Allow a bit of time after the sores go away before you start kissing again.

- Be extremely cautious if you have casual sex. Not every partner will feel obligated to tell you that he or she may have an STI. Protecting yourself against an infection is up to you.

- Wash your hands immediately with soap and water after any form of sexual contact.

- If you have herpes, reduce the risk of a herpes episode by avoiding excessive stress, sunlight, or whatever else appears to trigger a herpes outbreak in you.

- If you have questionable sores or lesions, seek medical help at once. Do not be afraid to name your sexual contacts.

- Since the herpes organism dies quickly upon exposure to air, toilet seats, soap, and similar sources are not likely means of transmission.

- If you have herpes, be responsible in your sexual contacts with others. If you have herpes lesions that might put your partner at risk, let that person know. Although it is not necessary to announce openly a herpes problem, use common sense in determining the appropriate time and place for a candid herpes discussion with your partner.

# ACQUIRED IMMUNE DEFICIENCY SYNDROME (AIDS)

**Acquired immune deficiency syndrome (AIDS)** is aptly named because it is a disease that is <u>a</u>cquired. Since the virus suppresses the immune system, it is termed <u>i</u>mmuno and renders the body immune's system deficient, therefore <u>d</u>eficiency is the third word. Finally, because the symptoms of AIDS all occur together, it is called a <u>s</u>yndrome.[26]

Since 1981, when the first case of AIDS was diagnosed, the numbers of AIDS-diagnosed individuals and of persons infected with **human immunodeficiency virus (HIV)** have skyrocketed, in North America and worldwide. Few regions of the world have been spared. It has been estimated that more than 21 million people have died as a result of AIDS and that 57 million individuals had been infected with HIV.[27] Individuals living in countries in southern and central Africa and South Asia account for three-quarters of these infections.[28]

The first case of AIDS in Canada was reported in 1982. Since HIV testing began in Canada in November 1985, there have been 57,674 positive HIV tests. The actual number of individuals in Canada living with HIV is expected to be higher than this number because not all individuals infected with HIV are actually tested for it.[29] It is estimated that approximately 2,500 new cases will be identified each year. Of the positive new cases each year, approximately 75 percent are men.[30] It should be pointed out there has been a disproportionate rise in the number of women testing positive for HIV since 1995, when fewer than 10 percent of new cases were found in women. Even though ethnic status is not available on approximately one-third of all positive HIV reports, disproportionate increases in newly identified cases have been found among black Canadians (15.5 percent) and Aboriginal Canadians (14.8 percent).[31]

The Focus on Canada box gives a detailed picture of the global face of AIDS.

## How HIV Is Transmitted

HIV typically enters one person's body when another person's infected body fluids (semen, vaginal secretions, blood, etc.) gain entry through a breach in body defences. Mucous membranes of the genital organs and the anus provide the easiest route of entry. If there is a break in the mucous membranes (as can occur during sexual intercourse, particularly anal intercourse), the virus enters and begins to multiply. After initial infection, the HIV typically begins to multiply rapidly in the body, invading the bloodstream and cerebrospinal fluid. It progressively destroys helper T-lymphocytes, weakening the body's resistance to disease. The virus also changes the genetic structure of the cells it attacks. In response to this invasion, the body quickly begins to produce antibodies.

Despite some rather hysterical myths, HIV is not a highly contagious virus. Countless studies of people living in households with a person with HIV/AIDS have turned up no documented cases of HIV infection due to casual contact.[32] Other investigations provide overwhelming evidence that insect bites do not transmit the virus. In fact, the virus is actually quite selective in the way it transmits itself from person to person.

### Engaging in High-Risk Behaviours

HIV is not a disease of certain groups. People are not predestined to get the disease because they belong to a group or associate with a group. Thus, HIV is not a gay disease, or a disease of minority groups, or Haitians, or any other class of people. It is a disease of certain high-risk behaviours. If you engage in the behaviours, you increase your risk for the disease. If you don't engage in the behaviours, your risk is minimal. Promiscuous sex—in males and females of all ages, races, ethnic groups, sexual orientations, and socioeconomic conditions—is the

**Genital herpes:** STI caused by herpes simplex virus type 2.

**Acquired immune deficiency syndrome (AIDS):** Extremely virulent sexually transmitted infection that renders the immune system inoperable.

**Human immunodeficiency virus (HIV):** The slow-acting virus that causes AIDS.

# State of the HIV/AIDS Epidemic

HIV/AIDS is a global threat that knows no boundaries. Epidemiological evidence shows that the developing world is bearing the brunt of the epidemic; more than 95 percent of new infections in 2000 were in developing countries. Sub-Saharan Africa accounts for a full 70 percent of the world's HIV-positive population, but the disease is also gaining strength in East Asia. Rates in Eastern Europe, the Middle East, Latin America, and the Caribbean are also on the rise. The Public Health Agency of Canada estimates from 2004 show that the impact of the epidemic is increasing in Canada.

An estimated 40 million people worldwide are living with HIV, more than 17.6 million of whom are women. In 2000, about 5 million people became infected, 800,000 of them children. Since the epidemic began, AIDS has killed 24.8 million people, a significant majority of them in Sub-Saharan Africa. Last year alone, AIDS claimed 3 million lives. HIV/AIDS has also orphaned more than 13 million children under the age of 15.

Health Canada estimates show that at the end of 2004, 57,674 people had tested positive for the HIV virus in Canada. Further, the number of new HIV infections per year has increased since 1999, from approximately 4,200 to 5,000. Not only had the number of positive HIV tests risen, the composition of these new infections changed. This prevalence data clearly illustrates

the changing face of the Canadian HIV epidemic, highlighting a potential resurgence of the epidemic among men who have sex with men and an increasingly urgent situation among Aboriginal and black Canadian populations. Although the estimates show a reduction among injection drug users, the number of new infections per year in this group is still unacceptably high.

Source: State of the HIV/AIDS Epidemic: Health Canada Online, Health Canada, 2002 and Public Health Agency "HIV and AIDS in Canada. Surveillance Report to Surveillance and Rick Assessment December 2004" Division, Centre for Infections Prevention Control, Public Health Agency of Canada. 2004. Reproduced with the permission of the Minister of Public Works and Government Services Canada, 2006.

greatest threat. Anyone who engages in unprotected sex at any time with a person who has engaged in high-risk behaviours is at risk. A celibate or monogamous gay man or a drug-injecting woman who never shares her needles is at very low risk for HIV. But a person who has had sex with someone who has, even once, had sex with an injecting drug user could be infected. You can't tell by looking at someone; you can't tell by questioning, unless the person has been tested recently and is HIV-negative. So, what should you do? The Building Communication Skills box offers some direct advice.

Of course, the best method of protection is abstinence. If you don't exchange body fluids, you won't get the disease. As a second line of defence, if you decide to be intimate, the best option is to use a condom. The following activities are high-risk behaviours.

## Exchange of Body Fluids

The exchange of HIV-infected body fluids during sexual intercourse is the greatest risk factor. Substantial research indicates that blood, semen, and vaginal, cervical, and anal secretions are the major fluids of concern. Although the virus was found in one person's saliva (out of 71 people in a study population), most health officials state that saliva is not a high-risk body fluid.

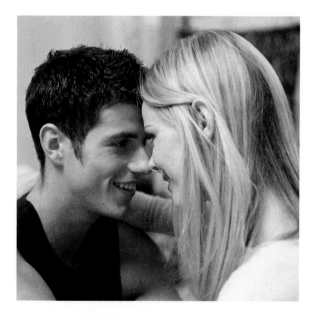

*You can't tell if someone has an STI, including HIV, just by looking at them. Being open and honest with your partners (and expecting the same from them) about sexual history and STI and HIV testing is an important part of prevention.*

But the fact that the virus has been found in saliva does provide a good rationale for using caution when engaging in deep, wet kissing.

# Communicating with Your Partner about STIs

The more people know about sexually transmitted infections and the more they internalize personal susceptibility, the greater the chance that they will adopt safer behaviours. Yet, despite large-scale public awareness and education programs, infection continues. Many medical, education, and youth officials feel that the major obstacle to preventing STIs among young people is the discomfort most feel about discussing personal needs and feelings regarding these infections and practising safer sex behaviours. For many young people, discussing STI status and safer sex practices, such as condom use, can be uncomfortable. Some fear that raising the issue suggests lack of trust in the partner; others worry that safer behaviours will ruin their sexual enjoyment; and still others fail to recognize their personal vulnerability. As a result, a great many put themselves at risk for infection rather than hurt the other person's feelings. Therefore, a major goal in the fight against STIs is to improve one-on-one communication between young people. The following tips can help open the lines of communication.

- Remember you have a responsibility to your partner to disclose your status. You also have a responsibility to yourself to do what needs to be done to stay healthy and infection free. Do not be afraid to ask your partner's STI status. If either person's status is unknown, suggest going through the testing together—before engaging in any sexual activity—as a means of sharing something important with each other.

- Be direct, honest, and determined in talking about sex before you become involved. Do not act silly or evasive. Get to the point, ask clear questions, and do not be put off receiving a response. Remember, a person who does not care enough to talk about sex probably does not care enough to take responsibility for his or her actions.

- Discuss the issues without sounding defensive or accusatory. Develop a personal comfort level with the subject prior to raising the issue with your partner. Be prepared with complete information and articulate your feelings clearly. Reassure your partner that your reasons for desiring abstinence or safer sex arise from respect rather than distrust. Sharing feelings is easier in a calm, suspicion-free environment in which both people feel comfortable.

- Encourage your partner to be honest and to share feelings. This will not happen overnight. If you have never had a serious conversation with this person before you get into an intimate situation, you cannot expect honesty and openness when the lights go out.

- Analyze your own beliefs and values ahead of time. The worst thing you can do is to get yourself into an awkward situation before you had time to think about what is important to you and what you believe in. Know where you will draw the line on certain actions, and be very clear with your partner about what you expect. If you believe that using a condom is necessary, make sure you communicate this to your partner.

- Decide what you will do if your partner does not agree with you. Anticipate your partner's potential objections or excuses and prepare your responses accordingly.

- Ask questions about past history. Although it may seem as though you are prying into another person's business, your health future depends upon knowing basic information about your partner's past. An idea of your partner's past sexual practices and use of injected drugs is valuable. Again, it is important to let your partner know why you are concerned and that you are not inquiring due to jealousy or other ulterior motives.

- Ask about the significance of monogamy in your partner's relationships. A basic question to ask before becoming involved in a regular sexual relationship is: "How important is a committed relationship to you?" You will need to decide early how important this relationship is to you and how much you are willing to work at arriving at an acceptable compromise on lifestyle.

Initially, public health officials also included breast milk in the list of high-risk fluids because a small number of infants apparently contracted HIV while breast-feeding. Subsequent research has indicated that HIV transmission could have been caused by bleeding nipples rather than actual consumption of breast milk. Infection through contact with feces and urine is believed to be highly unlikely (though technically possible).

## Receiving a Blood Transfusion Prior to 1986

A small group of people became infected with HIV as a result of a blood transfusion before 1986. Since then, the Canadian Red Cross (Canada's blood supply is now controlled by Canadian Blood Services) implemented a stringent testing program for all donated blood. Because of these massive screening efforts, the risk of receiving HIV-infected blood or any other blood-borne pathogen is almost nonexistent.

### Injecting Drugs

Another source of infection is sharing or using HIV-contaminated needles. Injection drug use (IDU) has increasingly been a route of HIV transmission in Canada. In 1999, the percentage of new HIV infections in Canada estimated as a result of IDU was 34 percent. With increased attention focused on preventing HIV transmission in IDU, the percentage of new infections attributed to drug users dropped to slightly less than 30 percent in 2002.[33]

While illegal drug users are the people we usually think of in this category, it is important to remember that others may also share needles—for example, individuals with type 1 diabetes who inject insulin. People who share needles and engage in sexual activities with members of high-risk groups, such as those who exchange sex for drugs, increase their risks dramatically. Any needle prick with an HIV-contaminated needle provides a risk of infection. Thus, tattooing, body piercing, and any practice using unsterilized needles presents a potential risk.

### Mother-to-Infant Transmission (Perinatal)

Infants may contract HIV from their infected mothers while in the womb or while passing through the vaginal tract during delivery.

## Symptoms of the Disease

A person may go for months or years after acquiring HIV before any significant symptoms appear. The incubation time varies greatly from person to person. Children have shorter incubation periods than adults. Newborns and infants are particularly vulnerable to HIV infection because they are not fully immunocompetent (that is, their immune system is not fully developed) until they are 6 to 15 months old. New information suggests that some very young children show the "adult" progression of the disease. In adults, the average length of time it takes the virus to cause the slow, degenerative changes in the immune system that result in AIDS is eight to ten years. During this time, the person may experience a large number of opportunistic infections (infections that gain a foothold when the immune system is not functioning effectively). Colds, sore throats, fever, tiredness, nausea, night sweats, and other generally non-life-threatening conditions commonly appear.

## Testing for HIV Antibodies

Once antibodies have begun to form in reaction to the presence of HIV, a blood test known as the **ELISA** test may detect their presence. If sufficient antibodies are present, this test will be positive. When a person who previously tested *negative* (no HIV antibodies present) has a subsequent test that is *positive*, seroconversion is said to have occurred. In such a situation, the person would typically take another ELISA test, followed by a

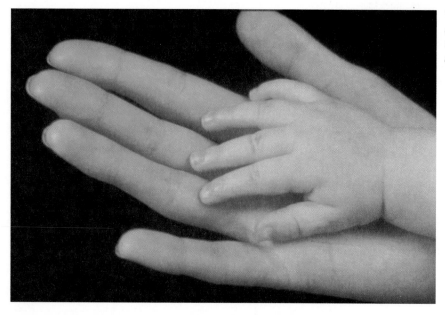

*Women carry not only the burden of their own health, but frequently that of a child infected before birth or at the time of delivery.*

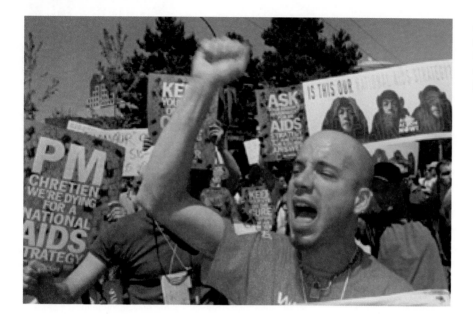

*Numerous demonstrations by gay activists have successfully called attention to the need for AIDS research and treatment programs.*

more expensive, more precise test known as the **Western blot** to confirm the presence of HIV antibodies.

Although the ELISA is viewed as quite accurate, it is a conservative test in that it errs on the side of caution, meaning it produces a large number of *false positive results*. It was deliberately designed to do this because it was intended as a test for screening the nation's blood supply. There have also been instances of *false negative results*. Some health professionals believe there are chronic carriers of HIV who, for unknown reasons, continually show false negative results on the ELISA and the Western blot test. False-negative HIV tests raise serious concerns about risks for these people's sexual partners. It should be noted that these tests are not AIDS tests per se. Rather, they detect antibodies for the disease, indicating the presence of HIV in the person's system. Whether or not the person will develop AIDS depends to some extent on the strength of the immune system. However, the vast majority of infected people do develop some form of the disease.

As testing for HIV antibodies improves, scientists have explored ways of making it easier for individuals to be tested. Health officials distinguish between reported and actual cases of HIV infection because it is believed that many HIV-positive people avoid being tested. One reason is fear of knowing the truth. Another is the fear of recrimination from employers, insurance companies, and health professionals. However, early detection and reporting are important, because immediate treatment for someone in the early stages of HIV infection is critical and necessary to attempt to prevent further spread of the virus.

## WHAT WOULD YOU DO?

Do you favour mandatory reporting of HIV and AIDS? Why or why not? Would you be less likely to have an HIV test if you knew that your name and vital statistics would be "on file" if you tested positive? Why or why not?

## Preventing HIV Infection

Although scientists have been searching for more than a decade for a vaccine to protect people from HIV infection, they have had no success so far. The only effective prevention strategies known relate to the means by which people contract HIV. HIV infection and AIDS are not uncontrollable conditions. You can reduce your risks by making responsible choices in your sexual and drug use behaviours. The Skills for Behaviour Change box suggests ways to reduce your risk for contracting HIV.

Because the status of your immune system is an important factor in whether you are susceptible to any of the STIs, it is important that you do everything possible to protect yourself. Adequate physical activity, a healthy dietary intake, sufficient sleep, stress management, vaccinations, and other preventive maintenance activities can do a great deal to ensure your long-term health.

**ELISA:** Blood test that detects the presence of antibodies to HIV.

**Western blot:** More precise test than the ELISA to confirm presence of HIV antibodies.

# Reducing Your Risks for HIV Disease

Contracting HIV is not uncontrollable. HIV cannot, like cold or flu viruses, be caught casually. The transmission of HIV depends upon specific behaviours. Therefore, HIV infection can be prevented. The following list offers ways to reduce your risk.

- Avoid casual sexual partners. Ideally, have sex only in a long-term, mutually monogamous relationship and with a partner whose HIV status is negative.

- Avoid unprotected intimate sexual activity with people whose present or past behaviours put them (and thus you) at risk for infection. Do not be afraid to ask intimate questions about your partner's sexual history and past injection drug use. You expose yourself to your partner's history whenever you choose to have sexual relations. Postpone sexual involvement until you are assured that he or she is not infected.

- Sexually active adults not in a lifelong monogamous relationship should practise safer sex by using latex condoms. Remember, however, that condoms do not provide 100-percent protection.

- Never share injecting needles with anyone for any reason.

- Never share any devices through which the exchange of blood could occur, including needles, razors, tattoo instruments, any body-piercing instruments, and any other sharp objects.

- Avoid injury to body tissue during sexual activity. HIV can enter the bloodstream through microscopic tears in anal or vaginal tissues.

- Avoid unprotected oral sex or any sexual activity in which semen, blood, or vaginal secretions could penetrate mucous membranes through breaks in the membrane. Always use a condom or a dental dam during oral sex.

- Avoid using drugs that may dull your senses and affect your ability to make decisions about responsible precautions with potential sex partners.

- Wash your hands before and after sexual encounters. Urinate after sexual relations and, if possible, wash your genitals.

- Although total abstinence is the only absolute means of preventing the sexual transmission of HIV, abstinence can be a difficult choice to make. If you are in doubt about the potential risks of having sex, consider other means of intimacy, at least until you can ensure your safety. Enjoyable and safer alternatives include massage, dry kissing, hugging, holding and touching, and masturbation (alone or with a partner).

- When receiving care from medical professionals such as dentists or doctors, make sure they take appropriate precautions to prevent potential transmission, including washing their hands and wearing gloves and masks. Be sure that all equipment used for treatment is properly sterilized.

- If you are worried about your own HIV status, have yourself tested rather than risk infecting others.

- If you are a woman and HIV-positive, you should take the steps necessary to ensure that you do not become pregnant.

- If you suspect that you may be infected or if you test positive for HIV antibodies, do not donate blood, semen, or body organs.

# NONINFECTIOUS DISEASES

Typically, when we think of the major ailments and diseases affecting people today, we think of "killer" diseases such as cancer and heart disease. Although these diseases capture much of the media attention, other forms of chronic disease cause substantial pain, suffering, and disability. Fortunately, the majority of these diseases can be prevented or their onset delayed.

To prevent the development of certain noninfectious and chronic diseases, we must identify the major common characteristics. They are not transmitted by any pathogen or by any form of personal contact. They usually develop over a long period of time, and they cause progressive damage to human tissues. Although these conditions normally do not result in death, they do lead to illness and suffering for many people. Lifestyle and personal health habits appear to be major contributing factors to the general increase observed in the incidence of chronic diseases in Canada in recent years. Education, reasonable changes in lifestyle behaviours, and public health efforts aimed at prevention and control could minimize the effects of many of these diseases.

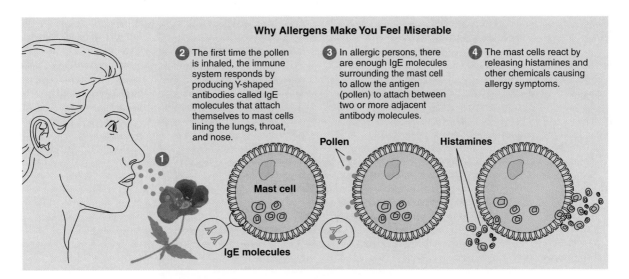

**Why Allergens Make You Feel Miserable**

**2** The first time the pollen is inhaled, the immune system responds by producing Y-shaped antibodies called IgE molecules that attach themselves to mast cells lining the lungs, throat, and nose.

**3** In allergic persons, there are enough IgE molecules surrounding the mast cell to allow the antigen (pollen) to attach between two or more adjacent antibody molecules.

**4** The mast cells react by releasing histamines and other chemicals causing allergy symptoms.

Pollen

Histamines

Mast cell

IgE molecules

## FIGURE 13.3
Steps of an Allergy Response

# RESPIRATORY DISORDERS

## Allergy-Induced Problems

An **allergy** occurs as a part of the body's attempt to defend itself against a specific *antigen* or *allergen* by producing specific antibodies. When foreign pathogens such as bacteria or viruses invade the body, the body responds by producing antibodies to destroy them. Under normal conditions, the production of antibodies is a positive element in the body's defence system. However, for unknown reasons, in some people the body overreacts by developing an overly elaborate protective mechanism against relatively harmless allergens or antigens. The resultant *hypersensitivity reaction* to specific allergens or antigens in the environment is fairly common, as anyone who has awakened with a runny nose or itchy eyes will testify. Most commonly, these hypersensitivity, or allergic, responses occur as a reaction to environmental antigens such as moulds, animal dander (hair and dead skin), pollen, ragweed, or dust. Once excessive antibodies to these antigens are produced, they trigger the release of **histamines,** chemical substances that dilate blood vessels, increase mucous secretions, cause tissues to swell, and produce other allergy-like symptoms (see Figure 13.3).

Although many people think of allergies as childhood diseases, in reality allergies tend to become progressively worse with time and with increased exposure to allergens. In these circumstances, allergic responses become chronic in nature, and treatment becomes difficult. Many people take allergy shots to reduce the severity of their symptoms. In most cases, once the offending antigen has disappeared, allergy-prone people suffer few symptoms. Although allergies

can cause numerous problems, one of the most significant effects is on the immune system.

## Hay Fever

Perhaps the best example of a chronic respiratory disease is **hay fever.** Usually considered a seasonally related disease (most prevalent when ragweed and flowers are blooming), hay fever is common throughout the world. Hay fever attacks, characterized by sneezing and itchy, watery eyes and nose, cause a great deal of misery for countless people. Hay fever appears to run in families, and research indicates that lifestyle is not as great a factor in developing hay fever as it is in other chronic diseases. Instead, an overzealous immune system and an exposure to environmental allergens including pet dander, dust, pollen from various plants, and other substances appear to be the critical factors that determine vulnerability. For some people, a change in setting may help; for others, medical assistance in the form of injections or antihistamines may provide the only possibility of relief.

## Asthma

Unfortunately for many hay fever sufferers, their condition is often complicated by the development of

**Allergy:** Hypersensitive reaction to a specific antigen or allergen in the environment in which the body produces excessive antibodies to that antigen or allergen.

**Histamines:** Chemical substances that dilate blood vessels, increase mucous secretions, and produce other allergy-like symptoms.

**Hay fever:** A chronic respiratory disorder most prevalent when ragweed and flowers bloom.

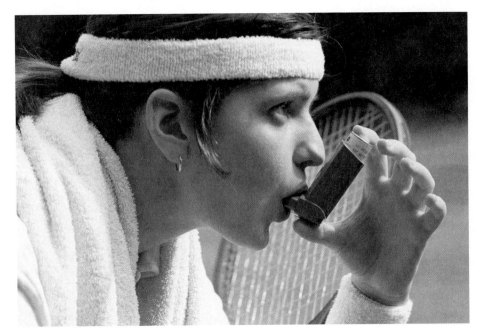

*Asthma attacks can be brought on by something as commonplace as physical activity. This does not mean that individuals with asthma shouldn't participate in sports or other physical activities, but rather that they should create a plan that takes into account their limitations.*

another chronic respiratory disease, **asthma.** Asthma is characterized by attacks of wheezing, difficulty breathing, shortness of breath, and coughing spasms. Although most asthma attacks are mild, they can trigger bronchospasms (contractions of the bronchial tubes in the lungs) of such a severe nature that, unless treatment is rapid, death may occur. Between attacks, most people have few symptoms.

In the majority of cases, asthma first occurs in children under the age of ten, afflicting males nearly twice as often as females. Although many children outgrow the condition, a number of them continue to experience asthma as adults.

Although exposure to allergens such as dust, pollen, and animal dander may trigger many asthmatic episodes, emotional factors and excessive anxiety or stress can also trigger an attack. *Exercise-induced asthma (EIA)* is a type of asthma that has gained increasing attention. Friends who bow out of a long run or a tennis game by claiming to be allergic to exercise may not be joking.

Relaxation techniques appear to help some individuals who have asthma. Drugs may be necessary for serious cases. Doctors warn against using over-the-counter inhalers without medical advice: some over-the-counter products can have serious side effects, depending on the type of asthma and other drugs used. Determining the specific allergen that provokes asthma attacks and taking steps to reduce your exposure, adjusting for triggers such as physical activity or stress, and finding the most effective medications are big steps in asthma prevention and control.

## Emphysema

**Emphysema** involves the gradual destruction of the alveoli (tiny air sacs) of the lungs. As the **alveoli** are destroyed, the affected person finds it more and more difficult to exhale. The individual typically struggles to take in a fresh supply of air before the air held in the lungs has been expended. The chest cavity gradually begins to expand, producing the barrel-shaped chest characteristic of individuals with chronic emphysema.

The exact cause of emphysema is uncertain. There is, however, a strong relationship between the development of emphysema and long-term cigarette smoking and exposure to air pollution. Individuals with emphysema often suffer discomfort over a period of many years. What we all take for granted—the easy, rhythmic flow of air in and out of our lungs—becomes a continuous struggle for people with emphysema. Inadequate oxygen supply, combined with the stress of overexertion on the heart, eventually takes its toll on the cardiovascular system and leads to premature death. Unfortunately, little can be done to reverse the effects of emphysema.

## Chronic Bronchitis

Although often dismissed as "smoker's cough" or a bad case of the common cold, **chronic bronchitis** may be a serious, if not life-threatening, respiratory disorder. In this ailment, the bronchial tubes become so inflamed and swollen that normal respiratory function is impaired. Symptoms of chronic bronchitis include a productive cough and shortness of breath that persist for several weeks over the course of the year. Cigarette smoking is the major risk factor for this disease, although fumes, dust, and particulate matter in the air are also contributing factors. Individuals with chronic bronchitis must often use respiratory devices similar to those used by individuals with emphysema. They must also avoid things—such as cigarette smoking—that contributed to the development of bronchitis. Bronchitis coupled with a severe cold may be serious enough to warrant immediate medical attention.

# NEUROLOGICAL DISORDERS

## Headaches

Almost all of us have experienced the agony of at least one major headache in our lives, whether it is the mild, throbbing variety or the severe, pounding ache that makes us nauseated or dizzy. Not all headaches are equal, and more important, it's possible that not all headaches have the same cause. However some experts suggest that all serious headaches share the same basic causes but fall along a spectrum, with ordinary tension headaches at one end and full-blown migraines at the other.[34] Headaches may result from dilated blood vessels within the brain, underlying organic problems, or excessive stress and anxiety. The following are the most common forms of headaches and the most effective methods of treatment.

### Tension Headaches

Tension headaches are generally caused by muscle contractions or tension in the neck or head. This tension may be caused by actual strain placed on the neck or head muscles due to overuse, static positions held for long periods of time, or tension triggered by stress. Research indicates that tension headaches may be a product of a more "generic mechanism" in which chemicals deep inside the brain may cause the muscular tension, pain, and suffering often associated with an attack. Triggers for this chemical assault may be red wine, lack of sleep, fasting, menstruation, or other factors, and the same symptoms (sensitivity to light and sound, nausea, and/or throbbing pain) may be characteristic of different types of headaches. Symptoms may vary in intensity and duration. Relaxation, hot water treatment, and massage have surfaced as the new "holistic treatments," while Aspirin, Tylenol, and Advil are the old standby forms of pain relief.

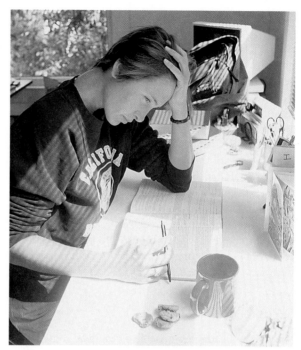

*Tension headaches are triggered by many factors, including lack of sleep, stress, and strain on head and neck muscles.*

### Migraine Headaches

If you've ever experienced pulsating pain on one side of the head in combination with dizzy spells, nausea, and intolerance for light and noise, you are probably one of those who suffer from **migraines,** a type of headache that has severe debilitating symptoms. Many migraine sufferers feel excruciatingly painful, recurring headaches that last for minutes, hours, or even days and possibly some temporary visual impairment. Symptoms vary greatly by individual and attacks typically last anywhere from 4 to 72 hours, with distinct phases. In about 15 percent of cases, migraines are preceded by a sensory warning sign known as an aura, such as flashes of light, flickering vision, blind spots, or tingling in the arms or legs, or sensations of odour or taste. Symptoms of migraine include excruciating pain behind or around

**Asthma:** A chronic respiratory disease characterized by attacks of wheezing, shortness of breath, and coughing spasms.

**Emphysema:** A respiratory disease in which the alveoli become distended or ruptured and no longer functional.

**Alveoli:** Tiny air sacs of the lungs.

**Chronic bronchitis:** A serious respiratory disorder in which the bronchial tubes become so inflamed and swollen that respiratory function is impaired.

**Migraine:** A condition characterized by localized headaches that result from alternating dilation and constriction of blood vessels.

one eye and usually on the same side of the head. In some people, there is sinus pain, neck pain, or an aura without headache. Usually migraine incidence peaks in young adulthood (ages 20–45), the prime years for post-secondary students.[35]

Migraines may occur when blood vessels dilate in the membrane that surrounds the brain. Historically, treatments have centred on reversing or preventing this dilation. Critics of this theory question why only blood vessels of the head dilate in these circumstances. Other researchers believe that migraines are started by disturbances that keep the pain-regulating chemical serotonin from doing its job.

When true migraines occur, relaxation is only minimally effective as a treatment. Often, strong pain-relieving drugs prescribed by a physician are necessary.

## Secondary Headaches

Secondary headaches arise as a result of some other underlying condition. An example is a person with a severe sinus blockage that causes pressure in the sinus cavity. This pressure may induce a headache. Hypertension, allergies, low blood sugar, diseases of the spine, the common cold, poorly fitted dentures, problems with eyesight, and other types of pain or injury can trigger this condition. Relaxation and pain relievers are of little help in treating secondary headaches. Rather, medications or other therapies designed to relieve the underlying organic cause of the headache must be included in the treatment regimen.

## Psychological Headaches

With this type of headache, the "it's all in your head" diagnosis may, in fact, be correct. Rather than having a physical cause, psychological headaches stem from anxiety, depression, and other emotional factors. Psychological headaches result from the stress of emotional disturbances, particularly depression. Unlike tension headaches, no muscles or blood vessels appear to be involved, thereby making relaxation and painkillers ineffective as treatment. Only therapy designed to treat the underlying depression or emotional problem appears to be effective in reducing this kind of headache.

# Seizure Disorders

The word **epilepsy** is derived from the Greek *epilepsia*, meaning "seizure." Reports of epilepsy appeared in Greek medical records as early as 300 B.C. Ancient peoples interpreted seizures as invasions of the body by evil spirits or as punishments by the gods. Although much of the mystery surrounding epileptic seizures has been solved in recent years, the stigma and lack of understanding remain.

These disorders are generally caused by abnormal electrical activity in the brain and are characterized by loss of control of muscular activity and unconsciousness. Symptoms vary widely from person to person.

There are several forms of seizure disorders. The most common are:

1. *Grand mal, or major motor seizure:* These seizures are often preceded by a shrill cry or a seizure aura (body sensations such as ringing in the ears or a specific smell or taste that occurs prior to a seizure). Convulsions and loss of consciousness generally occur and may last from 30 seconds to several minutes or more. Keeping track of the length of time elapsed is one aspect of first aid.
2. *Petit mal, or minor seizure:* These seizures involve no convulsions. Rather, a minor loss of consciousness that may go unnoticed occurs. Minor twitching of muscles may take place, usually for a shorter time than grand mal convulsions.
3. *Psychomotor seizure:* These seizures involve mental processes and muscular activity. Symptoms may include mental confusion and a listless state characterized by activities such as lip smacking, chewing, and repetitive movements.
4. *Jacksonian seizure:* This is a progressive seizure that often begins in one part of the body, such as the fingers, and moves to other parts, such as the hand or arm. Usually only one side of the body is affected.

In the majority of cases, people with seizure disorders can lead normal, seizure-free lives under medical supervision. Epilepsy is seldom fatal. The greatest risk for individuals with epilepsy whose seizures are uncontrolled is motor vehicle or other accidents. Public ignorance about these disorders is one of the most serious obstacles confronting individuals with seizure disorders. Improvements in medication and surgical interventions to reduce some causes of seizures are among the most promising treatments today.

## WHAT WOULD YOU DO?

Do you suffer from recurrent headaches or other neurological problems? What do you do to relieve the symptoms? Have you addressed the underlying causes? If not, why not? What actions might you take to prevent headaches?

# SEX-RELATED DISORDERS

## Fibrocystic Breast Condition

**Fibrocystic breast condition** is a common, non-cancerous problem among women in Canada. Symptoms range in severity from a small palpable lump to large masses of irregular tissue found in both breasts. The underlying causes of the condition are unknown. Although some experts believe it is related to hormonal changes during the normal menstrual cycle, many women report their conditions neither worsen nor improve during their cycles. In fact, in most cases, the condition appears to run in families and to become progressively worse with age, regardless of pregnancy or other hormonal disruptions. Although the majority of these cyst formations consist of fibrous tissue, some are filled with fluid. Treatment often involves removal of fluid from the affected area or surgical removal of the cyst itself.

## Premenstrual Syndrome (PMS)

**Premenstrual syndrome (PMS)** refers to as many as 150 possible physical and emotional symptoms that occur prior to menstruation in some women and vary from woman to woman and from month to month. These symptoms usually appear a week to ten days preceding the menstrual period and may include depression, tension, irritability, headaches, tender breasts, bloated abdomen, backache, abdominal cramps, acne, fluid retention, diarrhea, and fatigue. It is believed that women with PMS develop a predictable pattern of symptoms during the menstrual cycle and that the severity of their symptoms may be influenced by external factors, such as stress.

Women usually experience PMS for the first time after the age of 20, and it may remain a regular part of their reproductive life unless they seek treatment. For many women, the first day of their period brings immediate relief. For others, the depressive symptoms persist all month and are simply heightened before the menstrual period.

Most authorities believe that the most plausible cause of PMS is a hormonal imbalance related to the rise in estrogen levels preceding the menstrual period. This theory is substantiated by the fact that women with PMS given prescriptions for progesterone often experience relief of symptoms. Critics of this theory argue that controlled research has not yet been conducted on the effects of progesterone on PMS.

Common treatments for PMS include hormonal therapy in addition to drugs and behaviours designed to relieve the symptoms. These include Aspirin for pain, diuretics for fluid retention, decreases in caffeine and salt intake, increases in complex carbohydrate intake, stress-reduction techniques, and physical activity.

## Endometriosis

Whether the incidence of **endometriosis** is on the rise or whether the disorder is simply attracting more attention is difficult to determine. Women who develop endometriosis tend to be between the ages of 20 and 40. Symptoms include severe cramping during and between menstrual cycles, irregular periods, unusually heavy or light menstrual flow, abdominal bloating, fatigue, painful bowel movements with periods, painful intercourse, constipation, diarrhea, menstrual pain, infertility, and low back pain. What is this disease? What causes it? What are the common methods of treatment?

Although much remains unknown about the causes of endometriosis, we do know that the disease is characterized by the abnormal growth and development of endometrial tissue (the tissue lining the uterus) in regions of the body other than the uterus. Among the most widely accepted theories concerning the causes of endometriosis are the transmission of endometrial tissue to other regions of the body during surgery or through the birthing process; the movement of menstrual fluid backward through the fallopian tubes during menstruation; and abnormal cell migration through body-fluid movement. Women with cycles shorter than 27 days and those with flows lasting over a week are at increased risk. The more aerobic physical activity a woman engages in and the earlier she starts, the less likely she is to develop endometriosis.

Treatment of endometriosis ranges from bed rest and reduction in stressful activities to **hysterectomy** (the removal of the uterus) or the removal of one or both ovaries and the fallopian tubes. In some areas, where the rate of hysterectomy is high, physicians have been criticized for overreliance on this procedure. More conservative treatments that involve dilation and curettage, surgically scraping endometrial tissue

---

**Epilepsy:** A neurological disorder caused by abnormal electrical brain activity; can be accompanied by altered consciousness or convulsions.

**Fibrocystic breast condition:** A common, noncancerous condition in which a woman's breasts contain fibrous or fluid-filled cysts.

**Premenstrual syndrome (PMS):** A series of physical and emotional symptoms that may occur in women prior to their menstrual periods.

**Endometriosis:** Abnormal development of endometrial tissue outside the uterus resulting in serious side effects.

**Hysterectomy:** Surgical removal of the uterus.

off the fallopian tubes and other reproductive organs, and combinations of hormone therapy have become more acceptable. Hormonal treatments include gonadotropin-releasing hormone (GnRH) analogues, various synthetic progesterone-like drugs (Provera), and oral contraceptives.

# DIGESTION-RELATED DISORDERS

## Diabetes

According to the Canadian Diabetes Association more than 2 million Canadians have **diabetes;** approximately 10 percent of all cases are type 1 diabetes and 90 percent are type 2.[36] Aboriginal people are three to five times more likely to develop type 2 diabetes than the general population. It is further estimated that by the end of the decade 3 million Canadians will have diabetes. An increase in prevalence is expected because (1) the population is aging, (2) obesity rates are rising, (3) 77 percent of new Canadians come from high-risk groups for developing type 2 diabetes (that is, Hispanic, Asian, South Asian, or African descent), and (4) there is a growing incidence of type 2 diabetes in children and high-risk populations. Further, it should be pointed out that approximately one-third of persons with diabetes are undiagnosed.[37]

Contrary to popular belief, diabetes does not result from eating too much sugar, although it does relate to insulin and the body's ability or inability to use sugar. In healthy people, the *pancreas,* a powerful enzyme-producing organ, produces the hormone **insulin** in sufficient quantities to allow the body to use or store glucose (blood sugar). When this organ fails to produce enough insulin to regulate sugar metabolism, or when the body fails to use insulin effectively, diabetes occurs. Individuals with diabetes exhibit **hyperglycemia,** or elevated blood sugar levels, and high glucose levels in their urine. Other symptoms include excessive thirst, frequent urination, hunger, tendency to tire

easily, wounds that heal slowly, numbness or tingling in the extremities, changes in vision, skin eruptions, and, in women, a tendency toward vaginal yeast infections.

Many individuals with diabetes remain unaware of their condition until they begin to show overt symptoms. How does a person develop diabetes? The more serious form, known as type 1 (insulin-dependent) diabetes or diabetes mellitus, usually begins early in life. Individuals with Type 1 diabetes typically depend on insulin injections or oral medications for the rest of their lives, because insulin is not present in their bodies. Non–insulin dependent diabetes (formally termed adult-onset), or type 2 diabetes, in which insulin production is deficient, tends to develop in later life. Individuals with type 2 diabetes can often control the symptoms of their disease with minimal medical intervention through a healthy dietary intake, weight control, and regular physical activity. Following this regimen, they may be able to avoid oral medications or insulin indefinitely.

Diabetes tends to run in families, and a tendency to being overweight, coupled with inactivity, dramatically increases a person's risk. Older persons and mothers of babies weighing over 4 kilograms also run an increased risk. Approximately 80 percent of all patients are overweight at the time of diagnosis. Weight loss and regular physical activity are important factors in lowering blood sugar and improving the efficiency of cellular use of insulin. Both can help to prevent overwork of the pancreas and the development of diabetes. People who develop diabetes today have a much better prognosis than those who developed it 20 or 25 years ago.

Many physicians attempt to control diabetes with a variety of insulin-related drugs. Most of these drugs are taken orally, although self-administered hypodermic injections are prescribed when oral treatments are inadequate. Recent breakthroughs in individual monitoring and the implanting of insulin monitors and insulin infusion pumps that regulate insulin intake "on demand" have provided many individuals with diabetes the opportunity to lead normal lives. Other individuals with diabetes find they can control their diabetes by eating foods rich in complex carbohydrates, low in sodium, and high in fibre, by losing weight, and by getting regular physical activity.

## Colitis and Irritable Bowel Syndrome (IBS)

**Ulcerative colitis** is a disease of the large intestine in which the mucous membranes of the intestinal walls become inflamed. Individuals with severe cases may have as many as 20 bouts of bloody diarrhea a day.

Colitis can also produce severe stomach cramps, weight loss, nausea, sweating, and fever. What causes colitis? We are not sure. Although some experts believe that it occurs more frequently in people with high stress levels, this theory is controversial. Hypersensitivity reactions, particularly to milk and certain foods, have also been considered as a possible cause. It is difficult to determine the cause of colitis because the disease goes into unexplained remission and then recurs without apparent reason. This pattern often continues for years and may be related to the later development of colorectal cancer. Because the cause of colitis remains unknown, treatment focuses exclusively on relieving the symptoms.

Effective measures include increasing fibre intake and taking anti-inflammatory drugs, steroids, and other medications designed to reduce inflammation and soothe irritated intestinal walls.

Many people develop a condition related to colitis known as **irritable bowel syndrome (IBS),** in which nausea, pain, gas, diarrhea, or cramps occur after eating certain foods or when a person is under unusual stress. IBS symptoms commonly begin in early adulthood. Symptoms may vary from week to week and can fade for long periods of time only to return. The cause of IBS is unknown, but researchers suspect that people with IBS have digestive systems overly sensitive to what they eat and drink, to stress, and to certain hormonal changes. They may also be more sensitive to pain signals from the stomach. Stress management, relaxation techniques, regular physical activity, and a healthy dietary intake can bring IBS under control in the vast majority of cases.

## Diverticulosis

**Diverticulosis** occurs when the walls of the intestine become weakened for undetermined reasons and small pea-sized bulges develop. These bulges often fill with feces and, over time, become irritated and infected, causing pain and discomfort. If this irritation persists, bleeding and chronic obstruction may occur, either of which can be life-threatening. If you have a persistent pain in the lower abdominal region, seek medical attention at once.

## Peptic Ulcers

An ulcer is a lesion or wound that forms in body tissue as a result of some form of irritant. A **peptic ulcer** is a chronic ulcer that occurs in the lining of the stomach or the section of the small intestine known as the *duodenum*. It had long been thought to be caused by the erosive effect of digestive juices on these tissues.

Research indicates that most peptic ulcers result from an infection from a common bacteria, *Helicobacter*

*pylori,* and require powerful antibiotics to treat them. This is a dramatic departure from the typical treatment using acid-reducing drugs known as H2 blockers, such as cimetidine (Tagamet) or ranitidine (Zantec). The new treatment recommends a two-week course of antibiotics. H2 blockers are still used in ulcer cases in which excess stomach acid or overuse of drugs such as Aspirin and ibuprofen have caused the irritation.

Ulcers appear to run in families and to be more prevalent in people who are highly stressed over long periods of time and who consume high-fat foods or excessive alcohol. People with ulcers should avoid high-fat foods, alcohol, and substances such as Aspirin that may irritate organ linings or cause increased secretion of stomach acids and thereby exacerbate this condition. In some cases, surgery has been necessary to relieve persistent symptoms.

## Gallbladder Disease

Gallbladder disease, also known as *cholecystitis*, occurs when the gallbladder has been repeatedly irritated by chemicals, infection, or overuse, thus reducing its ability to release bile for the digestion of fats. Usually, gallstones, consisting of calcium, cholesterol, and other minerals, form in the gallbladder itself. When the individual eats foods high in fats, the gallbladder contracts to release bile; these contractions cause pressure on the stone formations. One of the characteristic symptoms of gallbladder disease is acute pain in the upper right portion of the abdomen after eating fatty foods. This pain, which can last several hours, may feel like a heart attack or an ulcer attack and is often accompanied by nausea.

Not all gallstones cause acute pain. In fact, small stones that pass through one of the bile ducts and become lodged may be more painful than gallstones that are the size of golf balls. Many people find out that

**Diabetes:** A disease in which the pancreas fails to produce enough insulin or the body fails to use insulin effectively.

**Insulin:** A hormone produced by the pancreas; required by the body for the metabolism of carbohydrates.

**Hyperglycemia:** Elevated blood sugar levels.

**Ulcerative colitis:** An inflammatory disorder that affects the mucous membranes of the large intestine, producing bloody diarrhea.

**Irritable bowel syndrome (IBS):** Nausea, pain, gas, or diarrhea caused by certain foods or stress.

**Diverticulosis:** A condition in which bulges form in the walls of the intestine; results in irritation and infection of the intestine.

**Peptic ulcer:** Damage to the stomach or intestinal lining, usually caused by digestive juices.

they have gallstones only after undergoing ultrasound and diagnostic X-rays to rule out other conditions. The absence of symptoms is significant because gallstones are considered a predisposing factor for gallbladder cancer.

Current treatment of gallbladder disease usually involves medication to reduce irritation, restriction of fat consumption, and surgery to remove the gallstones. New medications designed to dissolve small gallstones are currently used with some patients. In addition, some doctors use a technique known as lithotripsy, in which a series of noninvasive shock waves break up small stones. Lasers and laparoscopic surgery now reduce the risks associated with large surgical incisions.

## WHAT WOULD YOU DO?

What role does improved dietary intake and regular physical activity have in reducing your risks for and symptoms of the above diseases? Are you or any of your family members at risk for these problems? What actions can you take today that will reduce your risks?

# MUSCULOSKELETAL DISEASES

Most of us will encounter some form of chronic musculoskeletal disease during our lifetime. Some form of arthritis will afflict half of us over 65; low back pain hits most of us at some point in our life. While these diseases are found throughout the world, the treatments differ.

## Arthritis

**Arthritis** is much more than occasional aches or pains; it is a serious and urgent problem in Canada. Currently, more than four million Canadians suffer from some form of arthritis, and more than 600,000 Canadians are disabled by it.[38]

**Osteoarthritis** is a progressive deterioration of bones and joints associated with the "wear and tear" theory of aging. More recent research indicates that as joints are used, they release enzymes that digest cartilage while other cells in the cartilage try to repair the damage. When the enzymatic breakdown overpowers cellular repair, the pain and swelling characteristic of arthritis may occur. Weather extremes, excessive strain, and injury often lead to osteoarthritis flare-ups. But a specific precipitating event does not seem to be

necessary. It is estimated that 85 percent of Canadians will be affected by osteoarthritis by age 70.[39] Although age and injury are undoubtedly factors in the development of osteoarthritis, heredity, abnormal use of the joint, dietary intake, abnormalities in joint structure, and impaired blood supply to the joint may also contribute. Osteoarthritis of the hands seems to have a particularly strong genetic component. Extreme disability as a result of osteoarthritis is rare. However, when joints become so distorted that they impair activity, surgical intervention is often necessary. Joint replacement and bone fusion are common surgical repair techniques. For most people, anti-inflammatory drugs and pain relievers such as Aspirin and cortisone-related agents ease discomfort. In some, applications of heat, mild physical activity, and massage may also relieve the pain.

**Rheumatoid arthritis** is similar but far more serious than osteoarthritis. Rheumatoid arthritis is an inflammatory joint disease that can occur at any age, but most commonly appears between the ages of 20 and 45. It is three times more common among women than men during early adulthood but equally common among men and women in the over-70 age group. Symptoms may be gradually progressive or sporadic, with occasional unexplained remissions.

Rheumatoid arthritis typically attacks the synovial membrane, which produces the lubricating fluids for the joints. Advanced rheumatoid arthritis often involves destruction of the bony ends of joints. The remedy for this condition is typically bone fusion, which leaves the joint immobile. In some instances, joint replacement may be a viable alternative.

Although the exact cause of this form of arthritis is unknown, some experts theorize that it is an autoimmune disorder, in which the body responds as if its own cells were the enemy, eventually destroying the affected body parts. Other theorists believe that rheumatoid arthritis is caused by some form of invading microorganism that takes over the joint. Certain toxic chemicals and stress have also been mentioned as possible causes.

Regardless of the cause, treatment of rheumatoid arthritis is similar to that for osteoarthritis. Emphasis is placed on pain relief and attempts to improve the functional mobility of the patient. In some instances, immunosuppressant drugs are also given to reduce the inflammatory response.

Fibromyalgia is a chronic, painful rheumatological-like disorder. Symptoms include widespread pain; stiffness and numerous tender points; weakness; swelling; and neurovascular complaints including coldness, numbness, tingling, mottled skin, headaches, auditory sensitivity, irritable bowel syndrome, sleep disorders, depression, and dysmenorrhea. The cause of fibromyalgia remains a mystery, with many theories under investigation. Acute sleep disturbances, muscular irregularities, and forms of psychopathological disturbance have been considered as possible culprits. What is known is that the disease primarily affects women (particularly in their 30s and 40s), that the disease causes more chronic pain and debilitation than other musculoskeletal disorders, and that significant research must be conducted before an effective, long-term treatment will be available.

## Systemic Lupus Erythematosus (SLE)

**Lupus** is a disease in which the immune system attacks the body, producing antibodies that destroy or injure organs such as the kidneys, brain, and heart. The symptoms vary from mild to severe and may disappear for periods of time. A butterfly-shaped rash covering the bridge of the nose and both cheeks is common. Nearly all individuals with SLE have aching joints and muscles, and 60 percent develop redness and swelling that moves from joint to joint. Extensive research has not yet found a cure for this sometimes fatal disease.

## Low Back Pain

Most people (about 80 percent) will experience low back pain at some point during their life. Although some of these low back pain (LBP) episodes may result from muscular damage and be short-lived and acute, others may involve dislocations, fractures, or other problems with spinal vertebrae or discs and be chronic or require surgery. LBP is epidemic throughout the world.

### Risk Factors for Low Back Pain

Health experts believe that the following factors contribute to LBP:

- advancing age
- body types
- poor posture
- poor muscular strength and endurance
- psychological factors
- occupational risks

### Preventing Back Pain and Injury

Almost 90 percent of all back problems occur in the lumbar spine region (lower back). Consciously protecting this region of the body from blows, excessive strain, or sharp twists when muscles are not warmed up is essential. You can reduce many problems by consciously attempting to maintain good posture when sitting, standing, and sleeping.

In addition, physical activity, particularly activities that strengthen the abdominal muscles and the muscles that support the spine and stretch the back muscles, are important. It is also important to sleep on a supportive mattress, to work in an ergonomically friendly environment (supportive chair with feet flat on the floor, computer at eye level, keyboard appropriately placed, etc.), to lift heavy objects with your knees rather than your back, to avoid high-heeled and otherwise poorly-fitting shoes, and to engage in regular physical activity. If you injure your back, be sure to consult with at least two different experts in rehabilitation and therapy to determine your best options. Consult an exercise physiologist, biomechanist, ergonomist, physical therapist, or physician specializing in bone and joint injuries for recommended physical activities.

# OTHER MALADIES

During the last decade or so, numerous afflictions have surfaced that seem to be products of our times. Some of these health problems relate to specific groups of people, some are due to technological advances, and some are unexplainable. Still other diseases have been present for many years and continue to cause severe disability (see Table 13.5). Among conditions that have received attention in recent years are chronic fatigue syndrome and disorders related to the use of video display terminals.

## Chronic Fatigue Syndrome (CFS)

In the late 1980s, a characteristic set of symptoms was noted that included chronic fatigue, headaches, fever, sore throat, enlarged lymph nodes, depression, poor memory, general weakness, nausea, and symptoms remarkably similar to mononucleosis. Researchers initially believed that individuals were really talking about a series of symptoms caused by the Epstein-Barr virus, the same virus as mononucleosis. In some

---

**Arthritis:** Painful inflammatory disease of the joints.

**Osteoarthritis:** A progressive deterioration of bones and joints associated with the "wear and tear" theory of aging.

**Rheumatoid arthritis:** A serious inflammatory joint disease.

**Lupus:** A disease in which the immune system attacks the body, producing antibodies that destroy or injure organs such as the kidneys, brain, and heart.

TABLE 13.5

**Other Modern Afflictions**

| Disease | Description | Treatment |
|---|---|---|
| Parkinson's disease | Disease affecting mostly people over the age of 55. Symptoms include tremors, rigidity, slowed movement, loss of autonomic movements, and difficulty walking. | Unknown cause makes prevention difficult. Tranquillizers are useful in controlling nerve responses. |
| Multiple sclerosis | Disease that affects women more than men. Precise cause uncertain. Symptoms include vision problems, tingling and numbness in extremities, chronic fatigue, and neurological impairments. | Medication to control symptoms and slow progression of the disease. Stress management may be helpful. |
| Cystic fibrosis | Inherited disease occurring in 1 out of every 1,600 births. Characterized by pooling of large amounts of mucus in lungs, digestive disturbances, and excessive sodium excretion. Results in premature death. | Most treatments are geared toward relief of symptoms. Antibiotics are administered for infection. Recent strides in genetic research suggest better treatments and potential cure in the near future. |
| Sickle cell disease | Inherited disease affecting mostly blacks. Disease affects hemoglobin, forming sickle-shaped red blood cells that interfere with oxygenation. Results in severe pain, anemia, and premature death. | Reduce stress and attend to minor infections immediately. Seek genetic counselling. |
| Cerebral palsy | Disorder characterized by the loss of voluntary control over motor functioning. Believed to be caused by a lack of oxygen to the brain at birth, brain disorders or an accident before or after birth, poisoning, or brain infections. | Follow preventive actions to reduce accident risks; improved neonatal and birthing techniques. |
| Graves' disease | Thyroid disorder characterized by swelling of the eyes, staring gaze, and retraction of the eyelid. Can result in loss of sight. The cause is unknown and it can occur at any age. | Medication may help control symptoms. Radioactive iodine supplements also may be administered. |

instances, the symptoms were so severe that individuals required hospitalization. Since those initial studies, researchers have all but ruled out the possibility of a mysterious form of the Epstein-Barr virus. Despite extensive testing, no viral cause has been found.

Today, in the absence of a known pathogen, many researchers believe that the illness, now commonly referred to as chronic fatigue syndrome (CFS), may have strong psychosocial roots.

The diagnosis of chronic fatigue syndrome depends on two major criteria and eight or more minor criteria. The major criteria are debilitating fatigue that persists for at least six months and the absence of diagnoses of other illnesses that could cause the symptoms. Minor criteria include headaches, fever, sore throat, painful lymph nodes, weakness, fatigue after physical activity, sleep problems, and rapid onset of these symptoms. Because an exact cause is not apparent, treatment of CFS focuses on improved dietary intake, rest, counselling for

# Managing Your Disease Risks

Infectious diseases pose serious challenges throughout the world. In particular, sexually transmitted infections, including HIV, present an increasing health risk to young people. Infectious diseases can be prevented by practising safe and responsible behaviours. In addition, many noninfectious diseases can be prevented or their onset delayed by making positive personal health choices.

## MAKING DECISIONS FOR YOU

Protecting yourself from infectious diseases is not always easy. Because most pathogens are microscopic, exposure to one can occur without your knowledge. Therefore, you need to be aware of your risks. What can you do to improve your own awareness of your potential exposure to disease-causing pathogens?

What are some actions you can take to reduce your risk of contracting a sexually transmitted infection? What steps could you take right now to ensure the sexual health of your partners? Finally, if you thought you had been exposed to HIV, would you seek testing?

## CHECKLIST FOR CHANGE: MAKING PERSONAL CHOICES

- Be aware of factors that threaten your health. Know your disease and immunization history.
- Take the precautions needed to protect yourself from exposure to infectious pathogens.
- Know the health status of your intimate partners.
- Communicate openly and honestly with your partners about your feelings regarding sexual intimacy.
- Wash your hands frequently and thoroughly with soap and water.
- Limit travel to places where outbreaks of infectious diseases have not been controlled.
- Maintain a healthy routine of adequate sleep, good dietary intake, and regular physical activity.
- Cook foods at their appropriate temperatures. Keep hot foods hot, and cold foods cold.
- Recognize the symptoms that indicate a possible infection and seek treatment immediately.
- Recognize your responsibility for the health of others.
- Behave in sexually responsible ways.
- Limit your sexual partners.
- Limit alcohol or other drug use during intimate sexual encounters.
- Assess your level of risk for acquiring an STI, including HIV.
- Respect the rights and needs of individuals affected by an infectious disease.

- Adopt personal health habits that will reduce your risk of a chronic disease.
- Identify actions you can take today to reduce your risks for the diseases and disorders discussed in this chapter.

## CHECKLIST FOR CHANGE: MAKING COMMUNITY CHOICES

- Does your student health service offer testing for all STIs, including HIV?
- Do you support government spending for HIV research and health promotion?
- Does your local school system offer a sex education curriculum including discussion about how to stop the spread of STIs, including HIV?
- If you worked for a government agency charged with helping people improve their personal health habits, what approaches would you take?
- Have you done anything to support campaigns raising money for research into chronic illnesses?
- What role should businesses play in improving employee health? Should the federal government provide tax credits to help businesses support employee health?

## CRITICAL THINKING

You have been in a relationship for several months that has grown from a nice friendship to a state of passionate sexual intimacy. During this time, a close and trusting bond has also developed. You have remained monogamous and believe that your partner has as well, although you have never discussed it. Nor has any discussion arisen about each other's sexual history or HIV status. You have been involved in sexual relationships in the past and have never been tested for HIV antibodies, and you're quite certain your partner is experienced as well. You trust your partner but recognize that, without complete information, you are both at risk for HIV infection. You want to take some precautionary steps but worry about insulting your partner's feelings.

Use the DECIDE model described in Chapter 1 to decide what you would do in this situation. Develop several different strategies and approaches for reaching the desired result.

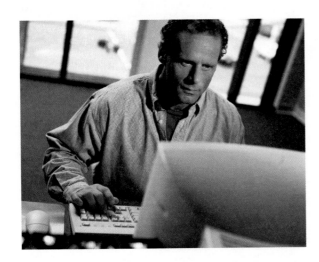

*Working in front of a computer for several hours a day can put you at risk for eyestrain and back, neck, shoulder, and wrist pain.*

depression, judicious physical activity, and development of a strong support network.

## Job-Related Disorders

During the last decade, a new potential health risk for computer users has been the topic of growing debate. Adverse health effects have been noted in people who work at computer video display terminals (VDTs) for several hours per day. Many post-secondary students are regular high-volume users of VDTs and are therefore at risk.

Most of these problems relate to eyestrain and discomfort in the low back, neck, shoulders, and wrists. Questions about the danger posed by radiation from the electrical fields produced within the circuits of the VDT and about the potential effects on pregnant women and their fetuses remain unanswered.

**Carpal tunnel syndrome** is a common occupational injury in which the median nerve in the wrist becomes irritated, causing numbness, tingling, and pain in the fingers and hands. This condition is worsened by the repetitive typing motions made by computer users and is often classified as a common repetitive motion injury. For those who must work on a computer for hours at a time, day after day, ergonomists recommend regular breaks. Remove your hands from the keyboard to move them about every 20 minutes; stretch other body parts such as the neck and shoulders periodically. Physically remove yourself from your computer at least once every hour for several minutes, perhaps walking around the room or doing some simple stretches. Paying attention to the design, height, and support of your chair, and placing your keyboard at a comfortable angle and height, can save countless hours of suffering—though they do not remove the need to get up and move every so often.

**Carpal tunnel syndrome:** A common occupational injury in which the median nerve in the wrist becomes irritated, causing numbness, tingling, and pain in the fingers and hands.

# SUMMARY

- The major uncontrollable risk factors for contracting infectious diseases are heredity, age, and environmental conditions. The major controllable risk factors are stress, dietary intake, inactivity, insufficient sleep, poor hygiene, and drug use and other high-risk behaviours.

- The major pathogens are bacteria, viruses, fungi, protozoa, parasitic worms, and rickettsia.

- Your body uses a number of defence systems to keep pathogens from invading. The skin is our major protection, helped by enzymes. The immune system creates antibodies to destroy antigens. In addition, fever and pain play a role in protecting the body. Vaccines bolster the body's immune system against specific diseases.

- Sexually transmitted infections are spread through vaginal, oral, and anal sex, hand–genital contact, and sometimes through mouth-to-mouth contact. Major STIs include chlamydia, pelvic inflammatory disease, gonorrhea, syphilis, pubic lice, venereal warts, candidiasis, trichomoniasis, and herpes.

- Acquired immune deficiency syndrome (AIDS) is caused by the human immunodeficiency virus (HIV). HIV is not confined to certain high-risk groups. Your risk for HIV infection can be reduced by not engaging in risky sexual activities or sharing needles.

- Headaches may be caused by a variety of factors, the most common of which are tension, dilation and/or contraction of blood vessels in the brain, chemical influences on muscles and vessels that cause inflammation and pain, and underlying physiological and psychological disorders.

- Several modern maladies affect only women. Fibrocystic breast condition is a common, noncancerous buildup of irregular tissue. Premenstrual syndrome (PMS) is the name given to a wide variety of symptoms related to the menstrual cycle. Endometriosis is the buildup of endometrial tissue in regions of the body other than the uterus.
- Pathogens, problems in enzyme or hormone production, anxiety or stress, functional abnormalities, and other problems are often listed as probable causes of digestive disorders.
- Musculoskeletal diseases such as arthritis, lower back pain, repetitive motion injuries, and other problems cause significant pain and disability in millions of people.

# DISCUSSION QUESTIONS

1. What is a pathogen? What are the similarities and differences between pathogens and antigens? What are the risk factors that can threaten your health? What factors are controllable?

2. What is the difference between natural and acquired immunity?

3. Identify five sexually transmitted infections. Identify their symptoms in men and women. How do they develop? How are they treated? What are their potential long-term risks?

4. Why might it be inappropriate to identify groups as at high risk for HIV infection? Why might HIV infection be better referred to as a sexually transmissible infection than as a sexually transmitted infection?

5. What are some of the major noninfectious chronic diseases affecting Canadians today? What are the common risk factors? How are they treated?

6. List the common respiratory diseases affecting Canadians. Which of these diseases have a genetic basis? An environmental basis? An individual basis?

7. Compare and contrast the different types of headaches, including their symptoms and treatments. What can be done to prevent them? Treat them?

8. Do you believe that PMS is a disorder or disease or simply a catchall name for many naturally occurring events in the menstrual cycle? Why?

9. What are the medical risks of fibrocystic breast condition and endometriosis? How can they be treated? Prevented?

10. Describe the symptoms and treatment of diabetes. How can type 2 diabetes be prevented?

11. How can you tell whether your stomach is reacting to final exams or telling you that you have a serious medical condition?

# APPLICATION EXERCISE

Reread the What Do You Think? scenario at the beginning of this chapter and answer the following questions.

1. What was your initial reaction to this scenario? Why?

2. What are some legal issues that could arise or that already exist regarding all infectious diseases, including STIs? Why do the rights of all the individuals involved in relationships need to be considered?

3. What services exist on your campus for people living with HIV infection or AIDS? What services focus on informing people about sexually transmitted infections?

# HEALTH ON THE NET

Sexuality and You
**www.sexualityandu.ca**

Public Health Agency of Canada
**www.phac-aspc.gc.ca**

Canadian Diabetes Association
**www.diabetes.ca**

World Health Organization
**www.who.int**

# CHAPTER 14

# LIFE'S TRANSITIONS

*The Aging Process*

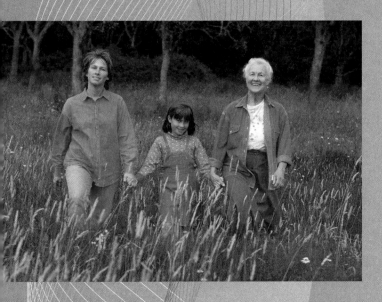

# CHAPTER OBJECTIVES

- Define aging, and explain the related concepts of biological, psychological, social, legal, and functional age.

- Explain the impact on society of the growing population of the elderly, including considerations of economics, health care, housing and living arrangements, and ethical and moral issues.

- Discuss the biological and psychosocial theories of aging and examine how knowledge of these theories may have an impact on your aging process.

- Identify the major physiological and mental changes that occur as a result of the aging process.

- Discuss the unique health challenges faced by the elderly.

- Define death using different criteria and explain why people deny death.

- Describe the stages of the grieving process and several strategies for coping more effectively.

- Describe the ethical concerns that arise from the concepts of the right to die and rational suicide.

Bonnie, aged 82, is a springboard diver. She walks 10 blocks every morning to the city pool, where she practises her diving and swims to stay in shape. Erin, aged 79, is an internationally recognized expert in family dysfunction. She travels extensively, giving several lectures a week, volunteering her services to community groups and maintaining an active social life. Stewart, aged 83, is a master's level marathoner. He lifts weights regularly, runs or rides a bike, and hikes the hills and valleys around his home when he is not training for his next race. He is a professional writer and recently learned how to run the latest versions of software programs on his computer. He keeps in touch with his children and grandchildren using various modes of electronic communication.

■ What do all these people have in common? Are these people atypical? Why or why not? What factors do you think contributed to their healthy aging? Do you know any elderly people like them? How do these people compare to your grandparents?

In a society that appears to worship youth, researchers have begun to offer good—even revolutionary—news about the aging process. Growing old does not have to mean declining physical and mental health. Health promotion, disease prevention and wellness-oriented activities can prolong vigour and productivity, even among those who may not have always led a model lifestyle or made healthy choices a priority. Getting older can mean getting better in many ways—particularly socially, psychologically, spiritually, and intellectually.

The manner in which you view aging (either as a natural part of living or as an inevitable move toward disease and death) is an important factor in how successfully you will adapt to life's transitions. If you view these transitions as periods of growth, as changes that will lead to improved mental, emotional, spiritual, and physical phases in your development as a human being, your journey through even the most difficult times may be easier. Explore your own knowledge of aging in the Rate Yourself box.

Getting older is something that cannot be avoided, despite the perennial human quest for a fountain of youth. Since you can't stop the process, why not resolve to have a positive aging experience by improving your understanding of the various aspects of aging, taking steps toward maximizing your potential, and learning to adapt and develop strengths you can draw on over a lifetime? **Aging** has traditionally been described as the patterns of life changes that occur in members of all species as they grow older. Some believe that it begins at the moment of conception. Others contend that it starts at birth. Still others believe that true aging does not begin until we reach our 40s. Typically, experts and laypersons alike have used chronological age to assign a person to a particular life-cycle stage. However, people of different chronological ages view age very differently. To the 4-year-old, a university or college student seems quite old. To the 20-year-old, parents in their 40s are over the hill. Have you ever heard your 65-year-old grandparents talking about "those old people down the street"? Views of aging are also coloured by occupation. For example, a professional linebacker may find himself too old to play football in his mid-30s. Although some baseball players have continued to demonstrate high levels of skill into their 40s, most players are considering other careers by the time they reach 40. Airline pilots and police officers are often retired in their 50s, while professors, senators, and prime ministers may work well into their 70s. Perhaps our traditional definitions of aging need careful re-examination.

# REDEFINING AGING

Discrimination against people based on age is known as **ageism.** When directed against the elderly, this type of discrimination carries with it social ostracism and negative portrayals of older people. A developmental task approach to life-span changes tends to reduce the potential for ageist or negatively biased perceptions about what occurs as a person ages chronologically.

The study of individual and collective aging processes, known as **gerontology,** explores the reasons for aging and the ways in which people cope with and adapt to this process. Gerontologists have identified several types of age-related characteristics that should be used to determine where a person is in terms of biological, psychological, social, legal, and functional life-stage development:[1]

■ *Biological age* refers to the relative age or condition of the person's organs and body systems. Arthritis and other chronic conditions often accelerate biological age.

■ *Psychological age* refers to a person's adaptive capacities, such as coping abilities and intelligence,

**Aging:** The patterns of life changes that occur in members of all species as they grow older.

**Ageism:** Discrimination based on age.

**Gerontology:** The study of our individual and collective aging processes.

# Aging Quiz

Test your knowledge of healthy aging by taking the following test. Answer true or false to each statement. The answers are listed below

1. Men usually outlive women.
2. If your parents had Alzheimer's disease, you will also get it.
3. Dietary intake and physical activity can reduce the risk of developing osteoporosis.
4. Heart disease affects women as much as men.
5. The older you get, the less sleep you need.
6. People should watch their weight as they age.
7. People take more medications as they age.
8. As your body changes with age, so does your personality.
9. Intelligence declines with age.
10. Most older people live alone.
11. Most people become "senile" if they live long enough.
12. Physical strength tends to decline with age.
13. Most seniors limit their travel to be closer to home.
14. Seniors have the lowest income of all adult groups.
15. Most older adults have no interest in, or capacity for, sexual relations.
16. People tend to become more religious with age.
17. People tend to change their driving habits as they age.
18. Older people are more likely to commit suicide than younger people.
19. Many older people are preoccupied with death.
20. Most seniors who are new to Canada speak neither English nor French.

## ANSWERS

1. **False**. Women have an average life expectancy greater than men. In 1996, a 65-year old woman could expect to live an additional 19.8 years, approximately four years longer than her male counterpart.
2. **False**. Between 90 and 95 percent of people with Alzheimer's disease have a form of the disease not necessarily linked to family history. Only 5 percent of Alzheimer's cases are a result of a genetic link.
3. **True.** Bone loss can be reduced by eating foods rich in calcium (for example, milk and other dairy products, dark green, leafy vegetables, canned salmon, sardines, and tofu) and engaging in regular, weight-bearing physical activity, such as walking and resistance training.
4. **True**. Heart disease is one of the leading causes of death for men and women.

5. **False**. Although quality of sleep declines when we age, required sleep time does not. Further, sleep tends to get more fragmented as we get older.
6. **True**. Older people need fewer calories because of decreases in metabolic function and physical activity. If an involuntary weight gain or loss of 5 kg or more occurs in six months, a physician should be consulted.
7. **True**. Most Canadian seniors take some form of prescription or over-the-counter medication. Further, older seniors (85+) are more likely than younger seniors (65–74) to take more than one medication (65 vs. 52 percent).
8. **False**. Other than personality changes associated with Alzheimer's disease and other forms of dementia, personality does not change appreciably as you age.
9. **False.** Although studies show that the elderly have a slower reaction time and take longer to learn something new, their intellect is maintained and can be improved as they get older.
10. **False.** The majority of Canadian seniors (69 percent) live with their family or extended family.
11. **False**. Dementia (senility is not the correct term) is not a normal part of aging. One in 50 seniors between the ages of 65 and 74, one in nine seniors between the ages of 75 and 84, and one in three seniors over the age of 85 will develop dementia.
12. **True**. Physical strength does decrease with age—as does the quality of the muscles. Decreases in strength can be reduced by regular participation in physical activity, including resistance training.
13. **False**. In fact, some seniors are more likely to travel abroad than younger adults.
14. **True.** In 1997, 19 percent of all seniors (65+) had an income below the low-income cut-off. Women (24 percent) are more likely than men (11.7 percent) to have a low income.
15. **False.** Aging does not equate to a loss of interest in or capacity for sex.
16. **False**. Despite a perception that people tend to become more religious with age, this is not true. This perception may reflect a difference between generations rather than a characteristic of aging.
17. **True.** To accommodate the changes associated with aging many seniors modify their driving behaviour by planning their trips, driving less, limiting highway travel, and avoiding driving in bad weather or at night.

and to the person's awareness of his or her individual capabilities, self-efficacy, and general ability to adapt to a given situation.

- *Social age* refers to a person's habits and roles relative to society's expectations. People in a particular life stage often share similar tastes in music, television shows, and decor.

- *Legal* or *chronological age* is probably the most common definition of age in Canada. Legal age is based on chronological years and is used to determine such things as voting rights, driving privileges, drinking age, eligibility for Old Age Security and Canada Pension Plan benefits, and a host of other rights and obligations.

- *Functional age* refers to the ways in which people compare to others of a similar age. It is difficult to separate functional aging from other types of aging, particularly chronological and biological aging.

# WHAT IS NORMAL AGING?

Contemporary gerontologists have begun to analyze the vast majority of people who continue to live full and productive lives throughout their later years. In the past, our youth-oriented society has viewed the onset of the physiological changes that occur with aging as something to be dreaded. The aging process was seen primarily from a pathological (disease) perspective, and therefore as a time of decline; the focus was not on the gains and positive aspects of normal adult development throughout the life span. Many of these positive developments occur in the areas of emotional and social life as older adults learn to cope with and adapt to the many changes and crises that life has in store for them.

Gerontologists have devised several categories for specific age-related characteristics. For example, people who reach the age of 65 are considered to fit the general category of old age. They receive special consideration in the form of government assistance programs such as the old age pension.

People aged 65 to 74 are viewed as the **young-old;** those aged 75 to 84 are the **middle-old** group; those 85 and over are classified as the **old-old.**

You should note that chronological age is not the only component considered when objectively defining aging. The question is not how many years a person has lived, but how much life a person has packed into those years. This quality-of-life index, combined with the inevitable chronological process, appears to be the best indicator of the "aging gracefully" phenomenon. The eternal question then becomes, "How can I age gracefully?" Most experts agree that the best way to experience a productive, full, and satisfying old age is to take appropriate action to lead a productive, full, and satisfying life prior to old age. Essentially, older people are the product of their lifelong experiences, moulded over years of happiness, heartbreak, and day-to-day existence.

## WHAT WOULD YOU DO?

How do you define aging? What factors influence the aging process? Which of these factors do you have the power to change through the behaviours that you engage in right now?

## Who Are the Elderly?

Contrary to popular belief, the elderly are not and never will be the "forgotten minority." The 65-and-over age group will unquestionably continue to be a major force in the social, political, and economic plans of the nation because of their sheer numbers (see Table 14.1) and buying power. Canadian seniors are living longer lives in better health than in the past. By the year 2010, a whole generation of 1960s "flower children," who once proclaimed that no one over 30

**Young-old:** People aged 65 to 74.

**Middle-old:** People aged 75 to 84.

**Old-old:** People 85 and over.

**TABLE 14.1**

Canada's Elderly

| Age | Total | Men | Women |
|-----|-------|-----|-------|
| 65–69 | 1,193,500 | 574,400 | 619,100 |
| 70–74 | 1,042,600 | 488,600 | 554,000 |
| 75–79 | 864,300 | 377,700 | 486,500 |
| 80–84 | 625,300 | 241,700 | 383,600 |
| 85–89 | 322,500 | 107,100 | 215,400 |
| 90 and over | 169,500 | 44,600 | 125,000 |

Source: Statistics Canada. "Population by Sex and Age Group," retrieved on May 16, 2006, from www40.statcan.ca/101/cst01/ demo10a.htm.

could be trusted, will be turning 65. Whereas people aged 65 and older made up less than 10 percent of the population in 1981, they are projected to make up more than 20 percent by 2031. In 2005, it was estimated that 4.22 million Canadians, or 13 percent of the population, were 65 years of age or older (see Table 14.2).[2]

For a more detailed profile of today's elderly, download "Canada's Aging Population," a report prepared by Health Canada in collaboration with the Interdepartmental Committee on Aging and Seniors Issues, at www.globalaging.org/elderrights/world/canada.pdf.

# THEORIES ON AGING
## Biological Theories

Explanations about the biological causes of aging include:

- The *wear-and-tear theory*, which states that, like everything else in the universe, the human body wears out. Inherent in this theory is the idea that the more you abuse your body, the faster it will wear out.

- The *cellular theory*, which states that at birth we have only a certain number of usable cells, and these cells are genetically programmed to divide or reproduce only a limited number of times. Once these cells reach the end of their reproductive cycle, they begin to die and the organs they make up begin to show signs of deterioration. The rate of deterioration varies from person to person, and the impact of the deterioration depends on the system involved.

- The *autoimmune theory*, which attributes aging to the decline of the body's immunological system. Studies indicate that as we age, our immune systems become less effective in fighting disease. Lifestyle can contribute negatively to this process in bodies subjected to too much stress, lack of sleep, a poor dietary intake, inactivity, and so on. Although autoimmune diseases occur in all age groups, some gerontologists believe that they increase in frequency and severity with age.

**TABLE 14.2**

Age Structure of Population, Medium-Growth Scenario (in millions)

| Age | 1996 | 2000 | 2006 | 2016 | 2026 | 2036 | 2051 |
|-----|------|------|------|------|------|------|------|
| 0 to 14 | 5,992 | 5,869 | 5,527 | 5,241 | 5,382 | 5,203 | 5,053 |
| 15 to 64 | 20,098 | 21,018 | 22,400 | 23,477 | 23,056 | 22,765 | 22,440 |
| 65 and over | 3,582 | 3,863 | 4,302 | 5,702 | 7,753 | 9,067 | 9,366 |
| Total | 29,672 | 30,750 | 32,229 | 34,420 | 36,191 | 37,035 | 36,860 |

| **Percentage** | | | | | | | |
|-----|------|------|------|------|------|------|------|
| **Age** | **1996** | **2000** | **2006** | **2016** | **2026** | **2036** | **2051** |
| 0 to 14 | 20.2 | 19.1 | 17.1 | 15.2 | 14.9 | 14.0 | 13.7 |
| 15 to 64 | 67.7 | 68.3 | 69.5 | 68.2 | 63.7 | 61.5 | 60.9 |
| 65 and over | 12.1 | 12.6 | 13.3 | 16.6 | 21.4 | 24.5 | 25.4 |

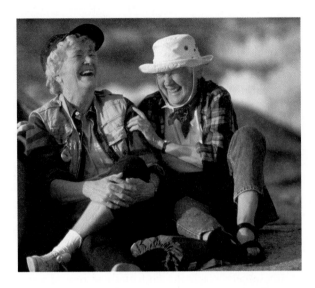

*For many, the secret to aging well is to remain physically active and enjoy the company of good friends.*

- The *genetic mutation theory,* which proposes that the number of cells exhibiting unusual or different characteristics increases with age. Proponents of this theory believe that aging is related to the amount of mutational damage within the genes. The greater the mutation, the greater the chance that cells will not function properly, leading to eventual dysfunction of body organs and systems.

## Psychosocial Theories

Numerous psychological and sociological factors also have a strong influence on the manner in which people age. Psychologists have formulated theories of personality development that encompass the human life span. These theories emphasize adaptation and adjustment. In the developmental model, it is noted that people must progress through eight critical stages during their lifetime. If a person does not receive adequate stimulation or develop effective methods of coping with life's stresses from infancy onward, problems are likely to develop later in life. According to this theory, attitudes, behaviours, and beliefs related to maladjustments in old age are often a result of problems encountered in earlier stages of a person's life. Specifically, the developmental theory focuses on the crucial issues of middle and old age because it is believed that during these periods people face a series of increasingly stressful tasks. Those who are poorly adjusted psychologically or who have not developed appropriate coping skills are likely to undergo a painful aging process.

A key element in these theories is the incorporation of age-related factors into lifelong behaviour patterns. Both models (biological and psychosocial) stress that successful aging involves maintaining emotional as well as physical well-being. Most probably, a combination of psychosocial and biological factors and environmental "trigger mechanisms" causes each of us to age in a unique manner. The question then arises as to what is considered normal in the aging process. How much change is inevitable and how much can be avoided or delayed?

# CHANGES IN THE BODY AND MIND

Answers to the question of what is "typical" or "normal" when applied to aging are highly speculative. In order to assess the typical aging process, we should probably ask ourselves what we can reasonably expect to happen to our bodies as we grow older. It is important to keep in mind that despite physical changes that occur, 76 percent of seniors 65 to 74 years old and 68 percent of seniors over 75 years of age reported their health to be "good," "very good," or "excellent."[3]

## Physical Changes

Although the physiological consequences of aging differ in their severity and timing from person to person, there are standard changes that occur.

### The Skin

As we age, the skin becomes thinner and loses elasticity, particularly in the outer surfaces. Fat deposits, which add to the soft lines and shape of the skin, begin to diminish. Starting at about age 30, lines develop on the forehead as a result of smiling, squinting, and other facial expressions. These lines become more pronounced, with added "crow's-feet" around the eyes, during the 40s. During a person's 50s and 60s, the skin begins to sag and lose colour, leading to pallor in the 70s. Body fat in underlying layers of skin continues to be redistributed away from the limbs and extremities into the trunk region of the body. Age spots become more numerous because of excessive pigment accumulation under the skin. The sun tends to increase pigment production, leading to more age spots.

### Bones and Joints

Throughout the life span, your bones are continually changing because of the accumulation and loss of minerals. By the third or fourth decade of life, bone mineral loss often exceeds bone mineral accumulation, resulting in a deterioration of bone tissue in which bones become fragile and brittle and thus at an increased risk of fracture. This loss of bone mineral content (particularly calcium) occurs in men and women, although it tends to occur at a faster rate in women. Loss of bone mineral content can contribute to **osteoporosis,** a condition characterized by weakened, porous, and fractured bones.

Although many people consider osteoporosis a disease of the elderly, it is actually a progressive disorder with roots firmly established in childhood and adolescence. When you hear of osteoporosis, you likely envision a slumped-over individual with a characteristic "dowager's hump" in the upper back, but this is the rare extreme. Bone loss occurs over many years and may be without symptoms until fractures occur. The spine, hips, and wrists are the most common sites of fractures, though other bones of the body may be involved.[4]

Osteoporotic fractures of the hip, vertebrae, proximal humerus, pelvis, and wrist increase in incidence with age and are more common among women. It is estimated that one in four women aged 60 years and over will have an osteoporotic fracture.[5] Further, about one-third of all women aged 65 and over are afflicted with vertebral osteoporosis. About 70 percent of all fractures among those in individuals over the age of 45 result from osteoporosis. Several risk factors for developing osteoporosis have been identified:[6]

- *Sex:* Women's risk is four times greater than men's. Their peak bone mass is lower than men's, and they experience an accelerated rate of bone loss after menopause.

- *Age:* After the third and fourth decade of life, all individuals lose bone mass and are more susceptible—particularly if sedentary.

- *Low bone mass:* Low bone mass is one of the strongest predictors of osteoporosis. Measurement of bone density is an important aspect of risk assessment. Low bone mass is often a result of inadequate bone-growth stimulation (inactivity), poor dietary intake (lack of total calories and insufficient calcium intake), estrogen suppression (delayed onset of menarche, amenorrhea), and smoking.

- *Early menopause:* The early occurrence of menopause, whether natural or caused by surgery, means that the positive effects of estrogen are lost for a longer period of time. (Decreases in sex hormones—estrogen in females and testosterone in males—appear to increase risk for the disease.) Menstrual disturbances, such as those caused by anorexia nervosa or bulimia nervosa or excessive exercise without an adequate dietary intake, may similarly result in an early loss of bone mineral.

- *Thin, small-framed body:* Petite, thin women usually have a relatively low bone mass and are therefore at greater risk for osteoporosis. (This is one of the few health areas in which being larger and even slightly overweight is an advantage.)

- *Race:* Whites and Asians are at higher risk of developing osteoporosis than blacks because blacks have greater bone density on average. Black women have about half the incidence of hip fractures of white women.

- *Lack of calcium:* A lifetime of low calcium intake (well below the DRI [dietary reference intake] and below the natural loss of calcium of 300 to 400 milligrams per day) may result in a lower than expected peak bone mineral content and above-average loss of bone mineral content throughout adulthood.

- *Lack of physical activity:* Immobilized, bedridden, or very inactive people usually have less muscle and bone mass.

- *Cigarette smoking:* It is thought that smoking suppresses estrogen, thereby reducing bone mineral accrual.

- *Alcohol and/or caffeine:* Excessive use is linked to the development of osteoporosis.

- *Heredity:* Hereditary factors may play a role in the development of osteoporosis.

The goal of treatment and prevention of osteoporosis is to decrease the likelihood and severity of bone fractures. Currently accepted treatments of established osteoporosis include adequate calcium intake, daily weight-bearing physical activity approved by a physician, fall-prevention measures, and use of the hormones estrogen (in individuals not at high risk for certain forms of cancer) and calcitonin.[7] One study indicated that increasing calcium intake to 1,380 milligrams per day—an amount that exceeds the current DRI for calcium—reduces bone loss and increases bone mineralization in women aged 58 to 77.[8] Other therapies for osteoporosis, such as sodium fluoride, various metabolites of vitamin D, and bisphosphonates, are under investigation.[9]

The most effective method of preventing osteoporosis is to develop strong, dense bones during growth. Critical to developing strong bones is sufficient calcium intake during childhood and young adulthood[10] as well as weight-bearing or weight resistance (that is, bone-growth-stimulating) physical activity. For adolescent males and females (ages 15 to 18 years), an adequate

**Osteoporosis:** A degenerative bone disease characterized by loss of bone mineral density resulting in fragile bones with an increased fracture risk.

intake of calcium is 1,300 mg per day.[11] Children and adolescents should also obtain 30 minutes of vigorous-intensity and 60 minutes of moderate-intensity physical activities most every day of the week.[12] Once strong bones are developed, the next critical step is to maintain them and delay the onset of bone mineral loss. This can most effectively be done by maintaining a healthy dietary intake and remaining physically active. Regular physical activity of weight-bearing joints, maintenance of muscular strength and flexibility, and an adequate intake of calcium are probably your best routes of osteoporosis prevention during early, middle, and late adulthood.

Another bone condition that affects a large number of people is *osteoarthritis*, a progressive breakdown of joint cartilage. Osteoarthritis becomes more common with age and is a leading cause of disability.

## The Head

With age, features of the head enlarge and become more noticeable. Increased cartilage and fatty tissue cause the nose to grow 1.25 cm wider and another 1.25 cm longer. Earlobes get thicker and grow longer, while overall head circumference increases 0.6 cm per decade, even though the brain itself shrinks.

## The Urinary Tract

One problem often associated with aging is **urinary incontinence,** which ranges from passing a few drops of urine while laughing or sneezing to having little or no control over when and where urination takes place. This condition affects 22 percent of older men and 35 percent of older women.[13] Incontinence poses major social, physical, and emotional problems for the elderly. Embarrassment and fear of wetting oneself may cause an older person to become isolated and avoid social functions. Caregivers may become frustrated. Prolonged wetness and the inability to properly care for oneself can lead to irritation, infections, and other problems. However, incontinence is not an inevitable part of the aging process. Most cases are caused by highly treatable underlying neurological problems that affect the central nervous system, medications, infections of the pelvic muscles, weakness in the pelvic walls, or other problems. When the problem is treated, incontinence usually vanishes.[14]

## The Heart and Lungs

Resting heart rate stays about the same during a person's life, but stroke volume (the amount of blood the muscle pumps per beat) diminishes as heart muscles deteriorate. Vital capacity, or the amount of air that moves when you inhale and exhale at maximum effort, also declines with age. Aerobic physical activity can do a great deal to reduce deterioration in heart and lung function.

## Eyesight

By the age of 30, the lens of the eye begins to harden, causing specific problems by the early 40s. The lens begins to yellow and loses transparency, while the pupil of the eye begins to shrink, allowing less light to penetrate. Activities such as reading become more difficult, particularly in dim light. By age 60, depth perception declines and farsightedness often develops. A need for glasses usually develops in the 40s that evolves into a need for bifocals in the 50s and trifocals in the 60s. **Cataracts** (clouding of the lens) and **glaucoma** (elevation of pressure within the eyeball) become more likely. There may eventually be a tendency toward colour-blindness, especially for shades of blue and green. **Macular degeneration** is the breakdown of the light-sensitive part of the retina responsible for the sharp, direct vision needed to read or drive. Its effects can be devastating to independent older adults.

## Hearing

The ability to hear high-frequency consonants (for example, *s, t,* and *z*) diminishes with age. Much of the actual hearing loss is in the ability to distinguish extreme ranges of sound versus normal conversational tones.

## Taste

The sense of taste begins to decline as a person gets older. At age 30, each tiny elevation on the tongue (called papilla) has 245 taste buds. By the age of 70, each has only 88 left. The mouth gets drier as salivary glands secrete less fluid. The ability to distinguish sweet, sour, bitter, and salty diminishes. Elderly people often compensate for their diminished sense of taste by adding excessive salt, sugar, and other flavour enhancers to their food.

## Smell and Touch

The sense of smell also diminishes with age. As a result of this loss, coupled with the loss of the sense of taste, food is often less appealing to older people. This lack of appeal may be one factor in seniors' tendency to be malnourished. Pain receptors also become less effective. The tactile senses decline.

## Mobility

Nearly half of older Canadians report some disability, usually related to mobility and agility; one-third require help with housework and shopping. Incidence and severity of disability increase with age.[15]

## Sexual Changes

As people age, they experience noticeable changes in sexual function. The degree and rate of change varies greatly from person to person. As men age, the following changes generally occur:

- The ability to obtain and maintain an erection is diminished.
- The length of the refractory period between orgasms increases.
- The orgasm itself grows shorter in duration.

Women experience the following changes as they age:

- Menopause usually occurs between the ages of 45 and 55. Women may experience such symptoms as hot flashes, mood swings, weight gain, development of facial hair, and other hormone-related problems.
- The walls of the vagina become less elastic, and the epithelium thins, making intercourse more painful.
- Vaginal secretions diminish, particularly during sexual activity.
- The breasts decrease in firmness. Loss of fat in various areas leads to fewer curves, with a decrease in the soft lines of the body contours.

While these physiological changes may sound discouraging, the fact is that many older people remain sexually active all their lives.[16] Indeed, one study refuted long-held beliefs that sexual desire decreases as we age. In this study, nearly half the population over 60 years of age engaged in sexual activity at least once a month, and 40 percent would like to have sex more frequently than they currently do.[17]

## Body Comfort

Because of the loss of body fat, thinning of the epithelium, and diminished glandular activity, elderly people experience greater difficulty in regulating body temperature. This change means that their ability to withstand extreme cold or heat may be limited, thus increasing their risks of hypothermia, heat stroke, and heat exhaustion.

Many of these changes are exacerbated by poor nutrition. For a variety of reasons, getting adequate nutrition is a problem for many seniors. Using assessments based on risk factors associated with malnutrition, 40 to 50 percent of community-dwelling seniors seem to have a moderate to high risk of becoming malnourished, especially among those who live alone. The limited data on frailer seniors suggest that the picture is much worse. Poor nutrition worsens the impact of chronic disease, reduces resistance to infections, slows healing, and increases use of the healthcare system. Identifying seniors at risk for malnutrition is key to their empowerment to strive to maintain an optimal quality of life and to sustain successful aging.[18]

### WHAT WOULD YOU DO?

Of the health conditions listed in this section, which ones can you prevent? Which ones can you delay? What actions can you take now?

## Mental Changes

### Intelligence

Stereotypes concerning inevitable intellectual decline among the elderly have been largely refuted. Research demonstrated that much of our previous knowledge about elderly intelligence was based on inappropriate testing procedures. Given an appropriate length of time, elderly people may learn and develop skills in a similar manner to younger people. Researchers also determined that what many elderly people lack in speed of learning they make up for in practical knowledge—that is, the "wisdom of age."

### Memory

Have you ever wondered why your grandfather seems unable to remember what he did last weekend even though he can graphically depict the details of a social event that occurred 40 years earlier? This phenomenon is not unusual among the elderly. Research indicates that although short-term memory may

**Urinary incontinence:** The inability to control urination.

**Cataracts:** Clouding of the lens that interrupts the focusing of light on the retina, resulting in blurred vision or eventual blindness.

**Glaucoma:** Elevation of pressure within the eyeball, leading to hardening of the eyeball, impaired vision, and possible blindness.

**Macular degeneration:** Disease that breaks down the macula, the light-sensitive part of the retina responsible for sharp, direct vision.

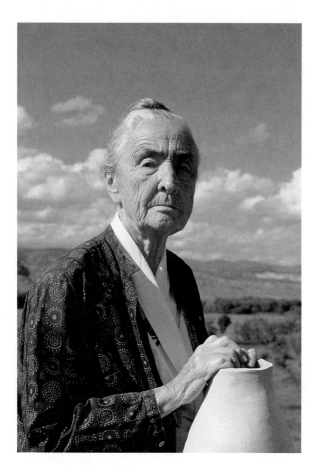

*Georgia O'Keeffe retained her intellectual and artistic abilities into old age.*

fluctuate on a daily basis, the ability to remember events from past decades seems to remain largely unchanged.

## Adaptability

Although it is widely believed that people become more like one another as they age, nothing could be further from the truth. Having lived through a multitude of experiences and faced diverse joys, sorrows, and obstacles, the typical elderly person has developed unique methods of coping. These unique adaptive variations make for interesting differences in how the elderly confront the many changes brought on by the aging process. As a group, the elderly are extremely heterogeneous.

## Depression

Most adults continue to lead healthy, fulfilling lives as they grow older. Some research indicates, however, that depression may be the most common psychological problem facing older adults. Still, those aged 25 to 44 years have greater depression rates (approximately 10 percent) than those older than 65 (5 percent).[19]

## Dementia

Over the years, the elderly have often been the victims of ageist attitudes. People chronologically old were often labelled "senile" whenever they displayed memory failure, errors in judgment, disorientation, or erratic behaviours. (The term *senile* is seldom used today except to describe a very small group of organic disorders.) Today, scientists recognize that these same symptoms can occur at any age and for various reasons, including disease or the use of OTC and prescription drugs. When the underlying problems are corrected, the memory loss and disorientation also improve.

## Alzheimer's Disease

Dementias are progressive brain impairments that interfere with memory and normal intellectual functioning. Although there are many types of **dementia,** one of the most common forms is **Alzheimer's disease.** Currently, Alzheimer's afflicts an estimated 1 in 20 people between the ages of 65 and 75 and 1 in 5 people over the age of 80. The total number of Alzheimer's sufferers seems almost certain to increase. Estimates are that dementia could triple by 2031.[20] This possibility represents a real economic burden for the future. While the disease is associated in most people's minds strictly with the elderly, it has been diagnosed in people as young as their late 40s. In fact, about 5 percent of all cases occur before age 65.

Alzheimer's refers to a degenerative disease of the brain in which nerve cells stop communicating with one another. Ordinarily, brain cells communicate by releasing chemicals that allow the cells to receive and transmit messages for various behaviours. In Alzheimer's patients, the brain doesn't produce enough of these chemicals, cells can't communicate, and eventually the cells die. This degeneration happens in the sections of the brain that affect memory, speech, and personality, leaving the parts that control other bodily functions, such as heartbeat and breathing, working fine. Thus, the mind begins to go as the body lives on. It all happens slowly and progressively, and it may be as long as 20 years before symptoms are noticed. Alzheimer's is generally detected first by family members, who note memory lapses and personality changes. Medical tests rule out underlying causes and certain neurological tests confirm the diagnosis.

What are the symptoms of Alzheimer's? Alzheimer's disease is characteristically diagnosed in three stages. During the first stage, symptoms include forgetfulness, memory loss, impaired judgment, increasing inability to handle routine tasks, disorientation, lack of interest in one's surroundings, and depression. These symptoms

# Canada's Aging Population Runs Greater Dementia Risk

*by Steven Wharry, Canadian Medical Association Journal*

The Alzheimer Society of Canada is warning that the number of Canadians battling dementia is set to explode as the population ages.

Steve Rudin, executive director of the Alzheimer Society told *CMAJ* that a study published this summer in *Neurology* predicts that about 109,000 Canadians will develop dementia in the next year alone, while the total number of those suffering from the syndrome will reach 364,000.

"These numbers are very alarming and with this huge number of new cases the implications for our health care system are profound," said Rudin. "The financial and social costs risk being overwhelming."

The estimates are based on data from the Canadian Study of Health and Aging (CSHA) report, which dementia experts warn contain some dire predictions: in 2011 new cases of dementia are expected to reach 145,300 a year; the total number of cases will be 475,000; by 2031 there will be an estimated 778,000 Canadians with Alzheimer's disease and related dementias.

Rudin states that long-term care facilities and services to help these individuals and that initiatives such as a national home care program need to be examined to help families cope with caring for stricken family members.

"The population in the 85-plus age group is the fastest growing segment of the population," states Joan Lindsay, co-investigator of the CSHA study and chief of the Aging Related Diseases Division of Health Canada. "The increase in the numbers of people with dementia is a direct result of the growth in the 'oldest of the old' segment of our population."

Dementia is a syndrome that includes loss of memory, judgment, reasoning, and ability to function. Alzheimer's disease is a degenerative brain disorder that destroys vital brain cells. The cause is unknown and the Alzheimer Society and other organizations continue to fund research aimed at finding a cure.

"Given the vast numbers of people predicted to get this disease, it's even more urgent for us to find a cause and a cure," said Rudin. "We must also develop better methods for diagnosis, caregiving and providing needed services."

accelerate in the second stage, which also includes agitation and restlessness (especially at night), loss of sensory perceptions, muscle twitching, and repetitive actions. Many patients become depressed and there is a tendency to be combative and aggressive. In the final stage, disorientation is often complete. The person becomes completely dependent on others for eating, dressing, and other activities. Identity loss and speech problems are common symptoms. Eventually, control of bodily functions may be lost.

Once Alzheimer's disease strikes, the victim's life expectancy is cut in half. Treatment includes several prescription drugs. Some physicians prescribe vitamin E because it may help protect brain cells from free radical damage. Researchers are examining anti-inflammatory drugs, theorizing that Alzheimer's may develop in response to an inflammatory ailment. Others are focusing on stimulating the brains of those prone to Alzheimer's, believing that as people learn more connections between brain cells are formed that may offset those that are lost.

# HEALTH CHALLENGES OF THE ELDERLY

The elderly are disproportionately victimized by a number of societally induced problems. Other problems result when people do not develop the ability to cope with life's hurdles. Still other problems come from a perceived loss of control over the circumstances of their lives by the elderly—who watch loved ones die, are forced to retire, face problems with personal health, and confront an uncertain economy on a fixed income. If you develop certain

**Dementia:** Refers to mental deterioration; loss of memory and judgment and orientation problems.

**Alzheimer's disease:** A chronic condition involving changes in nerve fibres of the brain that results in mental deterioration.

skills in your earlier years and acquire strong social supports, you may significantly reduce your risk for problems in old age.

## Alcohol Use and Abuse

A person prone to alcoholism during the younger and middle years is more likely to continue drinking during his or her later years. The older individual addicted to alcohol is no more common than the younger person, despite the stereotype of the old, lost soul hiding his or her sorrows in a bottle. Often when people think they see a drunken older person, they are really seeing a confused individual who has taken too many prescription drugs and is experiencing some form of drug interaction.

Alcohol abuse is five times more likely in older men than in older women. Yet, as many as half of all older men and even more older women do not drink at all. Those who do drink consume less than younger persons, at only five to six drinks per week.

## Prescription Drug Use: Unique Problems for the Elderly

It is extremely rare for elderly people to use illicit drugs, but some do overuse, and grow dependent upon, prescription and OTC drugs. Beset with numerous aches, pains, and inexplicable as well as diagnosable maladies, some elderly people take between four and six prescription drugs a day. Reported numbers of drugs taken are substantially higher for residents of healthcare institutions, but this may be because drugs that many of us purchase over the counter, such as ASA, are counted in the total numbers.

Anyone who combines different drugs runs the risk of dangerous drug interactions. The risks of adverse effects are even greater for people with circulation impairments and declining kidney and liver functions. Elderly people displaying symptoms of these drug-induced effects, which may include bizarre behaviour patterns or an appearance of being out of touch, are often misdiagnosed as experiencing dementia rather than examined for underlying causes and treated.

## Over-the-Counter Remedies

Although today's elderly appear to be more receptive to medical treatment than the elderly of previous generations, a substantial segment of the over-60 population avoid orthodox medical treatment, viewing it as only a last resort. As might be expected, ASA and laxatives head the list of commonly used OTC medications

for relief of arthritic pain and the irregular bowel activity sometimes experienced by the elderly.

## Physical Activity

An inevitable physical change the body undergoes as it ages is **sarcopenia,** age-related declines in muscle mass. The less muscle you have the less energy you will burn, even while resting. The lower your metabolic rate, the more likely you will gain weight. Regular moderate-intensity physical activity that gets your heart beating faster will help to reduce the expected age-related declines in quality and quantity of muscle. Further, regular strength training will increase (or maintain) muscle mass, boost metabolism, strengthen your bones, prevent osteoporosis, and in general help you to feel better and function more efficiently.

Canada's Physical Activity Guide to Healthy Living for Older Adults (available at www.healthcanada.ca/paguide) recommends that older adults choose a variety of endurance, flexibility, and strength and balance activities such that they accumulate 30 to 60 minutes of moderate-intensity physical activity most days of the week.[21] It is further noted that these activities can be accumulated up to 10 minutes at a time.

## Dietary Concerns

As with many bodily processes, the digestion of food begins to slow with age. Nevertheless, the body still requires nutrients consumed in moderate quantities and in the right combination. Certain nutrients are especially important to healthy aging:

- *Calcium:* Many elderly people do not consume adequate calcium, or they may take it as an individual supplement without vitamin D, which is necessary for calcium absorption in the body. Adequate calcium intake should be part of a lifelong regimen of preventive health care to reduce loss of bone mineral content. Over the age of 50, a calcium intake of 1,200 mg per day is recommended.[22]

- *Vitamin D:* As noted above, Vitamin D is essential to enable adequate calcium absorption. As people age, particularly in their 50s and 60s, they do not absorb vitamin D as readily from foods.

- *Protein:* As older adults become concerned about cholesterol and fatty foods, and as their budgets shrink, one nutrient often cut back is protein. It costs more, takes longer to cook, and has that "fat" stigma associated with animal products. Many older people cut back on protein to a point below the DRIs. Because protein is necessary to maintain muscle mass, deficiencies can spell trouble.

## Baby Boomers Sport Waistline Woes

In Andrew Wister's new book (*Baby Boomer Health Dynamics: How Are We Aging?* UTP, 2005), he calls obesity "the new tobacco." Despite today's baby boomers making many healthier lifestyle choices such as not smoking, reducing alcohol consumption, and engaging in physical activity or exercise, they are not aging any better than their forefathers 25 years ago. One thing boomers experience at a much higher rate than their forefathers is obesity. In fact, the number of people classified as obese has doubled in the past 15 years. Clearly the lifestyle improvements have not been sufficient to counteract the quantity and quality of our food consumption.

To examine the exercise–obesity paradox, Wister, Chair of the Department of Gerontology at Simon Fraser University, analyzed data from six Canadian health surveys. From these analyses, it was noted that 25 percent of the energy we take in (i.e., calories) comes from the "other" food group of Canada's Food Guide to Healthy Eating. Twenty percent of all meals were eaten outside the home, many at fast food restaurants which continue to serve exceedingly large portions. Further, it was noted that as many as 27 percent of people eat at least one meal per week in their car.

These changes have a direct impact on individual and national levels of obesity. Given the sheer number of boomers, combined with an increase in the number classified as obese, our healthcare system is likely to become overburdened in the coming years as the boomers age.

Source: Adapted from Centre on Aging, "Research through the Life Course," *The Bulletin* 14.1 (January 2006): 12. Retrieved on May 16, 2006, from www.coag.uvic.ca.

## Sex Issues: Caring for the Elderly

According to the most recent census data, elderly women fill a disproportionate place in Canadian society. In 2005, for example, 56.5 percent of seniors were women.[23] This difference in the number of older women increases with age. In the same year, women made up 58.4 percent of seniors aged 75 to 84, and 69.2 percent of seniors aged 85 or older. It is also a relatively new phenomenon—as recently as 1950, there were more senior men than women.[24] Because women live longer then men on average, elderly women are more likely than elderly men to be living alone, and thus to lack the support in the home that helps keep older people independent. Women over age 75 were the largest consumers of home-care services, with 20 percent reporting using these services.[25]

The rate of institutionalization is twice as high among older people without a spouse as for married older people; for one thing, a married person has a built-in potential caretaker. Further, women are more likely than men to experience poverty and multiple chronic health problems, a situation referred to as **comorbidity.** Consequently, more elderly women than men are likely to need assistance from children, other relatives, friends, and neighbours.

### WHAT WOULD YOU DO?

Why are women often the primary caregivers for aging spouses or other family members? What problems can such caregiving bring? How can caregivers cope with the stresses of their situation?

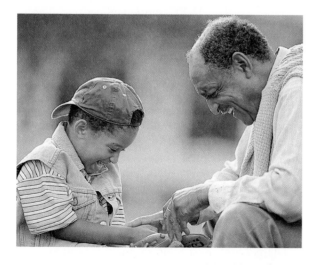

*Learning to cope with challenges and changes early in life develops attitudes and skills that contribute to a full and satisfying old age.*

**Sarcopenia:** Age-related declines in the quality and quantity of muscle mass.

**Comorbidity:** The presence of a number of diseases at the same time.

# UNDERSTANDING DEATH AND DYING

Death eventually comes to everyone. This can be a depressing thought, but each of us must accept the inevitable. The acceptance of death helps us shape our attitudes about the importance of life. Throughout history, humans have attempted to determine the nature and meaning of death. The questioning continues today. Although we will touch on moral, spiritual, and philosophical questions about death, we will not explore such issues in depth. Rather, our primary focus is to present dying and death as a normal part of life and to discuss how we can cope with it.

Confrontations with death elicit different feelings depending on many factors, including age, religious beliefs, family orientation, health, personal experience, and the circumstances of the death itself. To cope effectively with dying and death, we must address the individual needs of those involved. Why is it that we wish to deny, or even postpone, death? Let's begin by investigating what death means, at least in medical terms.

## Defining Death

**Dying** is the process of decline in body functions resulting in the death of an organism. **Death** can be defined as the "final cessation of the vital functions" and refers to a state in which these functions are "incapable of being restored."[26] This definition has become more significant as medical and scientific advances have made it increasingly possible to postpone death.

Although irreversible cessation of circulatory and respiratory functions acceptably defines death, irreversible cessation of brain function is also equivalent to death even though the heart continues to beat while the individual is on a respirator.

In 1968, following the publication of the Harvard Criteria for the diagnosis of brain death, the Canadian Medical Association (CMA) provided guidelines, revised in 1974 and 1975. In 1976, guidelines were established in the United Kingdom, and in 1981, revised guidelines were published in the *Journal of the American Medical Association*. Brain death must be determined clinically by an experienced physician in accordance with accepted medical standards.[27]

The following definitions facilitate classification of various phases of biological death:

- *Cell death:* The gradual death of a cell after all metabolic activity has ceased. The rate of cellular death varies according to the type of tissue involved. For example, higher-functioning brain cells die five to eight minutes after respiration ceases; striated muscle cells die two to four hours later; kidney cells die after about seven hours; and epithelial cells (hair and nails) die several days later. Rigor mortis, the temporary stiffening of muscles, is associated with cell death.

- *Local death:* The death of a body part or portion of an organ without the death of the entire organism. For example, a kidney may fail, part of the heart muscle may die, or a limb or section of intestine may die as a result of loss of circulation.

- *Somatic death:* The death of the entire organism, as opposed to death of a part of an organ or an extremity.

- *Apparent death:* The cessation of vital physiologic functions, particularly spontaneous cardiac and respiratory activities, which produces a state simulating actual death but from which recovery is possible through resuscitative efforts.

- *Functional death:* Extensive and irreversible damage to the central nervous system, with respiration and circulatory function maintained by artificial means.

- *Brain death:* The cessation of brain function, as evidenced by loss of all reflexes and electrical activity of the brain or by irreversible coma. Brain death is confirmed by an **electroencephalogram (EEG)** reading of electrical activity of brain cells.

The Canadian Medical Association has established the following criteria for the clinical diagnosis of brain death:[28]

1. An etiology has been established capable of causing brain death, and potentially reversible conditions have been excluded (drug intoxication, treatable metabolic disorders, core temperature less than 32.2°C, shock, and peripheral nerve or muscle dysfunction due to disease or neuromuscular-blocking drugs).

2. The patient is in deep coma and shows no response within the cranial nerve distribution to stimulation of any part of the body. In particular, there should be no motor response within the cranial nerve distribution to stimuli applied to any body regions. There should be no spontaneous or elicited movements arising from the brain. However, various spinal reflexes may persist in brain death.

3. Brain-stem reflexes are absent. Pupillary light and corneal, vestibulo-ocular, and pharyngeal reflexes must be absent. The pupils should be midsize or larger and must be unresponsive to light. Care should be taken that atropine or related drugs that could block the pupillary response to light have not been given to the patient.

4. The patient does not breathe when taken off the respirator for an appropriate time.
5. The conditions listed above persist when the patient is reassessed after a suitable interval to ensure that the nonfunctioning state of the brain is persistent and to reduce the possibility of observer error.

The CMA also suggests that a physician consult with another experienced physician before determining death.

**WHAT WOULD YOU DO?**

How long do you think you will live? Do you have concerns about the quality of your life up until you die? What can you do now and in the future to obtain not only a long life, but also a healthy quality of life?

## Denying Death

We can look at our attitudes toward death as falling on a continuum. At one end of the continuum, death is viewed as the enemy of humankind. Medical science has tended to promote this idea of death. At the other end of the continuum, death is accepted and even welcomed.[29] For people whose attitudes fall at this end, often people with a deep religious faith or spiritual belief, death is a passage to a better state of being. Most of us perceive ourselves somewhere in the middle of this continuum. From this perspective, death is a bewildering mystery that elicits fear and apprehension as well as profoundly influencing our attitudes, beliefs, and actions throughout our lives.

In Canada, a high level of discomfort is associated with dying and death. As a result, we often avoid speaking about them. You may also be denying death if you:

■ avoid people who are grieving after the death of a loved one so you won't have to talk about it

■ fail to validate a dying person's situation by talking to the person as if nothing were wrong

■ substitute euphemisms for the word death (a few examples are "passing away," "kicking the bucket," "no longer with us," "going to heaven," or "going to a better place")

■ give false reassurances to dying people by saying things like "everything is going to be okay"

■ shut off conversation about death by silencing people trying to talk about it

■ avoid touching a dying person

Although some experts indicate that the denial of death has always been a predominant characteristic of our society, we must keep in mind that social attitudes change over time. The miraculous feats of science and medicine during the first half of the century created an attitude closer to death-defying than to death-denying. However, the pendulum appears to be swinging back. Today, a growing number of people are rejecting "high-tech" death—death postponed through the use of life-support technology—in favour of more personal, and perhaps more humane, alternatives. The concept of death as an enemy may be giving way to acceptance of dying as a natural part of life.

# THE PROCESS OF DYING

Dying is a complex process that includes physical, intellectual, social, spiritual, and emotional dimensions. Accordingly, we must consider the process of dying from several perspectives. The preceding section primarily examined the physical indicators of death. It is also essential to consider the emotional aspects of dying and "social death" in establishing an appreciation for the multifaceted nature of life and health.

## Coping Emotionally with Death

Science and medicine have enabled us to understand changes associated with growth, development, aging, and social roles throughout the life span, but they have not revealed the nature of death. This may partially explain why the transition from life to death evokes so much mystery and emotion. Although emotional reactions to dying vary, there seem to be many similarities in this process.

Much of our knowledge about reactions to dying stems from the work of Elisabeth Kübler-Ross, a major figure in modern **thanatology,** the study of death and dying. In 1969, Kübler-Ross published *On Death and Dying*, a sensitive analysis of the reactions of terminally ill patients. This pioneering work encouraged the development of death education as a discipline and prompted efforts to improve the care of dying patients. In her book, Kübler-Ross identified five psychological stages that terminally ill patients often

**Dying:** The process of decline in body functions resulting in the death of an organism.

**Death:** The "final cessation of the vital functions" and the state in which these functions are "incapable of being restored."

**Electroencephalogram (EEG):** A device that measures the electrical activity of brain cells.

**Thanatology:** The study of death and dying.

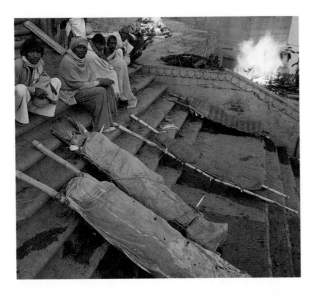

*In some cultures death is not feared but viewed as a passage to a better state of being that is to be celebrated.*

experience as they approach death: denial, anger, bargaining, depression, and acceptance. Health professions immediately embraced this "stage theory" and hastily applied it in clinical settings. However, research evidence supporting the concept of stages of grief is neither extensive nor convincing. Although it is normal to grieve when a severe loss has been sustained, some people never go through this process and instead remain emotionally calm. Others pass back and forth between the stages.

A summation of the five stages follows:

- *Denial:* ("Not me, there must be a mistake.") This is usually the first stage, experienced as a sensation of shock and disbelief. A person intellectually accepts his or her impending death but rejects it emotionally. The individual is too confused and stunned to comprehend "not being" and thus rejects the idea. Within a relatively short time, the anxiety level may diminish, enabling the individual to sort through the powerful web of emotions.

- *Anger:* ("Why me?") Anger is another common reaction to the realization of imminent death. The person becomes angry at having to face death when others, including loved ones, are healthy and not threatened. The dying person perceives the situation as "unfair" or "senseless" and may be hostile to friends, family, physicians, or the world in general.

- *Bargaining:* ("If I'm allowed to live, I promise . . .") This stage generally occurs at about the middle of the progression toward acceptance of death. During this stage, the dying person may resolve to be a better person in return for an extension of life or may secretly pray for a short reprieve from

death in order to experience a special event, such as a family wedding or birth.

- *Depression:* ("It's really going to happen to me and I can't do anything about it.") Depression eventually sets in as vitality diminishes and the person begins to experience distressing symptoms with increasing frequency. The individual's deteriorating condition becomes impossible for him or her to deny, and feelings of doom and tremendous loss may become unbearably pervasive. Feelings of worthlessness and guilt are also common in this depressed state because the dying person may feel responsible for the emotional suffering of loved ones and the arduous but seemingly futile efforts of caregivers.

- *Acceptance:* ("I'm ready.") This is often the final stage. The individual stops battling with emotions and becomes very tired and weak. The need to sleep increases, and wakeful periods become shorter and less frequent. With acceptance, the person does not "give up" and become sullen or resentfully resigned to death, but rather becomes passive. According to one dying person, the acceptance stage is "almost void of feelings. . .as if the pain had gone, the struggle is over, and there comes a time for the final rest before the long journey."[30] As he or she lets go, the dying person may no longer welcome visitors and may not wish to engage in conversation. Death usually occurs quietly and painlessly while the individual is unconscious.

Subsequent research indicated that each individual has a distinct mix and process of grieving. A person may move from denial to depression, to anger, to denial again, and so on. Even if it is not accurate in all its particulars, Kübler-Ross's theory offers valuable insights for those seeking to understand or cope with the process of dying.

## WHAT WOULD YOU DO?

What do you think of the stages of grief? Why? Have you ever lost someone close to you and experienced any of these stages? Do you know of anyone else's experience with death or dying? Did he or she experience these stages?

## Social Death

The need for recognition and appreciation within a social group is nearly universal. Although the size and nature of the social group may vary widely, the need to belong exists in all of us. Loss of value or of appreciation by others can lead to **social death,** an often irreversible situation in which a person is not treated like an active member of society. Dramatic examples of social death include the exile of nonconformists from their native countries or the excommunication of dissident members of religious orders. More often, however, social death is inflicted by avoidance of social interaction. Numerous studies indicate that people are treated differently when they are dying. The isolation that accompanies social death in terminally ill patients may be promoted by the following:[31]

- The dying person is referred to as if he or she were already dead.

- The dying person may be inadvertently excluded from conversations.

- Dying patients are often moved to terminal wards and given minimal care.

- Bereaved family members are avoided, often for extended periods, because friends and neighbours are afraid of feeling uncomfortable in the presence of grief.

- Medical personnel may make degrading comments about patients in their presence.

A decrease in meaningful social interaction often strips dying and bereaved people of recognition as valued members of society at a time when belonging is critical. Some dying people choose not to speak of their inevitable fate in an attempt to make others feel more comfortable and thus preserve vital relationships.

## Near-Death Experiences

We cannot speak of the process of dying without mentioning near-death experiences. Thousands of similar reports have been given by people who have almost died or who were actually pronounced dead but subsequently recovered. The descriptions of feelings, perceptions, and visions associated with being near death have many common features. Three phases have been identified in a large number of near-death accounts: resistance, life review, and transcendence. During the initial phase, resistance, the dying person is aware of extreme danger and struggles desperately to escape from the unseen threat. Many people report a sensation of expanding fear. The second phase, life review, has been described as a feeling of being outside one's body and beyond danger. During this period, the dying person feels a sensation of security while observing his or her physical body from an emotionally detached perspective. The dying person's life experiences may also seem to pass by in rapid review. The last phase, transcendence, is characterized by a reported feeling of euphoria,

contentment, and even ecstasy. Some people recall a sensation of being unified with nature and of having an awareness of infinity. In February 2000 Pam Barrett, long-time leader of the Alberta New Democratic Party, abruptly resigned from politics after a near-death experience due to an allergic reaction. She termed the experience "a spiritual awakening," and said that it had forced her to reevaluate all aspects of her life.

## Coping with Loss

The losses resulting from the death of a loved one may be extremely difficult to cope with. The dying person, as well as close family and friends, frequently suffers emotionally and physically from the impending loss of critical relationships and roles. Words used to describe feelings and behaviours related to losses resulting from death include *bereavement, grief, grief work,* and *mourning.* These terms are related but not identical. An understanding of them may help you to understand the emotional processes associated with loss and the cultural constraints that often inhibit normal coping behaviours (see Figure 14.1).

**Bereavement** is generally defined as the loss or deprivation experienced by a survivor when a loved one dies. Because relationships vary in type and intensity, reactions vary. The death of a parent, spouse, sibling, child, friend, or pet will result in different kinds of feelings. In the lives of the bereaved or of close survivors, "holes" will be left by the death of loved ones. We can think of bereavement as the awareness of these holes. Time and courage are necessary to fill these spaces.

When a person experiences a loss that cannot be openly acknowledged, publicly mourned, or socially supported, coping may be much more difficult. This type of grief is referred to as **disenfranchised grief.**[32] Some examples of a death that may lead to disenfranchised grief include:

- *Death of a divorced spouse:* Unresolved anger and hurt along with fond memories are conflicting feelings that may prevent the satisfactory resolution of feelings surrounding the ex-spouse's death.

- *Death of a secret lover:* When a lover dies and no one but the partner knew of the relationship, grief is often hidden. Examples would include a partner

**Social death:** An irreversible situation in which a person is not treated like an active member of society.

**Bereavement:** The loss or deprivation experienced by a survivor when a loved one dies.

**Disenfranchised grief:** Grief concerning a loss that cannot be openly acknowledged, publicly mourned, or socially supported.

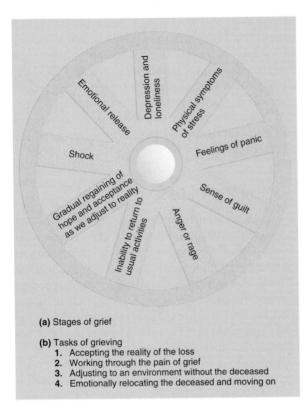

**(a) Stages of grief**

**(b) Tasks of grieving**
1. Accepting the reality of the loss
2. Working through the pain of grief
3. Adjusting to an environment without the deceased
4. Emotionally relocating the deceased and moving on

## FIGURE 14.1

### The Stages and Tasks of Grief

(a) People react differently to losses, but most eventually adjust. Generally, the stronger the social support system, the smoother the progression through the stages of grief.
(b) Worden's developmental tasks associated with grief are another way to understand the grieving process.

in an extramarital relationship or a lover of a gay person who is not openly gay.

- *Death of a gay lover:* Homosexuals may find it difficult to mourn the deaths of their lovers when they themselves are not accepted by their own families or the families of their lovers. The situation can be even more difficult if the lover has died of AIDS, because of the unjust stigma and discrimination associated with this disease.

A special case of bereavement occurs in old age. Death is an intrinsic part of growing old. The longer we live, the more deaths we are likely to experience. These deaths include physical, social, spiritual, and emotional losses as our bodies deteriorate and more and more of our loved ones die. The theory of *bereavement overload* has been proposed to explain the effects of multiple deaths and the accumulation of sorrow in the lives of some elderly people. This theory suggests that the gloomy outlook, disturbing behaviour

patterns, and apparent apathy that characterize these people may be related more to bereavement overload than to intrinsic physiological degeneration in old age.[33]

**Grief** is a mental state of distress that occurs in reaction to significant loss, including one's own impending death, the death of a loved one, or a quasi-death experience. Grief reactions include any adjustments needed for one to "make it through the day" and may include changes in patterns of eating, physical activity, sleeping, working, and even thinking.

The term **mourning** is often incorrectly equated with the term *grief*. As we have noted, *grief* refers to a wide variety of feelings and actions that occur in response to bereavement. *Mourning*, in contrast, refers to culturally prescribed and accepted time periods and behaviour patterns for the expression of grief. In Judaism, for example, "sitting *shivah*" is a designated mourning period of seven days that involves prescribed rituals and prayers. Depending on a person's relationship with the deceased, various other rituals may continue for up to a year.

By accepting dying as a part of the continuum of life, many people are able to make necessary readjustments after the death of a loved one. This holistic concept, which accepts dying as a part of the total life experience, is shared by believers and nonbelievers.

## What Is "Normal" Grief?

Grief responses vary widely from person to person. Despite these differences, a classic acute grief syndrome often occurs when a person acknowledges a death. This common grief reaction can include the following:

- periodic waves of physical distress lasting from 20 minutes to an hour
- a feeling of tightness in the throat
- choking and shortness of breath
- a frequent need to sigh
- a feeling of emptiness in the abdomen
- a feeling of muscular weakness
- an intense feeling of anxiety described as actually painful

Other common symptoms of grief include insomnia, memory lapse, loss of appetite, difficulty in concentrating, a tendency to engage in repetitive or purposeless behaviours, an "observer" sensation or feeling of unreality, difficulty in making decisions, lack of organization, excessive speech, social withdrawal or

# Bereavement and Grief

Each of us uses various methods to relieve sorrow and bereavement. The stress caused by grief affects people mentally and physically. If an individual is having an especially difficult time dealing with grief, he or she may become depressed or physically ill. There are a number of feelings that people experience while coming to terms with a loss, including:

- shock, numbness, bewilderment, a sense of disbelief, and possibly denial
- feelings of emptiness and intense suffering
- dreams or hallucinations that their loved one is still alive
- feelings of despair as one comes to terms with the loss
- feelings of sadness and the inability to feel pleasure
- tense, restless anxiety alternated with lethargy and fatigue
- avoiding reminders of the deceased alternated with reclaiming memories
- sadness mixed with anger
- self-blame for treating the deceased badly

Physical symptoms of grief include weakness, sleep disturbances, loss of appetite, headaches, back pain, indigestion, shortness of breath, heart palpitations, and occasional dizziness and nausea.

## WHY WE GRIEVE

All cultures have various rituals to mourn the passing of a loved one. Mourning customs help to confirm social bonds, reorder personal relationships, and establish a new identity for the bereaved. Within our society, people often die in hospitals or away from their families. These changes to the social fabric have made it difficult for some to see death as a natural part of life, and to come to terms with the death of a loved one. Friends and social groups are especially important for helping the bereaved readjust to their loss and move on with their life.

## WHAT YOU CAN DO TO HELP THE BEREAVED

People who have experienced a death need sympathetic company, reassurance, and willingness among or by others to listen. What the bereaved say they want most are offers of specific practical support, expressions of concern, and the presence of people close to them. Statements such as "time heals" and vague offers of help that never materialize have been found to be more annoying than helpful. People should not try to discourage expressions of grief or shut off discussions about the person who died, since that is part of the healing process. Understanding that this is a highly emotional time for the bereaved and assuring them that their anger, guilt, and other feelings are normal and part of the grieving process is the most supportive thing you can do.

Source: Copyright © Canadian Mental Health Association, Ontario Division, Fact Sheet: Bereavement and Grief, www.ontario.cmha.ca. All rights reserved.

hostility, guilt feelings, and preoccupation with the image of the deceased. Susceptibility to disease increases with grief and may even be life-threatening in severe and enduring cases.

# Coping with Grief

A bereaved person may suffer emotional pain and exhibit a variety of grief responses for many months after the death of a loved one. The rate of the healing process depends on the amount and quality of "grief work" that a person does. **Grief work** is the process of integrating the reality of the death with everyday life and learning to feel better. Often, the bereaved person must deliberately and systematically work at reducing denial and coping with the pain that results from memories of the deceased. This process takes time and requires emotional effort.

# Worden's Model of Grieving Tasks

William Worden, a researcher into the death process, developed an active grieving model suggesting four developmental tasks to complete in the grief work process (refer to Figure 14.1):[34]

1. *Accept the reality of the loss.* This task requires acknowledging and realizing that the person is dead. Traditional rituals, such as the funeral, help many bereaved people move toward acceptance.

**Grief:** The mental state of distress that occurs in reaction to significant loss, including one's own impending death, the death of a loved one, or a quasi-death experience.

**Mourning:** The culturally prescribed behaviour patterns for the expression of grief.

**Grief work:** The process of accepting the reality of a person's death and coping with memories of the deceased.

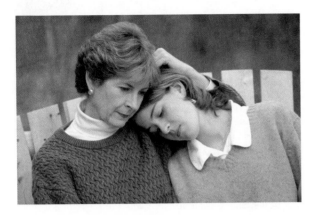

*Teenage suicide, a tragically growing cause of death for young people, affects many people, but siblings and friends—who generally have little experience with death—are especially challenged in coping with their grief.*

2. *Work through to the pain of grief.* It is necessary to acknowledge and work through the pain associated with loss or it will manifest itself through other symptoms or behaviours.

3. *Adjust to an environment in which the deceased is missing.* The bereaved may feel lonely and uncertain about a new identity without the person who has died. This loss confronts them with the challenge of adjusting to their own sense of self.

4. *Emotionally relocate the deceased and move on with life.* Individuals never lose memories of a significant relationship. They may need help in letting go of the emotional energy that used to be invested in the person who has died, finding an appropriate place for the deceased in their emotional lives.

Models of the grief process can be viewed as "generalized maps"—each theory is an attempt by an investigator to understand and guide grieving people through their pain. However, each individual will travel through grief at his or her own speed using an appropriate route.

## When an Infant or a Child Dies

The death of a child is terribly painful for the whole family. For several reasons, the siblings of the deceased child have a particularly hard time with grief work. Bereaved children usually have limited experience with death and therefore have not learned how to deal with it. Children may feel uncomfortable talking about death, they may have difficulty understanding it, and they may also receive less social support and sympathy than their

parents. Because so much attention and energy are devoted to the deceased child, the surviving children may also feel emotionally abandoned by their parents.

### WHAT WOULD YOU DO?

Can you remember an experience of grief when a loved one or pet died? Try to remember the emotional and physical symptoms that you experienced. Do you think this experience helped you grow as a person and contributed to your personal well-being and philosophy of life?

## Quasi-Death Experiences

Social and emotional support for the bereaved in the aftermath of death is supported by many cultures. Typically, however, there is little support for many other significant losses in life. Losses that in many ways resemble death and carry with them a heavy burden of grief include a child running away from home, an abduction or kidnapping, a divorce, a move to a distant place, a move to a senior care facility, the loss of a romance or an intimate friendship, retirement, job termination, finishing a "terminal" academic degree, or ending an athletic career.

These **quasi-death experiences**[35] resemble death in that they involve separation, termination, loss, and a change in identity or self-perception. If grief results from these losses, the pattern of the grief response will probably follow the same course as responses to death. Factors that may complicate the grieving process associated with quasi-death experiences include uncomfortable contact with the object of loss (for example, an ex-spouse) and a lack of adequate social and institutional support.

# LIFE-AND-DEATH DECISION MAKING

Life-and-death decisions are serious, complex, and often expensive. We will not attempt to present the "answers" to death-related moral and philosophical questions. Instead, we offer topics for your consideration. We hope that discussion of the needs of the dying person and the bereaved will help you to make difficult decisions in the future. Among problematic or controversial issues are questions concerning the right to die and euthanasia.

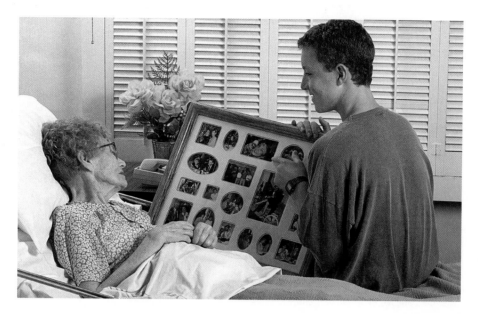

*Many terminally ill people spend their last days in a hospice where maximum involvement of loved ones is emphasized.*

Increasingly, Canadians living with terminal or life-threatening diagnoses are demanding to make decisions about their own lives. Options include pain and symptom management, extended palliative care, active and passive forms of euthanasia, and suicide.

The need to consider right-to-die issues accompanies the development of new reproductive technologies, increases in terminal AIDS cases, and a visible increase in public media coverage of actual cases in Canada and the United States. The right to self-determination is situated within the context of society, health and illness, and human rights and freedoms. Considerations of the economic, social, spiritual, and moral impact of the individual's choice are often involved in decision making. A *living will*, discussed in the Taking Charge box, is one way in which people may express their wishes about life-and-death choices.

**Dyathanasia** is a form of "mercy killing" in which someone plays a passive role in the death of a terminally ill person. This passive role may include withholding life-prolonging treatments or withdrawing life-sustaining medical support, thereby allowing the person to die. A recent study shows that withholding food and water from terminally ill patients may actually ease their suffering. **Euthanasia** is the active form of "mercy killing." An example of euthanasia is direct administration of a lethal drug overdose with the objective of hastening the death of a suffering person. Euthanasia is illegal and considered murder. After years of legal run-ins, the infamous American euthanasia proponent Dr. Jack Kevorkian was convicted of murder for assisting in euthanasia ("assisted suicide") in the late 1990s. Nevertheless, euthanasia continues to occur. In fact, some experts believe that some doctors induce euthanasia upon the request of the patient. This type of euthanasia is accomplished by administering large doses of painkillers that depress the central nervous system to the extent that basic life-sustaining regulatory centres cease to function. The heart stops beating, breathing ceases, and total brain death follows shortly.

## WHAT WOULD YOU DO?

Are there any end-of-life situations in which you would ask a physician to help you die? Why or why not? Are there any life-saving techniques that you would rather not be performed on you? Why or why not? How would you feel about carrying out someone else's wishes from a living will?

**Quasi-death experiences:** Losses or experiences that resemble death in that they involve separation, termination, significant loss, a change of personal identity, and grief.

**Dyathanasia:** The passive form of "mercy killing" in which life-prolonging treatments or interventions are not offered or withheld, thereby allowing a terminally ill person to die naturally.

**Euthanasia:** The active form of "mercy killing" in which a person or organization knowingly acts to hasten the death of a terminally ill person.

# Palliative Care

The needs of terminally ill patients are different from those of other patients. They require another approach and different services defined by different criteria. *Palliative care* is a compassionate form of health care for patients approaching the end of their life. Pain and symptom management and social, psychological, and spiritual support are components of palliative care. We need to understand more fully the meaning that death and dying have to seniors, and how to provide effective pain management for seniors experiencing the symptoms of several health conditions simultaneously.

Different models of care have been explored all over the world: St. Christopher's in London, the Maison Michel Sarrazin in Quebec, and the Elizabeth Bruyère Centre in Ottawa, for example, are highly specialized in pain control and offer supportive care and attention to dying patients. Friends and family are welcome at all times and special training is given to volunteers who can then assist the patients, their families, and the caregivers on staff.

In-home palliative care services are provided in collaboration with a care facility. If treatment is balanced, this type of service can ensure the full continuum of care and nurturing needed to allow terminally ill individuals to remain in their familiar surroundings for as long as possible. The family also needs to be supported and kept informed by being given clear explanations and directives. For individuals to derive maximum benefits from this situation, the home atmosphere needs to be calm and serene, and services must be of the same quality as those offered in hospital. If you are terminally ill, you can make your wishes regarding your care known in several ways:

- If you are facing a life-threatening illness, you should talk over your wishes with your family and let them know what you want.

- You can also put your wishes in writing so that, in the event you are unable to say what you want, your family and health-care providers will know. Such documents are called advance directives or living wills (see the Taking Charge box). You should seek advice within your community about advance directives, as the laws concerning them vary from province to province.

- Your public library may have material on palliative care. You can also call help lines, such as the Canadian Palliative Care Association at 1-800-668-2785 or 613-241-3663, or the Cancer Information Service at 1-888-939-3333 or 905-387-1153.

Sources: "Seniors & Palliative Care," *Expressions: Newsletter of the National Advisory Council on Aging* 11.3 (Health Canada Division of Seniors and Aging, Spring 1998); "Palliative Care: Info Sheet For Seniors," 1998, www.hc-sc.gc.ca/english/care/pallative.html#skipnav; "1999 and Beyond: Challenges of an Aging Canadian Society," National Advisory Council on Aging.

# The Living Will

A living will is a written document in which you set out your wishes for health care in the event that, some time in the future, you are unable to consent to treatment. Living wills deal with health care. They do not deal with property or assets. Living wills are only important if you are unable to consent and you have a terminal illness or are seriously injured and unlikely to recover. In such cases medical staff will need to know what measures you would wish them to take to care for you.

There are no guarantees that every term of the living will be followed. Family members or your proxy in consultation with medical staff will have to make the decision taking in all the existing circumstances, including your expressed wishes. (A proxy is someone you have appointed to make decisions about your health care should you become unable to consent.) A living will may ease the emotional burden from family members or your proxy if they have to make decisions about your health. Many families consider a living will morally binding, especially if you have discussed it with them beforehand.

It is not a request to take positive steps to end your life. Euthanasia, or mercy killing, as it is sometimes called, is the term used when someone takes steps to end your life in order to relieve suffering. Assisted suicide is a term used when someone, at your request, takes steps to end your life, because your illness or condition prevents you from committing suicide. Euthanasia and assisted suicide are illegal under Canadian criminal law.

The living will must have your name and address and the date. It should clearly identify what kind of life-sustaining treatments you would want in certain circumstances should you be incapable of consenting at the time. You must sign the living will and date it. Your signature should be witnessed by two adults. They should give their addresses. If you do not already have a proxy, you may also want to include the appointment of someone to consent to treatment on your behalf should you become unable. You should choose someone whom you trust to carry out your wishes. The person must be aged 19 or over but does not have to be your next of kin.

Source: The Legal Information Society of Nova Scotia (LISNS), *Living Wills*, www.legalinfo.org.

# SUMMARY

- Aging can be defined in terms of biological, psychological, social, legal, or functional age.
- The rising number of elderly (people age 65 and older) will have a growing impact on our society in terms of economy, health care, housing, and ethical considerations.
- Two broad groups of theories—biological and psychosocial—purport to explain the physiological and psychological changes that occur with aging.
- Aging changes the body and mind in many ways. Physical changes occur in the skin, bones and joints, head, urinary tract, heart and lungs, senses, mobility, sexual functioning, and temperature regulation. Major physical concerns are osteoporosis and urinary incontinence. Potential mental problems include depression and Alzheimer's disease.
- Special challenges for the elderly include prescription drug and OTC interactions, physical activity and dietary concerns, and issues regarding caregiving.
- Death can be defined biologically in terms of the final cessation of vital functions. Various classes of death include cell, local, somatic, apparent, functional, and brain death.
- Death is a multifaceted process and individuals may experience emotional stages of dying including denial, anger, bargaining, depression, and acceptance. Social death results when a person is no longer treated as living. Grief is the state of distress felt after a loss—whether the loss is the death of a loved one or a quasi-death experience. Children, too, need to be helped through the process of grieving.
- The right to die involves ethical, moral, spiritual, and legal issues. Dyathanasia involves passive help in suicide for a terminally ill patient; euthanasia involves direct help.

# DISCUSSION QUESTIONS

1. Discuss the various definitions of aging. At what age would you place your parents or grandparents in each category?
2. As the elderly population grows, what implications are there for you? Would you be willing to pay higher taxes to support social programs for the elderly?
3. List the major physiological changes that occur with aging. Which of these, if any, can you change? Slow down? Specifically address dietary intake and physical activity in your response.
4. Explain the major health challenges that the elderly face. What advice would you give to your grandparents before they took a prescription or OTC drug?
5. List the varied definitions of death. How do they relate to one another?
6. Discuss why so many of us deny death. How could death become a more acceptable topic to discuss?

7. What are the stages that terminally ill patients theoretically experience? Do you agree with the five-stage theory? Explain why or why not.

8. Debate whether assisted suicide should be legalized for the terminally ill. What restrictions would you include in a law?

# APPLICATION EXERCISE

Reread the What Do You Think? scenario at the beginning of the chapter and answer the following questions.

1. Do you think the individuals in the scenario are normal for their age? What is normal for a particular age? How is "normal" defined?

2. What changes have made it easier for elderly people to lead healthy lives? What changes have made it more difficult?

# HEALTH ON THE NET

Active Living Coalition for Older Adults (ALCOA)
**www.alcoa.ca**

Centre on Aging—University of Victoria
**www.coag.uvic.ca**

Health Canada—The Division of Aging and Seniors
**www.hc-sc.gc.ca/seniors-aines**

Ontario Gerontology Association
**http://ontgerontology.on.ca**

Canadian Association on Gerontology
**www.cagacg.ca**

Advocacy Centre for the Elderly
**www.advocacycentreelderly.org**

# CHAPTER 15

# ENVIRONMENTAL HEALTH

*Thinking Globally,*
*Acting Locally*

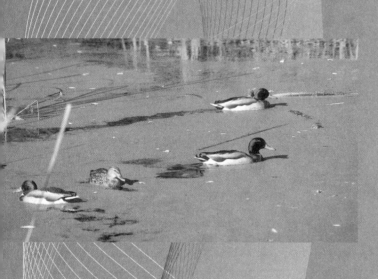

## CHAPTER OBJECTIVES

- Identify the problems associated with current levels of global population growth specific to developed, developing, and least developed nations.

- Describe the major causes of air pollution, including photochemical smog and acid rain.

- Identify the global consequences of the accumulation of greenhouse gases and of ozone depletion.

- Identify sources of water pollution and the specific contaminants often found in water.

- Describe the physiological consequences of noise pollution.

- Distinguish between municipal solid waste and hazardous waste.

- Summarize the health concerns associated with ionizing and nonionizing radiation.

In 1971, three friends in Vancouver (Jim Bohlen, Paul Cote, and Irving Stowe) and their wives decided to take a boat to protest a nuclear test by the United States on Amchitka Island in Alaska, located on a major fault line. Initially calling themselves the Don't Make a Wave Committee, they renamed their organization Greenpeace to better proclaim their purpose: to create a green and peaceful world. Although they were arrested, and the bomb was detonated, the opposition to the Amchitka tests became so strong that the president of the United States had to cancel the program the following year. The island was eventually turned into a bird sanctuary. Greenpeace today adheres to the belief that motivated that original voyage: that determined individuals can alter the actions and purposes of even the most powerful by "bearing witness"—that is, by drawing attention to an abuse of the environment through their unwavering presence at the scene, whatever the risk.

■ What can we as individuals do to stop pollution and its attendant problems? What factors put environmental groups at odds with government and industry?

Human health, well-being, and survival are ultimately dependent on the integrity of the planet. Today the natural world is under attack from the pressure of the number of people who live in it and the wide range of their activities. Even though Canada has made measurable environmental progress in recent years, our environmental achievements allow no room for complacency. An informed citizenry with a strong commitment to caring for the environment is essential to the survival of our planet.

Canadians' concern about the environment has intensified since the initial outpouring on the first Earth Day in April 1970. The federal, provincial/territorial, and municipal governments share responsibility for the environment. Public health agencies are becoming more responsive to public concerns regarding the environment. While Canadians get most of their environmental information from the media, the majority look to public health professionals for answers to their concerns.

Many approaches are taken to address environmental health issues that involve health agencies, in defining the problems and seeking solutions.[1] This is supported by thousands of individual Canadians changing their habits and working for the environment.

People are exposed to contaminants in water, air, food, and soil in various ways:[2]

■ Ingesting food, water, soil, objects, or liquids containing contaminants. The mouth, throat, stomach, and intestines can absorb ingested materials rapidly and at different rates, depending on the contaminant.

■ Inhalation of a contaminated gas or vapour, or of airborne particles. This includes small amounts of soil and dust inhaled into the lungs. The lungs often absorb gasses and vapours quickly and efficiently.

■ Dermal (skin) contact with contaminants in water, soil, or air. Some contaminants are absorbed through the skin, while in other cases the skin acts as an efficient barrier. In the case of radioactivity, exposure can occur through penetration of the skin by radioactivity in the atmosphere or released from radionuclides in the air or on the ground. The radionuclide does not actually need to be in contact with the skin.

See Figure 15.1 for a diagram of major exposure pathways.

# OVERPOPULATION

Our most challenging environmental problem is population growth. The anthropologist Margaret Mead wrote, "Every human society is faced with not one population problem but two: how to beget and rear enough children and how not to beget and rear too many."[3]

The United Nations report "World Populations Prospects: The 2004 Revision" provided a world's population estimate of 6.5 billion people for July 1, 2005.[4] Compared to the estimate made for 2000, this is an increase of 380 million people, equivalent to a gain of 76 million people per year. Despite the decreases in fertility projected for 2005 to 2050, the world population is expected to reach 9.1 billion people by 2050 and will be increasing by 34 million persons per year.

The majority (that is, 95 percent) of the population growth occurs in the developing world.[5] In fact, by 2050 the population of the more developed countries is expected to decline by one million persons per year. At the same time, the developing world will add 35 million people annually, with the least developed countries experiencing an annual increase of 22 million people. These projections result in population estimates that will more than double for the 50 least developed countries, passing 0.8 billion in 2005 and 1.7 billion in 2050. The population is expected to

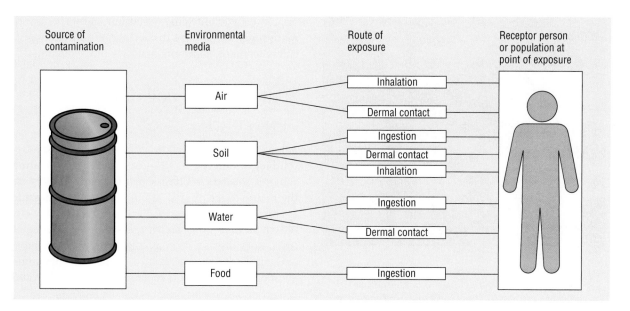

FIGURE 15.1

Major Pathways of Human Exposure to Environmental Contaminants

triple between 2005 and 2050 in Afghanistan, Burkina Faso, Burundi, Chad, Congo, the Democratic Republic of Congo, the Democratic Republic of Timor-Leste, Guinea-Bissau, Liberia, Mali, Niger, and Uganda. On the other hand, the population of 51 countries or areas, including Germany, Italy, Japan, the Baltic States, and most of the successor states of the former Soviet Union, are expected to be lower in 2050 than in 2005. Given these findings, nine countries are expected to account for half the world's projected population increase. In order of population growth, these countries are India, Pakistan, Nigeria, the Democratic Republic of China, Bangladesh, Uganda, the United States of America, Ethiopia, and China.

Estimates for population growth are highly dependent upon predicted fertility rates.[6] In the projections presented previously, worldwide average fertility was expected to slowly decrease from 2.6 to slightly over 2 children per woman in 2050. A fertility path half a child above or below the estimates would result in a world population in 2050 of 10.6 billion or 7.6 billion, respectively. Global fertility has decreased from 5 children per woman in 1950 to 2.65 children per woman in 2000–05. In developed countries fertility is currently 1.56 children per woman and is expected to increase to 1.84 children per woman by 2045–50. In the least developed countries, fertility is currently 5 children per woman and is expected to drop to 2.57. In the rest of the developing world, fertility is currently 2.58 children per woman and is expected to decrease to 1.92 children per woman by 2045–50.

Another factor to consider with world population is life expectancy. Current world life expectancy at birth is 65.4 years.[7] World life expectancy for 2045–50 is predicted to be 75.1. Individuals living in more developed regions have a much longer life expectancy in 2000–05 at 75.6 years, and a predicted life expectancy in 2045–50 of 82.1 years. In the least developed countries, an individual's current life expectancy is 51.0 years. In other less developed countries, current life expectancy is 66.1 years. In 2045–50, individuals in the least developed countries are expected to live 66.5 years, while those living in less developed countries are predicted to live 76.3 years. As a result of increases in life expectancy, the world population is expected to age. Currently, in developed countries 20 percent of the population is over the age of 60 years; this is expected to increase to 32 percent. In the developing world, only 8 percent of the current population is over the age of 60 years, with a projected increase to 20 percent by 2050.

As the global population expands, so does the competition for the earth's resources. Environmental degradation caused by loss of topsoil, pesticides, toxic residues, deforestation, global warming, air pollution, and acid rain seriously threatens the food supply and undermines world health. However, population doesn't tell the whole story. North Americans consume more energy and raw materials per person than people from other regions of the world. Many of these resources come from other countries, and our consumption is depleting the resource balances of those countries. Therefore, we must start by living environmentally conscious lives.

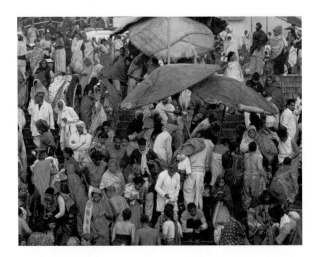

*As world population increases, the world's resources cannot keep up. In fact, in many parts of the world, governments struggle to meet the needs of their increasing number of citizens.*

# AIR POLLUTION

As our population has grown, so have the number and volume of the environmental pollutants that we produce. Concern about air quality prompted Parliament to pass the Clean Air Act in 1970. This was consolidated in 1985 into the Canadian Environmental Protection Act (CEPA). CEPA was further updated and revised in 1999 and came into effect March 31, 2000.[8] The Canadian Environmental Assessment Act (CEAA) provides a legal basis for federal environmental assessment and came into force on January 19, 2005.[9] Various agreements (that is, high-level commitments entered into by two or more parties that identify the actions, roles, and commitments of the parties involved in dealing with environmental pollution) have also been established. The Canada-Wide Accord on Environmental Harmonization, Pollution Prevention Policy Agreement, Comprehensive Air Quality Management Framework for Canada, and the Canada–United States Air Quality Agreement are examples of current agreements in place within the Canadian government and between the Canadian and U.S. governments.[10] These acts and agreements cover pollution prevention, managing toxic substances, clean air and water, controlling pollution and waste, information gathering, and the setting of guidelines and enforcement of environmental laws and regulations.

## Sources of Air Pollution

### Sulphur Dioxide

Sulphur dioxide is a yellowish-brown gas that is a by-product of burning fossil fuels. Electricity generating stations, smelters, refineries, and industrial boilers are the main source points. In humans, sulphur dioxide aggravates symptoms of heart and lung disease, obstructs breathing, and increases the incidence of respiratory diseases such as colds, asthma, bronchitis, and emphysema. It is toxic to plants, destroys some paint pigments, corrodes metals, impairs visibility, and is a precursor to acid rain.

### Particulates

Particulates are tiny solid particles or liquid droplets suspended in the air. Cigarette smoke releases particulates. They are also by-products of some industrial processes and the internal combustion engine. Particulates can in and of themselves irritate the lungs and carry heavy metals and carcinogenic agents deep into the lungs. When combined with sulphur dioxide, they exacerbate respiratory diseases. Particulates can also corrode metals and obscure visibility.

### Carbon Monoxide

Carbon monoxide is an odourless, colourless gas that originates primarily from motor vehicle emissions. Carbon monoxide interferes with the blood's ability to absorb and carry oxygen and can impair thinking, slow reflexes, and cause drowsiness, unconsciousness, and death. When inhaled by a pregnant woman, it may threaten the growth and mental development of the fetus. Long-term exposure can increase the severity of circulatory and respiratory diseases.

### Nitrogen Dioxide

Nitrogen dioxide is an amber-coloured gas emitted by coal-powered electrical utility boilers and by motor vehicles. High concentrations of nitrogen dioxide can be fatal. Lower concentrations increase susceptibility to colds and flu, bronchitis, and pneumonia. Nitrogen dioxide is also toxic to plant life and causes a brown discolouration of the atmosphere. It is a precursor of ozone and, along with sulphur dioxide, of acid rain.

### Ozone

**Ozone** is a form of oxygen produced when nitrogen dioxide reacts with hydrogen chloride. These gases release oxygen, which is altered by sunlight to produce ozone. In the lower atmosphere, ozone irritates the mucous membranes of the respiratory system, causing coughing and choking. It can impair lung functioning, reduce resistance to colds and pneumonia, and aggravate heart disease, asthma, bronchitis, and pneumonia. This ozone corrodes rubber and paint and can injure or kill vegetation. It is also one of the irritants found in smog. A Canadian study concluded that there is no safe level of human exposure to ground-level ozone.[11]

The natural ozone found in the upper atmosphere, however, serves as a protective layer against heat and radiation from the sun. This atmospheric layer, called the ozone layer, is discussed later in the chapter.

### Lead

Lead is a metal pollutant found in the exhaust of motor vehicles powered by fuel containing lead and in the emissions from lead smelters and processing plants. It also often contaminates drinking water systems in homes with plumbing installed before 1930. Lead affects the circulatory, reproductive, and nervous systems. It can also affect the blood and kidneys and accumulate in bone and other tissues. Lead is particularly detrimental to children and fetuses. It can cause birth defects, behavioural abnormalities, and decreased learning abilities.

### Hydrocarbons

Hydrocarbons encompass a wide variety of chemical pollutants in the air. Sometimes known as volatile organic compounds (VOCs), **hydrocarbons** are chemical compounds containing different combinations of carbon and hydrogen. The principal source of polluting hydrocarbons is the internal combustion engine. Most automobile engines emit hundreds of different types of hydrocarbon compounds. By themselves, hydrocarbons seem to cause few problems, but when they combine with sunlight and other pollutants they form such poisons as formaldehyde, various ketones, and peroxyacetylnitrate (PAN), all of which are respiratory irritants. Hydrocarbon combinations such as benzene and benzopyrene are carcinogenic. In addition, hydrocarbons play a major part in the formation of smog.

## Photochemical Smog

**Photochemical smog** is a brown, hazy mix of particulates and gases that forms when oxygen-containing compounds of nitrogen and hydrocarbons react in the presence of sunlight. Photochemical smog is sometimes called *ozone pollution* because ozone is created when vehicle exhaust reacts with sunlight. Such smog is most likely to develop on days when there is little wind and high traffic congestion. In most cases, it forms in areas that experience a **temperature inversion,** a weather condition in which a cool layer of air is trapped under a layer of warmer air, preventing the air from circulating. When gases such as the hydrocarbons and nitrogen oxides are released into the cool air layer they cannot escape, and thus they remain suspended until wind conditions move away the warmer air layer. Sunlight filtering through the air causes chemical changes in the hydrocarbons and nitrogen oxides, which results in smog. Smog is more likely to be produced in valley regions blocked by hills or mountains.

The most noticeable adverse effects of exposure to smog are difficulty in breathing, burning eyes, headaches, and nausea. Long-term exposure to smog poses serious health risks, particularly for children, the elderly, pregnant women, and people with chronic respiratory disorders such as asthma and emphysema. According to the Canadian Lung Association, continued exposure accelerates aging of the lungs and increases susceptibility to infections by hindering the functions of the immune system.

## Acid Rain

**Acid rain** is precipitation that falls through acidic air pollutants, particularly those containing sulphur dioxides and nitrogen dioxides. This precipitation, in the form of rain, snow, or fog, has a more acidic composition than unpolluted precipitation. When introduced into lakes and ponds, acid rain gradually acidifies the water. When the acid content of the water reaches a certain level, plant and animal life cannot survive. Ironically, acidified lakes and ponds become a crystal-clear deep blue, giving an illusion of beauty and health.

### Sources of Acid Rain

More than 95 percent of acid rain originates in human actions, chiefly the burning of fossil fuels. When industries burn fuels, the sulphur and nitrogen

---

**Ozone:** A gas formed when nitrogen dioxide interacts with hydrogen chloride.

**Hydrocarbons:** Chemical compounds that contain carbon and hydrogen.

**Photochemical smog:** The brownish-yellow haze resulting from the combination of hydrocarbons and nitrogen oxides.

**Temperature inversion:** A weather condition occurring when a layer of cool air is trapped under a layer of warmer air.

**Acid rain:** Precipitation contaminated with acidic pollutants.

# It's Not Easy Being Green

Circle the number of each item that describes what you have done or are doing to help the environment

1. When walking, cycling, camping, or spending time at beaches, I never leave anything behind.

2. I ride my bike, walk, carpool, or use public transportation whenever possible.

3. I have written my municipal, provincial, and federal representatives about environmental issues.

4. I avoid turning on the air conditioner or increasing the heat whenever possible.

5. My shower has a low-flow shower head.

6. I do not run the water while brushing my teeth, shaving, or hand-washing clothes.

7. I take short showers instead of baths.

8. My sink taps have aerators installed in them.

9. I have a water displacement device in my toilet.

10. I snip or rip plastic six-pack rings before I throw them out.

11. I choose recycled and recyclable products as often as possible.

12. I avoid noise pollutants. (I sit away from speakers at concerts, select an apartment away from busy streets or airports, and so on.)

13. I make sure my car is tuned and has functional emission control equipment.

14. I try to avoid known carcinogens such as vinyl chloride, asbestos, benzene, mercury, X-rays, and so on.

15. When shopping, I choose products with the least amount of packaging and I reuse shopping bags.

16. I dispose of hazardous materials (old car batteries, used oil or antifreeze) at gas stations or other appropriate sites.

17. If or when I have children, I will use cloth rather than disposable diapers.

18. I store food in glass jars or other reusable containers and waxed paper rather than in plastic wrap.

19. I use as few paper products as possible.

20. I take my own bag along when I go shopping.

21. I avoid products packaged in plastic and unrecycled aluminum.

22. I recycle newspapers, glass, cans, and other recyclables.

23. I run the clothes dryer only as long as it takes my clothes to dry.

24. I turn off lights and appliances when they are not in use.

25. I compost my organic wastes.

## SCORING AND INTERPRETATION

Count how many items you have circled. Ideally, you should be doing all these things, but if you are trying to do at least some, you can score yourself as follows:

**20–25:** Good contributions to maintaining the environment.

**14–19:** Moderate contributions to maintaining the environment.

**Below 13:** Need to consider the recommendations made in this chapter to help the environment.

---

in the emissions combine with the oxygen and sunlight in the air to become sulphur dioxide and nitrogen oxides (precursors of sulphuric acid and nitric acids, respectively). Small acid particles are then carried by the wind and combine with moisture to produce acidic rain, snow, or fog. Because of higher concentrations of sunlight in the summer months, rain is more strongly acidic in the summertime. Additionally, the rain or snow that falls at the beginning of a storm is more acidic than that which falls later. Southern Ontario experiences some of the highest concentrations of acid aerosols in North America.[12]

## Effects of Acid Rain

The damage caused to lake and pond habitats is not the worst of the problems created by acid rain. Each year, acid rain is also responsible for the destruction of millions of trees in forests in Europe and North America. Scientists concluded that 75 percent of Europe's forests are now experiencing damaging levels of sulphur deposition by acid rain. Forests in every country on the continent are affected.[13]

Doctors believe that acid rain also aggravates and may even cause bronchitis, asthma, and other respiratory problems. In Southern Ontario, several air pollution epidemiological studies demonstrated that increases in acid aerosols and ground-level ozone positively correlate with increased hospital admissions due to respiratory problems.[14] People with emphysema and those with a history of heart disease may also suffer from exposure to acid rain. In addition, it may be hazardous to a pregnant woman's unborn child.

Acidic precipitation can cause metals such as aluminum, cadmium, lead, and mercury to **leach** (dissolve and filter) out of the soil. If these metals make their way into water or food supplies (particularly fish), they can cause cancer in humans who consume them.

Acid rain is also responsible for crop damage, which, in turn, contributes to world hunger. Laboratory experiments showed that acid rain reduced seed yield by up to 23 percent. Actual crop losses are reported with increasing frequency. In May 1989, China's Hunan Province lost an estimated $260 million worth of crops and seedlings to acid rain. Similar losses have been reported in Chile, Brazil, and Mexico.[15] Another consequence of acid rain is the destruction of public monuments and structures, with billions of dollars in damage each year.[16]

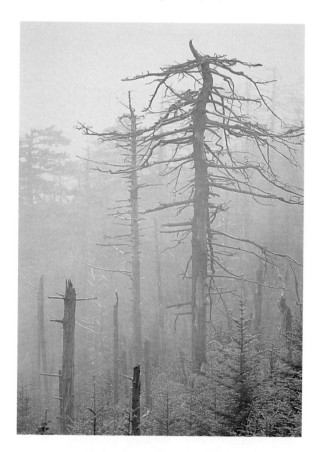

*Acid rain has many harmful effects on the environment and poses numerous health hazards, including the risk of cancer from heavy metals that can make their way into the food chain.*

# Indoor Air Pollution

In the last several years, a growing body of scientific evidence indicates that the air within homes and other buildings can be 10 to 40 times more hazardous than outdoor air even in the most industrialized cities. Research also indicates that some of the most vulnerable people, particularly the young, the elderly, and the chronically ill, often spend more than 90 percent of their time indoors.[17]

There are 20 to 100 potentially dangerous compounds in the average home. Most indoor pollution comes from sources that release gases or particles into the air. Inadequate ventilation, particularly in heavily insulated buildings with airtight windows, may increase pollution by not allowing in outside air. Some sources, such as building materials, furnishings, and household products such as air fresheners, release pollutants continuously. Others release pollutants intermittently. Several factors affect risk including age, pre-existing medical conditions, individual sensitivity, room temperature and humidity, and functioning of the liver, immune, and respiratory systems.[18]

Prevention should focus on three main areas: source control (eliminating or reducing individual contaminants), ventilation improvements (increasing the amount of outdoor air coming indoors), and air cleaners (removing particulates from the air).[19] Indoor air pollution comes primarily from woodstoves, furnaces, asbestos, passive smoke, formaldehyde, radon, and household chemicals. Mould may also be a significant source.

## Wood Stove Smoke

Wood stoves emit significant levels of particulates and carbon monoxide in addition to other pollutants, such as sulphur dioxide. If you rely on wood for heating, make sure that your stove is properly installed, vented, and maintained. Proper adjustments and emission controls taken to recombust potential pollutants can also help to reduce pollution levels from wood stoves. Burning properly seasoned wood reduces the amount of particulates released into the air.

## Furnaces

People who rely on oil- or gas-fired furnaces also need to make sure that these appliances are properly installed, ventilated, and maintained. Inadequate cleaning and maintenance can lead to a build-up of carbon monoxide in the home, which can be deadly.

**Leach:** A process by which chemicals dissolve and filter through soil.

## Asbestos

Asbestos is another indoor air pollutant that poses serious threats to human health. **Asbestos** is a mineral commonly used in insulating materials in buildings constructed before 1970. When bonded to other materials, asbestos is relatively harmless, but if its tiny fibres become loosened and airborne, they can embed themselves in the lungs and cannot be expelled. Their presence leads to cancer of the lungs, stomach, and chest lining, and is the cause of a fatal lung disease called mesothelioma.

## Passive Smoke

Typically, **passive smoke** is commonly encountered as secondhand or sidestream smoke at home. Similar to active smoking, lengthy exposure to passive smoke can cause serious negative health effects. Non-smokers who live with smokers are at a higher risk for heart disease and some cancers. Passive smoke is a major cause of respiratory problems, especially in infants and children who live with a smoker. Though widespread bans are now in place limiting smokers from lighting up in restaurants and in the workplace, many people are still susceptible to passive smoke at home. Avoiding regular exposure to secondhand tobacco smoke will greatly reduce your risks of heart and lung disease.

## Formaldehyde

**Formaldehyde** is a colourless, strong-smelling gas present in some carpets, draperies, furniture, particle board, plywood, wood panelling, countertops, and many adhesives. It is released into the air in a process called outgassing. Outgassing is greatest in new products, but the process can continue for many years. Exposure to formaldehyde can cause respiratory problems, dizziness, fatigue, nausea, and rashes. Long-term exposure can lead to central nervous system disorders and cancer. If you experience symptoms of formaldehyde exposure, have your home tested by a municipal, regional, or provincial health agency.

## Radon

**Radon,** an odourless, colourless gas, is the natural by-product of the decay of uranium and radium in the soil. Radon may penetrate homes through cracks, pipes, sump pits, and other openings in the foundation. At toxic levels, it can cause lung cancer. However, Health Canada does not consider radon pollution a widespread problem in Canadian homes. In fact, studies indicate that less than one-tenth of one percent of all homes in Canada—fewer than 8,000 out of a total of eight million—could have levels of radon sufficiently high to warrant efforts aimed at lowering the level. Population studies based on a survey of 14,000 homes in 19 Canadian cities did not show a correlation between radon levels in homes and lung cancer.[20]

## Household Chemicals

Cleansers and other cleaning products should be used only in well-ventilated rooms. Further, regular cleaning will reduce the need to use potentially harmful cleaning products. Cut down on dry cleaning, as the chemicals used by many cleaners can cause cancer. If your newly cleaned clothes smell of dry cleaning chemicals, either return them to the cleaner or hang them in the open air until the smell is gone. Avoid the use of household air freshener products containing the carcinogenic agent dichlorobenzene.

### WHAT WOULD YOU DO?

Has the Canadian federal government taken strong enough environmental measures to protect its citizens? What about the provincial governments? What is the obligation of developing and developed countries to reduce air pollution? What is your role as a concerned citizen? What efforts could you make?

# OZONE LAYER DEPLETION

We earlier defined *ozone* as a chemical produced when oxygen interacts with sunlight. Close to the earth, ozone creates health problems such as respiratory distress. Farther away from the earth, it forms a protective membrane-like layer in the earth's stratosphere—the highest level of the earth's atmosphere, located from 20 to 50 kilometres above the earth's surface. The ozone layer in the stratosphere protects the planet and its inhabitants from ultraviolet B (UV-B) radiation, a primary cause of skin cancer. Ultraviolet B radiation may also damage DNA and be linked to weakened immune systems in humans and animals.

In the early 1970s, scientists began to warn of a depletion of the earth's stratospheric ozone layer. Special instruments developed to test atmospheric contents indicated that specific chemicals used on the earth contributed to the rapid depletion of this vital protective layer. These chemicals are called **chlorofluorocarbons (CFCs)** (see Figure 15.2). In 1979, a satellite measurement showing a large hole in the ozone layer over Antarctica shocked scientists. Since then, satellite measurements of the ozone layer have regularly shown increases in the size of the hole. As a

# A Breath of Fresh Air: Made in Canada Solutions to Meet Canada's Environmental Challenges

Although the Government of Canada is viewed as a leader on environmental sustainability issues and a strong promoter of sustainable development opportunities, there remains a large number and variety of issues for Canada to deal with. Current efforts aimed at protecting the health and well-being of Canadians and their communities from air pollution have not matched our reputation. Since ratifying the Kyoto Protocol, Canada's greenhouse gas emissions are up 24 percent—a far cry from the target of 6 percent below 1990 levels. Further, Canada ranked 28th overall out of 30 countries on 29 environmental indicators in the "Maple Leaf in the OECD: Comparing Progress Toward Sustainability" report. More specifically, Canada ranked 26th in greenhouse gas emissions, 29th in water consumption, 27th in pollution from sulphur oxides, and 26th on species at risk.

As a result, we need to take action; we need to clean the air we breathe. It is critical that we act. It is critical that we act now. In a report from a 2004 British Columbia Provincial Officer of Health, it was estimated that air pollution would cause between 140 and 400 premature deaths, 700 to 2,100 hospital stays, and between 900 and 2,700 emergency room visits per year.

Further, the direct and indirect costs of air pollution are staggering. In Ontario for 2005 these costs were estimated to be $374 million due to lost productivity and work time, $507 million for indirect healthcare costs, $537 million in pain and suffering, and $6.4 billion in social welfare due to premature death.

There were 53 smog advisory days in Ontario, 24 in Quebec, and three in the Atlantic Provinces in the summer of 2005. Ten winter smog advisories were also issued in Quebec, and five more in Ontario.

Given these findings, the solutions proposed must address greenhouse gases and air pollution—not each separately, as has been done in the past. Thus, the federal government will develop—in conjunction with the provinces and territories, municipalities, and aboriginal communities—a new Canadian Clean Air Act. Canadians will be encouraged "to get out of their cars and get onto public transit by providing a federal tax credit to offset part of the costs of monthly transit passes. Increasing the use of public transit will help reduce traffic congestion in Canadian cities, reduce greenhouse gases and fight pollution." Those who cannot get out of their cars will be encouraged to use cleaner fuel.

It is expected that offering these cleaner choices and inviting Canadians to work with the government in making solutions will result in a cleaner Canada and lead to a cleaner world.

Source: Adapted from Environment Canada's "A Breath of Fresh Air: Made in Canada Solutions to Meet Canada's Environmental Challenges," speaking notes for an address by the Honourable Rona Ambrose, Minister of the Environment of Canada, Vancouver B.C., March 31, 2006. Retrieved on May 19, 2006, from www.ec.gc.ca/minister/speeches/2006/ 060331_s_e.htm. Reproduced with the permission of the Minister of Public Works and Government Services Canada, 2007.

result, Canada banned the production of CFCs in 1993 and their importation in 1996. Methyl chloroform was also banned in 1996.

## Global Warming

More than 100 years ago, scientists theorized that carbon dioxide emissions from fossil-fuel burning would create a buildup of greenhouse gases in the earth's atmosphere and that this accumulation would have a warming effect on the earth's surface. The century-old predictions are now coming true, with alarming effects. Average global temperatures are higher today than at any time since global temperatures were first recorded, and the change in atmospheric temperature may be taking a heavy toll on humans and crops. Climate researchers predicted in 1975 that the buildup of greenhouse gases would produce life-threatening natural phenomena, including drought, severe forest fires, flooding, extended heat waves over large areas of the earth, and killer hurricanes. Figure 15.3 illustrates the complex interactions and the influence of climate change on human health.

**Asbestos:** A substance that separates into stringy fibres and lodges in lungs, where it can cause various diseases.

**Passive smoke:** Secondhand or sidestream cigarette smoke.

**Formaldehyde:** A colourless, strong-smelling gas released through outgassing; causes respiratory and other health problems.

**Radon:** A naturally occurring radioactive gas resulting from the decay of certain radioactive elements.

**Chlorofluorocarbons (CFCs):** Chemicals that contribute to the depletion of the ozone layer.

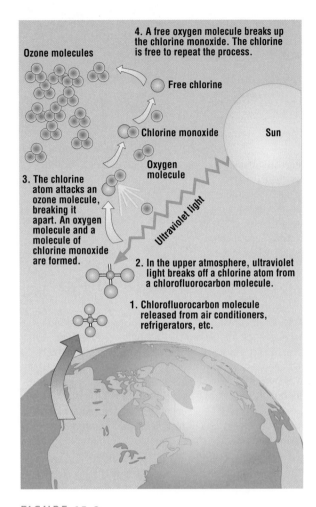

FIGURE 15.2

This diagram shows the depletion of the stratospheric ozone layer.

Text in Figure 15.2:

4. A free oxygen molecule breaks up the chlorine monoxide. The chlorine is free to repeat the process.

Ozone molecules

Free chlorine

Chlorine monoxide

Sun

Oxygen molecule

Ultraviolet light

3. The chlorine atom attacks an ozone molecule, breaking it apart. An oxygen molecule and a molecule of chlorine monoxide are formed.

2. In the upper atmosphere, ultraviolet light breaks off a chlorine atom from a chlorofluorocarbon molecule.

1. Chlorofluorocarbon molecule released from air conditioners, refrigerators, etc.

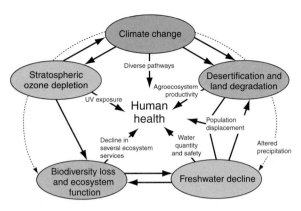

Text in Figure 15.3:

Climate change

Stratospheric ozone depletion

Diverse pathways

Agroecosystem productivity

Desertification and land degradation

UV exposure

Human health

Population displacement

Decline in several ecosystem services

Water quantity and safety

Altered precipitation

Biodiversity loss and ecosystem function

Freshwater decline

FIGURE 15.3

Large-scale and global environmental hazards to human health include climate change, stratospheric ozone depletion, loss of biodiversity, changes in hydrological systems and the supplies of fresh water, land degradation, and stresses on food-producing systems.

Source: World Health Organization, www.who.int/globalchange/en/.

The potential consequences of global warming are dire. The rising atmospheric concentration of greenhouse gases may be the most economically disruptive and costly change set in motion by our modern industrial society. Ozone causes damage to leaf tissue, inhibiting photosynthesis, the process by which plants use light energy for growth. Some forest species at risk include northern red oak, eastern white pine, black oak, and sugar maple. Ground-level ozone has been linked to the forest decline observed in Germany and other European countries.[21]

## Reducing Air Pollution

Canada's air pollution problems are rooted in our energy, transportation, and industrial practices. Comprehensive national strategies are required to reduce air pollution and clean the air for future generations. We must support policies that encourage the use of renewable resources such as solar, wind, and water power as the providers of most of the world's energy.[22] Our atmosphere has no borders.

Most experts agree that shifting away from gas-powered automobiles as the primary source of transportation is the only way to reduce air pollution significantly, which would reduce the greenhouse effect and, consequently, global warming. Some cities have taken steps in this direction by setting high parking fees, imposing bans on city driving, and establishing high road-usage tolls. Further, community governments should be encouraged to provide convenient, inexpensive, and easily accessible public transportation for citizens.

**Greenhouse gases** include carbon dioxide, CFCs, ground-level ozone, nitrous oxide, and methane. They become part of a gaseous layer that encircles the earth, allowing solar heat to pass through and then trapping that heat close to the earth's surface. The most predominant of these gases is carbon dioxide, which accounts for 49 percent of all greenhouse gases. Eastern Europe and North America are responsible for approximately half of all carbon dioxide emissions. Since the late nineteenth century, carbon dioxide concentrations in the atmosphere have increased 25 percent, with half of this increase occurring since the 1950s. Not surprisingly, these greater concentrations coincide with world industrial growth.

Rapid deforestation of the tropical rainforests of Central and South America, Africa, and Southeast Asia is also contributing to the rapid rise in the presence of greenhouse gases. Trees take in carbon dioxide, transform it, store the carbon for food, and then release oxygen into the air. Thus, as we lose forests we lose the capacity to dissipate carbon dioxide.

Auto makers must be encouraged to manufacture automobiles that provide good fuel economy and low rates of toxic emissions. Incentives given to manufacturers to produce such cars, tax breaks for purchasers who buy them, and "gas-guzzler" taxes on inefficient vehicles are three promising suggestions that may effectively help to reduce air pollution.

## WHAT WOULD YOU DO?

What products would you be willing to stop using in order to protect the ozone layer? What motivations lead to deforestation of the rain forests? What could be done to address these problems?

# WATER POLLUTION

Seventy-five percent of the earth is covered with water in the form of oceans, seas, lakes, rivers, streams, and wetlands. Beneath the landmass are reservoirs of groundwater. We draw our drinking water from either this underground source or surface freshwater sources. The status of our water supply reflects the pollution level of our communities and, ultimately, the whole earth.

The federal government passed the Canada Water Act in 1970 and created the Department of the Environment in 1971, entrusting the Inland Waters Directorate with providing national leadership for freshwater management. Under the Constitution Act (1867), the provinces are "owners" of the water resources and have wide responsibilities in their day-to-day management. The federal government has certain specific responsibilities relating to water, such as fisheries and navigation, as well as exercising certain overall responsibilities such as the conduct of external affairs.[23]

## Water Contamination

Any substance that gets into the soil has the potential to get into the water supply. Contaminants from industrial air pollution and acid rain eventually work their way into the soil and then into the groundwater. Pesticides sprayed on crops wash through the soil into the groundwater. Spills of oil and other hazardous wastes flow into local rivers and streams. Underground storage tanks for gasoline may develop leaks. The list continues.

Pollutants can enter waterways through a number of routes. These routes may be divided into two general categories: *point-source* and *non-point-source*.

Pollutants that enter a waterway at a specific point through a pipe, ditch, culvert, or other such conduit are referred to as **point-source pollutants.** The two major sources of this type of pollution are sewage treatment plants and industrial facilities.

**Non-point-source pollutants**—commonly known as *runoff* and *sedimentation*—seep into waterways from broad areas of land rather than through a discrete pipe or conduit. It is currently estimated that 99 percent of the sediment in our waterways, 98 percent of the bacterial contaminants, 84 percent of the phosphorus, and 82 percent of the nitrogen come from non-point sources.[24] Non-point-source pollution results from a variety of human land-use practices. It includes soil erosion and sedimentation, construction wastes, pesticide and fertilizer runoff, urban street runoff, wastes from engineering projects, acid mine drainage, leakage from septic tanks, and sewage sludge.[25] (See Figure 15.4.)

### Septic Systems

Bacteria from human waste can leach into the water supply from improperly installed septic systems. Toxic chemicals disposed of directly into septic systems can also get into the groundwater supply.

### Landfills

Landfills and dumps generate a liquid called leachate, a mixture of soluble chemicals that come from household garbage, office, biological, and industrial waste. If a landfill has not been properly lined, leachate trickles through its layers of garbage and eventually into the water supply.

### Gasoline and Petroleum Products

Underground storage tanks for gasoline and petroleum products are common; most are located at gasoline filling stations. A number of these underground tanks are thought to be leaking.[26] Most of these tanks were installed 30 to 35 years ago. They were made of fabricated steel that was unprotected from corrosion. Over time, pinpoint holes developed in the steel and the petroleum products stored in the tanks leaked into the groundwater. The most common way to detect the presence of petroleum products in the water supply is

**Greenhouse gases:** Gases that contribute to global warming by trapping heat near the earth's surface.

**Point-source pollutants:** Pollutants that enter waterways at a specific point.

**Non-point-source pollutants:** Pollutants that seep into waterways from broad areas of land.

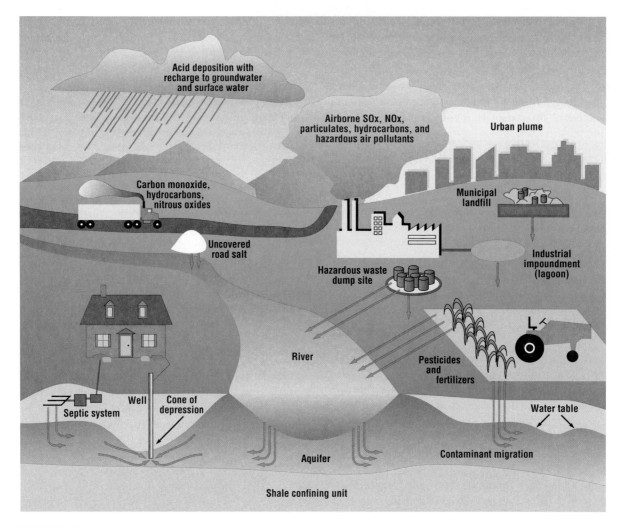

FIGURE 15.4

Sources of Groundwater Contamination

to test for benzene, a component of oil and gasoline. Benzene is highly toxic and associated with the development of cancer.

### Dioxins

**Dioxins** are chlorinated hydrocarbons contained in herbicides (chemicals that are used to kill vegetation) and produced during certain industrial processes. Dioxins have the ability to bioaccumulate and are much more toxic than PCBs (see below).

## Chemical Contaminants

Most chemicals designed to dissolve grease and oil are called *organic solvents*. These extremely toxic substances, such as carbon tetrachloride, tetrachloroethylene, and trichloroethylene (TCE), are used to clean clothing, painting equipment, plastics, and metal parts. Many household products, such as stain and spot removers, degreasers, drain cleaners, septic system cleaners, and paint removers, also contain these toxic chemicals.

Organic solvents work their way into the water supply in different ways. Consumers often dump leftover products into the toilet. Industries pour leftovers into large barrels, which are then buried. After a while, the chemicals eat their way out of the barrels and leach into the groundwater system.

A related group of toxic substances contains chlorinated hydrocarbons. The most notorious of these substances are the polychlorinated biphenyls (PCBs), their cousins the *polybromated biphenyls (PBBs)*, and the *dioxins*.

### PCBs

**Polychlorinated biphenyls (PCBs)** are fire-resistant and stable at high temperatures and therefore were used for many years as insulating materials in high-voltage electrical equipment such as transformers. PCBs bioaccumulate, meaning that the body does not excrete them but stores them in fatty tissues and the liver. PCBs are associated with birth defects, and exposure to them is known to cause cancer. PCBs have not been manufactured in North America since the late 1970s, but millions of kilograms of PCBs have been dumped into landfills and waterways, where they continue to pose an environmental threat.[27]

The long-term effects of bioaccumulation of these toxic substances include possible damage to the immune system, increased risk of infection, and elevated risk of cancer. Exposure to high concentrations of PCBs or dioxins for a short period of time can also have severe consequences, including nausea, vomiting, diarrhea, painful rashes and sores, and chloracne, an ailment in which the skin develops hard, black, painful pimples that may never go away.

## Pesticides

**Pesticides** are chemicals designed to kill insects, rodents, plants, and fungi. Canadians use millions of kilograms of pesticides each year, with only 10 percent actually reaching the targeted organisms. The remaining pesticides settle on the land and in the water. Pesticide residues also cling to many fresh fruits and vegetables and are ingested when people eat these items. Most pesticides accumulate in the body. Potential hazards associated with long-term exposure to pesticides include birth defects, cancer, liver and kidney damage, and nervous system disorders.

## Trihalomethanes

Most Canadians drink water treated with chlorine to kill harmful bacteria. *Trihalomethanes (THMs)* are synthetic organic chemicals formed at water treatment plants when the added chlorine reacts with natural organic compounds in the water. Any drinking water supply that has been chlorinated is likely to contain THMs, which include such substances as chloroform, bromoform, and dichlorobromomethane. Chloroform in high doses is known to cause liver and kidney disorders, central nervous system problems, birth defects, and cancer. Recent research indicates that THM concentrations can be substantially reduced by adjusting the chlorine dose, improving filtration practices to remove organic material, or adding chlorine after filtration rather than before.[28]

## Lead

Lead might be ingested in household water if the house is an older one with lead pipes. Water, particularly acidic water, will leach some of the lead from the pipes. One way to reduce the possibility of ingesting lead if it does exist in your home's water system is to run tap water for several minutes before taking a drink or cooking with it to flush out water that has been standing overnight. Although leaded paints and ceramic glazes also pose health risks, particularly for small children who put painted toys in their mouths, the use of leads in such products has been effectively reduced in recent years.

---

### WHAT WOULD YOU DO?

What can you do to ensure clean water in your home? In your community? What personal actions can you take to conserve water? What measures can you take to avoid excessive exposure to pesticides?

---

# NOISE POLLUTION

Loud noise has become commonplace. We are often painfully aware of construction crews working on our streets, jet airplanes roaring overhead, stereos blaring next door, and trucks rumbling down nearby freeways. Our bodies have definite physiological responses to noise, and noise can become a source of physical and mental distress.

Prolonged exposure to some noises results in hearing loss. Short-term exposure reduces productivity, concentration levels, and attention spans, and may affect mental and emotional health. Symptoms of noise-related distress include disturbed sleep patterns, headaches, and tension. Physically, our bodies respond to noises in a variety of ways. Blood pressure increases, blood vessels in the brain dilate, and vessels in other parts of the body constrict. The pupils of the eye dilate. Cholesterol levels in the blood rise and some endocrine glands secrete additional stimulating hormones, such as adrenaline, into the bloodstream.

At this point, it is necessary to distinguish between sound and noise. Sound is anything that can be heard. Noise is sound that can damage the hearing or cause mental or emotional distress. When sound becomes distracting or annoying, it becomes noise.

Unfortunately, despite gradually increasing awareness that noise pollution is more than just a nuisance,

---

**Dioxins:** Highly toxic chlorinated hydrocarbons contained in herbicides and produced during certain industrial processes.

**Polychlorinated biphenyls (PCBs):** Toxic chemicals once used as insulating materials in high-voltage electrical equipment.

**Pesticides:** Chemicals that kill pests.

governments have given noise-control programs low priority. In order to prevent hearing loss, it is important that you take it upon yourself to avoid exposure to excessive noise. Playing stereos in your car and home at reasonable levels, wearing earplugs when you use power equipment, and establishing barriers (closed windows, etc.) between you and noise will help keep your hearing intact.

# LAND POLLUTION

Many areas in North America currently face serious problems in safely and effectively managing their garbage.

## Solid Waste

**Municipal solid waste** is outstripping available landfill sites, and the opening of new landfill sites is usually controversial, as people become more aware of the hazards they pose to nearby land and water. Toronto has had to scramble in the last few years to find communities in other parts of Ontario that would take its overflow garbage.

Part of the answer is increased commitment to reducing, reusing, and recycling. Experts believe that as much as 90 percent of our garbage is ultimately reusable or recyclable.

## Hazardous Waste

The large number of **hazardous waste** dump sites in the United States indicates the severity of the toxic chemical problem in North America. American manufacturers generate more than one tonne of chemical waste per person per year (approximately 250 million tonnes). Three industrial groups produce most of this waste: chemicals and allied products, metal-related industries, and petroleum and coal products.[29]

The Canadian Environmental Protection Agency (CEPA) has established an overall program to deal with hazardous wastes. The CEPA divides hazardous materials into two groups. Persistent, bioaccumulative,

toxic hazardous wastes that are primarily the result of human activity will be targeted for virtual elimination from the environment; substances that do not meet these criteria are candidates for full life-cycle management to prevent or minimize their release into the environment.[30]

Industry education and cooperation are important in achieving a safer environment. In cooperation with provincial and municipal authorities, the following procedures have been put in place:

- Many wastes are now banned from land disposal or are treated in such a way that their toxicity is reduced before they are dumped in land disposal sites.

- Hazardous-waste handlers must now clean up contamination resulting from past waste management practices as well as from current activities.

- CEPA is exploring ways to create economic incentives to encourage ingenuity in waste minimization practices and recycling.

# RADIATION

A substance is considered radioactive when it emits high-energy particles from the nuclei of its atoms. There are three types of radiation: alpha particles, beta particles, and gamma rays. Alpha particles are relatively massive particles not capable of penetrating human skin. They pose health hazards only when inhaled or ingested. Beta particles are capable of slight penetration of the skin and are harmful if ingested or inhaled. Gamma rays are the most dangerous radioactive particles because they can pass right through the skin, causing serious damage to organs and other vital structures.

## Ionizing Radiation

Exposure to ionizing radiation is an inescapable part of life. **Ionizing radiation** is caused by the release of particles and electromagnetic rays from atomic

# A Brief History of the Kyoto Protocol

The Kyoto Protocol represents a crucial first step in the world's fight to stop climate change. The Kyoto Protocol is signed by 128 nations, and commits participating industrialized countries to cut deadly greenhouse gas emissions by 5 percent between 2008 and 2012. These are the highlights leading up to the Kyoto Protocol.

### 1972—1st Earth Summit In Stockholm, Sweden

World leaders announced their intention to hold a gathering every ten years to determine the health of the planet.

### 1988—The International Panel on Climate Change was created by the UN to find scientific answers to climate change

It released its first report in 1990, stating that it believed the planet was warming, that human activity was causing this warming, but that it needed to do more research to be certain.

### 1988—Toronto Conference on the Changing Atmosphere

Former prime minister Brian Mulroney and former Norwegian prime minister Gro Harlem Bruntland hosted one of the world's first major scientific conferences on climate change. It called for a 20 percent cut to 1988 greenhouse gas emissions by 2005 and called the effect of climate change, "second only to global nuclear war."

### 1992—2nd Earth Summit, Rio de Janeiro, Brazil

The largest gathering of world leaders ever, the Earth Summit created the United Nations Framework Convention on Climate Change, also known as the Rio Convention. This convention called on the world to stabilize 1990 greenhouse gas emissions by 2000.

Canada and the United States signed and ratified this convention. Former U.S. president George Bush Sr. negotiated an agreement to allow developing nations to increase emissions, the reason they are not included in the Kyoto Protocol. The treaty is legally binding on countries that ratified it.

### 1995—COP I In Berlin, Germany

Each year, the countries that ratified the Rio Convention held a Conference of Parties (COP). The first of these happened in 1995 and reviewed the adequacy of the Rio Convention's goal of stabilizing greenhouse gas emissions.

### 1995—The IPCC's Second Report

The IPCC released its second report saying "the balance of evidence" pointed to a "discernable human influence on the global climate system."

### 1997—COP III in Kyoto, Japan

After reviewing the original targets of the Rio Convention and finding them too weak, the countries came up with new targets. Now, 1990 greenhouse gas emissions would be cut by 5 percent between 2008 and 2012. Though 5 percent is a global target, different countries have different targets. The European Union's target is an 8 percent cut (Germany committed to a 25 percent cut and the U.K. to 15 percent). The United States had a target of 7 percent and Canada a target of 6 percent.

### 1998—COP IV in Buenos Aires, Argentina

Here, the Buenos Aires Plan of Action was developed to decide how the Kyoto mechanism (emissions trading, carbon sinks, clean development in the developing world, etc.) would be implemented. The countries agreed the mechanism through which targets would be achieved would be finalized by COP VI, or by 2000.

### 2001—COP V1/2 in Bonn, Germany

Just before dawn on July 29, 2001, 180 countries (that is, the whole world except for the United States and Australia) agreed to the rules for implementing the Kyoto Protocol. Now each country must officially ratify the accord.

### 2002—Update

Canadian Parliament ratified Canada's participation in the agreement. Currently, Canada produces less than 2 percent of total greenhouse-gas emissions. The United States, the largest producer of greenhouse-gas emissions, decided not to ratify the accord.

Source: Reprinted courtesy of Greenpeace Canada, www.greenpeace.ca.

---

nuclei during the normal process of disintegration. Some naturally occurring elements, such as uranium, emit radiation. Other radiation-producing elements, such as deuterium, develop as part of the decay process of uranium or are created by scientists in laboratories. Radiation, whether naturally occurring or

**Municipal solid waste:** Includes wastes such as durable goods, nondurable goods, containers and packaging, food wastes, yard wastes, and miscellaneous wastes from residential, commercial, institutional, and industrial sources.

**Hazardous waste:** Solid waste that, due to its toxic properties, poses a hazard to humans or to the environment.

human-made, can damage the genetic material in the reproductive cells of living organisms. It can also cause mutations, miscarriages, physical and mental deformities, cancer, eye cataracts, gastrointestinal illnesses, and shortened life expectancies.

Scientists cannot agree on a safe level of radiation. Reactions to radiation differ from person to person. Exposure is measured in radiation absorbed doses, or rads (also called roentgens). Recommended maximum "safe" dosages range from 0.5 to 5 rads per year. Approximately 50 percent of the radiation we are exposed to comes from natural sources, such as building materials. Another 45 percent comes from medical and dental X-rays. The remaining 5 percent comes from computer display screens, microwave ovens, television sets, luminous watch dials, and radar screens and waves. Most of us are exposed to far less radiation than the "safe" maximum dosage per year.

Radiation can cause damage at dosages as low as 100 to 200 rads. At this level, signs of radiation sickness include nausea, diarrhea, fatigue, anemia, sore throat, and hair loss. Death is unlikely at this dosage.

At 350 to 500 rads, the previously mentioned symptoms increase in severity, and death may result because the radiation hinders bone marrow production of the white blood cells we need to protect us from disease. Dosages above 600 to 700 rads are invariably fatal. The effects of long-term exposure to relatively low levels of radiation are unknown. Some scientists believe that such exposure can cause lung cancer, leukemia, skin cancer, bone cancer, and skeletal deformities.

## Nonionizing Radiation

The lower-energy portions of the electromagnetic spectrum, ranging from lower-energy ultraviolet radiation down through infrared, radar, radio, and the electric and magnetic fields associated with many household appliances and electric power lines, are **nonionizing radiation.** Although the biological effects of ionizing radiation have been recognized for some time, we still do not know very much about the effects of certain types of nonionizing

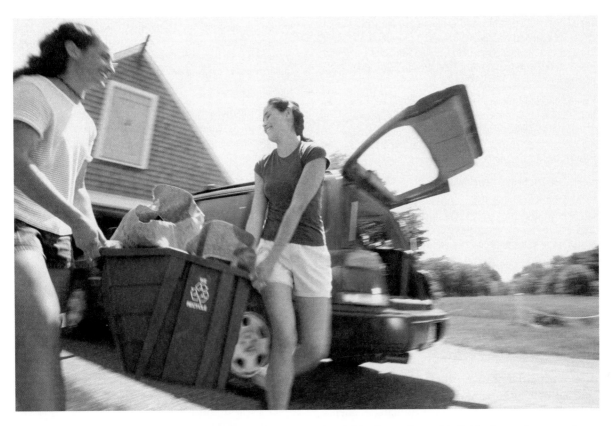

*While we may feel that many of the environmental problems facing the world today are beyond individual control, we can play a significant role in keeping our own little part of it clean, green, and beautiful.*

radiation—in particular, the photons associated with electric and magnetic fields. Techniques for assessing radiation from many such sources are still evolving.[31]

## Nuclear Power Plants

Nuclear power plants account for less than one percent of the total radiation we are exposed to. Other producers of radioactive wastes include medical facilities that use radioactive materials for treatment and diagnostic procedures and nuclear weapons production facilities.

Proponents of nuclear energy believe that it is a safe and efficient way to generate electricity. Initial costs of building nuclear power plants are high, but actual power generation is relatively inexpensive. A 1,000-megawatt reactor produces enough energy for 600,000 homes and saves 1,590 million litres of fossil fuels each year. In some areas where nuclear power plants were decommissioned, electricity bills tripled when power companies turned to hydroelectric or fossil fuel sources to generate electricity.

Nuclear reactors also discharge fewer carbon oxides into the air than fossil fuel–powered generators. Advocates believe that conversion to nuclear power could help slow the global warming trend.[32] Over the past 15 years, carbon emissions were reduced by 298 million tonnes, or five percent.

All these advantages of nuclear energy must be weighed against the disadvantages. First, disposal of nuclear wastes is extremely problematic for the entire world. Additionally, the chances of a reactor core meltdown pose serious threats to a plant's immediate environment and to the world in general.

A nuclear **meltdown** occurs when the temperature in the core of the reactor increases enough to melt the nuclear fuel and the containment vessel that holds it. Most modern facilities seal their reactors and containment vessels in concrete buildings with pools of cold water on the bottom. Then, if a meltdown occurs, the building and the pool should prevent the escape of radioactivity.

Human error and mechanical failure were the reported causes of the 1986 reactor core fire and explosion at the Chernobyl nuclear power plant in Russia. In just 4.5 seconds, the temperature in the reactor rose to 120 times normal, causing an explosion. Eighteen people were killed immediately, 30 died later from radiation sickness, and 200 others were hospitalized for severe radiation sickness. Officials evacuated people living nearby the plant. Some medical workers estimate that the eventual death toll from radiation-induced cancers topped 100,000. Direct costs of the disaster were more than $13 billion,

including lost agricultural output and the cost of replacing the power plant.

Opponents of nuclear energy believe that there is no safe place to dispose of, contain, or store our escalating supply of nuclear waste.

---

### WHAT WOULD YOU DO?

How much exposure do you have to ionizing and nonionizing radiation a year? What measures could you take to reduce this exposure? Do you believe the advantages outweigh the disadvantages of nuclear power? Why or why not?

---

## Food Quality

For most Canadians, food accounts for 80 to 95 percent of their daily intake of the most persistent toxic contaminants, while air contributes 10 to 15 percent and drinking water contributes very little. Compared with other countries Canada's food is some of the safest, but contamination remains a concern. Aside from microbial contamination, as discussed in Chapter 7, environmental contamination can occur in several fashions. Chemical contaminants can enter the food supply through uptake from water or soil, and by air deposition on leaves and fruit. Some contaminants can bioaccumulate to become more toxic when at the top of the food chain, as with mercury concentration in game fish in a number of Canadian water systems. Also, chemicals used in food production and handling can leave residues on food products, for example the hormones and antibiotics used to increase meat and dairy production, or the substances used to preserve freshness or enhance flavour.[33] Refer back to "Food Safety: Increasing Concerns" in Chapter 7 for steps you can take to reduce your risk.

---

**Ionizing radiation:** Radiation produced by photons having high enough energy to ionize atoms.

**Nonionizing radiation:** Radiation produced by photons associated with lower-energy portions of the electromagnetic spectrum.

**Meltdown:** An accident that results when the temperature in the core of a nuclear reactor increases sufficiently to melt the nuclear fuel and the containment vessel housing it.

# Managing Environmental Pollution

Environmental health begins at home. We all have to overcome our inertia and make sacrifices that contribute to the good of the planet. By understanding how political and economic issues affect the environment, we can pressure corporations and elected representatives to change policies harmful to the environment. For example, environmentalists pressured the World Bank to stop issuing development loans leading to the destruction of rainforests. Discussing issues with lawmakers and making decisions at the polls are two ways you can influence environmental policy.

## MAKING DECISIONS FOR YOU

One of the biggest decisions we make as consumers is whether to pay more for environmentally safe products. As a student on a tight budget, are you willing to pay more for products such as environmentally friendly soap and laundry detergent? If so, how much more? If not, are you willing to buy a less environmentally unfriendly product? While it's not likely that you can increase your budget enough to buy all environmentally safe products, you can start now. Think about the products you buy: Which could you substitute with more environmentally friendly brands?

## CHECKLIST FOR CHANGE: MAKING PERSONAL CHOICES

- Do you vote? Do you know the difference between rhetoric and reality when it comes to environmental issues?

- Do you conserve water? Do you fix leaky taps quickly? Do you wash only full loads? Do you overwater lawns or gardens?

- Do you think before you buy? Do you buy products in recyclable packaging? Do you reuse containers rather than buy new ones?

- Do you think before you throw household chemicals away? Make sure you finish them, give them away, or save them for a household hazardous waste collection instead. Consider nonhazardous substitutes.

- Do you recycle used oil? Oil dumped down storm drains or on the ground can pollute streams, killing insects, fish, birds, and wildlife.

- Do you recycle tin cans, glass, newspaper, paper, plastic, and cardboard?

- Have you considered turning in people who litter?

- Have you considered walking, riding the bus, using your bike, or carpooling whenever possible?

- Have you thought about the amount of fertilizers and pesticides you use? Rain can wash them off lawns and carry them into lakes and streams. Always use low-phosphorus fertilizers.

- Do you ask yourself if you really need a product before you buy it?

- Do you consider whether a product is practical and durable, well-made, and of timeless design?

- Do you buy used and rebuilt products whenever possible? Do you resell your unused items at yard or garage sales (your trash may be someone else's treasure) or donate them to charities?

- Do you compost leaves, clippings, and kitchen scraps?

## CHECKLIST FOR CHANGE: MAKING COMMUNITY CHOICES

- Do you work in your community to help create and enforce laws that protect drinking water and that prohibit the manufacture, use, storage, transport, or disposal of hazardous substances in your water supply area?

- Do you volunteer to take part in cleanup activities in your community?

- Does your community have a hazardous materials ordinance?

## CRITICAL THINKING

Your health teacher is leading a protest next week to the corporate headquarters of "one of the country's worst polluters." You are told not only that this company has a terrible record of point- and non-point-source pollutants, but also that the "corporate bigwigs refuse to do anything about it." After hearing the brief appeal to join the protest, you decide it's your duty as a citizen to go. As your teacher hands out maps to the protest site, you realize that the company in question is your employer! Now you're really confused: your company claims to have spent billions of dollars to reduce pollution and considers itself an innovator in cleaning up sites it polluted in the past. You are upset because only one side of the story is being told. Should you speak up in class?

Using the DECIDE model in Chapter 1, decide what you would do. First, decide why you are upset. Then decide what you would like to accomplish by speaking up. In addition, consider the best setting to communicate your message to your teacher (in class, during office hours, by e-mail, etc.).

# SUMMARY

- Population growth is the single largest factor affecting the demands made on the environment. Demand for food, products, and energy—as well as places to dispose of waste—places great strains on the earth's resources.

- The primary constituents of air pollution are sulphur dioxide, particulate matter, carbon monoxide, nitrogen dioxide, ozone, lead, and hydrocarbons. Air pollution takes the forms of photochemical smog and acid rain, among others. Indoor air pollution is caused primarily by wood stove smoke, furnace emissions, asbestos, passive smoke, formaldehyde, and radon. Pollution is depleting the earth's protective ozone layer, causing global warming.

- Water pollution can occur either through point sources (direct entry through a pipeline, ditch, etc.) or non-point sources (runoff or seepage from a broad area of land). Major contributors to water pollution include dioxins, pesticides, trihalomethanes, and lead.

- Noise pollution affects our hearing and produces other symptoms such as reduced productivity, reduced concentration, headaches, and tension.

- Solid waste pollution includes household garbage, plastics, glass, metal products, and paper; limited landfill space creates problems. Hazardous waste is toxic and its improper disposal creates health hazards for those in surrounding communities.

- Ionizing radiation results from the natural erosion of atomic nuclei. Nonionizing radiation is caused by the electric and magnetic fields around power lines and household appliances, among other sources. The disposal and storage of radioactive wastes from nuclear power plants and weapons production pose serious potential problems for public health.

# DISCUSSION QUESTIONS

1. Describe the issues surrounding global population and how they differ among the developed, developing, and least developed countries.

2. Explain the ways in which the expanding global population affects the environment.

3. List the primary sources of air pollution, acid rain, and indoor air pollution. What can be done individually and collectively to reduce each type of pollution?

4. What are the environmental consequences of global warming? What can we as Canadian citizens do to help slow the deforestation of tropical rainforests? How might the Kyoto Protocol help in the fight to stop climate change?

5. Explain point- and non-point sources of water pollution. Discuss how water pollution can be reduced or prevented altogether. What personal actions can you as a student take?

6. List the loudest sounds you encountered in the last week (rock concert, construction, airplanes, etc.). How many could have been avoided? What could be done to ease the strain of the unavoidable noises?

7. Given all the open land in Canada, do you think solid waste disposal is a problem? Why or why not?

8. Are the advantages of nuclear power worth the risks involved with storing nuclear waste? Put another way, if you live near a nuclear power plant, would you be willing to pay two or three times as much for electricity in order to have the nuclear power plant closed? Why or why not?

# APPLICATION EXERCISE

Reread the What Do You Think? scenario at the beginning of the chapter and answer the following questions.

1. How much progress can be made in the fight against environmental polluters by community action? What alternatives, if any, might be more effective?

2. What are an industry's responsibilities to its neighbours?

# HEALTH ON THE NET

Atomic Energy Canada Limited
**www.aecl.ca**

Environment Canada
**www.ec.gc.ca**

WHO Environmental Health
**www.who.int/health_topics/environmental_health/en**

Canadian Environmental Assessment Agency
**www.ceaa-acee.gc.ca**

The United Nations, World Population
**www.un.org/popin**

# CHAPTER 16

# CONSUMERISM

*Using Healthcare Products and Services*

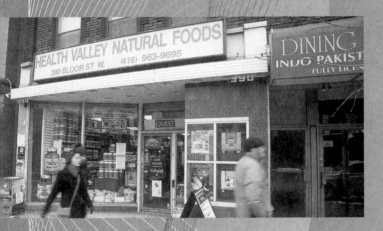

## CHAPTER OBJECTIVES

- Outline a method for making informed choices, including evaluating online medical resources.

- Explain when self-diagnosis and self-care are appropriate, when you should seek medical care, and how to assess health professionals.

- Compare and contrast allopathic and nonallopathic medicine, including the types of treatments that fall into each category.

- Discuss the types of health care available in Canada, including types of medical practices, hospitals, and clinics.

- Examine the current problems associated with our healthcare system, including access, quality, and fraud.

- Understand the HSO model of health care.

Roberta is a slightly older-than-average college student. She has a history of chronically painful menstrual periods and excessive bleeding. She seeks care from a gynecologist, who immediately tells her that she must have a hysterectomy. Because she believes that this is the most drastic option, has not yet had children, and does not want to risk early menopause, Roberta seeks a second opinion from the gynecologist's colleague. Without giving her much of an exam, the second doctor agrees with the first, so she seeks yet another opinion—but this time from a gynecologist outside the original group's practice. This third doctor adamantly disagrees with the first two and suggests a more conservative treatment not involving surgery.

■ Which doctor's advice should Roberta follow? Is it appropriate to seek more than one opinion? Is it appropriate to seek more than two opinions? How much say should the individual have in his or her course of treatment? How can a consumer determine what "quality health care" is?

There are many reasons for you to be an informed healthcare consumer. Most important, you have only one body, and it is no one's top priority to maintain but yours. It is your responsibility to take. Doing everything you can to stay healthy and to recover rapidly when you do get sick will enhance every other part of your life. Canada's history has brought about a commitment to share the liability of illness and injury among the entire population because our healthcare system is based on shared values of equity, fairness, compassion, and respect for the dignity of all.[1] This is not the case in all countries.

In the 1990s, the federal government cut its healthcare transfer payments to the provinces in stages from a 50–50 share to 15–85 share as part of its deficit reduction strategy. This shift had a profound impact on the provinces and territories, which are responsible for providing health care. In 2002, the Commission on the Future of Healthcare in Canada made recommendations aimed at sustaining our publicly funded health system by balancing investments in prevention and health maintenance with those directed to care and treatment.[2] As head of the Commission, Roy Romanow recommended comprehensive changes to ensure that our healthcare system would be sustained for years to come.

As we continue to scrutinize the evolution of our healthcare system, certain trends are emerging— including a shift from centralized governing bodies to regional health authorities, a growing shift in emphasis from institutionally focused care to community-based care, decision making based on need and the best available evidence, and funding of health services at sustainable levels.[3] Despite these changes, health care remains very important to Canadians. In fact, as recently as October 2004, 63 percent of individuals polled indicated that health care should receive the greatest attention from our country's leaders.[4] At the same time, approximately 20 percent and fewer than 10 percent of those polled thought education and the economy, respectively, should be the main issue for Canada's leaders.

Even though our society tends to treat health as a social good to which everyone is entitled, you must still be knowledgeable about what resources are available and at times you must be assertive in order to obtain services in your best interests. Almost all Canadians obtain some type of health services each year. When asked in 2003, 80 percent of teens and adults said they had consulted a physician in the past year and 84 percent reported taking a prescription or nonprescription medication.[5] Fewer received services from a dental professional (64 percent) or chiropractor or other complementary or alternative healthcare provider (12 percent). Still fewer used a telephone health line (10 percent) or had an overnight stay in a hospital (8 percent).

As you may already know, medical and healthcare services are much harder to evaluate than are, say, clothing or fruit and vegetables. That said, of the care received in the past 12 months, 85 percent of Canadians in 2003 were very or somewhat satisfied.[6] Further, most Canadians aged 15 or older rated the quality of care as excellent or very good. Although men and women across the country report similar levels of satisfaction overall regarding their health care, women were significantly more satisfied with the care they received from their physicians. In response to questions about access to health care, most Canadians (84 percent) did not have difficulty in accessing care.[7] The most common challenges to accessing health care were waiting too long to get an appointment, waiting too long in doctors' offices, and problems in contacting a physician.

The federal and provincial governments have responded to the need to adapt the system to today's realities in several ways, notably by:[8]

■ adopting a "determinant of health" framework that recognizes that while health care is obviously an important contributor to health, its role must be placed in context as only one component of a much broader set of determinants of health

■ shifting the emphasis of the healthcare system away from institutionally based delivery models (that is, physicians and hospital-based care) to integrated community-based models that place increased emphasis on prevention and health promotion

- developing strategies for the coordinated management of the healthcare workforce, including the remuneration, geographical distribution, and appropriate use of various healthcare providers

This chapter will help you to become proactive in making decisions that affect your health and health care. Our healthcare system is a shared responsibility among the federal, provincial, and territorial governments. It includes hospitals, home-care agencies, long-term care facilities, and people (physicians, nurses, social workers, healthcare providers).[9] In 2004, total health expenditure was $130 billion for a broad range of services—millions of physician visits, immunizations, prescriptions, lab tests, and hospital stays.[10] Many different companies aggressively market health products and services to the public. Even medical professionals sometimes feel overwhelmed, confused, and frustrated by the choices. So if you've experienced these feelings, you are not alone. However, there is much you can do to become an informed, responsible consumer of healthcare products and services.

# MAKING INFORMED HEALTHCARE CHOICES

Perhaps the single greatest difficulty that we face as consumers is the sheer magnitude of choices available. Informed consumers are aware that there is always more to learn. Because there are so many charlatans competing for a share of the lucrative healthcare market, and because misinformation is so common, wise consumers use every means at their disposal to ensure that they are acting responsibly in their own healthcare choices. Check out your own knowledge in the Rate Yourself self-assessment.

## Evaluating Online Medical Resources

The internet has increasingly become a source of health information for many Canadians. How can we be sure that the information we read is credible? The National Centre for Complementary and Alternative Medicine suggests that we ask ourselves the following questions:[11]

- **Who runs the site?** Any good site will make it easy for you to find out who is responsible for the information presented on it.
- **Who pays for the site?** The source for the website's funding should be clearly stated. You should know how a website pays for its existence. Does it sell advertising? Is it sponsored by a pharmaceutical

company? The source of funding may influence how information is presented.

- **What is the purpose of the site?** This is related to who runs and pays for the site. The site's purpose should be clearly stated and help you in evaluating the trustworthiness of the information included.
- **Where does the information come from?** If the information does not come from the website creator, the original source(s) should be identified.
- **What is the basis of the information?** In addition to providing a complete citation list, the site should describe what the materials presented are based upon. Facts and figures presented should have credible references. Opinions should be set apart from evidence-based information.
- **How is the information selected?** Was the presented material peer-reviewed? That is, did other appropriate health professionals review the material prior to posting?
- **How current is the information?** Good health websites are reviewed and updated on a regular basis to ensure the information presented is current. It should be clearly stated when the website was most recently updated.
- **How does the site choose links to other sites?** Credible websites have policies regarding what links they will establish.
- **What information about you does the site collect, and why?** Websites routinely track the paths visitors take to determine usage rates. Some websites may ask you to subscribe or become a member. This may be to collect a user fee or to assist in collecting information relevant to your concerns. Any credible website will tell you why it is requesting information.
- **How does the site manage interaction with visitors?** A credible site will provide a way for you to contact the site owner if you have any problems, questions, or feedback.

## Financing Health Care

Canada has a predominantly publicly funded, privately delivered healthcare system that rests on an interlocking set of ten provincial and three territorial health insurance plans. Known to Canadians as Medicare, the system provides access to universal, comprehensive coverage for medically necessary hospital, inpatient, and outpatient physician services. This structure results from the constitutional assignment of jurisdiction over most aspects of health care to provincial governments. The system is referred to as a "national" health insurance system because all

# How Good a Healthcare Consumer Are You?

Select the response that best describes your typical health behaviours. After completing this survey, total your points and assess your competence regarding healthcare products and services.

1. I never act this way
2. I sometimes act this way
3. I act this way most of the time
4. I always act this way

1. When moving to a new location, I seek recommendations from friends and ask for referrals from physicians who treated me in the past, before I get ill.    1  2  3  4
2. I schedule an interview with healthcare professionals prior to treatment to determine if I am comfortable with them.    1  2  3  4
3. I ask about costs of healthcare procedures.    1  2  3  4
4. I carefully assess my symptoms and go to the doctor only when necessary.    1  2  3  4
5. I get second opinions when I am unsure of what my physician tells me.    1  2  3  4
6. I ask my physician why a test is given and what my options are before I allow that test to be performed.    1  2  3  4
7. I follow recommended guidelines for health exams, inoculations, and self-care.    1  2  3  4
8. Whenever I receive a prescription drug, I follow the directions exactly, including finishing the medication in the prescribed time period.    1  2  3  4
9. I am aware of differences in prices at various pharmacies and comparison-shop whenever possible.    1  2  3  4
10. When my peers make obviously incorrect statements about "health alternatives," I tactfully point out their errors.    1  2  3  4
11. I am aware of my body and seek medical care quickly when unusual changes occur.    1  2  3  4
12. I attempt to obtain my health information from reputable sources.    1  2  3  4
13. I carefully scrutinize health-related advertisements and news items.    1  2  3  4
14. I read the labels of health products and follow instructions carefully.    1  2  3  4

## INTERPRETING YOUR SCORE

**14–19**  Health consumer skills dangerously weak

**20–29**  Health consumer skills below average

**30–44**  Health consumer skills about average, not adequate for many situations

**45–56**  Very good health consumer skills.

## BEYOND INTERPRETATION

- Given your results above, where do you need the most improvement?
- What can you do to improve in these areas?

---

provincial or territorial hospital and medical insurance plans are linked through adherence to national principles set at the federal level. The provinces and territories plan, finance, and evaluate the provision of hospital, physician, and allied health care, some aspects of prescription care, and public health.[12] Figure 16.1 details how health care is funded.

## Accepting Responsibility for Your Health Care

While income is generally not a barrier to universally insured medical services, disparities in access to uninsured health services remain. Most agree that dental care, vision care, and counselling services are not "frills." For many people, access to these services is essential to basic health, yet many have restricted or no access to these services because of lack of private or publicly assisted insurance.[13]

Even though most health care you need is publicly funded, you still need to learn how, when, and where to enter the system and how to obtain the care you need without incurring unnecessary risk or wasting valuable resources. Acting responsibly in times of illness can be difficult, but the person best able to act on your behalf is you. Being knowledgeable about self-care and its limits is critical for responsible consumerism.

## Why Some False Claims May Seem True

Many marketing strategies revolve around trendy news items. A good example of this is the current concern about trans fat. Whereas food ads and product

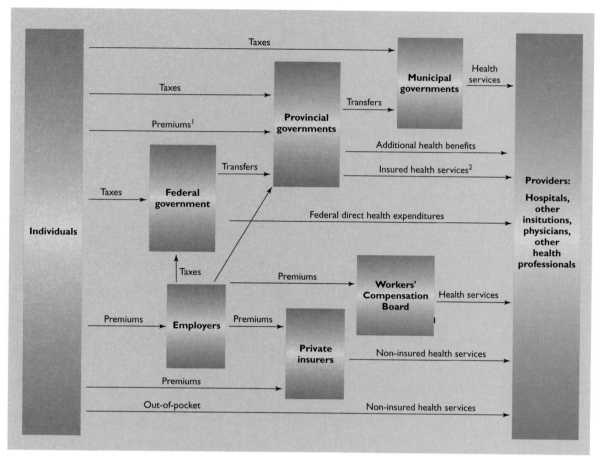

1. Two provinces, British Columbia and Alberta, levy health premiums.
2. Medically necessary hospital and physician services.

FIGURE 16.1

The Funding Structure of the Health System in Canada

Source: Health Canada, 1998. © Minister of Public Works and Government Services Canada, 2006.

labels previously focused heavily on "low calories," "low cholesterol" or "low fat," they now emphasize "0 trans fat." Many of these products, despite having 0 grams of trans fat, have high levels of saturated fats—another of the fats that put an individual at risk for heart disease. When it comes to gathering health information, it is your responsibility to approach advertisers' claims with a "buyer beware" mindset firmly in place.

The same skepticism should be used when evaluating advertising for medical cures. Because of Canadian restrictions and limitations on pharmaceutical advertising, we have not experienced as much of this as Americans have, whose laws in this regard are not as stringent. People often fall victim to false healthcare claims because they mistakenly believe that a product or provider has helped them. This belief often arises from two conditions: spontaneous remission and the placebo effect.

## Spontaneous Remission

It is commonly said that if you treat a cold, it will disappear in a week, but if you leave it alone, it will last seven days. A **spontaneous remission** from an ailment refers to the disappearance of symptoms without any apparent cause or treatment. Many illnesses, like the common cold and even back strain, are self-limiting and will improve in time, with or without treatment. Other illnesses, such as multiple sclerosis and some cancers, are characterized by alternating periods of severe symptoms and sudden remissions. Because of this phenomenon, people seeking profit may exploit consumers by claiming that their particular treatment, procedure, or drug cured the condition.

**Spontaneous remission:** The disappearance of symptoms without any apparent cause or treatment.

People experiencing spontaneous remissions can easily attribute their "cure" to a treatment, drug, or provider that had no real effect on the disease or condition.

### Placebo Effect

The **placebo effect** is an apparent cure or improved state of health brought about by a substance, product, or procedure that has no therapeutic value. It is not uncommon for patients to report improvements based on what they expect, desire, or were told would happen after taking simple sugar pills believed to be powerful drugs. About 10 percent of the population is believed to be exceptionally susceptible to the power of suggestion; the remainder may be influenced to varying degrees. Those most susceptible to the placebo effect may be victimized by aggressive marketing of products and services. Although the placebo effect is often harmless, it does account for the expenditure of millions of dollars on worthless health products and services every year. Further, people who mistakenly use placebos when medical treatment is needed are not likely to get better.

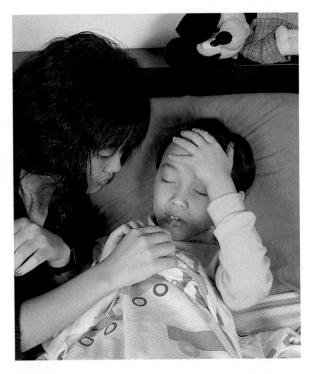

*For parents, knowing when to seek help for a sick child is often a challenge since young children are unable to assess their own symptoms and may not be able to describe them adequately.*

# SELF-HELP OR SELF-CARE

Self-care is a composite of individual identity and specific attitudes and behaviours associated with looking after the "self."[14] Self-care and informal caregiving are widespread phenomena. As medical technologies become more sophisticated and as healthcare consumers become better informed, individuals can perform many healthcare tasks that were formerly the exclusive responsibility of formal caregivers in institutional settings.[15] They can also interpret basic changes in their physical and emotional health and treat minor afflictions without seeking professional help. Self-care consists of knowing your body, recognizing its signals, and taking appropriate action to stop the progression of illness or injury or to improve your overall health.

## When to Seek Help

Effective self-care requires understanding when you should seek professional medical attention rather than treat a condition on your own. Generally, you should consult a physician if you experience any of the following:

- a serious accident or injury
- sudden or severe chest pains resulting in difficulty breathing

- trauma to the head or spine accompanied by a persistent headache, blurred vision, loss of consciousness, vomiting, convulsions, or paralysis
- sudden high fever or recurring high temperature (over 38.5°C for adults and 39.5°C for children) or sweats
- tingling sensation in the arm accompanied by slurred speech or impaired thought processes
- adverse reactions to a drug or insect bite (shortness of breath, severe swelling, itchiness, or dizziness)
- unexplained bleeding or loss of bodily fluid from any body opening
- unexplained sudden weight loss
- persistent or recurrent diarrhea or vomiting
- blue-coloured lips, eyelids, or nail beds
- any lump, swelling, thickness, or sore that does not subside or that grows for over a month
- any marked change in or pain accompanying bowel or bladder habits
- yellowing of the skin or the whites of the eyes
- any unusual symptom that recurs over time
- signs that suggest possible pregnancy

# Being Proactive in Your Health Care

Your personal involvement in your wellness is critical. Taking a proactive approach to practising preventive behaviours can go a long way toward giving you a long and healthy life. Sometimes, however, regardless of the steps you take to care for yourself, you still get sick. At such a time, it is important that you continue to be actively involved in your care. The more you know about your body and the factors that affect your health, the better able you will be to communicate complete information to your doctor. It also helps you to make informed decisions and to recognize when a certain treatment may not be right for you. The following points may be helpful:

- Know your and your family's medical history.
- Be knowledgeable about your condition—causes, physiological effects, possible treatments, prognosis. Don't rely on the doctor for this information. Do some research.
- Bring a friend or relative along for medical visits to help you review what the doctor says and possibly write down the doctor's answers to your questions.
- Ask the practitioner to explain the problem and appropriate treatments, tests, and drugs in a clear and understandable way. Ask for clarification if you do not understand.
- If the doctor prescribes medications, ask for their generic names so that you can pay less for them.
- Ask for a written summary of the results of your visit and any lab tests.
- If you have any doubt about the doctor's recommended treatment, seek a second opinion.

Afterward:

- Write down an account of what happened and what was said. Be sure to include the names of the doctor and all other people involved in your care, the date, and the place.
- Shop around drugstores for the best prices in the same way that you would when shopping for clothes.
- When filling prescriptions, ask to see the pharmacist's package inserts that list medical considerations concerning the prescribed drug and any possible interactions.
- Have clear instructions written on the label to avoid risk to others who may take the drug in error.

Doctors are human, just like you. Their decisions are based on the best information they have available to them and may be influenced by a number of factors—workload, limited information, personal views. Therefore, in addition to following the practical steps listed above, being proactively involved in your health care also means that you should be aware of your rights as a patient. The following are the basic rights of all individuals seeking care from a healthcare professional. You have the right to:

1. Informed consent. Before receiving any care, you have the right to be fully informed of what is planned, the risks and potential benefits, and possible alternative forms of treatment, including the option of no treatment. Your consent must be voluntary and without any form of coercion. It is critical that you read consent forms carefully and amend them as necessary before signing.

2. Know whether the treatment you are receiving is standard or experimental. In experimental conditions, you have the legal and ethical right to know if the study is one in which some people receive treatment while others do not and if a drug is used in the research project for a purpose not approved by the Health Protection Branch of Health Canada.

3. Privacy, which includes protecting your right to make personal decisions concerning all reproductive matters.

4. Refuse or stop treatment at any time.

5. Receive care.

6. Access your medical records and to confidentiality of your records.

7. Seek the opinions of other healthcare professionals regarding your condition.

With the vast array of home diagnostic devices currently available, it appears to be relatively easy for most people to take care of themselves. But a strong word of caution is in order: although many of these devices are valuable for making an initial diagnosis, home health tests cannot fully substitute for regular, complete examinations by a trained practitioner. The Skills for Behaviour Change box offers valuable information about taking an active part in your health care.

## Assessing Health Professionals

Suppose you decide that you do need medical help. You must then identify what type of medical help you need and where to obtain it. Initially, selecting a doctor

**Placebo effect:** An apparent cure or improved state of health brought about by a substance or product with no medicinal value.

may seem a simple matter, yet many people have no idea how to assess the qualifications of a medical practitioner.

Knowledge of traditional medical specialties and alternative medicine is critical to making an intelligent selection. You also need to be aware of criteria for evaluating a health professional. Studies indicate that many people's greatest concerns when choosing a doctor have less to do with medical qualifications than with availability and personality. While a warm and caring personality is certainly a valuable attribute, doctors who lack in bedside manner may, in fact, be better trained and qualified than more cordial practitioners. That said, it is still critical to find a physician who is willing and able to listen to your concerns. Carefully consider the following factors about all prospective healthcare providers:

- What professional educational training do they have? What licence or board certification do they hold?

- Are they affiliated with an accredited medical facility or institution? The Canadian Council on Health Facilities Accreditation requires these institutions to verify all education, licensing, and training claims of their affiliated practitioners.

- Do they indicate clearly how long a given treatment may last, or do they have you returning week after week with no apparent end in sight?

- Do their diagnoses, treatments, and general statements appear to be consistent with established scientific theory and practice?

- Do they listen to you, appear to respect you as an individual, and give you time to ask questions?

Asking the right questions at the right time may save you personal suffering. Many individuals find that writing their questions down ahead of time helps them to get all their inquiries answered. You should not accept a defensive or hostile response; asking questions is your right as a patient. The Building Communication Skills box discusses finding a personal physician in more detail.

### WHAT WOULD YOU DO?

If you had the choice of seeing a practitioner of your own sex and ethnic background, would you? Why or why not? Do you think it would make a difference in how comfortable you may feel sharing personal or embarrassing but relevant health information? Why or why not? Have you ever had difficulty finding a practitioner with whom you are comfortable?

# CHOICES OF MEDICAL CARE

Familiarizing yourself with the various health professions and health subspecialties will help you choose the right provider for your needs. There are more than 59,000 physicians in Canada today. Those you are most familiar with probably subscribe to allopathic medical procedures. Most people believe that **allopathic medicine,** or traditional, Western medical practice, is based on scientifically validated methods, but you should consider the fact that only about 20 percent of all allopathic treatments have been proven clinically effective in research trials.

Many standard procedures focus on addressing a patient's symptoms, not necessarily the problem causing the symptoms. Medical practitioners who adhere to allopathic principles are bound by a professional code of ethics.

## Traditional (Allopathic) Medicine

Selecting a **primary care practitioner**—a medical practitioner whom you can go to for routine ailments, preventive care, general medical advice, and appropriate referrals—is not an easy task, particularly given the shortage of general practitioners in various parts of Canada. The primary care practitioner for most people is a family practitioner. Others use nontraditional providers as their primary source of care. The common denominator is continuity in services over a period of time. Having a "usual source of care" is important to the quality of care you receive.

Some of what is done in medicine either does not improve health outcomes or creates *iatrogenic disease* (illness caused by the medical treatment itself). An essential part of medical care is informed consent. This refers to your right to have explained to you—in plain language you can understand—all possible side effects, benefits, and consequences of a specific procedure and treatment regimen as well as available alternatives to it. It also means that you have the right to refuse a specific treatment or to seek a second or even third opinion from unbiased, noninvolved healthcare providers.[16]

**Allopathic medicine:** Traditional, Western medical practice; based, in theory, on scientifically validated methods and procedures.

**Primary care practitioner:** A medical practitioner who treats routine ailments, advises on preventive care, gives general medical advice, and makes appropriate referrals when necessary.

# Finding a Personal Physician

Consider the following situation. Mary wakes one morning with a chest cold. Within several days, the cold has worsened and she thinks she may have developed bronchitis. Mary knows she should see a doctor but she doesn't have a primary care physician, so she decides to let the cold take its course, without seeing someone. The next day, after a night of very laboured breathing, Mary gives in, looks up the name of a walk-in clinic in the phone book, and calls for an appointment.

Unfortunately, a great many people hesitate about seeking early care because they don't have a physician. The treatment Mary receives will probably be fine. But she will know nothing about the doctor and will be taking a chance on whether she will feel comfortable being treated by him or her. If Mary had had a primary care physician, she could have called him or her up as soon as her symptoms worsened.

One of the most important decisions a person or family has to make is choosing a primary care physician. Your physician plays a critical role in the prevention and treatment of illnesses. When you are ill or develop symptoms that need attention, having someone to contact in whom you have confidence can relieve a great deal of anxiety. Yet, despite the importance of identifying and regularly visiting a primary care physician, a great many people wait until they are ill to seek a doctor. Depending on the severity of the illness, waiting this long can limit a person's options. Selecting a doctor long before the development of an illness allows you the opportunity to identify and interview several doctors in order to find the one that will best fit your needs and with whom you feel the most comfortable. In Canada, you may have easier access to a primary care physician (general or family practitioner) if another family member visits that practitioner or if you are new to the area. It may be difficult to change doctors if you are remaining in the same location. This difficulty makes it all the more important to properly assess a doctor at the outset. (Another issue to keep in mind is that there is a physician shortage in many areas in Canada, with some physicians not taking new patients.)

The following procedure can help you with this process.

1. First, consider the following questions:
   - Would you feel more comfortable with a male or female health professional? Why?
   - Is age an important factor to you? Why?
   - Do you have a pre-existing condition for which specialization may be helpful?
   - Do you prefer to see primarily one physician or are you comfortable visiting a service with a team of doctors (like what you would find in a health clinic)?

2. Next, assemble a list of names of doctors in your area. Names of potential physicians can be identified by:
   - Asking friends and colleagues for recommendations. These are often your best sources of information about a doctor's availability and promptness as well as overall general concern.
   - Calling the local medical association, local health advocacy groups (many communities provide references as a service), or the local hospital for names of doctors accepting new patients.
   - Researching medical directories at your local library. The *Canadian Medical Directory,* for example, includes information about every physician who belongs to the CMA (Canadian Medical Association).

3. Call the offices of the physicians on your list and explain that you are seeking a primary care physician. Ask the receptionist about the doctor's hospital affiliation, office hours, and the kind of coverage the physician has for emergency situations that occur outside normal office hours. Take into consideration the receptionist's tone and how your questions are answered. Find out how much time is allotted for appointments (30 to 45 minutes for a routine physical is average).

4. Narrow the list to two or three physicians and make appointments for brief consultations.

5. While visiting with each doctor, you should find answers to the following questions:
   - Is the doctor's educational and experiential background appropriate?
   - While visiting, do you feel that he or she cares about you as a person?
   - Do you feel relaxed in his or her presence?
   - Does he or she make you feel rushed?
   - Are you encouraged to ask questions and are answers explained clearly?
   - Does the physician use a lot of medical jargon? If so, how does that make you feel?
   - Does the doctor use a condescending tone?
   - Does the physician attend to you personally or does he or she serve primarily as a "gatekeeper" to specialists?

6. Develop some direct questions about treatment that will help to identify the person's philosophy on care. For example, you could ask how the physician would treat a terminally ill patient or about his or her willingness to accommodate your religious feelings.

7. Once you choose a physician, get the most from your visits by maintaining an open line of communication. You can do this by:
   - Always being prepared for an appointment. Know your medical and family history and be very specific and detailed about the symptoms you may be experiencing.
   - Not bringing up irrelevant questions regarding your partner's, children's, or parent's health when the appointment is about you. If these individuals need an appointment, book one for them too. Do not try to get two appointments in during one booked time.

- Being an educated patient. Expect and insist on a diagnosis explained in a way that you fully understand. Never leave your doctor's office with questions unanswered.
- Taking a proactive role in your health care. Treatment will work only if you follow it. Listen to and follow instructions, find

out when you can call with follow-up questions, and be sure that the doctor reports any test results to you promptly. "No news is good news" is not an appropriate adage to follow.
- Communicating your needs to the doctor. If you have concerns about communication or treatment, speak up.

## WHAT WOULD YOU DO?

Have you ever taken a list of questions to your practitioner's office? If you have, were your questions answered fully? Did you feel intimidated or rushed? Do you think people have the right to question their practitioners' judgment? Why or why not?

Informed consent gives you the right to ask:

- What will happen if I choose not to have a particular test or treatment?

- Can other tests be performed instead? What are their risks? Why should I choose this test instead of one of the alternatives?

- How often has the doctor performed this test, surgery, or procedure, and with what proportion of success?

- Are the risks from the treatment greater than the risks from the condition?

- What are the side effects of the diagnostic tests? Can these side effects be prevented, treated, or reduced?

- Does this procedure require an overnight stay at a hospital or can it be performed in a doctor's office?

- Why has this test been ordered? What is the doctor trying to find or exclude?

- Are these medications necessary? What are their possible side effects? What will happen if I decide not to take them? What alternatives are available? Is there a generic version that costs less? Will they interact with the other drugs I currently consume (other prescription or OTC drugs, caffeine, alcohol)?

- What caused me to have this problem? What can I do to prevent if from happening again?

## Allied Professionals

Canada lags behind other countries in creative use of allied health professionals. The official recognition of midwifery has occurred very recently and in only a few provinces. The use of nurse practitioners is relatively

rare except in isolated northern communities, and the Dentacare Program in Saskatchewan, which relied mostly on dental therapists, folded.[17]

**Nurses** are highly trained and strictly regulated health practitioners who provide a wide range of services for patients and their families, including patient education, counselling, community health and disease prevention information, and administration of medications. They have the designation RN (registered nurse). Although nurses may work in health service organizations (HSOs), clinics, doctors' offices, student health centres, nursing homes, public health departments, schools, businesses, and other healthcare settings, many are employed in the hospital setting. There has been an increasing trend away from hospital-based employment as the demand for nurses in other settings has increased.

Nurse practitioners are professional nurses with advanced training obtained through either a master's degree program or a specialized nurse practitioner program. Nurse practitioners have the training and authority to conduct diagnostic tests and prescribe medications. They work in a variety of settings, particularly in hospitals, clinics, and client homes. They have become an increasingly popular source of health care in recent years. Nurses may also earn a bachelor of science and nursing degree (B.Sc.N.), a master of science and nursing (M.Sc.N.), or a research-based Ph.D. in nursing.

## Nonallopathic Medicine

While people in other parts of the world consider **nonallopathic medicine** the "traditional" form of treatment, in North America we tend to think of nonallopathic medicine as "alternative medicine." As the government, private payers, and consumers evaluate the costs, effectiveness, and quality of traditional health care, many have found it wanting. The two core services under the Canada Health Act, hospital and physician services, count for 43 percent of the total health spending of $130 billion in 2004.[18] Although these two core services account for a smaller part of the total healthcare spending than in the past, they have increased more than 51 percent since 1994. However, it should be pointed out that the increase in spending on public health and administration (6 percent of the total) has outpaced increases for hospital and physician services. Further, the cost of prescription and OTC drugs has been the fastest-growing component of the total bill. As a result of dissatisfaction with traditional methods of care and the financing of the healthcare system, each year more and more people seek nonallopathic or alternative medical care from providers other than licensed medical doctors. One survey found that 7 percent of Canadians aged 12 and over used alternative health services. If this category is expanded to include complementary and alternative treatments such as herbal remedies, the figure rises to 42 percent.[19] See Figure 16.2 for the types of practitioners used.

Numerous nonallopathic alternatives are available. Many people turn to nonallopathic medicine only after more traditional methods have failed to improve their conditions. Because they are often "providers of last resort," these unconventional treatments may appear to produce more negative outcomes overall than traditional medicine. This has given them a bad reputation even though it was the failure of traditional medicine that sent many patients to nonallopathic practitioners in the first place. Although some alternative therapies are controversial and may be

dangerous, many offer significant benefits at reasonable costs. It is the consumer's job to ascertain the credentials of nonallopathic practitioners, because not all are licensed or regulated; this job of verifying credentials may be even more difficult than it is in traditional medicine.

As with any type of therapy, you must be assertive and directly ask providers of nonallopathic medicine about their training, licensing (if relevant to their field), and affiliations. You should also ask them how many patients with your specific complaint they have treated. The greatest danger in seeking the assistance of an alternative medical practitioner is that it may keep you from obtaining effective conventional treatment (if any is available).

## Chiropractic Treatment

**Chiropractic medicine** has been practised for more than 100 years; allopathic medicine and chiropractic medicine were in direct competition more than a century ago.[20] Although there have always been some medical doctors who worked collaboratively with chiropractic doctors, their number has recently increased. Some chiropractic treatments are covered by provincial health insurance, and many private insurance companies will now pay for chiropractic treatment if a medical doctor recommends it.

Chiropractic medicine is based on the idea that a life-giving energy flows through the spine via the nervous system. If the spine is subluxated (partly misaligned or dislocated), that force is disrupted. Chiropractors use a variety of techniques to manipulate the spine back into alignment so the life-giving energy can flow unimpeded through the nervous system. It has been established that their treatment is effective for chronic low back pain, neck pain, and headaches.

The average chiropractic training program requires four years of intensive courses in biochemistry, anatomy, physiology, diagnostics, pathology, nutrition, and related topics, combined with hands-on clinical training. Currently, there is only one school in Canada where you can learn to become a chiropractor, Canadian Memorial Chiropractic College, and it is located in Toronto. Many chiropractors continue their

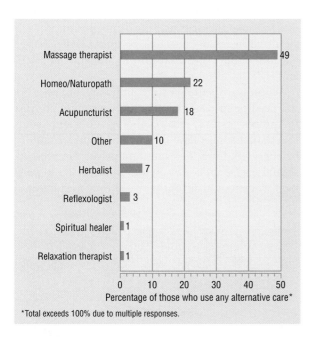

Massage therapist — 49
Homeo/Naturopath — 22
Acupuncturist — 18
Other — 10
Herbalist — 7
Reflexologist — 3
Spiritual healer — 1
Relaxation therapist — 1

Percentage of those who use any alternative care*

*Total exceeds 100% due to multiple responses.

FIGURE 16.2

Percentage of Canadians Aged 12+ Who Use Alternative Healthcare Practitioners, by Type, Canada, 1996–97.

Source: Adapted from the Statistics Canada Publication, *National Population Health Survey Overview*, Catalogue No. 82–567, released July 29, 1998.

**Nurse:** Health practitioner who provides many services and may work in a variety of settings.

**Nonallopathic medicine:** Medical alternatives to traditional, allopathic medicine.

**Chiropractic medicine:** A form of medical treatment that emphasizes the manipulation of the spinal column.

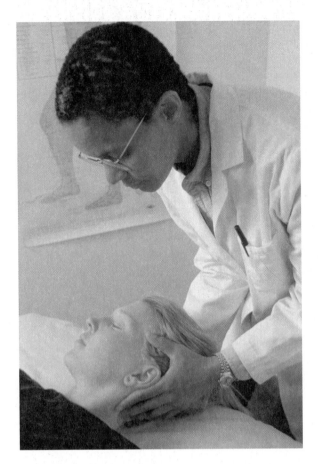

*A chiropractor treats a patient using a variety of techniques to manipulate the spine into alignment.*

training to obtain specialized certification—for example, in women's health, gerontology, or pediatrics.

You should investigate and question a chiropractor as carefully as you would a medical doctor. As with many healthcare professionals, you may note vast differences in technique among specialists. It is recommended that you choose a chiropractor who follows standard chiropractic regimens for treating musculoskeletal conditions.

### Massage Therapy

Massage therapy refers to the assessment and treatment of the body's soft tissues.[21] More specifically, massage therapy is used to treat soft-tissue injuries and dysfunctions (whiplash, sprains, strains, muscle spasms), diseases and disorders (osteoarthritis, rheumatoid arthritis, bronchitis), painful conditions such as low back or neck pain, and conditions with psychological implications such as stress, anxiety, or depression. The Canadian Massage Therapy Alliance recommends a two-year intensive program, equivalent to approximately 2,200 hours of training. All provinces and territories have different requirements

to become a registered massage therapist. Check out the Canadian Massage Therapist Alliance website at www.cmta.ca for the specific requirements related to where you live.

### Acupuncture and Acupressure

Acupuncture is the ancient (more than 2,000 years old) Chinese art of inserting fine needles at points on the skin that fall along 14 major meridians, or pathways of energy (called *qi*), that flow through the body. These points and meridians are thought to be associated with particular internal organs and bodily functions. Proponents of acupuncture believe that the vital forces of life—the yin and the yang—are restored to equilibrium when these points are stimulated. Acupuncture has been effective for treating chronic pain and for blocking acute pain briefly.[22] Acupuncturists treat complaints as diverse as back and neck pain, menstrual cramps, morning sickness, addiction, asthma, infections, and arthritis. They also help women in labour and people who want to quit smoking.

The Acupuncture Foundation of Canada Institute teaches licensed health practitioners about acupuncture. Some licensed M.D.s and chiropractors have also trained in acupuncture. If you decide to have acupuncture, it is very important to ensure the needles the acupuncturist uses are disposable or properly sterilized using an autoclave, because needles reused without proper sterilization can transmit hepatitis and HIV.

Acupressure is similar to acupuncture, but does not use needles. Instead, the practitioner applies pressure to points critical to balancing yin and yang. Practitioners must have the same basic understanding of energy pathways as acupuncturists. Acupressure should not be applied by an untrained person to pregnant women or to anyone with a chronic condition.

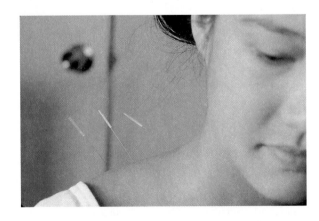

*Many have found acupuncture an effective treatment for a variety of complaints.*

## Herbalists and Homeopaths

Herbalists practise *herbal medicine,* which is based on the medicinal qualities of plants or herbs. Homeopaths also use herbal medicine (as well as minerals and chemicals), but at the root of their practice is the theory that administering extremely diluted doses of potent natural agents that produce disease symptoms in healthy persons will cure the disease in the sick. Herbal and homeopathic medicines are common in Europe and Asia, but are not nearly as accepted in Canada.

Although plants have been used for medicinal purposes for centuries and form the basis of many modern "wonder drugs," herbal medicine should not be taken lightly. Because something is natural does not necessarily mean that it is safe. Many plants are poisonous, and others can be toxic if consumed in high doses. One of the greatest dangers with this kind of therapy is that practitioners who mix their own tonics do not use standardized measures. It is therefore imperative that you carefully investigate the chemical properties of herbs yourself before you ingest them.

## Naturopathy

Naturopaths believe that illness results from violations of natural principles of life in modern societies. They view diseases as the body's effort to ward off impurities and harmful substances from the environment. Naturopathic treatment uses substances and forces found in nature: water, magnets, gravity, heat, crystals and minerals, herbs, and even the sun. Practitioners argue that returning to a natural, purified state will restore health.

Few naturopathic claims have been substantiated. Although many naturopaths use the title "doctor," the vast majority are not M.D.s, and many have very little health training. Thorough training is provided at three naturopathic medical schools in the United States and Canada, and those who receive a naturopathic doctor (N.D.) degree from one of these schools have been through a four-year graduate program that emphasizes humanistically oriented family medicine. If you decide to be treated by a naturopath, you should carefully check his or her credentials.

## Other Alternative Therapies

Many other therapies exist, including reflexology (zone therapy), iridology (light therapy), aromatherapy, and auramassage. Some of these may work, but they have yet to be substantiated scientifically. Others may be harmful to your health or delay you from seeking more efficacious forms of care. Until you can sort through the proliferation of new therapies, it's a good idea to follow the maxim "buyer beware."

## Types of Medical Practices

Many healthcare providers have found it essential to combine resources into a **group practice,** which can be single- or multi-specialty. Physicians share their offices, equipment, utility bills, and staff costs. Proponents of group practice maintain that it reduces unnecessary duplication of equipment and improves the quality of health care through peer review. **Solo practitioners** are medical providers who practise independently of others.

## Hospitals and Clinics

Hospitals and clinics provide a range of healthcare services. These include emergency treatment, diagnostic tests, and inpatient and outpatient (ambulatory) care.

There are several ways to classify hospitals: by profit status (nonprofit or for-profit), by ownership (private, public), by specialty (children's, chronic care, psychiatric, general, acute), by teaching status (teaching-affiliated or not), and by size. **Nonprofit (voluntary) hospitals** have traditionally been run by religious or other humanitarian groups. Before universal health care, such hospitals often cared for patients whether they could pay or not. Today, some hospitals retain religious ties and orientations; others are run by independent hospital boards. **For-profit (proprietary) hospitals** are few and far between in Canada. They do not receive tax breaks and tend to focus on particular specialties.

More treatments or services, including surgery, are delivered on an **outpatient (ambulatory) care** basis

**Group practice:** A group of physicians who combine resources including offices, equipment, and staff, to render care to patients.

**Solo practitioner:** Physician who renders care to patients independently of other practitioners.

**Nonprofit (voluntary) hospitals:** Hospitals funded by taxes.

**For-profit (proprietary) hospitals:** Hospitals that provide a return on earnings to the investors.

**Outpatient (ambulatory) care:** Treatment that does not involve an overnight stay in a hospital.

# Health Care in Canada 2005: Executive Summary

Consistently identified as a top issue for Canadians, access to care is a priority from coast to coast. What matters most differs between regions of the country and over time—sometimes the focus is on wait times for hip replacements, sometimes finding a family doctor is a priority—but the underlying challenge is shared. Reflecting this reality, Canada's first ministers put timely access to quality care for all at the top of their agenda in the recent *Ten-Year Plan to Strengthen Health Care*.

The goal of *Health Care in Canada 2005* is to provide a window into today's $130 billion health system by highlighting what we know and don't know about access to care and other emerging issues. This year's report focuses on the relationship between surgical volumes and patient outcomes.

## WHAT THE RESEARCH SAYS

Many studies across a variety of procedures, diseases, and healthcare settings have shown that patients treated in centres with higher numbers of cases are less likely to die after surgery. A new systematic review commissioned for this report—the largest ever conducted—found 161 journal articles on this topic published worldwide between 1979 and the spring of 2004. In more than two-thirds (68 percent) of the analyses, the greater the volume of procedures performed by a hospital or a physician, the better the outcomes. In a further 31 percent, the relationship between volumes and outcomes was either not statistically significant or was undetermined. Only a few analyses (1 percent) showed a significant association between higher volumes and poorer patient outcomes.

There are two theories often used to explain why higher volumes are associated with better outcomes. The first is that "practice makes perfect." That is, high volume centres may have more experienced teams and a broader range of resources. The second is that these hospitals and care providers have better outcomes because physicians tend to refer more patients to centres of excellence. This theory is known as "selective referral." Regardless of which theory is correct (or if both have some merit), much remains to be learned about the nature of the link between volumes and outcomes and the potential effects of consolidating care in centres of excellence.

## NEW FINDINGS FOR CANADA

The bulk of existing volume-outcome research (about 80 percent of studies) comes from the United States. To further explore the relationship in Canada, we studied the risk of dying in hospital within 30 days of admission for nine different types of surgery. Our analyses covered more than 180,000 surgeries performed between 1998–1999 and 2003–2004 (excluding procedures in Quebec and parts of Manitoba). Adjusted mortality rates ranged from 0.2 percent to 5.9 percent.

The results confirm that hospitals that perform higher numbers of selected procedures tend to have better outcomes for some types of surgery, but the nature and strength of the relationship varies. In three of the nine selected procedures, we found a steady drop in the risk of death with higher volumes, after taking patient characteristics and the year the procedure was performed into account. For example, for every 10 additional procedures performed in a hospital, the risk of mortality was 44 percent lower for esophagectomies (complete or partial surgical removal of the esophagus) and 46 percent lower for pancreatic cancer surgery. A smaller, but still statistically significant, effect was also seen for angioplasty (1 percent reduction). For the six other procedures, either no statistically significant relationship was observed, or a difference was seen only between hospitals performing the highest and lowest volumes of surgery.

## CONSOLIDATING CARE: TRADE-OFFS TO BE MADE?

Across the country, decisions are being made to concentrate care in centres of excellence—or not to—on a regular basis. For both relatively rare operations and more common procedures, there are large variations in the number of hospitals performing different types of surgery. Many hospitals conduct a very small number of procedures. A much smaller number of centres perform higher volumes of surgery. Cardiac surgery is among the most highly concentrated, reflecting decisions in many parts of the country to consolidate care within high-volume centres.

The issues involved in deciding how and when to consolidate care are clearly complex. The "right" balance likely varies from procedure to procedure and place to place. The potential travel burden for patients and families is just one of many factors that may weigh in the balance. A new survey of adults aged 20 and older across the country found that many respondents would prefer to have surgery at a hospital close to their home. But if forced to choose, quality was more important than closeness. Only 9 percent of those surveyed were primarily concerned with how close to home they received their care. More valued having a surgeon recommended by their family doctor (42 percent) or the number of similar procedures the surgeon had performed in the past (41 percent). However, less than half (38 percent) of those who actually had a procedure in the past two years said that they had been aware of the number of procedures that their surgeon had performed recently.

## MONITORING KEY TRENDS

Almost all Canadians receive some type of health services each year. Visiting a doctor and taking medication are the most common types of care. In 2003, 80 percent of teens and adults said that they had consulted a physician in the past year. About the same number (84 percent) reported having taken prescription or non-prescription medication.

In addition to the detailed analyses of this year's focus topic, *Health Care in Canada 2005* highlights broad trends related to these and other health services.

Two chapters profile health expenditures. Findings include:

- Canada spent an estimated $130 billion on health care in 2004. That's approximately $4,078 per Canadian. The amount spent represents about 10 percent of Canada's gross domestic product, placing us fifth among OECD countries in 2002.

- Both public and private health expenditures are higher than in the past, but recent public-sector spending growth has outpaced that of the private sector.

- Hospitals, drugs, and physician services are the three largest categories of expenditures. In 2004, hospitals accounted for an estimated $39 billion—about 30 percent of all healthcare expenditures. Hospital spending has grown an average of 7 percent per year since 1975. Retail spending on prescribed drugs, over-the-counter medications, and personal health supplies has doubled since 1996. It reached an estimated $21.8 billon in 2004, about 17 percent of total health expenditures.

There are about 59,000 physicians practising in Canada. Spending on physician services rose 4.8 percent between 2003 and 2004. Last year, it reached an estimated $16.8 billion or 13 percent of total health spending.

The report also looks at Canadians' views on health care. For example:

- Most Canadians give high marks to their care. A 2003 Statistics Canada survey found that 85 percent of Canadians were very or somewhat satisfied with the care they had received in the last year, about the same number as in 2000–2001.

- As in other countries, Canadians tend to give higher ratings to the care that they or their families receive than to the healthcare system in general. In 2004, only 1 percent to 3 percent of adults in Canada, Australia, New Zealand, the United Kingdom, and the U.S. said that their medical care in the past year was poor.

More (13 percent to 33 percent) said that their health system needed to be completely rebuilt. About one in seven Canadians

(14 percent) felt this way. This is down from 23 percent in 1998, but higher than the 1988 level of 5 percent.

In addition, *Health Indicators 2005* highlights how health, health care, and patient outcomes vary across the country. It offers comparative data on a range of health and health system indicators for health regions with a population of 75,000 or more and for provinces and territories, representing 95 percent of the Canadian population.

The thousands of Canadians who are wheeled into operating rooms every year all hope for good outcomes from surgery. Their age, state of health, and even where they live can make a difference. Other factors may also contribute to outcomes, including how early a diagnosis is made, the skills and experience of the healthcare team, and the setting in which the surgery takes place. In recent years, researchers in several countries have explored the relationship between surgical volume and patient outcomes. Many studies—across a variety of procedures, diseases, and healthcare settings—show improved clinical outcomes when patients are cared for by physicians or in hospitals performing a higher volume of procedures. The bulk of this research comes from the United States, but a few studies are from other countries. *Health Care in Canada 2005* provides new information on the relationship between volumes and outcomes of care in Canada.

Understanding this relationship, and what might be influencing it, is more than an academic question. There are practical implications for health policy and patient care that flow from this research and how results are interpreted. For example, policymakers may consider the results as they weigh decisions about where different types of care should be provided. Individual Canadians also indicate that they want information that will inform their own choices. This report is a first step in responding to both sets of information needs.

To download a copy of the full report, go to: http://secure.cihi.ca/cihiweb/dispPage.jsp?cw_page=download_form_e&cw_sku=05HCCPDF&cw_ctt=1&cw_dform=N

Source: Canadian Institute for Health Information, "Health Care in Canada 2005." Retrieved on May 19, 2006, from www.cihi.ca. The last two paragraphs of this box are extracted from the Introduction of *Health Care in Canada*; the rest is extracted from the Executive Summary.

(care which does not involve an overnight stay) by hospitals, traditional clinics, student health clinics, and nontraditional clinical centres. One type of ambulatory facility becoming common is the *surgicentre*—a place where minor, low-risk procedures such as vasectomies, tubal ligations, tissue biopsies, cosmetic surgery, abortions, and minor eye operations are performed.

Hospitals have made efforts to improve the quality of care and patient outcomes. Many hospitals are now designated as trauma centres. They have helicopters available to transport patients to the hospital quickly, specialty physicians who are in-house (not just on call) around the clock, and specialized diagnostic equipment. This combination of rapid transport and readily available specialty equipment and staff has dramatically reduced mortality rates for trauma patients. However, this same combination means that trauma centres are exceptionally expensive to run.

# PROMISES AND PROBLEMS OF OUR HEALTHCARE SYSTEM

Since the beginning, Canada's healthcare system has been a work in progress.[23] Over the past 40 years, reforms have been made and will continue to be made in response to changes within medicine and demands from society. Despite the various changes made over the years, the underlying concepts of Canada's healthcare system, known to Canadians as "Medicare," remains the same: universal coverage for medically necessary healthcare services provided on the basis of need, rather than the ability to pay.

Even though we have one of the best healthcare systems in the world, there are a number of problems with the system. First, several levels of government are involved in delivering healthcare services. The federal government provides monies that fund health care provided the provinces meet the guidelines. The federal government also funds and administers health programs for special groups such as First Nations peoples, war veterans, and prisoners. Using federal dollars, the provinces allot monies to health care. As governments struggle to reduce deficits, there is less money available at a time when healthcare costs continue to rise. Federal and provincial governments have been forced to limit healthcare spending, resulting in downsizing and restructuring. These organizational divisions and increased fiscal pressures have caused added tension between the federal and provincial governments over power, dollars, and responsibilities.

Physicians and provincial governments have also been in conflict. The provinces are responsible for medical programs and the allocation of dollars, while physicians control access to programs and institutions. Some provinces provide bonuses for physicians working in remote areas or reduce payments to physicians working in over-serviced areas. As well, other stakeholders such as midwives, nurses, and nutritionists vie for financial resources and recognition for their contribution to the health status of Canadians.

Another source of pressure for funding is the many voluntary organizations that help Canadians, some long-established. For example, the Canadian National Institute for the Blind has been in operation since before Confederation.

Health research is also supported by federal monies. Direct-care health services (hospitals and physicians, for example) must compete for dollars with research and prevention. Prevention runs a weak third, accounting for only about 5 percent of total health spending in 1996. Figure 16.3 shows Canada's place on a spectrum of public versus private health systems.

## Access

Your access to health care is determined by numerous factors, including the supply of providers and facilities and your health status. Doctors are not well distributed by specialty and geographic area. Some rural areas face constant shortages of physicians.

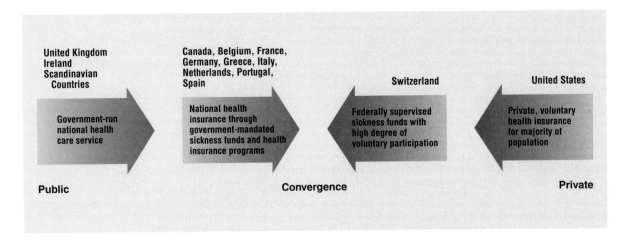

**United Kingdom, Ireland, Scandinavian Countries** — Government-run national health care service

**Canada, Belgium, France, Germany, Greece, Italy, Netherlands, Portugal, Spain** — National health insurance through government-mandated sickness funds and health insurance programs

**Switzerland** — Federally supervised sickness funds with high degree of voluntary participation

**United States** — Private, voluntary health insurance for majority of population

Public | Convergence | Private

### FIGURE 16.3

#### The Convergence of Public/Private Healthcare Systems

Source: Reprinted with permission from Gunter Becher, "European Health Issues," *Employee Benefits Journal* 38 (March 1993), published by the International Foundation of Employee Benefit Plans, Brookfield, WI.

## Quality Assurance

The Canadian healthcare system employs several mechanisms for ensuring quality services overall: education, licensure, certification or registration, accreditation, peer review, and, as a last resort, the legal system of malpractice litigation. Some of these mechanisms are mandatory before a professional organization may provide care, while others are purely voluntary. (Consumers should note that licensure, although provincially mandated for some practitioners and facilities, is only a minimum guarantee of quality.)

## Detecting Fraud and Abuse in the System

Becoming knowledgeable and acting responsibly when selecting healthcare providers and payers will reduce your likelihood of financial or physical abuse. Nevertheless, with the number of options in health products and services available, even the most careful consumer can be victimized. Individual provinces maintain boards for quality assurance in the medical system. If you find yourself in a situation you cannot deal with, remember that the Health Protection Branch of Health Canada, the provincial ministries of health, and the colleges of various professions are responsible for protecting you and other health consumers. Do not hesitate to contact them if you have suspicions about a provider, service, or product.

### WHAT WOULD YOU DO?

What do you think about Canada's healthcare system? Do you think it is in crisis? Why or why not? Do you think the current system of federal/provincial/territorial management works? Why or why not?

# HEALTH SERVICE ORGANIZATIONS: A NEW MODEL OF HEALTH CARE

The dominant model of medicine in Canada is fee-for-service. A practitioner, most often a physician, performs a service and bills the provincial health plan.

Planners have been searching for other models that would contain costs while providing improved services and encouraging prevention and shared responsibility. One model that has already been put in place is the health service organization (HSO). The patient registers with the organization, which is funded a set amount per patient per year (capitation), and is responsible for the patient's overall care. The originators of this model believed it would encourage practitioners and patients alike to emphasize prevention. There are currently 87 HSOs in Ontario alone, serving more than half a million patients. Many are run by community-based boards. In Ontario, the community health branch of the provincial Ministry of Health is responsible for the HSOs, and defines the program's objectives as:

- to create an atmosphere that supports physicians and other healthcare personnel, and that allows flexibility in responding to healthcare needs
- to develop a coordinated system of healthcare delivery that makes the most appropriate use of healthcare resources and is accessible, efficient, and economical
- to provide special attention to health maintenance and illness prevention
- to decrease institutional health care by giving emphasis to outpatient care, self-care, and home care

HSOs may offer a more comprehensive range of services than the conventional system. For example, counselling is available through HSOs as part of the service. If you live in Ontario your physician may be a member of an HSO, so additional services may be available at no cost to you.

### WHAT WOULD YOU DO?

How do health service organizations (HSOs) fit with Canada's model of health care, which focuses on universal care for all? Are you willing to pay to belong to an HSO? Why or why not?

# Canadians Open to Health User Fees, Poll Finds

Most Canadians are open to major changes to Medicare, including having to dig into their own pockets for services, as long as a single-tier, universally accessible system is preserved, a recent survey suggests.

The Environics Research poll of 2,000 health professionals and 3,300 other adults finds that most Canadians believe the healthcare system is in a state of crisis.

The greatest concern relates to the amount of time people have to wait for medical services. However, most people oppose ratcheting up government spending to solve the problems.

"People are saying, 'If the system is overloaded and it can't sustain itself, then I'm willing to pay a small user fee,'" said Diana MacDonald, a senior associate with Environics Research.

The poll found that 8 in 10 respondents want significant reforms to Medicare, but only 1 in 10 would approve of a system in which those who can afford to pay for medical services get better or faster care.

"People really do believe in universality," said MacDonald. "They don't want to see a private and a public system."

A minority of Canadians said they would be willing to pay higher taxes, but a majority said they favoured a variety of reforms, including measures that would reduce the need for large infusions of cash.

Overall, two-thirds of respondents said they were open to a range of strategies that would include user fees—as long as low-income Canadians were exempt—and more intensive use was made of nurses and other health practitioners instead of doctors.

However, 45 percent of those asked said they favoured market-oriented changes such as private delivery of health-care services, provided those services also remained publicly funded.

"We're always told that (people) are not open to a lot of reform, they want things as they are," said MacDonald. "But they are open to reform and we think that's startling."

Half said they favoured a greater emphasis on prevention and health promotion rather than relying on treating those already ill.

Environics billed the survey as the most comprehensive ever done in Canada of the attitudes and behaviours of the public and health professionals toward healthcare issues.

However, the company cited client confidentiality in refusing to release a breakdown of the actual questions posed or even a detailed breakdown of the results.

Source: The Canadian Press

# Managing Your Healthcare Needs

Throughout this text, we have emphasized behaviours important to keeping you healthy. But now you need to turn your attention to your potential attitudes and behaviours about when and how you need to seek medical attention. Most people wait until a problem arises to seek medical care and take the first available physician or medical facility. But by looking ahead to future needs, you can take charge of your choices and make positive moves toward getting better health care.

### MAKING DECISIONS FOR YOU

As you have seen in this chapter, many healthcare decisions are dictated by physicians and government agencies. Still many decisions rest with you.

### CHECKLIST FOR CHANGE: MAKING PERSONAL CHOICES

Considering the following questions may help you in obtaining excellent health care from your medical practitioner.

- How long did you have to wait before getting an appointment?
- How long did you have to wait in the waiting room before being seen?
- Do the clerical staff convey their concern for you when delays occur?
- Are there educational materials available in the waiting areas?
- Are the doctor's credentials clearly displayed?
- Does the physician treat you as if he or she is concerned about you?
- Do you feel comfortable discussing your problems with the physician?
- Are you confident that your doctor knows what he or she is talking about?
- Is the doctor willing to talk about issues such as credentials, hospital affiliations, and qualifications of referrals for special needs?
- Are you able to understand answers to your questions? Does the doctor seem interested in whether you understand?
- Seem willing to answer questions? Encourage you to ask questions?
- Does the physician tell you why one test is being given rather than another? About risks of the test? About preparation for the tests? About what to expect concerning certain results?
- Does the doctor support you in obtaining a second opinion, or does he or she seem irritated with such a request?
- If you became seriously ill and had to see a lot of this doctor, would you feel comfortable with him or her, or would you rather have someone else?

## CHECKLIST FOR CHANGE: MAKING COMMUNITY CHOICES

The following questions may help you in determining the level of healthcare service available in your community.

- What healthcare services are located in your community?
- How long has your doctor been practising in your community?
- How many hospitals are within a 30-minute drive of your home? Are any of them teaching hospitals?

# SUMMARY

- Advertisers of healthcare products and services use sophisticated tactics to attract your attention and get your business. Advertising claims sometimes appear to be supported by spontaneous remission (symptoms disappearing without any apparent cause) or the placebo effect (symptoms disappearing because you expect them to).

- Self-care and individual responsibility are key factors involved in reducing rising healthcare costs and improving health status. But you need to seek medical treatment in situations that are unfamiliar to you or that are emergencies. You should assess healthcare professionals using their qualifications, their record of treating your specific problem, and their ability to work with you.

- In theory, allopathic ("traditional") medicine is based on scientifically validated methods and procedures. Medical doctors, specialists of various kinds, nurses, and other healthcare professionals practise allopathic medicine. Many nonallopathic ("alternative") forms of health service—including chiropractic treatment, massage therapists, acupuncture, herbalists and homeopaths, and naturopathy—have proven effective for a variety of ailments.

- Healthcare providers may provide services as solo practitioners or in group practices (in which overhead is shared). Hospitals and clinics are classified by profit status, ownership, specialty, and teaching status.

- Problems experienced in the Canadian healthcare system concern demand for scarce dollars, balancing chronic care needs with more acute care facilities, and the shift away from a single-payer approach to a business mentality.

# DISCUSSION QUESTIONS

1. List some dubious claims made by healthcare products (such as fat-reducing creams, hair-growth tonics, muscle-building milkshakes, to name a few). Why do marketers use such claims to attempt to sell their products? Why do consumers buy such products?

2. List some conditions (resulting from illness or accident) for which you don't need to seek medical help. If the symptoms increase in severity, when would you seek medical attention? How do you decide to whom and where to go for treatment?

3. What are the differences in education between M.D.s and nonallopathic practitioners? Under what circumstances would you seek treatment from a nonallopathic practitioner? Which types of nonallopathic medicine appeal to you? Why? Which types of nonallopathic medicine do not appeal to you? Why not?

4. What are the pros and cons of group practices?

5. Discuss the problems of the Canadian healthcare system. If you were a Minister of Health, what would you propose as a solution? Which groups might oppose your plan? Which groups might support it?

6. Should governments dictate rates for various medical tests and procedures in an attempt to keep costs down?

# APPLICATION EXERCISE

Reread the What Do You Think? scenario at the beginning of the chapter and answer the following questions.

1. When you have a medical problem like Roberta's, how do you know if you are getting good advice?

2. Make up a list of questions for Roberta to ask each physician so that she has a better understanding of her diagnosis and the recommended treatment plan.

# HEALTH ON THE NET

Canadian Council on Health Services Accreditation
**www.cchsa.ca**

Canadian Institute for Health Information
**www.cihi.ca**

Health Canada—Commission on the Future of Health Care in Canada
**www.hc-sc.gc.ca/english/care/romanow/index.html**

Canadian Health Network
**www.canadian-health-network.ca**

Quackwatch
**www.quackwatch.com**

American Council on Science and Health
**www.acsh.org**

# NOTES

Note: All red numbers indicate Canadian references.

## CHAPTER 1

1. Statistics Canada, *Canada Year Book 1997* (Ottawa: Minister of Industry, Cat. No. 402-XPE, 1996) 116.

2. Statistics Canada, "Deaths," *The Daily*, Wednesday, December 21, 2005. Retrieved on May 31, 2006, from www.statcan.ca/Daily/English/051221/d051221b.htm.

3. C. F. Beckington, "The World Health Organization," in *World Health* (New York: Longman, 1975) 149.

4. World Health Organization, "Constitution of the World Health Organization," *Chronicles of the World Health Organization* (Switzerland: Geneva, 1947).

5. Rene Dubos, *So Human an Animal* (New York: Scribners, 1968) 15.

6. The Secretariat for the Intersectoral Healthy Living Network in partnership with the F/P/T Healthy Living Task Group and the F/P/T Advisory Committee on Population Health and Health Security (ACPHHS), "The Integrated Pan-Canadian Healthy Living Strategy 2005." Retrieved on May 31, 2006, from www.phac-aspc.gc.ca/hl-vs-strat/pdf/hls_e.pdf.

7. Public Health Agency of Canada, "Healthy Living: Frequently Asked Questions (FAQ)." Retrieved on May 31, 2006, from www.phac-aspc.gc.ca/hl-vs-strat/faq_e.html.

8. Ibid.

9. Ibid.

10. The Secretariat for the Intersectoral Healthy Living Network in partnership with the F/P/T Healthy Living Task Group and the F/P/T Advisory Committee on Population Health and Health Security (ACPHHS), op. cit.

11. Lisa Miller, "Medical Schools Put Women in Curricula," *Wall Street Journal*, May 24, 1994: B1, B7.

12. M. Eichler, A. L. Reisman, and E. M. Borins, "Gender Bias in Medical Research," *Women and Therapy* 12 (1992): 61–70.

13. Eichler et al., op. cit., 63.

14. M. DiMatteo, *The Psychology of Health, Illness, and Medical Care: An Individual Perspective* (Pacific Grove, CA: Brooks/Cole, 1994) 101–103.

15. Edward P. Sarafino, *Health Psychology* (New York: John Wiley & Sons, 1990) 189–191.

16. George D. Bishop, *Health Psychology* (Needham Heights, MA: Allyn & Bacon, 1994) 84–86.

17. I. Ajzen. "The Theory of Planned Behavior," *Organizational Behavior and Human Decision Processes* 50 (1991): 179–211.

18. A. Ellis and M. Bernard, *Clinical Application of Rational-Emotive Therapy* (New York: Plenum, 1985).

19. P. Watson and R. Tharp, *Self-Directed Behavior: Self-Modification for Personal Adjustment* (Pacific Grove, CA: Brooks/Cole, 1993) 13.

20. S. K. Powers, S. L. Dodd, A. M. Thompson, and C. C. Condon, *Total Fitness and Wellness,* Canadian ed. (Toronto: Pearson, 2006).

21. The Stanford DECIDE Drug Education Curriculum, Garfield Company, CA.

## CHAPTER 2

1. National Mental Health Association, *Mental Health* (Alexandria, VA: National Mental Health Association, 1988) 3–4; W. Menninger, "Emotional Maturity," in *A Psychiatrist for a Troubled World: Selected Papers of William Menninger,* ed. Bernard H. Hall (New York: Viking, 1967) 789–807; and Gerald Caplan, *Principles of Preventive Psychiatry* (New York: Basic Books, 1964).

2. Richard Lazarus, *Emotion and Adaptation* (New York: Oxford Press, 1991).

3. Christine Ritter, "Social Supports, Social Networks, and Health Behaviors," in *Health Behavior: Emerging Research Perspectives,* ed. David Gochman (New York: Plenum, 1988).

4. Lester Lefton, *Psychology,* 5th ed. (Boston: Allyn & Bacon, 1994) 626.

5. A. O'Connell and V. O'Connell, *Choice and Change: Psychology of Holistic Growth, Adjustment, and Creativity* (Englewood Cliffs, NJ: Prentice Hall, 1992).

6. J. A. Astin et al., "Mind-Body Medicine: State of the Science, Implications for Practice," *Journal of the American Board of Family Practice* 16 (2003): 131–147; J. Bishop et al., "Mindfulness: A Proposed Operational Definition," *Clinical Psychology* 11 (2004): 230–241.

7. Bishop et al., op. cit.

8. Ibid.

9. Ibid.

10. A. Astin et al., "Spirituality in Higher Education: A National Study of College Students' Search for Meaning and Purpose," Higher Education Research Institute, Graduate School of Education & Information Studies, UCLA, 2004, www.spirituality.ucla.edu.

11. Z. Segal et al., *Mindfulness-Based Cognitive Therapy for Depression: A New Approach to Preventing Relapse* (New York: Guilford Publications, 2001); M. Weiss, J. W. Nordlie, and E. P. Siegel, "Mindfulness-Based Stress Reduction as an Adjunct to Outpatient Psychotherapy," *Psychotherapy and Psychosomatics* 74.2 (2005): 108–112; J. Cohen-Katz et al., "The Effects of Mindfulness-Based Stress Reduction on Nurse Stress and Burnout, Part II: A Quantitative and Qualitative Study," *Holistic Nurse Practice* 1 (2005): 26–35; A. Tacon et al., "Mindfulness Meditation, Anxiety Reduction, and Heart Disease: A Pilot Study," *Family and Community Health* 26.1 (2003): 25–33.

12. D. Elkins, *Beyond Religion—A Personal Program for Building a Spiritual Life Outside the Walls of Traditional Religion* (Wheaton, IL: Quest Books, 1998).

13. Martin Seligman, *Learned Optimism* (New York: Knopf, 1990).

14. Ibid.

15. P. Zimbardo, A. Weber, and R. Johnson, *Psychology* (Boston: Allyn and Bacon, 2000) 403.

16. Excerpted by permission from the University of California at Berkeley Wellness Letter, July 1992, 3–4. © Health Letter Associates, 1992.

17. M. Lemonick, "The Biology of Joy," *Time* 165.3 (2005): A12–A14.

18. J. Kluger, "The Funny Thing about Laughter," *Time* 165.3 (2005): A25–A29.

19. Ibid.

20. R. Davidson, J. S. Maxwell, and A.J. Shockman, "The Privileged Status of Emotion in the Brain," *Proceedings of the National Academy of Sciences of the United States of America* 101.33 (2004): 11915–11916.

21. E. Diener and M. E. P. Seligman, "Beyond Money: Toward an Economy of Well-Being," *Psychological Science in the Public Interest* 5 (2004): 1–31; C. Peterson and M. Seligman, *Character Strengths and Virtues* (London: Oxford University Press, 2004).

22. B. Fredrickson, "Cultivating Positive Emotions to Optimize Health and Well-Being," *Prevention and Treatment* 3 (March 7, 2000), Article 0001a.

23. D. Grady, "Think Right, Stay Well," *American Health* xi (1992): 50–54.

24. J. M. Gottman and N. Silver, *The Seven Principles of Making Marriage Work* (New York: Crown Publishers Inc., 1999).

25. Grady, op. cit., 50–54.

26. Health Canada, "Message from the Minister of Health: National Mental Health Week: May 1–7, 2006." Retrieved on May 8, 2006, from www.hc-sc.gc.ca/ahc-asc/minist/health-sante/messages/2006_05_01_e.html.

27. Statistics Canada, "Risk of Depression, by Age Group and Sex, Household Population Aged 12 and Over, Canada, 2000/01." Retrieved on May 30, 2006, from dissemination. stat.ca/ English/freepubl/82-221-XIE/2005002/tables/html/1295.htm.

28. Adapted by permission of the author from Kathryn Rose Gertz, "Mood Probe: Pinpointing the Crucial Differences between Emotional Lows and the Gridlock of Depression," *Self* (November 1990): 165–168, 204.

29. The Canadian Mental Health Association, Ontario Division, Information Sheet: Understanding, 1999.

30. Levitan, "An Overview of Seasonal Affective Disorder," *Psychiatry Rounds*, Department of Pyschiatry, University of Toronto Centre for Addiction and Mental Health, October 2, No.7, 1998.

31. Ibid.

32. Ibid.

33. Statistics Canada, op. cit.

34. Statistics Canada, "Suicides, and Suicide Rate, by Sex and by Age Group." Retrieved on April 25, 2006, from www40.statcan.ca/l01/cst01/health01a.htm.

35. World Health Organization, "Self-Directed Violence." Retrieved on April 25, 2006, from www.who.int/violence_injury_prevention.

36. Royal Commission of Aboriginal Peoples, *Special Report on Suicide among Aboriginal People*, Minister of Supply and Services, Ottawa: 1995.

## CHAPTER 3

1. Hans Selye, *Stress without Distress* (New York: Lippincott, 1974) 28–29.

2. Charles Morris, *Understanding Psychology* (Englewood Cliffs, NJ: Prentice Hall, 1993) 471–473.

3. W. B. Kannel and E. D. Eaker, "Psychosocial and Other Features of Coronary Heart Disease: Insights from the Framingham Study," *American Heart Journal* 112.5 (1986): 1066–1073.

4. R. Ader and S. Cohen, "Psychoneuroimmunology: Conditioning and Stress," *Annual Review of Psychology* 44 (1993): 53–85.

5. N. Cohen, D. Tyrrell, and A. Smith, "Negative Life Events, Perceived Stress, Negative Affect, and Susceptibility to the Common Cold," *Journal of Personality and Social Psychology* 64 (1993): 131–140.

6. Ader and Cohen, op. cit., 53–85.

7. Ibid., 59.

8. Selye, op. cit., 28–29.

9. Thomas Holmes and Richard Rahe, "The Social Readjustment Rating Scale," *Journal of Psychosocial Research* (1967): 213–217.

10. Ibid., 214.

11. Richard Lazarus, "The Trivialization of Distress," in *Preventing Health Risk Behaviors and Promoting Coping with Illness*, ed. J. Rosen and L. Solomon (Hanover, NH: University Press of New England, 1985) 279–298.

12. Lester Lefton, *Psychology* (Boston: Allyn & Bacon, 1994) 471.

13. Ibid., 471.

14. R. C. Kessler, K. S. Kendler, A. C. Heath, M. C. Neale, and L. J. Eaves, "Social Support, Depressed Mood, and Adjustment to Stress: A Genetic Epidemiological Investigation," *Journal of Personality and Social Psychology* 62 (1992): 257–272.

15. Morris, op. cit., 447–448.

16. Meyer Friedman and Ray H. Rosenman, *Type A Behavior and Your Heart* (New York: Knopf, 1974).

17. R. Ragland and R. Brand, "Distrust, Rage May Be Toxic: Cores That Put Type A Person at Risk," *Journal of the American Medical Association* 261 (1989): 813, 814.

18. Philip L. Rice, *Stress and Health* (Monterey, CA: Brooks/Cole, 1992) 471.

19. Ibid.

20. Robert Eliot, *Is It Worth Dying For?* (New York: Bantam, 1984) 225.

## CHAPTER 4

1. World Health Organization: "Injuries and Violence Prevention." Retrieved on April 25, 2006, from www.who.int/violence_injury_prevention/violence/en/.

2. Jan J. M. van Dijk, Pat Mayhew, and Martin Killias, *Experiencing Crime across the World* (Deventer, the Netherlands: Kluwer Law and Taxation Publishers, 1990) 38.

3. Ibid., 78.

4. J. Frank, "Violent Youth Crime," *Canadian Social Trends* (Autumn 1992): 3.

5. W. Gleberzon, "Ethnicity and Violence: Racial Conflict in Vancouver" (unpublished, undated, on file at the Human Rights Library, Fauteux Hall, University of Ottawa) 7–8.

6. K. Adachi, *The Enemy That Never Was: A History of the Japanese Canadians* (Toronto: McClelland and Stewart, 1991).

7. M. Suderman and P. Jaffe, *Preventing Violence: School and Community-Based Strategies*, Health Canada, 1996.

8. Statistics Canada, "Homicide Offences, Number and Rate, by Province and Territory." Retrieved on April 25, 2006, from www40.statcan.ca/l01/cst01/legal12a.htm.

9. Statistics Canada, "Homicides by Method." Retrieved on April 25, 2006, from www40.statcan.ca/l01/cst01/legal01a.htm.

10. Statistics Canada, "Victims and Persons Accused of Homicide, by Age and Sex." Retrieved on April 25, 2006, from www40.statcan.ca/l01/cst01/legal10a.htm.

11. Ibid.

12. Canadian Firearms Program Statistics, "Statistics." Retrieved on April 25, 2006, from www.cfc-cafc.gc.ca/media/program_statistics/default_e.asp.

13. M. Asberg et al., "Psychology of Suicidal Behaviour," *Annals of the New York Academy of Sciences* 487 (1986).

14. B. L. Tanney, "Mental Disorders, Psychiatric Patients and Suicide," in *Assessment and Prediction of Suicide*, eds. R. Maris et al. (New York: Guilford Press, 1992).

15. I. Sakinofsky, "The Ecology of Suicide in the Provinces of Canada, 1967–71 to 1979–81," in *The Epidemiology of Psychiatric Disorders* ed. B. C. Cooper (Baltimore: Johns Hopkins, 1987).

16. World Health Organization, "Self-Directed Violence." Retrieved on April 25, 2006, from www.who.int/violence_injury_prevention.

17. Statistics Canada, "Suicides and Suicide Rate, by Sex and by Age Group." Retrieved on April 25, 2006 from www40.statcan.ca/l01/cst01/health01a.htm.

18. Ibid.

19. Health Canada, *Toward a Healthy Future: Second Report on the Health of Canadians,* a public policy report developed by the Federal, Provincial and Territorial Advisory Committee on Population Health (ACPH) in collaboration with Health Canada, Statistics Canada, the Canadian Institute for Health Information and a project team from the Centre for Health Promotion, University of Toronto. Health Canada, Ottawa: 1999, 23.

20. Ibid., 24.

21. Ibid., 24.

22. Child & Family Canada, Fact Sheet on Suicide.

23. World Health Organization, "Self-Directed Violence."

24. Statistics Canada, "Victims and Persons Accused."

25. Ibid.

26. Dianne Hendrick, "Youth Court Statistics," *Juristat* 19.2, Statistics Canada, Cat. No. 85-002-XPE, 1.

27. K. Stevenson et al., "Youth and Crime," *Canadian Social Trends* (Summer 1999), Statistics Canada, Cat. No. 11-008, 19.

28. Ibid., 17.

29. D. Patel, *Dealing with Interracial Conflict: Policy Alternatives* (Montreal: Institute for Research on Public Policy, 1980).

30. "Hate-Motivated Violence," ACJNet, www2.ca.nizkor.org/ftp.cgi/orgs/canadian/canada/ justice/hate-motivated-violence/hmv-002-02.

31. Linda McLeod, *Wife Battering in Canada: The Vicious Circle* (Ottawa: Canadian Advisory Council on the Status of Women, 1980).

32. K. Rodgers, "Wife Assault in Canada," *Canadian Social Trends* (Autumn 1994): 3.

33. Ibid.

34. "Wife Abuse Information," The National Clearinghouse on Family Violence, September 1995.

35. Solicitor General, *Family Violence: Not a Private Problem,* RCMP Policy, Public Education Doc. 1966.

36. A. Joerger et al., "Why Men Batter: Why Women Stay," *Community Safety Quarterly* 5 (1992): 22–23.

37. N. West, "Crimes against Women," *Community Safety Survey* 5 (1992): 1.

38. Statistics Canada, *Canadian Crime Statistics,* 1995, 60.

39. Statistics Canada, *Family Violence in Canada: A Statistical Profile,* Cat. No. 85-224.

40. Ibid.

41. H. Pan et al., "Physical Aggression in Early Marriage: Pre-relationship and Relationship Effects," *Journal of Consulting Psychology.*

42. G. Wilson et al., *Abnormal Psychology* (Boston, MA: Allyn & Bacon, 1996).

43. Ibid.

44. Ibid.

45. N. Trocomé, B. Fallon, B. MacLaurin, J. Daciuk, C. Felstiner, T. Black, L. Tonmyr, C. Blackstock, K. Barter, D. Turcotte, and R. Cloutier. "Canadian Incidence Study of Reported Child Abuse and Neglect—2003: Major Findings," Minister of Public Works and Government Services Canada, 2005.

46. World Health Organization: Communications and Public Relations, WHO Fact Sheet N150, March 1997.

47. A. Miller, "Newly Recognized Shattering Effects of Child Abuse," *Empathic Parenting* 1 & 2 (1992).

48. World Health Organization, WHO Fact Sheet N150.

49. Statistics Canada, "Selected Violations against the Person, by Gender of Victim and Accused, 1995," *Canadian Crime Statistics* (1995).

50. Health Canada, "Abuse and Neglect of Older Adults," Cat. No. H72-22/6-1998E.

51. Statistics Canada, *Family Violence in Canada.*

52. "Sex Offenders," *Juristat* 19.3, Statistics Canada Cat. No. 85-002-XPE 19, 3.

53. Statistics Canada, *Family Violence in Canada,* 86.

54. Health Canada, "Dating and Violence: Fact Sheet," February 1993.

55. A. Berkowitz, "College Men as Perpetrators of Acquaintance Rape and Sexual Assault: A Review of the Literature," *Journal of American College Health* 40 (1992): 177.

56. Ibid., 178.

57. D. Benson et al., "Acquaintance Rape on Campus: A Literature Review," *Journal of American College Health* 40 (1992): 158.

58. M. Whittaker, "The Continuum of Violence against Women: Psychological and Physical Consequences," *Journal of American College Health* 40 (1992): 151.

59. A. Mathews, "Campus Crime 101," *Eugene Register Guard,* March 1993: 2B.

60. T. Schneider, "Rape Prevention," *Community Safety Quarterly* (1992): 8–13.

61. Ibid., 12.

62. Ibid., 13.

63. Ibid.

64. Health Canada, *Health Aspects of Violence against Women,* Women's Health Forum, Ottawa, 1996.

## CHAPTER 5

1. MayoClinic.com, "Nurture Relationships: A Healthy Habit for Healthy Aging," 2003, Mayo Foundation for Medical Education and Research (MFMER), www.mayohealth.org; K. Uberg et al., "Supportive Relationships as a Moderator of the Effects of Peer Drinking on Adolescents," *Journal of Research on Adolescents* 15.1 (2005): 1–20.

2. C. Snapp and M. Leary, "Hurt Feelings among New Acquaintances: Moderating Effects of Interpersonal Familiarity," *Journal of Social and Personal Relationships* 18.3 (June 2001): 1344–1350.

3. V. Manusov and J. Harvey, eds., *Attribution, Communication Behavior and Close Relationships* (New York: Cambridge University Press, 2001).

4. J. Caputo, H. C. Hazel, and C. McMahon, *Interpersonal Communication* (Boston: Allyn & Bacon, 1994) 224.

5. Janet D. Woititz, *Struggle for Intimacy* (Pompano Beach, FL: Health Communications, 1985).

6. Sharon S. Brehm, *Intimate Relationships* (New York: McGraw-Hill, 1992) 4–5.

7. "Vanier Institute on the Family Mission Statement," *Canadian Social Trends* (Summer 1993), Statistics Canada, Cat. No. 11-008E, Ottawa: Ministry of Supply and Services.

8. J. Dunn, "Siblings and Development," *Current Directions in Psychological Science* 1 (1992): 6–11.

9. J. Turner and L. Rubinson, *Contemporary Human Sexuality* (Englewood Cliffs, NJ: Prentice Hall, 1993) 457.

10. Ibid.

11. E. Hatfield, "Passionate and Companionate Love," in *The Psychology of Love,* eds. R. J. Sternberg and M. Barnes (New Haven: Yale University Press, 1988) 191–217.

12. R. A. Baron and D. Byrne, *Social Psychology* (Boston: Allyn & Bacon, 1994) 318.

13. E. Hatfield and G. W. Walster, *A New Look at Love* (Reading, MA: Addison-Wesley, 1981).

14. Helen Fisher, *Anatomy of Love: The Natural History of Monogamy, Adultery, and Divorce* (New York: Norton, 1993).

15. A. Toufexis and P. Gray, "What Is Love? The Right Chemistry," *Time* (1993): 47–52.

16. Ibid., 49.

17. Fisher, op. cit.

18. C. McLoughlin, "Science of Love—Cupid's Chemistry," The Naked Scientists Online, 2003, www.thenakedscientist.com/HTML/Columnists/clairemcloughlincolumn1.htm.

19. "Science and Technology: I Get a Kick Out of You: The Science of Love," *The Economist* 370 (8362) (2004): 89.

20. Deborah Tannen, *You Just Don't Understand: Women and Men in Conversation* (New York: Ballantine, 1990).

21. M. McGill, *The McGill Report on Male Intimacy* (New York: Holt, Rinehart & Winston, 1985) 87–88.

22. Lillian Rubin, *Intimate Strangers* (New York: Harper and Row, 1983).

23. S. Hendricks and C. Hendricks, *Liking, Loving, and Relating,* 2nd ed. (Pacific Grove, CA: Brooks/Cole, 1992).

24. R. Landerman, M. Swartz, and L. George, "The Long-Term Effects of Childhood Exposure to Parental Drinking." Paper presented at the annual meeting of the American Public Health Association, Mental Health session, Washington, DC, 1992. See also A. Diaz, F. Yancovitz, N. Showers, and I. Epstein, "Predictors and Psychological Consequences of Disclosure of Incest by Female Adolescents." Paper presented at the annual meeting of the American Public Health Association, Mental Health session, Washington, DC, 1992.

25. M. Klausner and B. Hasselbring, *Aching for Love: The Sexual Drama of the Adult Child* (New York: Harper and Row, 1990).

26. Statistics Canada, "Population by Marital Status and Sex." Retrieved on May 9, 2006, from www.40.statcan.ca/l01/cst01/famil01.htm.

27. Statistics Canada, "Marriages by Province and Territory." Retrieved on May 9, 2006, from www.40.statcan.ca/l01/cst01/famil04.htm.

28. Statistics Canada, "Divorces by Province and Territory." Retrieved on May 9, 2006, from www.40.statcan.ca/l01/cst01/famil02.htm.

29. Statistics Canada, "2001 Census: Marital Status, Common-Law Status, Families, Dwellings and Households," *The Daily,* October 22, 2002.

30. Statistics Canada, "Changing Conjugal Life in Canada," *The Daily,* July 11, 2002.

31. Ibid.

32. Public Legal Association of Saskatchewan (PLEASASK), Living Common Law.

33. R. Friedman and J. Downey, "Homosexuality," *New England Journal of Medicine* 33 (1994): 923–928.

34. Statistics Canada, "Population by Marital Status and Sex".

35. J. Hirdes and P. Forbes, "Factors Associated with the Maintenance of Good Self-Rated Health," *Journal of Aging and Health* 5.1 (1993): 101–122.

36. Statistics Canada, "Divorces by Province and Territory," 35.

37. Writing Group for the Women's Health Initiative Investigators, "Risk and Benefits of Estrogen Plus Progestin in Healthy Postmenopausal Women: Principal Results from the Women's Health Initiative Randomized Controlled Trial," *Journal of the American Medical Association* 288.3 (2002): 321–333.

38. R. C. Friedman and J. I. Downey, "Homosexuality," *Journal of the American Medical Association* 331 (1994): 923–930.

39. Dorothy Tennov, *Love and Limerence* (Chelsea, MI: Scarborough House, 1989) 45–50.

40. Alex Comfort, *The Joy of Sex* (New York: Simon and Schuster, 1972) 14.

41. R. O'Carroll, "Sexual Desire Disorders: A Review of Controlled Treatment Studies," *The Journal of Sex Research* 28.19: 607–624.

42. National Kidney and Urological Diseases Information Clearinghouse, "Erectile Dysfunction," 2004, http://kidney.niddk.nih.gov/kudiseases/pubs/impotence/index.htm.

43. B. Handy, "The Potency Pill," *Time,* May 4, 1998: 50–57.

44. Arnot Ogden Medical Center, "Frequently Asked Questions," 1998, www.aomc.org/HOD2/general/ViagraFAQ.html.

45. C. Darling and J. Davidson, "Enhancing Relationships: Understanding the Feminine Mystique of Pretending Orgasm," *Journal of Sex and Marital Therapy* 12.19 (1986): 182–196.

# CHAPTER 6

1. Centers for Disease Control, *Contraceptive Options: Increasing Your Awareness* (Washington, DC: NAACOG, 1990).

2. University of Southern California School of Medicine, "Noncontraceptive Health Benefits," *Dialogues in Contraception* 3 (1990): 2.

3. D. E. Greydanus and R. B. Shearin, *Adolescent Sexuality and Gynecology* (Philadelphia: Lea & Febiger, 1990) 107.

4. Planned Parenthood, "Chronology of Court Cases: Dr. Morgentaler and Others."

5. Ibid.

6. Childbirth by Choice Trust, *Abortion in Canada Today: The Situation Province by Province* (1995).

7. Planned Parenthood, *Therapeutic Abortions* (1994).

8. Statistics Canada, "Induced Abortions by Area of Residence of Patients." Retrieved on May 12, 2006, from www40.statcan.ca/l01/cst01/health41a.htm?sdi=abortions.

9. Statistics Canada, "Pregnancy Outcome by Age Group (Induced Abortions)." Retrieved on May 12, 2006, from www40.statcan.ca/l01/cst01/hlth65c.htm?sdi=abortions.

10. K. Schmidt, "The Dark Legacy of Fatherhood," *U.S. News and World Report,* December 14, 1992: 94–95.

11. U.S. Department of Health and Human Services, *The Health Benefits of Smoking Cessation: A Report of the Surgeon General,* United States, Public Health Service, Office on Smoking and Health, Washington, DC: 1990.

12. American College of Obstetricians and Gynecologists, "Nutrition during Pregnancy," Patient Education Pamphlet (AP001), April 1992.

13. D. Hall and D. Kaufmann, "Effects of Aerobic and Strength Conditioning on Pregnancy Outcomes," *American Journal of Obstetrics and Gynecology* 157 (1987): 1199–1203.

14. J. D. Forrest, "Contraceptive Needs through Stages of Women's Reproductive Lives," *Contemporary OB/GYN* (Special Issue on Fertility) (1988): 12–22.

15. W. J. Millar, C. Nair, and S. Wadhera, "Declining Cesarean Section Rates: A Continuing Trend?" *Health Reports* 8.1 (1996): 17–24.

16. Statistics Canada, "Pregnancy Outcome by Age Group (Fetal Loss)." Retrieved on May 12, 2006, from www40.statcan.ca/l01/cst01/hlth65d.htm.

17. Public Health Agency of Canada, "Canadian Perinatal Surveillance System: Sudden Infant Death Syndrome." Retrieved on May 16, 2006, from www.phac.aspc.gc.ca/rhs-ssg/factshts/sids_e.html.

18. Ibid.

19. Public Health Agency of Canada, "Canadian Perinatal Surveillance System: Infant Mortality." Retrieved on May 16, 2006, from www.phac.aspc.gc.ca/rhs-ssg/factshts/mort_e.html.

20. University of Southern California of Medicine, *Dialogues in Contraception* 3 (1991): 2.

# CHAPTER 7

1. Health and Welfare Canada, *Food Guide Facts: Background for Educators and Communicators* (Ottawa: Minister of Supply and Services, Cat. No. H39-253/101-1992E, 1992).

2. Health Canada: Food and Nutrition, "Canada's Food Guides from 1942 to 1992." Retrieved on May 25, 2006, from www.hc-sc.gc.ca/fn-an/food-guide-aliment/hist/fg_history-histoire_ga_e.html#process.

3. Health Canada: Food and Nutrition, "Draft Food Guide Revision Project Timeline." Retrieved on May 25, 2006, from www.hc-sc.gc.ca/fn-an/food-guide-aliment/revision/fg_rev_pro_timeline-cal_rev_ga_e.html.

4. Health Canada: Food and Nutrition, "Revision of Canada's Food Guide to Healthy Eating." Retrieved on May 25, 2006, from www.hc-sc.gc.ca/fn-an/food-guide-aliment/revision/revision_fg-examen_ga_e.html.

5. Ibid.

6. Ibid.

7. J. Thompson, M. Manore, and J. Sheeska, *Nutrition: A Functional Approach*, Canadian edition (Toronto: Pearson Benjamin Cummings, 2007).

8. Ibid.

9. Ibid.

10. Janet Christian and Janet Gregor, *Nutrition for Living*, 4th ed. (Benjamin Cummings, 1994), 129.

11. Ibid., 129.

12. R. B. Kanarck and R. Kaufman, *Nutrition and Behavior* (New York: Van Nostrand Reinhold, 1991).

13. Thompson, Manore, and Sheeska, op. cit.

14. Ibid.

15. *University of California Wellness Letter*, April 1992, 4–6.

16. Thompson, Manore, and Sheeska, op. cit.

17. Ibid.

18. R. Mensink and M. Katan, "Effect of Dietary Trans-Fatty Acids on High-Density and Low-Density Lipoprotein and Cholesterol Levels in Healthy Subjects," *New England Journal of Medicine*, August 16, 1990.

19. G. Ruoff, "Reducing Fat Intake with Fat Substitutes," *American Family Physician* 43 (1991): 1235–1242.

20. R. Maddox and S. Maddox, "Reducing the Risk of Alzheimer's Disease," *U.S. Pharmacist* 30.3 (2005): 34–36; American Cancer Society (July 18, 2005), www.asc.com; National Women's Health Resource Center, "Women and Alzheimer's Disease," *National Women's Health Report* 26.6 (2004): 1–8; R. Mensink, "Metabolic and Health Effects of Fatty Acids," *Current Opinions in Epidemiology* 16.1 (2005): 27–30.

21. S. K. Powers, S. L. Dodd, A. M. Thompson, and C. C. Condon, *Total Fitness and Wellness*, Canadian edition (Toronto: Pearson Benjamin Cummings, 2006).

22. Thompson, Manore, and Sheeska, op. cit.

23. Ibid.

24. Ibid.

25. Christian and Gregor, op. cit., 56.

26. Thompson, Manore, and Sheeska, op. cit.

27. Ibid.

28. Ibid.

29. Ibid.

30. "Special Report: Irradiation Plants Geared to 'Zap' Meat and Poultry—Is It Safe?" *Tufts University Health and Nutrition Letter* 18.1 (2000): 4–7.

31. Centers for Disease Control and Prevention, "Food Borne Illnesses," 2002, www.cdc.gov; American Medical Association, "Diagnosis and Management of Foodborne Illness: A Primer for Physicians and Other Health Care Professionals," 2004, www.ama-assn.org/ama/org.

32. Ibid.

33. Ibid.

34. P. Morris, Y. Motarjemi, and F. Kaferstein, "Emerging Food-Borne Diseases," *World Health* 50 (1997): 16–22; Centers for Disease Control and Prevention, "Food Borne Illnesses."

35. L. Katzenstein, "Food Irradiation: The Story Behind the Scare," *American Health*, 60–80.

36. A. Hechtt, "Preventing Food-Borne Illnesses," *FDA Consumer Magazine*.

# CHAPTER 8

1. Statistics Canada, "Health Indicators." Catalogue No. 82-221-XIE. May 2002.

2. Philip Elmer-Dewitt, "Fat Times," *Time*, January 16, 1995: 60.

3. P. T. Katzmarzyk, "The Canadian Obesity Epidemic, 1985–1998." *Canadian Medical Association Journal* 166.8 (2002): 1039–1040.

4. R. M. Malina, C. Bouchard, and O. Bar-Or. *Growth, Maturation, and Physical Activity* (Champaign, IL: Human Kinetics, 2004).

5. Malina, Bouchard, and Bar-Or, op. cit.

6. Ibid.

7. C. J. Crespo and E. Smit, "Prevalence of Overweight and Obesity in the United States," in *Obesity: Etiology, Assessment, Treatment and Prevention* ed. R. E. Andersen (Champaign, IL: Human Kinetics, 2003).

8. B. A. Reeder, A. Senthilselvan, J-P. Després, A. Angel, L. Liu, H. Wang, and S. W. Rabkin, "The Association of Cardiovascular Disease Risk Factors with Abdominal Obesity in Canada," *Canadian Medical Association Journal* 157 (1997) (1 suppl): S39–S45.

9. Malina, Bouchard, and Bar-Or, op. cit.

10. Health Canada, "Canadian Guidelines for Body Weight Classifications in Adults," 2003. Retrieved July 21, 2004, from www.hc-sc.gc.ca/hpfb-dgpsa/onpp-bppn/weight_book_tc_e.html.

11. W. Sheldon, S. Stevens, and W. Tucker, *The Varieties of Human Physique* (New York: Harper and Row, 1940) 104.

12. Malina, Bouchard, and Bar-Or, op. cit.

13. A. Stunkard, *Psychiatric Update: American Psychiatric Association* (New York: Harper and Row, 1985) 87.

14. Claude Bouchard et al., "The Response to Long-Term Overfeeding in Identical Twins," *New England Journal of Medicine* 322 (1990): 1477–1488.

15. Ibid.

16. Albert Stunkard et al., "The Body-Mass Index of Twins Who Have Been Raised Apart," *New England Journal of Medicine* 322 (1990): 1483–1487.

17. Y. C. Chagnon, T. Rice, L. Perusse, I. B. Borecki, M. A. Ho-Kim, M. Lacaille, C. Pare, L. Bouchard, J. Gagnon, A. S. Leon, J. S. Skinner, J. H. Wilmore, D. C. Rao, and C. Bouchard, "Genomic Scan for Genes

Affecting Body Composition before and after Training in Caucasians from HERITAGE." *Journal of Applied Physiology* 90 (2001): 1777–1787.

18. P. Jaret, "The Way to Lose Weight," *Health* (January/February 1995): 52–59.

19. Ibid., 55.

20. Malina, Bouchard, and Bar-Or, op. cit.

21. Ibid.

22. F. Katch and W. McArdle, *Introduction to Nutrition, Exercise, and Health*, 4th ed. (Philadelphia: Lea & Febiger, 1992) 77.

23. L. A. Wadsworth, and A. MacQuarrie, "Nutrition Messages on Saturday Morning Children's Television: 1989–1998." *Canadian Journal of Dietetic Practice and Research* 63 (2002) (Supp): 105.

24. L. A. Wadsworth, and S. Berenbaum, "Textual Analyses of Nutrition Messages on Prime Time Television," *Canadian Home Economics Journal* 51 (2001): 13–18.

25. Philip Elmer-DeWitt, op. cit., 61.

26. S. Lichman et al., "Discrepancy between Self-Reported and Actual Caloric Intake and Exercise in Obese Subjects," *New England Journal of Medicine* 327 (1992): 1894–1897.

27. Kelly Brownell, "Comments on the Latest Study on Yo-Yo Diets by Steven N. Blair of the Institute for Aerobics Research in Dallas." Paper presented at the annual research meeting of the American Heart Association, Monterey, CA, January 1993.

28. Statistics Canada, "Health Indicators." Catalogue no. 82-221-X9. May 2002.

29. Canadian Fitness and Lifestyle Research Institute, "Survey Statistics Summaries—2004 Physical Activity Monitor." Retrieved on June 5, 2006, from www.cflri.ca/eng/statistics/index.php.

30. M. Boyle and G. Zyla, *Personal Nutrition* (St. Paul, MN: West Publishing, 1991) 21.

31. Surgeon General's Report on Physical Activity and Health, 1996; adapted from B. E. Ainsworth, W. L. Haskell, A. S. Leon et al., "Compendium of Physical Activities: Classification of Energy Costs of Human Physical Activities," *Medicine and Science in Sports and Exercise* 25.1 (2003): 71–80.

32. J. Robison et al., "Obesity, Weight Loss, and Health," *Journal of the American Dietetic Association* 93 (1993): 448.

33. Ibid., 448.

34. Simone French and R. Jeffery, "Consequences of Dieting to Lose Weight: Effects on Physical and Mental Health," *Health Psychology* 13.3 (1994): 195–212; G. Wilson, "Relation of Dieting and Voluntary Weight Loss to Psychological Functioning and Binge Eating," *Annals of Internal Medicine* 119 (1993): 727–730.

35. French and Jeffrey, op. cit., 195–196.

36. L. Lissner et al., "Variabilities in Body Weight and Health Outcomes in the Framingham Study," *New England Journal of Medicine* 324 (1991): 1839–1844; ibid., 197–198.

37. J. Horm and K. Anderson, "Who in America Is Trying to Lose Weight?" *Annals of Internal Medicine* 119 (1993): 672–676; ibid., 203.

38. K. D. Raine, "Determinants of Health Eating in Canada: An Overview and Synthesis" *Canadian Journal of Public Health* 96.3 (July/August 2005): S8–S14.

39. G. Terrence Wilson, Peter Nathan, K. Daniel O'Leary, and Lee Anna Clark, *Abnormal Psychology* (Boston: Allyn & Bacon, 1996).

40. Bulimia Anorexia Nervosa Association (Canada), www.bana.ca.

41. Ibid.

42. "Treating Eating Disorders," *Harvard Women's Health Watch* (May 1996): 4–5.

# CHAPTER 9

1. World Health Organization, "Health and Development through Physical Activity and Sport." *WHO/NHM/NPH/PAH/O3.2.* (Geneva: WHO Document Production Services, 2003).

2. C. Bouchard, R. J. Shephard, T. Stephens, J. R. Sutton, and B. D. McPherson, "Exercise, Fitness, and Health: The Consensus Statement," in *Exercise, Fitness, and Health: A Consensus of Current Knowledge* eds. C. Bouchard, R. J. Shephard, T. Stephens, J. R. Sutton, and B. D. McPherson (Champaign, IL: Human Kinetics, 1988) 4–27.

3. Statistics Canada, "Physical Activity, by Age Group and Sex, Household Population Aged 12 and Older." Retrieved on February 20, 2006, from www40.statcan.ca/l01/cst01/health46.htm?sdi=physical activity.

4. Canadian Fitness and Lifestyle Research Institute, "Survey Statistics Summaries—2004 Physical Activity Monitor." Retrieved on June 5, 2006, from www.cflri.ca/eng/statistics/index.php.

5. A. M. Thompson, P. D. Campagna, L. A. Rehman, R. J. L. Murphy, R. L. Rasmussen, and G. W. Ness, "Physical Activity and Body Mass Index in Grade 3, 7, and 11 Nova Scotia Students," *Medicine & Science in Sports & Exercise* 37.11 (2005): 1902–1908.

6. A. M. Thompson, M. L. Humbert, and R. L. Mirwald, "A Longitudinal Study of the Impact of Childhood and Adolescent Physical Activity Experiences on Adult Physical Activity Perceptions and Behaviours," *Qualitative Health Research* 13.3 (2003): 358–377.

7. The College of Family Physicians of Canada, "Exercise: A Healthy Habit to Start and Keep." Last modified October 31, 2002. Retrieved on February 9, 2003, from www.cfpc.ca/programs/education/pated/Exercise.asp.

8. Health Canada: Physical Activity Unit, "Helpful Definitions." Retrieved on August 23, 2004, from www.hc-sc.gc.ca/ hppb/fitness/definitions.html.

9. Statistics Canada, "At Risk of First or Recurring Heart Disease," 1998. Catalogue No. 82-003-XPB.

10. T. Baranowski, C. Bouchard, O. Bar-Or, et al., "Assessment, Prevalence, and Cardiovascular Benefits of Physical Activity and Fitness in Youth," *Medicine and Science in Sports and Exercise,* 24.6 (1992) (suppl.): S237–S247.

11. L. Bernstein et al., "Adolescent Exercise Reduces Risk of Breast Cancer in Younger Women," *Journal of the National Cancer Institute* (September 1994).

12. Baranowski, Bouchard, and Bar-Or, op. cit.

13. D. S. Freedman, W. H. Dietz, S. R. Srinivasan, et al, "The Relation of Overweight to Cardiovascular Disease Risk Factors among Children and Adolescents: The Bogalusa Heart Study," *Pediatrics* 103 (1999): 1175–1182.

14. A. V. Chobanian, G. L. Bakris, H. R. Black, W. C. Cushman, L. A. Green, J. L. Izzo, Jr., D. W. Jones, B. J. Materson, S. Oparil, and E. J. Roccella, "The Seventh Report of the Joint National Committee on Prevention, Detection, Evaluation, and Treatment of High Blood Pressure: The JNC-7 Report," *Journal of the American Medical Association* 289.19 (2003): 2560–2572. Erratum 2003: 290.2: 197.

15. W. L. Haskell, A. S. Leon, C. J. Caspersen, et al., "Cardiovascular Benefits and Assessment of Physical Activity and Physical Fitness in Adults," *Medicine and Science in Sports and Exercise* 24.6 (1992) (suppl.): S201–S220.

16. Haskell, Leon, Caspersen, et al., op. cit.

17. "Third Report of the National Cholesterol Education Program Expert Panel on Detection, Evaluation, and Treatment of High Blood Cholesterol in Adults," *Journal of the American Medical Association* 285.19 (2001): 1–19.

18. W. H. Ettinger, Jr., and R. F. Afable, "Physical Disability from Knee Osteoarthritis: The Role of Exercise as an Intervention," *Medicine and Science in Sports and Exercise* 26 (1994): 1435–1440.

19. P. A. Kovar, J. P. Allegrante, C. R. MacKenzie, et al., "Supervised Fitness Walking in Patients with Osteoarthritis of the Knee: A Randomized, Controlled Trial," *Annals of Internal Medicine* 116 (1992): 529–534; D. T. Felson, Y. Zhang, J. M. Anthony, et al., "Weight Loss Reduces the Risk of Symptomatic Knee Osteoarthritis in Women: The Framingham Study," *Annals of Internal Medicine* 116 (1992): 535–539.

20. H. M. Frost, "Skeletal Structural Adaptations to Mechanical Usage (SATMU): 1. Redefining Wolff's Law: The Bone Remodeling Problem," *The Anatomical Record* 226 (1990): 403–413.

21. B. L. Drinkwater, "Does Physical Activity Play a Role in Preventing Osteoporosis?" *Research Quarterly for Exercise and Sport* 65 (1994): 197–206.

22. National Institutes of Health, "Consensus Development Conference Statement on Diet and Exercise in Non-Insulin-Dependent Diabetes Mellitus," *Diabetes Care* 10 (1987): 639–644.

23. C. E. Tudor-Locke, R. C. Bell, and A. M. Meyers, "Revisiting the Role of Physical Activity and Exercise in the Treatment of Type II Diabetes," *Canadian Journal of Applied Physiology* 25.6 (2000): 466–492.

24. S. P. Helmrich, D. R. Ragland, and R. S. Paffenbarger, Jr., "Prevention of Non-Insulin-Dependent Diabetes Mellitus with Physical Activity," *Medicine and Science in Sports and Exercise* 26 (1994): 824–830.

25. R. Paffenbarger, R. Hyde, A. Wing, and C. Hsieh, "Physical Activity, All Cause Mortality, Longevity of College Alumni," *New England Journal of Medicine* 314 (1986): 605–613.

26. S. N. Blair, H. W. Kohl III, R. S. Paffenbarger, et al., "Physical Fitness and All-Cause Mortality: A Prospective Study of Healthy Men and Women," *Journal of the American Medical Association* 262.17 (1989): 2395–2401.

27. E. R. Eichner, "Infection, Immunity, and Exercise: What to Tell Patients?" *Physician and Sportsmedicine* (January 1993): 125–135.

28. D. C. Nieman, "Exercise, Immunity and Respiratory Infections," *Sports Science Exchange,* August 1992.

29. D. C. Nieman, L. M. Johanssen, J. W. Lee, et al., "Infectious Episodes in Runners before and after the Los Angeles Marathon," *Journal of Sports Medicine and Physical Fitness* 30 (1990): 316–328.

30. E. R. Eichner, op. cit.

31. Health Canada: Physical Activity Unit, op. cit.

32. Baranowski et al., op. cit.

33. Canadian Society for Exercise Physiology, *The Canadian Physical Activity, Fitness & Lifestyle Approach (CPAFLA): CSEP Health & Fitness Program's Health-Related Appraisal and Counselling Strategy,* 3rd edition (Ottawa: Canadian Society for Exercise Physiology, 2003).

34. E. Fox, R. Bowers, and M. Foss. *The Physiological Basis for Exercise and Sport* (Dubuque, IA: Brown and Benchmark, 1989).

35. B. Stamford, "Tracking Your Heart Rate for Fitness," *Physician and Sportsmedicine* (March 1993).

36. Public Health Agency of Canada, "Canada's Physical Activity Guide for Healthy Active Living." Ottawa.

37. Ibid.

38. P. D. Wood, "Physical Activity, Diet, and Health: Independent and Interactive Effects," *Medicine and Science in Sports and Exercise* 26 (1994): 838–843.

39. S. K. Powers, S. L. Dodd, A. M. Thompson, and C. C. Condon, *Total Fitness and Wellness,* Canadian edition (Toronto: Pearson, 2006).

40. P. A. Sienna, *One Rep Max: A Guide to Beginning Weight Training* (Indianapolis: Benchmark, 1989).

41. H. G. Knuttgen and W. J. Kraemer, "Terminology and Measurement in Exercise Performance," *Journal of Applied Sport Science Research* 1 (1987): 1–10.

42. W. J. Kraemer, "Involvement of Eccentric Muscle Action May Optimize Adaptations to Resistance Training," *Sports Science Exchange* (November 1992).

43. Sienna, op. cit.

44. W. J. Kraemer and N. A. Ratamess, "Fundamentals of Resistance Training: Progression and Exercise Prescription," *Medicine and Science in Sports and Exercise* 36.4 (2004): 674–688.

45. Kraemer and Ratamess, op. cit.

46. Kraemer, op. cit.

47. S. J. Hartley-O'Brien, "Six Mobilization Exercises for Active Range of Hip Motion," *Research Quarterly for Exercise and Sport* 51 (1980): 625–635.

48. D. M. Brody, "Running Injuries: Prevention and Management," *Clinical Symposia* 39 (1987).

49. J. C. Erie, "Eye Injuries: Prevention, Evaluation, and Treatment," *Physician and Sportsmedicine* (November 1991): 108–122.

50. R. C. Wasserman and R. V. Buccini, "Helmet Protection from Head Injuries among Recreational Bicyclists," *American Journal of Sports Medicine* 18 (1990): 96–97.

51. J. Andrish and J. A. Work, "How I Manage Shin Splints," *Physician and Sportsmedicine* (December 1990): 113–114.

52. Brody, op. cit.

53. American Academy of Orthopedic Surgeons, *Athletic Training and Sports Medicine,* 2nd ed. (Park Ridge, IL: AAOS, 1991).

54. B. Q. Hafen and K. J. Karren, *Prehospital Emergency Care and Crisis Intervention,* 4th ed. (Englewood Cliffs, NJ: Prentice-Hall, 1992).

55. J. S. Thornton, "Hypothermia Shouldn't Freeze Out Cold-Weather Athletes," *Physician and Sportsmedicine* (January 1990): 109–113.

## CHAPTER 10

1. Addiction Foundation of Manitoba, Mission Statement.

2. H. F. Doweiko, *Concepts of Chemical Dependency* (Pacific Grove, CA: Brooks/Cole, 1993) 9.

3. C. Nakken, *The Addictive Personality* (Center City, MN: Hazelden, 1988) 23.

4. V. Johnson, *Intervention: Helping Someone Who Doesn't Want Help* (Minneapolis, MN: Johnson Institute, 1986) 16–35.

5. Canadian Institute for Health Information. "Drug Expenditure in Canada 1985–2004, (Ottawa: 2005).

6. Canadian Institute for Health Information, op. cit.

7. Ibid.

8. Ibid.

9. Ibid.

10. E. Single et al. "The Relative Risks and Etiologic Fractions of Different Causes of Death and Disease Attributable to Alcohol, Tobacco, and Illicit Drug Use in Canada," *Canadian Medical Association Journal* 162.12 (2000): 1669–1675.

11. Canadian Foundation for Drug Policy, *Canada Drug Legislation Update* (Ottawa: 1997).

12. Health Canada, "A National Survey of Canadians' Use of Alcohol and Other Drugs: Prevalence of Use and Related Harms, (Ottawa: Canadian Centre on Substance Abuse, 2004) 1–12.

13. Canadian Centre on Substance Abuse and the Centre for Addiction and Mental Health, *Canadian Profile 1999,* CCSA and CAMH, Ottawa and Toronto: 1999, 139.

14. World Health Organization, "Other Psychoactive Substances." Retrieved on March 3, 2006 from www.who.int/substances_abuse/ facts/psychoactives/en/print.html.

15. Ibid.

16. Ibid.

17. Canadian Centre on Substance Abuse, "Substance Abuse Policy in Canada," presentation to the House Standing Committee on Health (October 8, 1996).

18. Centre for Addiction and Mental Health, "Do You Know . . . Cocaine, 2006." Retrieved on March 2, 2006, from www.camh.net/ About_Addiction_Mental_Health/Drug_and_Addiction_ Information/cocaine_dyk.html.

19. Centre for Addiction and Mental Health, op. cit.

20. Health Canada, op. cit.

21. Addiction Research Foundation, "Drug Abuse Update: Drugs and Driving" (Spring 1991).

22. Centre for Addiction and Mental Health, op. cit.

23. Ibid.

24. Centre for Addiction and Mental Health, "Do You Know . . . Amphetamines, 2004." Retrieved on March 2, 2006, from www.camh.net/About_Addiction_Mental_Health/Drug_and_Addiction_Information/amphetamines_dyk.html.

25. Centre for Addiction and Mental Health, "Do You Know . . . Methamphetamines, 2005." Retrieved on March 2, 2006, from www.camh.net/About_Addiction_Mental_Health/Drug_and_Addiction_Information/methamphetamine_dyk.html.

26. Centre for Addiction and Mental Health, "Do You Know . . . Cannabis, 2005." Retrieved on March 2, 2006, from www.camh.net/About_Addiction_Mental_Health/Drug_and_Addiction_Information/cannabis_dyk.html.

27. Health Canada, op. cit.

28. Centre for Addiction and Mental Health, "Do You Know . . . Cannabis, 2005."

29. R. Mathias, "Marijuana Impairs Driving-Related Skill and Workplace Performance," NIDA Notes 11.1 (January–February 1996): 6.

30. National Institute on Drug Abuse, "NIDA Capsules: Designer Drugs" (August 1989): 17–21.

31. Centre for Addiction and Mental Health, "Do You Know . . . Ecstasy, 2005." Retrieved on March 2, 2006, from www.camh.net/About_Addiction_Mental_Health/Drug_and_Addiction_Information/ecstasy_dyk.html.

32. Centre for Addiction and Mental Health, "Do You Know . . . Anabolic Steroids, 2003." Retrieved on March 2, 2006, from www.camh.net/About_Addiction_Mental_Health/Drug_and_Addiction_Information/anabolic_steroids_dyk.html.

33. Health Canada, "Canada's Drug Strategy," Cat. No. H390440/1998E, 25.

34. Canadian Council on Social Development, "Canadian Profile 1997: Alcohol, Tobacco & Other Drugs."

35. Statistics Canada, The Daily, Thursday, July 19, 2001.

# CHAPTER 11

1. Statistics Canada, "Control and Sale of Alcoholic Beverages," The Daily, September 8, 2005. Retrieved on March 8, 2006 from www.statcan.ca/Daily/English/050908/d050908b.htm.

2. Ibid.

3. Health Canada, "A National Survey of Canadians' Use of Alcohol and Other Drugs: Prevalence of Use and Related Harms," (Ottawa: Canadian Centre on Substance Abuse, 2004) 1–12.

4. Ibid.

5. Ibid.

6. Ibid.

7. Ibid.

8. Statistics Canada, op. cit.

9. Ibid.

10. Ibid.

11. Ibid.

12. Ibid.

13. Ibid.

14. Ibid.

15. World Health Organization, WHO Fact Sheet N127, August 1996, "Trends in Substance Use and Associated Health Problems." Retrieved from www.who.int/inf-fs/en/fact127.html.

16. E. Single et al., "The Relative Risks and Etiologic Fractions of Different Causes of Death and Disease Attributable to Alcohol, Tobacco, and Illicit Drug Use in Canada," Canadian Medical Association Journal 162.12 (2000): 1669–1675.

17. Addiction Research Foundation, Statistical Information Service.

18. Centre for Addiction and Mental Health, "Do You Know . . . Alcohol," 2003. Retrieved on March 2, 2006, from www.camh.net/About_Addiction_Mental_Health/Drug_and_Addiction_Information/alcohol_dyk.html.

19. Addiction Research Foundation, op. cit.

20. R. D. Moore and T. A. Pearsons, "Moderate Alcohol Consumption and Coronary Heart Disease: A Review," Medicine 65 (1986): 242–267; Y. Okamota et al., "Role of Liver in Alcohol-Induced Alteration of High Density Lipoprotein Metabolism," Journal of Laboratory Clinical Medicine 111 (1988): 484–485.

21. W. C. Willett et al., "Moderate Alcohol Consumption and the Risk of Breast Cancer," New England Journal of Medicine 316 (1987): 1174–1180.

22. B. Stade, W. J. Ungar, B. Stevens, J. Beyene, and G. Koren, "The Burden of Prenatal Exposure to Alcohol: Measurement and Cost," JFAS International 4 (2006): 1–14.

23. Ibid.

24. Ibid.

25. Statistics Canada, "Mortality: Summary List of Causes," 1995, Cat. No. 84-209, 14–15.

26. Centre for Addiction and Mental Health, "Do You Know . . . Alcohol, Other Drugs and Driving, 2003." Retrieved on March 2, 2006, from www.camh.net/About_Addiction_Mental_Health/Drug_and_Addiction_Information/alchohol_drugs_driving_dyk.html.

27. Single et al., op. cit.

28. F. K. Goodwin and E. M. Gause, "Alcohol, Drug Abuse, and Mental Health Administration," Prevention Pipeline 3 (1990): 19.

29. Kenneth Blum et al., "Allelic Association of Human Dopamine D2 Receptor Gene in Alcoholism," AMA 262 (1990): 2055–2059.

30. Ray and Ksir, Drugs, Society, and Human Behavior (St. Louis: Times Mirror/Mosby, 1990).

31. Statistics Canada, op. cit.

32. Eric Single, Lynda Robson, Xiaodi Xie, and Jürgen Rehm, The Costs of Substance Abuse in Canada (Ottawa: Canadian Centre on Substance Abuse, 1996).

33. J. Kinney and G. Leaton, Loosening the Grip: A Handbook of Alcohol Information, 4th ed. (St. Louis: Times Mirror/Mosby, 1991).

34. World Health Organization, Fact Sheet N154, "Tobacco Epidemic: Health Dimensions," revised May 1998.

35. Health Canada, "Canadian Tobacco Use Monitoring Survey (CTUMS) 2005." Retrieved on June 5, 2006, from www.hc-sc.gc.ca/hl-vs/tobac-tabac/research-recherche/stat/ctums-esutc/2005/wave-phase-1_summary-sommaire_e.html.

36. Ibid.

37. U.S. DHHS/Office on Smoking & Health, "Psychosocial Risk Factors for Initiating Tobacco Use," in Preventing Tobacco Use among Young People: A Report of the Surgeon General (Atlanta: 1994); U.S. DHHS/OSH, "Changes in Knowledge about the Determinants of Smoking Behaviour," in Reducing the Health Consequences of Smoking: 25 Years of Progress, U.S. Surgeon General, Washington, DC: 1989, 329–376; E. Fisher, Jr., E. Lichtenstein, and D. Haire-Joshu, "Multiple Determinants of Tobacco Use and Cessation," in Nicotine Addiction: Principles & Management, eds. C. T. Orleans and J. Slade, Jr. (New York: Oxford, 1993), 59–88; S. Spoke and Associates, A Literature Review on Smoking: The Social, Psychological and Physiological Influencers Affecting Decisions and Behaviour (Health Canada, OTC/HPB, March 1996).

38. P. Hilts, "Wide Peril Is Seen in Passive Smoking," *New York Times,* May 9, 1990: A25.

39. Ibid.

40. M. Dewey, *Smoke in the Workplace* (Toronto: N.C. Press, 1986) 14.

# CHAPTER 12

1. Statistics Canada, "At Risk of First or Recurring Heart Disease," 1998, Cat. No. 82-003-XPB.

2. Health Canada, Canadian Heart and Stroke Surveillance System (CHSSS), *The Changing Face of Heart Disease and Stroke in Canada, 2000,* a report prepared in collaboration with the Laboratory Centre for Disease Control, Health Canada; Statistics Canada; the Canadian Institute for Health Information; the Canadian Cardiovascular Society; the Canadian Stroke Society; and the Heart and Stroke Foundation of Canada. Heart and Stroke Foundation of Canada, Ottawa: October 1999.

3. Health Canada, *Heart Disease and Stroke in Canada,* 1995.

4. American Heart Association, *Heart and Stroke Facts 1995,* American Heart Association, Dallas, TX: 1995, 1.

5. Ibid., 2.

6. Ibid.

7. Heart and Stroke Foundation of Canada, "Risk Factors: Coronary Heart Disease Risk Factor." Retrieved on June 2, 2004, from http://ww1.heartandstroke.ca/Page.asp?PageID=110&ArticleID=589&Src=heart.

8. Heart and Stroke Foundation of Canada and ACTI-MENU, "Do You Have a Healthy Heart?" (Canada: ACTI-MENU, 1999).

9. Ibid.

10. Ibid.

11. Ibid.

12. Ibid.

13. Ibid.

14. Canadian Institute for Health Information, *Health Care in Canada 2003,* Canadian Institute for Health Information, Ottawa: 2003.

15. M. Barrow, *Heart Talk: Understanding Cardiovascular Diseases* (Gainsville, FL: Cor-Ed Publishing, 1992).

16. Ibid.

17. Ibid.

18. A. V. Chobanian, G. L. Bakris, H. R. Black, W. C. Cushman, L. A. Green, J. L. Izzo, Jr., D. W. Jones, B. J. Materson, S. Oparil, and E. J. Roccella, "The Seventh Report of the Joint National Committee on Prevention, Detection, Evaluation, and Treatment of High Blood Pressure: The JNC-7 Report," *Journal of the American Medical Association* 289.19: 2560–2572. Erratum 2003: 290.2: 197.

19. Canadian Institute for Health Information, op. cit.

20. Barrow, op. cit.

21. Heart and Stroke Foundation of Canada and ACTI-MENU, op. cit.

22. Statistics Canada, "High Blood Pressure, by Age Group and Sex, Household Population Aged 12 and Over, Canada, 2000/01." Retrieved on April 18, 2006, from www.statcan.ca/english/freepub/82-221-XIE/00502/tables/html/1265.htm.

23. B. A. Reeder, A. Senthilselvan, J-P. Després, A. Angel, L. Liu, H. Wang, and S. W. Rabkin, "The Association of Cardiovascular Disease Risk Factors with Abdominal Obesity in Canada," *Canadian Medical Association Journal* 157 (1 suppl.) (1997): S39–S45.

24. Health Canada, *Heart Disease and Stroke in Canada, 1997,* a report prepared in collaboration with Health Canada, the Laboratory Centre for Disease Control, Statistics Canada, and the University of Saskatchewan. Heart and Stroke Foundation of Canada, Ottawa: June 1997, 42.

25. R. Eliot, "Changing Behavior: A New Comprehensive and Quantitative Approach." Keynote address at the annual meeting of the American College of Cardiology on "Stress and the Heart," Jackson Hole, WY, July 3, 1987.

26. Statistics Canada, *Mortality, Summary List of Causes, 1995,* Cat. No. 84-209-XPB, Minister of Industry, Ottawa: 1997, 84–209.

27. Health Canada, *Toward a Healthy Future,* op. cit., 17.

28. Heart and Stroke Foundation of Canada, op. cit.

29. Heart and Stroke Foundation of Canada, "Women and Heart Health," March 1999, available online at: www.hc-sc.gc.ca/hl-vs/alt_formats/hpb-dgps/pdf/facts_heart.pdf.

30. D. Grady et al., "Cardiovascular Disease Outcomes during 6.8 Years of Hormone Therapy: Heart and Estrogen/Progestin Replacement Study Follow-up (HERS II)," *Journal of the American Medical Association* 288.1: 11–128.

31. National Institutes of Health, "Facts about Postmenopausal Hormone Replacement Therapy," October 2002. NIH Publication No. 02-5200.

32. American Heart Association, op. cit., 12.

33. Ibid, 12.

34. Heart and Stroke Foundation of Canada and ACTI-MENU, op. cit.

35. Ibid.

36. National Heart, Lung, and Blood Institute, *Heart Memo: The Cardiovascular Health of Women* (Bethesda, MD: NHLBI, 1995) 5.

37. American Heart Association, op. cit., 10.

38. Canadian Cancer Society/National Cancer Institute of Canada, *Canadian Cancer Statistics 2006,* CCS/NCIC, Toronto: 2006.

39. Ibid.

40. Ibid.

41. J. Peto, "Cancer Epidemiology in the Last Century and Next Decade," *Nature* 411 (2001): 390–395.

42. Canadian Cancer Society/National Cancer Institute of Canada, op. cit.

43. American Cancer Society, *Cancer Facts and Figures 2005,* American Cancer Society, Atlanta: 2005.

44. E. Calle et al., "Overweight, Obesity and Mortality from Cancer in a Prospectively Studied Cohort of U.S. Adults," *New England Journal of Medicine* 348.77: 1625–1638; L. Cooney and C. Gufer, "Hyperglycemia, Obesity, and Cancer Risk on the Horizon," *Journal of the American Medical Association* 293: 235–236.

45. T. G. Krontirus, "The Emerging Genetics of Human Cancer," *New England Journal of Medicine* 309 (1983): 404; A. G. Knudson, "Genetics of Human Cancer," *Annual Review of Genetics* 20 (1986): 23.

46. Canadian Cancer Society/National Cancer Institute of Canada, op. cit.

47. American Cancer Society, *Cancer Facts and Figures* 2005, op. cit., 1.

48. Ibid., 20.

49. P. Pisani, *Estimates of Number of Cancer Cases throughout the World Attributable to Infectious Diseases* (Lyon, France: IARC Press, 2004).

50. B. W. Stewart and P. Kleihues, eds., "Cancers of the Female Reproductive Tract," *World Cancer Report* (Lyon, France: IARC Press, 2003) 215–222.

51. American Cancer Society, *Cancer Facts and Figures 2005,* op. cit.

52. National Cancer Institute Statistics, "Breast Cancer Risk," *Health,* May/June 1994, 14.

53. National Cancer Institute of Canada, *Canadian Cancer Statistics 1999.*

54. American Cancer Society, Cancer Facts and Figures 2005, op. cit., 10.

55. Stewart and Kleihues, eds., op. cit.

56. American Cancer Society, *Cancer Facts and Figures 2005*, op. cit., 10.

57. Leslie Bernstein, Brian E. Henderson, Rosemarie Hanisch, Jane Sullivan-Halley, and Ronald K. Ross, "Physical Exercise and Reduced Risk of Breast Cancer in Young Women," *Journal of the National Cancer Institute* 86.18 (September 21, 1994): 1403–1408.

58. Canadian Cancer Society/National Cancer Institute of Canada, op. cit.

59. American Cancer Society, *Cancer Facts and Figures 2005*, op. cit., 9.

60. Ibid., 9.

61. Canadian Cancer Society/National Cancer Institute of Canada, op. cit.

62. Ibid.

63. American Cancer Society, *Cancer Facts and Figures 2005*, op. cit., 11–12.

64. Ibid., 15.

65. Canadian Cancer Society/National Cancer Institute of Canada, op. cit.

66. American Cancer Society, *Cancer Facts and Figures 2005*, op. cit., 15–16.

67. Ibid., 16.

68. Harvey A. Risch, Meera Jain, Loraine D. Marrett, and Geoffrey R. Howe, "Dietary Fat Intake and Risk of Epithelial Ovarian Cancer," *Journal of the National Cancer Institute* 86.18 (September 1994): 1409–1415.

69. American Cancer Society, *Cancer Facts and Figures 2005*, op. cit., 16.

70. Canadian Cancer Society/National Cancer Institute of Canada, op. cit.

71. American Cancer Society, *Cancer Facts and Figures 2005*, op. cit., 13.

72. Ibid., 13.

73. Ibid.

74. Ibid., 14.

75. Ibid.

76. Ibid.

# CHAPTER 13

1. World Health Organization, *Report on Infectious Disease: Removing Obstacles to Health Development*, World Health Organization, 1999.

2. Health Canada, *Prevention and Management of Infectious Diseases* (July 1995).

3. T. Shulman, J. Phair, and H. Sommers, *The Biological and Clinical Basis of Infectious Disease* (Philadelphia: W. B. Saunders, 1992); A. Benenson, *Control of Communicable Diseases in Man* (Washington, DC: American Public Health Association, 1990).

4. K. Nelson, C. Williams, and N. Graham, *Infectious Disease Epidemiology: Theory and Practice* (Gaithersburg, MD: Aspen, 2001) 17–39.

5. Health Canada, "Tuberculosis." Retrieved on April 21, 2006, from www.hc-sc.gc.ca/dc-ma.tuberulos/index_e.html.

6. *Canada Communicable Disease Report* 22.18 (September 15, 1996).

7. Health Canada, "Tuberculosis," op. cit.

8. Health Canada, "Vaccine-Preventable Diseases: Mumps." Retrieved on April 21, 2006, from www.hc-sc.gc.ca/im/vpd-mev/mumps_e.html.

9. Ibid.

10. World Health Organization, op. cit.

11. Health Canada, "Reported Cases and Rates of Notifiable STI from January 1 to June 30, 2005 and January 1 to June 30, 2004." Retrieved on April 21, 2006, from www.hc-sc.gc.ca/pphb-dgspsp/std-mts/stdcases-casmts/index/html.

12. T. Wong and D. Sutherland, "Canadian STI National Goals and Phase Specific Strategies," *Sexually Transmitted Infections* 78 (suppl. I), (2002): i189–i190.

13. Health Canada, "Reported Cases and Rates of Notifiable STI."

14. Ibid.

15. Noni E. MacDonald and Robert Brunham, "The Effects of Undetected and Untreated Sexually Transmitted Diseases: Pelvic Inflammatory Disease and Ectopic Pregnancy in Canada," *Canadian Journal of Human Sexuality* 6.2 (1997); SIECCAN: The Sex Information & Education Council of Canada.

16. "PID: Guidelines for Prevention, Detection, and Management," *Clinical Courier* 10 (1992): 1–5.

17. P. Marchbanks, N. Lee, and H. Peterson, "Cigarette Smoking as a Risk Factor for PID," *American Journal of Obstetrics and Gynecology* 162 (1990): 639–644; J. Kahn, C. Walker, and A. Washington, "Diagnosing Pelvic Inflammatory Disease," *Journal of the American Medical Association* 226 (1991): 2594–2604.

18. Health Canada, "Reported Cases and Rates of Notifiable STI."

19. Health Canada, Bureau of HIV/AIDS and STD and TB Update Series, "Gonorrhea in Canada," May 1999.

20. Health Canada, "Reported Cases and Rates of Notifiable STI."

21. Health Canada, *Canada Communicable Diseases Report* 23.12 (June 15, 1997).

22. Health Canada, Bureau of HIV/AIDS and STD and TB Update Series, "Syphilis in Canada," May 1999.

23. Health Canada, *Canada Communicable Diseases Report.*

24. S. Kroon, "Limiting the Continued Spread of Genital Herpes: Recommendations from the International Herpes Management Forum Management Strategies Workshop," *PPS Europe* (1994).

25. Marc Steben and Stephen L. Sack, "Genital Herpes: The Epidemiology and Control of a Common Sexually Transmitted Disease," *Canadian Journal of Human Sexuality.*

26. B. Strong, C. DeVault, B. Sayad, and W. Yarber. *Human Sexuality* (St. Louis: McGraw-Hill, 2005).

27. Health Canada, "HIV/AIDS." Retrieved on August 18, 2004, from www.hc-sc.gc.ca/datapcb/iad/ih_hivadis-e.htm.

28. World Health Organization, "AIDS Epidemic Update" (December 1999): 4.

29. Public Health Agency of Canada, Centre for Infectious Disease Prevention and Control, Surveillance and Risk Assessment Division, *HIV and AIDS in Canada: Surveillance Report to December 31, 2004*, Public Health Agency of Canada, Ottawa: April 2005.

30. Ibid.

31. Ibid.

32. National Institute of Allergy and Infectious Diseases, "HIV Infection and AIDS: An Overview," 2005, available online at: www.niaid.nih.gov/factsheets/hivinf.htm.

33. Public Health Agency of Canada, "HIV/AIDS Epi Update: May 2004: HIV/AIDS among Injecting Drug Users in Canada." Retrieved on April 24, 2006, from www.phac-aspc.gc.ca/publicat/epiu-aepi/epi_unpdate_may_04/11_e.html.

34. J. Allen, "Oh, My Aching Head," *Life* (1994): 66–76.

35. National Headache Foundation (NFH), "NFH Headache Fact Sheet," 2004, www.headaches.org.

36. Canadian Diabetes Association, "The Prevalence and Costs of Diabetes." Retrieved on June 2, 2006, from www.diabetes.ca/Section_About/prevalence.ca.

37. Health Canada, "Canadian Diabetes Strategy." Retrieved on November 13, 2002, from www.hc-sc.gc.ca/english/media/releases/1999/99135ebk3.htm; currently available online at: www.phac-aspc.gc.ca/ccdpc-cpcmc/diabetes-diabete/english/strategy/index.html.

38. The Arthritis Society, *Defining the Arthritis Crisis: Canadian Arthritis Bill of Rights* (2001).

39. Health Canada National Advisory Council on Aging, *How Many People Have Arthritis?* (1997).

# CHAPTER 14

1. B. Hayslip and P. Panek, *Adult Development and Aging* (New York: Harper and Row, 1992) 21.

2. Statistics Canada. "Population by Sex and Age Group." Retrieved on May 16, 2006, from www40.statcan.ca/l01/cst01/demo10a.htm.

3. National Advisory Council on Aging, "1999 and Beyond—Challenges of an Aging Canadian Society" (1999) 19.

4. National Osteoporosis Foundation, *Physicians' Resource Manual on Osteoporosis: A Decision-Making Guide,* 2nd ed. (National Osteoporosis Foundation, 1991); and National Dairy Council, "Calcium and Osteoporosis: New Insights," *Dairy Council Digest* 63 (1992): 1–6.

5. National Advisory Council on Aging, op. cit., 23.

6. U.S. Department of Health and Human Services, Public Health Service, National Institutes of Health, Osteoporosis Research, Education, and Health Promotion (NIH Publication No. 91-3216, September 1991) 2.

7. National Dairy Council, op. cit., 3; National Research Council, Food and Nutrition Board, *Recommended Dietary Allowances,* 10th ed., a report of the subcommittee on the 10th edition of the FDA's dietary allowances (Washington, DC: National Academy Press, 1989).

8. National Dairy Council, op. cit., 6.

9. U.S. Department of Health and Human Services, op. cit., 21–25.

10. Ibid., 6.

11. J. Thompson, M. Manore, J. Sheeska, *Nutrition: A Functional Approach,* Canadian edition (Toronto: Pearson, 2007).

12. Health Canada, "Canada's Physical Activity Guide for Youth," Cat. H39-611/2002-1E, 2002.

13. National Kidney and Urologic Diseases Information Clearinghouse, "Kidney and Urologic Diseases Statistics for the United States" (NIH Publication No. 04-3895), Retrieved in February 2004 from www.kidney.niddk.nih.gov/kudiseases/pubs/kustats/index.htm.

14. A. Ferrini and R. Ferrini, *Health in the Later Years* (Madison, WI: Brown and Benchmark, 1993) 281.

15. National Institute of Nutrition, *Food and Nutrition Opportunities in the Seniors' Market: A Situation Analysis—Executive Summary, March 1996.*

16. Philadelphia Corporation for Aging, "Older Adults and Sexuality," *Health Matters* 14.14 (August 2004), www.pcaphl.org/healthmatters/agingsexuality.pdf.

17. National Council on Aging, "Half of Older Americans Report They Are Sexually Active, 4 in 10 Want More Sex, Says New Survey," Retrieved on September 28, 1998, from http://ncoa.org/mews/archives.sexsurvey.htm.

18. National Institute of Nutrition, op. cit.

19. Health Canada, Depression Aging Vignettes #78, Division of Seniors and Aging, 1998, www.hc-sc.gc.ca/seniors-aines/seniors/pubs/vigdepre.htm#Dep 2.

20. National Advisory Council on Aging, op. cit., 23.

21. Public Health Agency of Canada, *Canada's Physical Activity Guide for Healthy Active Living for Older Adults* (Ottawa).

22. Thompson, Manore, Sheeska, op. cit.

23. Statistics Canada, op. cit.

24. Health Canada Division of Aging and Seniors, Statistical Snapshot #5, "More Women Than Men," September 1999.

25. Health Canada, *Toward a Healthy Future: Second Report on the Health of Canadians,* a public policy report developed by the Federal, Provincial and Territorial Advisory Committee on Population Health (ACPH) in collaboration with Health Canada, Statistics Canada, the Canadian Institute for Health Information and a project team from the Centre for Health Promotion, University of Toronto. Health Canada, Ottawa: 1999, 166.

26. *Oxford English Dictionary* (Oxford: Oxford University Press, 1969) 72, 334, 735.

27. Canadian Medical Association, "Guidelines for the Diagnosis of Brain Death," *Canadian Medical Association Journal* 136 (1987): 200A.

28. Ibid.

29. Lewis R. Aiken, *Dying, Death, and Bereavement,* 3rd ed. (Boston: Allyn & Bacon, 1994) 4.

30. Elisabeth Kübler-Ross, *On Death and Dying* (New York: Macmillan, 1969) 113.

31. Robert J. Kastenbaum, *Death, Society, and Human Experience,* 5th ed. (Boston: Allyn & Bacon, 1995) 95.

32. K. J. Doka, ed., *Disenfranchised Grief: Recognizing Hidden Sorrow* (Lexington, MA: Lexington Books, 1989).

33. Kastenbaum, op. cit., 336–337.

34. J. W. Worden, *Grief Counseling and Grief Therapy: A Handbook for the Mental Health Practitioner,* 3rd ed. (New York: Springer, 2001).

35. The term "quasi-death experience" was coined by J. B. Kamerman; see J. B. Kamerman, *Death in the Midst of Life* (Englewood Cliffs, NJ: Prentice Hall, 1988) 71.

# CHAPTER 15

1. Health Canada, "Health and Environment Handbook for Health Professionals," Cat. No. H46-2/98-211-2E, 1998, v.

2. Ibid., 81–82.

3. R. Caplan, *Our Earth, Ourselves* (New York: Bantam, 1990) 247.

4. United Nations, "World Population Prospects: The 2004 Revision." Retrieved on May 18, 2006, from http://esa.un.org/unpp/.

5. Ibid.

6. Ibid.

7. Ibid.

8. Environment Canada, "Canadian Environmental Protection Act, 1999 (CEPA, 1999)." Retrieved on May 19, 2006, from www.ec.gc.ca/CEPARegistry/the_act/.

9. Canadian Environmental Assessment Agency, "Introduction and Features: Canadian Environmental Assessment Act." Retrieved on May 19, 2006, from www.ceaa-acee.gc.ca/013/intro_e.htm.

10. Environment Canada, "Agreements." Retrieved on May 19, 2006, from www.ec.gc.ca/cleanair-airpur/Agreements-WS475C5F00-1_En.htm.

11. Environment Canada, "Canadian 1996 NOx/VOC Science Assessment, Executive Summary," www.ec.gc.ca/air/acid-rain_e.html.

12. Canadian Lung Association, *Why Care about the Air You Breathe?* (1991).

13. Lester Brown, "A New Era Unfolds," in *State of the World, 1993,* ed. Lester Brown (New York: Norton, 1993).

14. Canadian Lung Association, op. cit.

15. H. F. French, "Clearing the Air," in *State of the World, 1990,* 109.

16. U.S. Environmental Protection Agency, "Effects of Acid Rain," 2005, www.epa.gov/acidrain.

17. U.S. Environmental Protection Agency, "The Inside Story: A Guide to Indoor Air Quality" (EPA Document # 402-K-93-007), January 2002, http://epa.gov/iaq/pubs/insdet.html.

18. Ibid.

19. Ibid.

20. Health Canada, "Radon Information Sheet" (Minister of Supply and Services, 1989).

21. Canadian Lung Association, op. cit.

22. French, op. cit., 110.

23. Environment Canada, *Water Policy in Canada—Canada's Water* (March 1997).

24. A. Nadakavukaren, *Man and Environment: A Health Perspective* (Prospect Heights, IL: Waveland, 1990), 412–414.

25. R. Griffin, Jr., "Introducing NPS Water Pollution," *EPA Journal* 17 (1991): 6–9.

26. J. Naar, *Design for a Livable Planet* (New York: Harper and Row, 1990), 68.

27. A. Nadakavukaren, op. cit., 183.

28. Ibid., 447.

29. Ibid., 415.

30. Environment Canada, *Toxic Substances Management Policy*, Government of Canada, Ottawa: June 1995.

31. D. W. Moeller, *Environmental Health* (Cambridge, MA: Harvard University Press, 1992) 31.

32. C. Flavin, "Slowing Global Warming," in *State of the World, 1990*.

33. Health Canada, "Health and Environment Handbook," 125–126.

## CHAPTER 16

1. Canadian Institute for Health Information, *Canada's Health System* (1996).

2. Commission on the Future of Health Care in Canada. Media release: "Romanow Report Proposes Sweeping Changes to Medicare," November 28, 2002, available online at: www.hc-sc.gc.ca/english/care/romanow/hcc0403.html.

3. Health Canada, *Toward a Healthy Future: Second Report on the Health of Canadians*, a public policy report developed by the Federal, Provincial and Territorial Advisory Committee on Population Health (ACPH) in collaboration with Health Canada, Statistics Canada, the Canadian Institute for Health Information and a project team from the Centre for Health Promotion, University of Toronto. Health Canada, Ottawa: 1999, 136.

4. Canadian Institute for Health Information, "Health Care in Canada 2005." Retrieved on May 19, 2006, from www.cihi.ca.

5. Ibid.

6. Ibid.

7. Ibid.

8. Health Canada, "Canada's Health Care System," Cat. No. H39-502/1999, 7.

9. Public Health Agency of Canada, "Canadian Health Network: Health System." Retrieved on May 23, 2006, from www.canadian-health-network.ca/servlet/ ContentServer?cid=1047418085892&pagename= CHN-RCS%2FPage%2FGTPageTemplate&c=Page&lang=En.

10. Canadian Institute for Health Information, "Health Care in Canada 2005."

11. National Center for Complementary and Alternative Medicine, "Get the Facts: 10 Things to Know about Evaluating Medical Resources on the Web." Retrieved on May 23, 2006 from www.nccam.nih.gov.

12. Health Canada, *Toward a Healthy Future*, 1.

13. Health Canada, *Toward a Healthy Future*, 154.

14. Munroe Anne Johnston, *Gender and Self-Care in Undergraduate Students: A Qualitative Study* (Waterloo, ON: Wilfrid Laurier University, 1993) 12.

15. Health Canada, *Health Human Resources in Community-Based Health Care: A Review of the Literature*, a report prepared for the Federal/Provincial/Territorial Conference of Deputy Ministers of Health through the Advisory Committee on Health Human Resources (ACHHR). Health Promotion and Programs Branch, Health Canada, Ottawa: 1995, 51.

16. G. Annas, *The Rights of Patients: The Basic ACLU Guide to Patient Rights*, 2nd ed. (Chicago: Southern Illinois University Press, 1989) 105; J. A. Robertson, *The Rights of the Critically Ill* (New York: Bantam, 1983) 32–77.

17. Health Canada, *Health Human Resources*, 55.

18. Canadian Institute for Health Information, "Health Care in Canada 2005."

19. Health Canada, *Toward a Healthy Future*, 153.

20. P. Starr, *The Social Transformation of American Medicine* (New York: Basic Books, 1982) 127, 229.

21. Newfoundland and Labrador Massage Therapy Association, "Frequently Asked Questions about Massage Therapy." Retrieved on May 24, 2006, from www.nlmta.ca/res/index.html.

22. A. Toufexis, "Dr. Jacob's Alternative Mission: A New NIH Office Will Put Unconventional Medicine to the Test," *Time*, March 1, 1993: 43–44, 64–66.

23. Health Canada, "Health Care System." Retrieved on May 24, 2006, from www.hc-sc.gc.ca/hcs-sss/index_e.html.

# INDEX

opiates, 263–265
psychedelics, 265–266
steroids, 268–269
imagined rehearsal, 22
immune system
function of, 342–343
physical activity and, 225
psychosocial health and, 40–42
stress and, 57–58, 64
immunization schedule, 344
immunological competence, 335
immunotherapy, 329
in vitro fertilization, 162
incomplete proteins, 174
incubation period, 338
induction abortions, 146
infatuation, 105
infectious diseases
*see also* pathogens; sexually transmitted
infections (STIs)
body's defences, 341–343
and cancer, 321
current challenges, 336
overview of, 334
risk factors, 334–335
infectious mononucleosis, 339
infertility
causes of, 161
surrogate motherhood, 162
treatment for, 161–162
influenza, 338–339
inhalants, 253, 267–268
inhalation of drugs, 253
inhibited sexual desire, 127
inhibition interaction of drugs, 254
injection of drugs, 252
injuries
*see also* fitness injuries
prevention of, 91–92, 93
victims of, 92
Inland Waters Directorate, 407
insomnia, 39–40
insulin, 364
intelligence and aging, 381
interconnectedness, 34
intercourse, 125–126
interferon, 338
internal influences of psychosocial
health, 36–37
International Day for Evaluation of Abdominal
Obesity, 312
International Panel on Climate Change, 411
internet
online dating, 123
online medical resources, 419
intervention, 289

intimate relationships
*see also* committed relationships
barriers to, 106–107
characteristics of, 99–101
families, 101–102
friendships, 102
gender issues, 104–106
love, 103–104
partners and couples, 102–103
intolerance of drugs, 254
intramuscular injection, 252
intrauterine devices (IUDs), 141
intravenous injection, 252
Inuit, and cardiovascular disease, 312
inunction of drugs, 253
iron, 183–184
irritable bowel syndrome (IBS), 365
ischemia, 305
ISD, 127
isometric muscle contraction, 232

**J**

Japanese Canadians
internment, during World War II, 78
Vancouver riot (1907), 78, 80–81
jealousy, 107
Johnson, Ben, 268
*Journal of the American Medical Association*, 386
*Joy of Sex* (Comfort), 126

**K**

ketosis, 176, 214
Kevorkian, Jack, 393
Kübler-Ross, Elisabeth, 387–388
Kyoto Protocol, 405, 411

**L**

labour and delivery, 157–158
land pollution, 410
landfills, 407
laughter and psychosocial health, 42
Laval University, 312
laxatives, 257
LDLs. *See* lipoproteins
leaching of heavy metals, 403
lead, 401, 409
learned behaviour tolerance, 279
learned helplessness, 36–37
learned optimism, 37
Legionnaire's disease, 337
legislation
illicit drugs, 258, 270
same-sex marriage, 109
tobacco sales, 295
Lenton, Rhonda, 123
Lepine, Marc 81

## X

x-rays and pregnancy, 152
xanthines, 297

## Y

yo-yo diets, 208
youth(s)
   Aboriginal suicide rates, 79

and violence, 80
Yukon River Quest, 5
YWCA, 83

## Z

Zoloft, 44
Zone, 176

p. 1 Health Canada IMG027: Disk 8 Health Canada 8. Reproduced with permission of the Minister of Public Works and Government Services Canada, 2006; p. 3 Stock Boston/David Coleman; p. 4 CP/Jon Murray; p. 23 Michael Newman/PhotoEdit; p. 24 Offshoot Stock/Elena; p. 29 Firstlight.ca; p. 31 Getty Images/Lori Adamski; p. 40 PhotoEdit/Mark Richards; p. 42 Health Canada IMG069: Disk 52 Health Canada 8. Reproduced with permission of the Minister of Public Works and Government Services Canada, 2006; p. 43 Lawrence Manning/CORBIS; p. 47 CP/Ottawa Citizen/Wayne Cuddington; p. 55 Spike Mafford/Photodisc; p. 57 Digital Vision/Getty Images; p. 61 Photodisc/Getty Images; p. 73 Jason Homa/Getty Images; p. 77 Mary-Arthur Johnson/Taxi; p. 80 PhotoEdit/Mark Richards; p. 82 Bill Aron/PhotoEdit; p. 84 Woodfin Camp/Jacques; p. 90 William Thomas Cain/Getty Images; p. 97 Health Canada IMG007, Health Images Disk—Focus on Children, Health Canada 8. Reproduced with permission of the Minister of Public Works and Government Services Canada, 2006; p. 99 Charles Gupton/CORBIS; p. 101 Jose Luis Pelaez, Inc./CORBIS; p. 107 Getty Images/Gary Wolinsky; p. 114 Getty Images/Ziggy Kaluzny; p. 124 Black Star/Lisa Quinones; p. 125 Getty Images/Sarma Ozols; p. 132 Superstock; p. 133 Tony Stone Worldwide/Bruce Ayres; p. 139 Dorling Kindersley; p. 148 Bruce Ayres/Getty Images; p. 152 Photo Library/Maxx Images Inc.; p. 156 PhotoEdit/Tom McCarthy; p. 159 Health Canada IMG003, Health Images Disk—Focus on Children, Health Canada 8. Reproduced with permission of the Minister of Public Works and Government Services Canada, 2006; p. 165 Getty Images/Peter Cade; p. 168 Michael Keller/CORBIS; p. 173 A. Neste; p. 175 The Image Works/B. Daemmrich; p. 187 Photo Researchers/Will & Deni McIntyre; p. 192 The Image Works/J. Sohm; p. 197 © Jupiterimages Corporation; p. 201 (top) PhotoEdit/David Young-Wolff; p. 201 (bottom) Gilles Daigle/PhotoCanada Moncton; p. 209 Frank Siteman/Getty Images; p. 215 Photo Researchers/Biophoto Associates; p. 221 Paul Viant/Getty Images; p. 223 David Stoecklein/CORBIS; p. 228 © Jupiterimages Corporation; p. 232 Gilles Daigle/PhotoCanada Moncton; p. 234 Gilles Daigle/PhotoCanada Moncton; p. 235 (top) Stock Boston/Bob; p. 235 (bottom) PhotoDisc; p. 237 Mike Powell/Getty Images; p. 246 Health Canada IMG026: Disk 13 Health Canada 8. Reproduced with permission of the Minister of Public Works and Government Services Canada, 2006; p. 252 Bill Aron/PhotoEdit; p. 268 © Abhay Martin MD, Dermatlas, www.dermatlas.org; p. 274 Health Canada; p. 276 © Jupiterimages Corporation; p. 279 Firstlight.ca; p. 285 Chuck Savage/CORBIS; p. 293 Oral Health America; p. 301 Canadian Cancer Society; p. 306 © Tom Stewart/CORBIS; p. 311 Dennis MacDonald/PhotoEdit; p. 322 Stock Boston/Stacey Pick; p. 324 Dr. P. Marazzi/SPL/Photo Researchers; p. 333 Arthur Tilley/Taxi; p. 339 Don Klumpp/Firstlight.ca; p. 354 Steve Mercer/Getty Images; p. 356 Health Canada IMG018, Healthy Images Disk Vol. 2 Health Canada 8. Reproduced with permission of the Minister of Public Works and Government Services Canada, 2006; p. 357 Chuck Stoody/CP Photo Archive; p. 360 Paul Windsor/Taxi/Getty Images; p. 361 Elena Dorfman/Offshoot Inc.; p. 370 PhotoDisc; p. 373 © Larry Wells/Maxximages.com; p. 378 John Henley/CORBIS; p. 382 Photo Researchers/Joe; p. 385 Dan Bosler/Stone Allstock/Getty Images; p. 388 Arvind Garg/Photo Researchers; p. 392 Fredde Lieberman/Maxx Images Inc.; p. 393 David Young-Wolff; p. 397 Dick Hemingway; p. 400 Richard L'Anson/Lonelyplant Images/Getty Images; p. 403 Photo Researchers/Will & Deni McIntyre; p. 412 © Jupiterimages Corporation; p. 417 Dick Hemingway; p. 422 The Image Works/Epsin-Anderson; p. 428 (top) Novastock/The Stock Connection; p. 428 (bottom) The Image Works/W. Hill Jr.